CURRENT DIAGNOSIS IN NEUROLOGY

EDWARD FELDMANN, M.D.

Associate Professor of Neurology
Department of Clinical Neurosciences
Brown University School of Medicine
and Rhode Island Hospital
Providence, Rhode Island

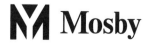 Mosby

St. Louis Baltimore Boston Chicago London Madrid Philadelphia Sydney Toronto

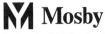

Dedicated to Publishing Excellence

Publisher: George Stamathis
Executive Editor: Susan M. Gay
Senior Managing Editor: Lynne Gery
Project Manager: Linda Clarke
Production Supervisor: Victoria Hoenigke
Manufacturing Supervisor: John Babrick

Copyright © 1994 by Mosby–Year Book, Inc.

Printed in the United States of America.

Mosby–YearBook, Inc.
11830 Westline Industrial Drive
St. Louis, Missouri 63146

NOTICE: The authors and publisher have made every effort to ensure that the patient care recommended
herein, including choice of drugs and drug dosages, is in accord with the accepted standards and practice at
the time of publication. However, since research and regulation constantly change clinical standards, the
reader is urged to check the product information sheet included in the package of each drug, which includes
recommended doses, warnings, and contraindications. This is particularly important with new or infrequently
used drugs.

ISBN 0-8016-6963-4
94 95 96 97 98 CL/MY 9 8 7 6 5 4 3 2 1

EDWARD AKELMAN, M.D.

Assistant Professor of Orthopaedic Surgery, Brown University School of Medicine; Chief, Division of Hand, Upper Extremity and Microvascular Surgery, Rhode Island Hospital, Providence, Rhode Island

DAVID L. BACHMAN, M.D.

Associate Professor of Neurology and of Psychiatry and Behavioral Sciences, and Director of Behavioral Neurology, Medical University of South Carolina, Charleston, South Carolina

JAMES L. BERNAT, M.D.

Professor of Medicine (Neurology), Dartmouth Medical School, Hanover, New Hampshire; Chief, Neurology Section, Veterans Affairs Medical Center, White River Junction, Vermont

DUANE S. BISHOP, M.D.

Associate Professor, Department of Psychiatry and Human Behavior, Brown University School of Medicine; Director, Rehabilitation Psychiatry, Rhode Island Hospital, Providence, Rhode Island

PETER McL. BLACK, M.D., Ph.D.

Franc D. Ingraham Professor of Neurosurgery, Harvard Medical School; Neurosurgeon-in-Chief, Brigham and Women's Hospital, and Children's Hospital, Boston, Massachusetts

GREGORY M. BLUME, M.D.

Resident in Neurology, University of Colorado Health Sciences Center, Denver, Colorado

GEORGE J. BREWER, M.D.

Professor, Departments of Human Genetics and Internal Medicine, University of Michigan Medical School, Ann Arbor, Michigan

JOSEPH P. BRODERICK, M.D.

Associate Professor of Neurology, University of Cincinnati College of Medicine, Cincinnati, Ohio

MARK B. BROMBERG, M.D., Ph.D.

Assistant Professor of Neurology, and Director, Motor Neuron Disease Clinic, University of Michigan Medical School, Ann Arbor, Michigan

MARK T. BROWN, M.D.

Assistant Professor of Medicine (Neurology), Duke University School of Medicine, Durham, North Carolina

ROBERT H. BROWN Jr., D. Phil., M.D.

Associate Professor of Neurology, Harvard Medical School; Associate Neurologist, Massachusetts General Hospital, and Director, Day Neuromuscular Research Laboratory, Boston, Massachusetts

JOHN C.M. BRUST, M.D.

Professor of Clinical Neurology, Columbia University College of Physicians and Surgeons; Director, Department of Neurology, Harlem Hospital Center, New York, New York

GREGORY K. CALL, M.D.

Assistant Professor of Neurology, University of Utah School of Medicine; University Hospital, Primary Children's Medical Center, Veterans Administration Medical Center, Salt Lake City, Utah

J. KEITH CAMPBELL, M.D., F.R.C.P. Ed.

Professor of Neurology, Mayo Medical School; Consultant in Neurology, Mayo Clinic, Rochester, Minnesota

JOHN J. CARONNA, M.D.

Professor of Clinical Neurology, and Vice-Chairman, Department of Neurology, Cornell University Medical College; Attending Neurologist, New York Hospital–Cornell Medical Center, New York, New York

RICHARD J. CASELLI, M.D.

Assistant Professor of Neurology, Mayo Medical School, Rochester, Minnesota; Consultant in Neurology, Mayo Clinic, Scottsdale, Arizona

MICHAEL CHERINGTON, M.D.

Clinical Professor of Neurology, University of Colorado School of Medicine; Chairman, Lightning Data Center, St. Anthony Hospital, Denver, Colorado

MARC I. CHIMOWITZ, M.B., Ch.B.

Assistant Professor of Neurology, and Director, Cerebrovascular Program, University of Michigan School of Medicine, Ann Arbor, Michigan

MONROE COLE, M.D.

Professor of Neurology, Case Western Reserve University School of Medicine; Neurologist, MetroHealth Medical Center, Cleveland, Ohio

CYNTHIA L. COMELLA, M.D.

Assistant Professor, Movement Disorders Section, Department of Neurological Sciences, Rush Medical College of Rush University; Attending Associate in Neurology, Rush-Presbyterian–St. Luke's Medical Center, Chicago, Illinois

JAMES J. CORBETT, M.D.

Professor of Neurology and Ophthalmology and Chairman of Neurology, The University of Mississippi School of Medicine; Attending Physician, University of Mississippi Medical Center, Jackson, Mississippi

PATRICIA K. COYLE, M.D.

Professor of Neurology, State University of New York at Stony Brook, Health Sciences Center School of Medicine; Director, Multiple Sclerosis Comprehensive Care Center, University Hospital, Stony Brook, New York

ROBERT B. DARNELL, M.D., Ph.D.

Assistant Professor and Head of Laboratory, The Rockefeller University, and Assistant Professor of Neurology and Neuroscience, Cornell University Medical College; Assistant Attending Neurologist, The New York Hospital, Affiliate Assistant Attending Neurologist, Memorial Sloan-Kettering Cancer Center, and Associate Physician, Rockefeller University Hospital, New York, New York

LARRY E. DAVIS, M.D.

Professor of Neurology and Microbiology, University of New Mexico School of Medicine; Chief, Neurology Service, Albuquerque Veterans Administration Hospital, Albuquerque, New Mexico

LISA M. DeANGELIS, M.D.

Associate Professor of Neurology, Cornell University Medical College; Associate Member, Department of Neurology, Memorial Sloan-Kettering Cancer Center, New York, New York

OSCAR H. DEL BRUTTO, M.D.

Chief of Neurology, Hospital Luis Vernaza, Guayaquil, Ecuador

ORRIN DEVINSKY, M.D.

Associate Professor of Neurology, New York University School of Medicine; Chief, Department of Neurology, and Director, Comprehensive Epilepsy Center, Hospital for Joint Diseases, New York, New York

SALVATORE DiMAURO, M.D.

Lucy G. Moses Professor of Neurology, Columbia University College of Physicians and Surgeons, New York, New York

JAMES O. DONALDSON, M.D.

Professor of Neurology, University of Connecticut School of Medicine, Farmington, Connecticut

DAVID A. DRACHMAN, M.D.

Professor and Chairman, Department of Neurology, University of Massachusetts Medical School; Attending Physician, Department of Neurology, University of Massachusetts Medical Center, Worcester, Massachusetts

EDWARD FELDMANN, M.D.

Associate Professor of Neurology, Department of Clinical Neurosciences, Brown University School of Medicine and Rhode Island Hospital, Providence, Rhode Island

ERNESTO FERNÁNDEZ-BEER, M.D.

Private Practice, Atlanta Neurological Institute, Riverdale, Georgia

JOSEPH H. FRIEDMAN, M.D.

Associate Professor, Department of Clinical Neurosciences, Brown University School of Medicine; Chief, Division of Neurology, Roger Williams Medical Center, and Director, Brown University Parkinson's Disease and Movement Disorders Unit, Providence, Rhode Island

KAREN FURIE, M.D.

Assistant Instructor, Department of Clinical Neurosciences, Brown University School of Medicine, Providence, Rhode Island

STEVEN L. GALETTA, M.D.

Associate Professor of Neurology, University of Pennsylvania School of Medicine, Philadelphia, Pennsylvania

ROBERT D. GERWIN, M.D.

Assistant Professor of Neurology, The Johns Hopkins University School of Medicine, Baltimore, Maryland

JAMES M. GILCHRIST, M.D.

Associate Professor of Neurology, Department of Clinical Neurosciences, Brown University School of Medicine; Director, Muscular Dystrophy Association Clinic, Rhode Island Hospital, Providence, Rhode Island

MICHAEL J. GLANTZ, M.D.

Assistant Professor, Departments of Oncology and Clinical Neurosciences, Brown University School of Medicine; Co-Director, Brain Tumor Program, Rhode Island Hospital, Providence, and Chief of Neurology, Memorial Hospital of Rhode Island, Pawtucket, Rhode Island

JOHN C. GODERSKY, M.D.

Private Practice, Anchorage Neurosurgical Associates, Anchorage, Alaska

RICHARD J. GOLDBERG, M.D.

Professor, Departments of Psychiatry and Human Behavior and Medicine, Brown University School of Medicine; Psychiatrist-in-Chief, Rhode Island Hospital and Women and Infants Hospital, Providence, Rhode Island

CAMILO R. GOMEZ, M.D.

Associate Professor of Neurology, St. Louis University School of Medicine; Director, The Souers Stroke Institute, St. Louis, Missouri

NEILL R. GRAFF-RADFORD, M.B.B.Ch., M.R.C.P. (UK)

Associate Professor, Mayo Medical School, Rochester, Minnesota; Consultant, Mayo Clinic, Jacksonville, Florida

ROBERT C. GRIGGS, M.D.

Chairman of Neurology, Edward A. and Alma Vollertsen Rykenboer Professor of Neurophysiology, and Professor of Neurology, Medicine, Pathology, Laboratory Medicine, and Pediatrics, University of Rochester School of Medicine, Rochester, New York

THOMAS J. GUILMETTE, Ph.D., A.B.P.P.

Clinical Assistant Professor, Department of Psychiatry and Human Behavior, Brown University School of Medicine; Director of Neuropsychology, Rhode Island Hospital, Providence, Rhode Island

BRIAN HAINLINE, M.D.

Assistant Professor of Neurology, New York University School of Medicine; Director, Clinical Neurology Service and Sports Neurology, Hospital for Joint Diseases, New York, New York

R. NORMAN HARDEN, M.D.

Director, Center for Pain Studies, Rehabilitation Institute of Chicago, Chicago, Illinois

LAWRENCE J. HAYWARD, M.D., Ph.D.

Fellow in Neurology, Massachusetts General Hospital, Harvard Medical School, Boston, Massachusetts

EDWARD B. HEALTON, M.D.

Associate Professor of Clinical Neurology, Associate Dean, and Assistant Vice President, Columbia University College of Physicians and Surgeons; Medical Director, Harlem Hospital Center, New York, New York

DAVE HOLLANDER, M.D., F.R.C.P.C.

Assistant Professor of Neurology, Tufts University School of Medicine; Associate Director, Neuromuscular Research Unit, New England Medical Center, Boston, Massachusetts

GREGORY L. HOLMES, M.D.

Associate Professor of Neurology, Harvard Medical School; Director, Epilepsy Program and Clinical Neurophysiology Laboratory, Children's Hospital, Boston, Massachusetts

LAWRENCE S. HONIG, M.D., Ph.D.

Clinical Assistant Professor of Neurology and Neurological Sciences, Stanford University School of Medicine; Attending Neurologist, Stanford University Medical Center, Stanford, California

WILLIAM G. JOHNSON, M.D.

Professor of Neurology, and Director, Neurogenetics Division, University of Medicine and Dentistry of New Jersey—Robert Wood Johnson Medical School; Attending Neurologist, Robert Wood Johnson University Hospital, New Brunswick, New Jersey

BARRY D. JORDAN, M.D.

Assistant Professor of Neurology, Cornell University Medical College; Medical Director, New York State Athletic Commission, Assistant Attending Neurologist, Hospital for Special Surgery and The New York Hospital, and Assistant Adjunct Physician, New York Eye & Ear Infirmary, New York, New York

CARLOS S. KASE, M.D.

Professor of Neurology, Boston University School of Medicine; Assistant Neurologist, Boston University Medical Center, Boston, Massachusetts

NEVILLE W. KNUCKEY, M.B.B.S., F.R.A.C.S.

Associate Professor, Department of Clinical Neurosciences, Brown University School of Medicine; Neurosurgeon, Rhode Island Hospital, Providence, Rhode Island

JEROME E. KURENT, M.D.

Associate Professor of Neurology, Medical University of South Carolina, Charleston, South Carolina; Fellow in Medicine (Geriatrics), 1993-95, Harvard Medical School, Boston, Massachusetts

PHILIP J. LANDRIGAN, M.D., M.Sc.

Ethel H. Wise Professor and Chairman, Department of Community Medicine, Mount Sinai School of Medicine of the City University of New York, New York, New York

MATT J. LIKAVEC, M.D.

Associate Professor of Neurosurgery, Case Western Reserve University School of Medicine; Associate Director of Neurosurgery, MetroHealth Medical Center, Cleveland, Ohio

JOHN LINDENBAUM, M.D.

Professor and Associate Chairman, Department of Medicine, Columbia University College of Physicians and Surgeons; Associate Director, Medical Service, and Attending Physician, The Presbyterian Hospital in the City of New York, and Attending Physician, Harlem Hospital Center, New York, New York

ALAN H. LOCKWOOD, M.D.

Professor of Neurology and Nuclear Medicine, State University of New York at Buffalo School of Medicine and Biomedical Sciences, Buffalo, New York

ERIC L. LOGIGIAN, M.D.

Assistant Professor of Neurology, Harvard Medical School; Director, Clinical Neurophysiology Laboratory, and Physician (Neurology), Brigham and Women's Hospital, Boston, Massachusetts

MARK LUCIANO, M.D., Ph.D.

Attending Staff, Neurosurgery, Cleveland Clinic, Cleveland, Ohio

DAVID R. LYNCH, M.D., Ph.D.

Instructor, Department of Neurology, University of Pennsylvania School of Medicine, Philadelphia, Pennsylvania

CHRISTINA M. MARRA, M.D.

Assistant Professor of Medicine (Neurology), University of Washington School of Medicine, Seattle, Washington

JOELLE MAST, Ph.D., M.D.

Assistant Professor of Pediatrics and Neurology, Cornell University Medical College; Assistant Attending, Pediatrics and Neurology, The New York Hospital, New York, New York

M. EILEEN McNAMARA, M.D.

Assistant Professor, Departments of Psychiatry and Neurology, Brown University School of Medicine; Director, Ambulatory EEG Program, Department of Psychiatry, Rhode Island Hospital, Providence, Rhode Island

AARON E. MILLER, M.D.

Professor of Clinical Neurology, State University of New York Health Science Center at Brooklyn College of Medicine; Director, Division of Neurology, Maimonides Medical Center, Brooklyn, New York

NEIL R. MILLER, M.D.

Professor of Neuro-ophthalmology, The Johns Hopkins University School of Medicine, Baltimore, Maryland

ROBERT G. MILLER, M.D.

Clinical Professor of Neurology, University of California, San Francisco, School of Medicine; Chairman, Department of Neurology, California Pacific Medical Center, San Francisco, California

PATRICIA M. MOORE, M.D.

Associate Professor of Neurology, Wayne State University School of Medicine; Vice Chief of Neurology, Harper Hospital, Detroit, Michigan

KEVIN D. MULLEN, M.B., F.R.C.P.I.

Associate Professor of Medicine, Case Western Reserve University School of Medicine; Consultant Gastroenterologist/Hepatologist, MetroHealth Medical Center, Cleveland, Ohio

THEODORE L. MUNSAT, M.D.

Professor of Pharmacology and Neurology, Tufts University School of Medicine; Director, Neuromuscular Research Unit, New England Medical Center, Boston, Massachusetts

RUTH NASS, M.D.

Associate Professor of Neurology, New York University School of Medicine, New York, New York

RICHARD K. OLNEY, M.D.

Associate Professor of Neurology, University of California, San Francisco, School of Medicine; Director, EMG Laboratory, University of California, San Francisco, Hospitals and Clinics, San Francisco, California

BRIAN R. OTT, M.D.

Assistant Professor, Department of Clinical Neurosciences, Brown University School of Medicine; Director, Alzheimer's Disease and Memory Disorders Unit, Neurology Division, Roger Williams Medical Center, Providence, Rhode Island

SUSAN C. PANNULLO, M.D.

Resident, Division of Neurosurgery, Department of Surgery, New York Hospital–Cornell University Medical Center; Fellow in Neuro-oncology, Department of Neurology, Memorial-Sloan Kettering Cancer Center, New York, New York

JOHN R. PARZIALE, M.D.

Clinical Assistant Professor of Rehabilitation Medicine, Brown University School of Medicine; Physiatrist-in-Chief, University Rehabilitation, East Providence, Rhode Island

WILLIAM W. PENDLEBURY, M.D.

Associate Professor of Pathology and Neurology, The University of Vermont College of Medicine; Director of Neuropathology, Medical Center Hospital of Vermont, Burlington, Vermont

KENNETH PERRINE, Ph.D.

Clinical Assistant Professor of Neurology, New York University School of Medicine; Chief of Neuropsychology, Hospital for Joint Diseases, New York, New York

HART PETERSON, M.D.

Clinical Professor of Neurology and of Neurology in Pediatrics, Cornell University Medical College; Attending Neurologist and Attending Pediatrician, The New York Hospital, and Attending Neurologist, Hospital for Special Surgery, New York, New York

R. MICHAEL POOLE, M.D.

Senior Instructor, Department of Neurology, University of Rochester School of Medicine; Attending Neurologist, Rochester General Hospital, Rochester, New York

ZIAD RIFAI, M.D.

Assistant Professor of Neurology, University of Rochester School of Medicine, Rochester, New York

GABRIËL J. E. RINKEL, M.D.

Assistant Professor of Neurology, University of Utrecht, Utrecht, The Netherlands

ALLAN E. RUBINSTEIN, M.D.

Associate Professor of Neurology, Mount Sinai School of Medicine of the City University of New York; Director, Mount Sinai Neurofibromatosis Center, and Medical Director, National Neurofibromatosis Foundation Center, New York, New York

THOMAS D. SABIN, M.D.

Professor of Neurology and Psychiatry, Boston University School of Medicine; Director, Neurological Unit, Boston City Hospital, Boston, Massachusetts

JEFFREY L. SAVER, M.D.

Assistant Professor of Neurology, Northwestern University Medical School; Assistant Director, Stroke Program, Northwestern Memorial Hospital, and Director, Stroke Service, Lakeside Veterans Administration Hospital, Chicago, Illinois

S. CLIFFORD SCHOLD Jr., M.D.

Professor and Chairman, Department of Neurology, The University of Texas Southwestern Medical School at Dallas; Chairman, Departments of Neurology, Parkland Memorial Hospital and Zale-Lipshy University Hospital, Dallas, Texas

ROBERT J. SCHWARTZMAN, M.D.

Professor and Chairman of Neurology, Jefferson Medical College of Thomas Jefferson University, Philadelphia, Pennsylvania

KAPIL D. SETHI, M.D., M.R.C.P. (U.K.)

Associate Professor of Neurology, Medical College of Georgia; Staff Physician, Veterans Hospital, and Director, Movement Disorders Clinic, Medical College of Georgia, Augusta, Georgia

WILLIAM A. SHEREMATA, M.D.

Associate Professor of Neurology, and Director, Multiple Sclerosis Center, University of Miami School of Medicine, Miami, Florida

LISA M. SHULMAN, M.D.

Clinical Fellow, Movement Disorders Center, Department of Neurology, University of Miami School of Medicine, Miami, Florida

RICHARD M. SILVER, M.D.

Professor of Medicine and Pediatrics, Medical University of South Carolina, Charleston, South Carolina

BARNEY J. STERN, M.D.

Associate Professor of Neurology, The Johns Hopkins University School of Medicine; Director, Division of Neurology, Department of Medicine, Sinai Hospital of Baltimore, Baltimore, Maryland

RICHARD L. STRUB, M.D.

Clinical Professor of Neurology, Tulane University School of Medicine; Chief of Neurology, Ochsner Clinic, New Orleans, Louisiana

LEWIS R. SUDARSKY, M.D.

Assistant Professor of Neurology, Harvard Medical School, Boston; Assistant Chief, Neurology Service, Veterans Administration Medical Center, West Roxbury, and Associate Physician in Neurology, Brigham and Women's Hospital, Boston, Massachusetts

CHARLES H. TEGELER, M.D.

Associate Professor of Neurology, Bowman Gray School of Medicine of Wake Forest University; Director, Neurosonology Laboratory, Wake Forest University Medical Center, Winston-Salem, North Carolina

ALLEN J. TEMAN, M.D.

Assistant Professor of Neurology, University of Miami School of Medicine, Miami, Florida

DAVID M. TREIMAN, M.D.

Professor of Neurology, University of California, Los Angeles, School of Medicine; Co-Director, Regional Epilepsy Center, Department of Veterans Affairs West Los Angeles Medical Center, Los Angeles, California

ROEKCHAI TULYAPRONCHOTE, M.D.

Clinical Instructor, St. Louis University School of Medicine; Cerebrovascular Fellow, Souers Stroke Institute, St. Louis, Missouri

KENNETH L. TYLER, M.D.

Associate Professor of Neurology, Medicine, and Microbiology-Immunology, University of Colorado School of Medicine; Neurologist, University Hospital and Denver Veterans Administration Medical Center, Denver, Colorado

JAN van GIJN, M.D., F.R.C.P.E.

Professor and Chairman, Department of Neurology, University of Utrecht; Head, Department of Neurology, University Hospital, Utrecht, The Netherlands

NAGAGOPAL VENNA, M.D.

Associate Professor of Neurology, Boston University School of Medicine; Director, Clinical Neurology, Boston City Hospital, Boston, Massachusetts

RUSSELL W. WALKER, M.D.

Associate Professor of Neurology, Cornell University Medical College; Associate Attending Neurologist, Memorial Sloan-Kettering Cancer Center, New York, New York

WILLIAM J. WEINER, M.D.

Professor of Neurology, and Director, Movement Disorders Center, University of Miami School of Medicine; Clinical Research Scholar, National Parkinson Foundation, Miami, Florida

PETER D. WILLIAMSON, M.D.

Professor of Medicine (Neurology), Dartmouth Medical School, Hanover, New Hampshire

JANET L. WILTERDINK, M.D.

Assistant Professor, Department of Clinical Neurosciences, Brown University School of Medicine; Attending Neurologist, Rhode Island Hospital, Providence, Rhode Island

ROBERT J. WITYK, M.D.

Instructor, Department of Neurology, The Johns Hopkins University School of Medicine; Physician, Division of Neurology, Department of Medicine, Sinai Hospital of Baltimore, Baltimore, Maryland

This book, the first of a new series on *Current Diagnosis* and an extension of the *Current Therapy* series, is designed to provide neurologic practitioners with a state of the art approach to the diagnosis of neurologic diseases. The format is to have a group of experienced physicians describe their approach to difficult and common diagnostic problems in neurology. This book is intended to be a practical aid for neurologists and neurology residents. It is also intended to be of value to internists and neurosurgeons as well as other physicians who care for patients with the diseases and conditions covered in this volume. The diseases in this book were selected because they were either commonly encountered in daily practice (headache), new and exciting conditions coming to the fore in clinical neurology (metabolic myopathies) or conditions traditionally known to be difficult to diagnose (dizziness). The table of contents makes it clear that the menu is diverse.

Pathophysiology and exhaustive lists of differential diagnoses are well covered in standard textbooks and are not repeated here. On the other hand, many physicians would like to know how to approach the diagnosis of a particular disease. Contributors have been selected based on experience and expertise with specific neurologic disorders. Emphasis is placed on the historical setting in which the diagnosis is suspected, the key physical signs and the laboratory tests necessary and sufficient for diagnosis. The differential diagnoses are practical, and common pitfalls in diagnostic approach are highlighted. Illustrations cover important diagnostic findings, as do summary tables and flow charts. A selected reference list is provided at the end of each chapter. Treatment is discussed only if empiric therapy helps establish a diagnosis. Otherwise, treatment of many of these conditions is described in detail in the companion volume to this text, *Current Therapy in Neurologic Diseases,* edited by Richard T. Johnson and John W. Griffin.

Edward Feldmann, M.D.

To Marcy

CONTENTS

MOVEMENT DISORDERS

EPILEPTIC DISORDERS

PSYCHOGENIC SEIZURES AND SYNCOPE

ORRIN DEVINSKY, M.D.

All that shakes is not epilepsy. The differential diagnosis of an epileptic seizure continues to challenge clinical neurologists. Paroxysmal changes in behavior result from a diverse group of medical, psychiatric, and neurologic disorders. These disorders may coexist in the same individual, further confounding accurate diagnosis.

The tremendous diversity of epileptic symptoms includes such vague phenomena as indescribable feelings, dizziness, lightheadedness, and other nonspecific symptoms such as nausea, chest discomfort, simple visual hallucinations, palpitations, fear, and sadness. Even those symptoms considered relatively specific for epilepsy, such as olfactory hallucinations, déjà vu, focal clonic jerking, and impairment of consciousness, can occur in patients with other disorders and even in healthy people. This is especially true of déjà vu and benign sleep jerks. Nonepileptic paroxysmal disorders are common and can mimic all forms of epileptic seizures (Table 1).

Correct diagnosis of paroxysmal disorders is essential. Failure to recognize seizures can prevent prompt diagnosis of treatable lesions such as an arteriovenous malformation prior to pregnancy or a low-grade tumor in childhood. Failure to diagnose may also fail to prevent death or injury from impaired consciousness or motor control while driving or operating dangerous equipment and may cause social, educational, and employment handicaps. In contrast, misdiagnosing other paroxysmal disorders as epilepsy can cause a long-standing stigma, with loss of self-esteem, employment opportunities, and driving privileges. The situation is compounded by failure to diagnose and treat the actual problem. This chapter reviews the clinical features of the two most common disorders that are confused with epilepsy: syncope and psychogenic seizures.

SYNCOPE

Syncope is common, causing more than 60 percent of episodes of brief loss of consciousness. Syncope is a transient loss of consciousness resulting from a transient, at least two-thirds reduction of cerebral blood flow. Vasovagal (vasodepressor) syncope is the most common cause, with neurogenic, orthostatic, and cardiac forms less frequent.

Differential diagnosis of syncope from seizure is a common problem. Both disorders are frequent and occur in all age groups. The diagnosis of syncope is supported if episodes: (1) are precipitated by anxiety or pain (e.g., venipuncture) or assumption of the upright position, (2) exclusively occur while standing or sitting, (3) are associated with facial pallor and diaphoresis, (4) are not associated with sustained tonic or clonic movements, bladder incontinence, or tongue or cheek bites, and (5) are not followed by postepisode confusion, lethargy, muscle soreness, and headache. Although incontinence strongly suggests a seizure (or convulsive syncope, as described below), if the bladder is unusually full when syncope occurs, there may be incontinence. While seizures often cause sinus tachycardia and rarely cause tachy- or bradyarrhythmias, loss of consciousness with documented bradycardia or tachyarrythmias should be considered a primary cardiac disorder until proven otherwise.

Prodromal symptoms such as abdominal sensations, (e.g., "butterflies" or nausea), flushing and warmth, dizziness and lightheadness, bilateral paresthesia, and feelings of fear and unreality occur with both syncope and epileptic seizures. Symptoms such as formed auditory or visual hallucinations, olfactory hallucinations, déjà vu, or focal sensory or motor phenomena strongly suggest partial seizures. A prodrome lasting several seconds followed by loss of consciousness for 15 to 60 seconds and followed by a rapid return to a normal level of attentiveness is typical of syncope. Such episodes are highly atypical for seizures. However, a brief or unwitnessed loss of consciousness followed by prolonged lethargy or an unnatural need to sleep strongly suggests a disorder other than simple syncope.

The greatest source of error in distinguishing seizures from faints is failure to recognize that brief tonic

Table 1 Nonepileptic Paroxysmal Disorders

I. Syncope
  A. Reflex
    1. Vasodepressor (vasovagal)
    2. Carotid sinus
    3. Glossopharyngeal
    4. Visceral stimuli
    5. Hyperventilation
  B. Respiratory
    1. Valsalva
    2. Cough
    3. Breath-holding spells (young children)
  C. Decreased systemic venous resistance—autonomic insufficiency
    1. Neurogenic
    2. Medication
  D. Hypovolemia/dehydration (orthostatic)
  E. Decreased left ventricular filling or emptying
    1. Pulmonary embolism
    2. Arrhythmias
    3. Aortic stenosis
    4. Myocardial infarction
    5. Mitral valve prolapse
  F. Cerebral ischemia
    1. Bilateral cervical arterial obstructions
    2. Vertebral-basilar migraine or transient ischemic attacks
    3. Sudden (plateau) waves of increased intracranial pressure
II. Cerebrovascular: transient ischemic attacks
III. Migraine
IV. Movement disorders
  A. Tics, Tourette syndrome
  B. Myoclonus
  C. Startle attacks
  D. Chorea and other dyskinesias
  E. Shuddering attacks
  F. Spasmus mutans
V. Sleep disorders
  A. Narcolepsy
  B. Night terrors
  C. Somnambulism
  D. Benign sleep jerks
  E. Restless legs
VI. Metabolic-toxic
  A. Hepatic or renal insufficiency
  B. Electrolyte disorders
  C. Endocrine
  D. Drug ingestion
VII. Visceral disorders (autonomic and affective symptoms; may cause loss of consciousness)
  A. Cardiac
  B. Gastrointestinal
VIII. Psychiatric disorders
  A. Panic disorder
  B. Somatization disorder
  C. Dissociative disorder
  D. Intermittent explosive disorder (episodic dyscontrol)
  E. Conversion disorder (psychogenic seizures and other symptoms)
IX. Malingering

or clonic movements often occur in syncope. These movements are often observed by witnesses, and their duration and intensity may be exaggerated. Observers commonly overestimate the duration of symptoms by two- to tenfold. Tonic and clonic movements during syncopal attacks are more common if the person is maintained in the upright or sitting position, which is often done by an observer attempting to prevent injury.

Falling to the ground serves an important compensatory role in syncope. It brings the head and the heart to the same level, facilitating blood flow to the brain. It is humbling to realize that when neurologists or internists at major teaching hospitals are shown a simultaneous video and electroencephalogram (EEG) of a young woman having a syncopal attack due to a bradyarrhythmia with brief tonic and clonic movements, the vast majority incorrectly diagnose epilepsy. In the real world, we are usually faced with partial and inaccurate observations.

Convulsive syncope refers to an episode of syncope in which the diminution of blood flow to the brain is more severe or prolonged. In such cases, the person, most often a child, has a tonic-clonic seizure due to the cerebral hypoxia. As discussed above, convulsive syncope often occurs when a person is maintained in the upright or sitting position. These tonic-clonic seizures are similar to those of primary epilepsy and can be associated with bladder incontinence, biting of tongue, lip, or cheek, muscle soreness, and postepisode confusion and lethargy. The differential diagnosis of epilepsy from convulsive syncope rests on the history. For example, a child with three tonic-clonic seizures occurring only in association with venipuncture or painful physical injury probably has convulsive syncope.

The history usually reveals the cause for loss of consciousness. Questions regarding the circumstances surrounding the attack, what occurred immediately before, during, and after the attack, and a history of similar episodes in other family members will often provide important diagnostic clues. Depending on the age of the patient and features of the attack, other paroxysmal behavioral disorders such as hyperventilation or narcolepsy should be considered and specific inquiries made.

The physical examination in patients with possible syncope includes a brief survey of general medical and neurologic systems and, specifically, palpation of the pulse and thyroid, measurement of orthostatic heart rate and blood pressure changes, and auscultation of the heart, lungs, and neck. Laboratory studies are often not necessary in obvious cases of vasovagal or orthostatic syncope in a young person. However, in any patient whose history and physical do not reveal the cause and in those over age 40 years old, an electrocardiogram (ECG) should be obtained. The QT interval must be measured. Patients with prolonged QT syndrome often present with syncope and later die during a subsequent attack. An ambulatory, 24-hour (Holter) ECG is helpful in evaluating patients with suspected arrhythmias. Routine or sleep deprived EEGs should be obtained when the history suggests an epileptic seizure. Unfortunately, a normal EEG is not uncommon in patients with epilepsy, especially in those with only one or infrequent seizures. Ambulatory, 24-hour EEG recordings can be useful in selected cases. This test should be reserved for those in whom there is a relatively strong suspicion of an epileptic seizure.

PSYCHOGENIC SEIZURES

Psychogenic (hysterical, pseudo, nonepileptic) seizures are among the most common forms of conversion disorder, occurring in approximately 15 percent of these patients. Conversion symptoms suggest a physical disorder but are due to psychological factors. Although sexual and physical abuse or a major life stress are often identified as the precipitating factor, in many cases no psychological cause can be identified. In many patients, prior abuse has been repressed and patients are unaware of its occurrence or magnitude. In contrast to patients with malingering and factitious disorder (Munchhausen syndrome), patients with psychogenic seizures and other conversion symptoms do not willfully feign epilepsy. When attacks develop or recur after minor head trauma, and litigation is pending or disability benefits are sought, intentional deceit should be considered.

The pathogenesis of psychogenic seizures is controversial, although psychiatrists postulate that most patients achieve either primary or secondary gain. In primary gain, an internal conflict or need is suppressed through the elaboration of a conversion symptom. For example, following rape or physical abuse, the rage and anger may be symbolically expressed as a seizure. In secondary gain, the seizure allows the patient to receive support and social services they might otherwise not obtain, or avoid unpleasant situations they would otherwise have to confront. In many cases, the mechanism underlying psychogenic seizures is never identified, because patients may be extremely resistant to psychiatric intervention. An amytal interview may be effective in uncovering repressed conflicts.

There are many pitfalls in the diagnosis of psychogenic seizures, and the diagnosis of psychogenic seizures and other forms of conversion disorder must be made with great care. Among patients diagnosed with conversion symptoms at major academic centers, 20 to 40 percent are subsequently found to have organic disorders such as epilepsy, lupus, or multiple sclerosis. On the other hand, conversion symptoms often go unrecognized. This is especially true for seizures. One must maintain a high degree of suspicion when seizures are refractory to therapy or when atypical features are present. Consider how most neurologists make the diagnosis of epilepsy: historically. In many cases, routine EEGs are normal or show nonspecific findings. A physician presented with the parents' eyewitness report of their 16-year-old daughter's episodes of right arm jerking movements, when routine and sleep deprived EEGs are normal, will likely make the diagnosis of partial epilepsy and will probably be correct. However, such a case could be a psychogenic seizure. Asking the parents to imitate or, even better, videotape the episode can provide important diagnostic information.

One common diagnostic error is the assumption that patients with psychogenic seizures have "hysterical" personality features. Histrionic (hysterical) personality traits (increased emotionality and attention-seeking behavior) and la belle indifference (inappropriate lack of concern) are incorrectly considered typical of hysterical (conversion) patients. The majority of patients with psychogenic seizures have neither of these features. Also, patients with attention-seeking behavior or indifference may have serious medical or neurologic disorders, as when a stoic person who avoids physicians is diagnosed with widely metastatic cancer. Another common error is to assume that episodes precipitated by stress are psychogenic. In some surveys, more than half of patients with epileptic seizures report that stress can precipitate or aggravate their disorder.

Clues to the diagnosis of psychogenic seizures are presented in Table 2. There is no single clinical finding that reliably allows one to distinguish psychogenic from epileptic seizures. A complete seizure history is essential. A careful description of the episode by the patient and a trustworthy witness should be obtained, but the recollections may be inaccurate or confusing. Beware of leading questions. When psychogenic seizures are considered, ask the patient to act out what occurred during the seizure. In some cases, you will be shocked to see the entire "tonic-clonic" seizure recalled from memory. It is also helpful to have witnesses imitate the behaviors they saw. Wild head movements, rapid kicking, and thrashing movements may be demonstrated, leading one to strongly suspect a psychogenic attack.

Important historical data to obtain include:

1. Precipitating features: e.g., sleep deprivation, stress, drugs
2. Suggestibility: ability to talk the subject into or out of a seizure
3. Mode of onset: gradual versus sudden
4. Duration: brief (ictal phase <5 minutes) versus prolonged
5. Stereotypy: episodes nearly identical versus frequently changing
6. Ictal features: typical versus atypical for partial or tonic-clonic seizures
7. Ability to recall events during the seizure
8. Bodily injury during the seizure: e.g., tongue or lip bites, laceration
9. Postictal state: confusion, lethargy, muscle soreness

The combination of several clinical features may allow a fairly confident diagnosis of psychogenic seizures. Attacks that are always precipitated by the same stressor, begin gradually with symptoms that wax and wane, last longer than 15 minutes, and are followed by a feeling of relief can be reliably diagnosed on historical grounds as nonepileptic. Unfortunately, the history is often unclear or includes features suggesting both epileptic and psychogenic seizures.

Psychogenic seizures are most often confused with complex partial seizures (CPS) and generalized tonic-clonic seizures (GTCS). CPS are usually accompanied by sudden involuntary changes in facial expression, e.g., blank stare or grimace, automatisms, and amnesia for the episode. Automatisms are stereotypical and classified

Table 2   Clinical Features of Psychogenic Seizures

Clinical Feature	Comment
Seizures induced by stress or specific settings (school, spouse)	Stress can precipitate epileptic seizures
Frequent seizures despite therapeutic AED levels	AED toxicity (especially phenytoin and carbamazepine) may exacerbate seizures or cause symptoms confused with seizure
Gradual onset of ictus	Epileptic seizures begin suddenly but are often preceded by auras (usually <1 min) or premonitory symptoms (e.g., irritability, depression; last hours)
Prolonged duration	Epileptic seizures usually last <5 min; any seizure type can be prolonged
Thrashing, struggling, crying, pelvic thrusting, side-to-side rolling, wild movements	Bizarre, complex automatisms occur with frontal lobe complex partial seizures
Intermittent, arrhythmic, out-of-phase jerking	During GTCS, jerking is rhythmic, in phase, and usually slows before stopping
Motor activity that stops and starts	Activity that waxes and wanes several times during the same spell is very rare in epilepsy; CPS status is often a series of discrete seizures
Bilateral motor activity with preserved consciousness	May occur with supplementary motor area seizures
Clinical features that fluctuate from one seizure to the next	Epileptic seizures are usually stereotypical
Lack of postictal confusion or lethargy after GTCS or CPS	May occur with frontal lobe and, less often, temporal lobe CPS
Postictal crying or shouting of obscenities	Aggressive verbal and physical behavior can occur if patients are restrained

AED = antiepileptic drug; GTCS = generalized tonic-clonic seizures; CPS = complex partial seizures.

into the following types, the first two being most common: (1) oral-alimentary (lip smacking, chewing, swallowing), (2) upper extremity–gestural (hand clasping, grabbing, picking, tapping, waving, dystonic posture), (3) lower extremity–ambulatory (walking, running, kicking, bicycling movements), (4) vocalizations (grunts, screams, repetition of words or phrases), and (5) sexual (pelvic thrusting, masturbatory movements). Postictal disorientation, confusion, and lethargy are common. Occasionally, complex partial status occurs and presents as prolonged confusion or bizarre behavior. In most cases, complex partial status consists in a series of CPS with the interseizure interval characterized by quiet or agitated confusion.

During psychogenic seizures, facial expression usually appears volitional, and the "automatic" behaviors seen are rarely characteristic of those found in CPS. Postictally, patients are often attentive and oriented and are able to recall the episode in detail. Some can imitate the ictal automatisms.

GTCS are characterized by sudden loss of consciousness, a tonic phase (single cry or shriek, adversive or extension movements of the head, tonic spasm of the appendicular and truncal muscles), followed by a clonic phase in which the bilateral, symmetrical (or nearly so) tonic contractions are interrupted by periods of relaxation. As the seizure ends, the rate of the clonic contractions gradually slows, and there is often a final, large clonic jerk followed by flaccidity and coma. The end of a GTCS is the most difficult part to imitate. In most psychogenic attacks, the rate of jerking increases and then suddenly stops. During and immediately after GTCS, memory, pupillary light and corneal reflexes, and responsiveness to noxious stimuli are absent. The ictal phase usually lasts less than 3 minutes, and the postictal phase often blends into sleep. Features that help distinguish psychogenic seizures from GTCS include the absence of (1) cyanosis, (2) injury (tongue or cheek biting, especially of the sides, or trauma), (3) incontinence, or (4) progressive slowing of clonic jerks. With psychogenic seizures that mimic GTCS, patients often recall events during the period of bilateral motor activity (beware of supplementary motor area seizures); jerking movements are out of phase (e.g., left arm extends the while the right arm flexes); motor activity stops and starts (as if the patient gets tired and takes a brief rest—imitation of the movement by a witness can help distinguish from clonic jerks); and there is often pelvic thrusting, rolling, or thrashing from side to side.

Some patients with psychogenic seizures have sophisticated medical knowledge. This information is acquired through a personal history of epilepsy, observing seizures in others, extensive reading, attending epilepsy self-help groups, and, not infrequently, having been previously diagnosed with psychogenic seizures by doctors who told them "what they did wrong." Occasionally patients may injure themselves or urinate during psychogenic GTCS or display typical automatisms during psychogenic CPS. I have seen patients with a negative provocation test later comment to a friend (on camera), "they thought they were going to fool me with that normal saline."

Another important caveat is that epileptic seizures can evoke bizarre behavior and a very great diversity of symptoms. Symptoms such as autoscopy (out-of-body experiences or seeing one's double), derealization, depression, fear, and laughing automatisms may be mistaken for primary psychiatric symptoms. Frontal lobe seizures are most often confused with nonepileptic attacks (see the chapter *Temporal and Extratemporal Lobe Seizures*). Also, patients with epilepsy can develop personality changes or depression that suggests psychiatric disease. Epilepsy and behavioral disorders are not mutually exclusive.

The EEG cannot be used in isolation to diagnose psychogenic seizures. A normal interictal EEG is not uncommon in patients with epilepsy. Conversely, the presence of interictal epileptiform activity does not confirm the diagnosis. True epileptiform discharges occur in 1 to 2 percent of the general population. In addition, patterns that are normal (mu rhythm, 14 and 6 Hz positive spikes, positive occipital sharp transients of sleep, lambda waves) or of uncertain clinical significance (benign epileptiform transients of sleep or small sharp spikes, rhythmic midtemporal discharge of drowsiness, a psychomotor variant, and wicket spikes) may be misinterpreted as supporting the diagnosis of epilepsy. Finally, because 10 to 40 percent of patients with psychogenic seizures have also had epileptic seizures, interictal or ictal epileptiform activity does not prove that all their seizures are epileptic.

Familiarity with EEG patterns during and after the ictus is essential for accurate diagnosis. Ictal recordings of (1) absence seizures always reveal generalized epileptiform discharges, almost always spike and wave discharges; (2) simple partial seizures often show no changes in the background activity, but focal epileptiform or rhythmic slowing may be found; (3) temporal lobe CPS most often show unilateral or bilateral rhythmic temporal slowing; (4) frontal lobe CPS show epileptiform transients, slow activity, or no background changes. The ictal and postictal EEG and GTCS is always abnormal. During the tonic phase, there is a buildup of generalized low-voltage fast activity that evolves into a high-voltage generalized polyspike discharge. With muscular relaxation in the clonic phase and postictally, there is generalized suppression of EEG activity. Muscle artifact often obscures cerebral electrographic seizure discharges during GTCS and less often, during CPS. Although not pathognomonic, absence of background depression or immediate return of the alpha rhythm after GTCS or a 1 minute or longer CPS strongly suggests a psychogenic seizure.

Simultaneous video-EEG monitoring has revolutionized our understanding of psychogenic seizures. Fifteen years ago, these spells were considered uncommon. They now appear epidemic. However, there is no evidence that the incidence has changed. Video-EEG monitoring has, however, allowed us to confidently make the diagnosis. Such studies have served to humble all experts. "Definitive" clinical diagnoses of psychogenic or epileptic seizures are not infrequently wrong. Patients who appear to be solid citizens without a sign of behavioral problems, have spells that are "classic" but are subsequently found to be psychogenic seizures. Unfortunately, many of these patients are only diagnosed after years or decades of antiepileptic drug therapy (often polytherapy with disabling doses), when they are referred for consideration of epilepsy surgery.

Video-EEG monitoring permits a simultaneous correlation of behavior (video and audio) and the EEG.

Attacks can be viewed in slow motion and replayed for careful study. When multiple attacks are recorded, stereotypy of features and duration can be determined. Further, in patients with multiple episode types, recorded seizures can be shown to family members or care givers for comparison with events observed outside the hospital.

Provocative testing with suggestion has been an invaluable tool in my experience. The test requires the physician to suggest to the patient that some provocation (placement of alcohol pads "over the carotid artery" or injection of normal saline) can cause seizures in people with epilepsy. I have found that when the patient and family are told what was done and why (to make a diagnosis and help the patient), the doctor-patient relationship is rarely harmed. When the relationship is damaged, it is often because of the diagnosis of psychogenic seizures, not because of how the diagnosis was made. Provocative testing is best performed during video-EEG monitoring so that if an episode occurs, it can be studied and later examined by family members to ensure that it is the same as those occurring outside the hospital. Provocative testing can be performed in the doctor's office, ideally with EEG monitoring. I find it helpful to have an "antidote" available to abort intense or prolonged attacks.

Serum prolactin levels increase after all GTCS, most CPS, and some SPS. Postictal levels (20 to 50 ng per milliliter) peak within 15 minutes after the seizure and return to baseline levels (5 to 10 ng per milliliter) after approximately 30 to 60 minutes. Prolactin levels are not significantly increased after psychogenic seizures. As with individual clinical and EEG criteria, absence of postictal prolactin elevation is not by itself a reliable indicator of a psychogenic seizure. Few have found prolactin levels to be practical and reliable in differentiating epileptic and nonepileptic seizures.

Head computed tomography or, preferably, magnetic resonance imaging should be obtained in patients with suspected epilepsy. Many patients with psychogenic seizures have epileptic seizures or other central nervous system disorders, and occasionally epileptic seizures produce bizarre features leading to a misdiagnosis of hysteria. Some findings such as arachnoid cysts may be confusing because such lesions can cause seizures. In the vast majority of these cases, however, the seizures are easily controlled with low therapeutic levels of a single antiepileptic drug.

SUGGESTED READING

Cohen RJ, Suter C. Hysterical seizures: Suggestion as a provocative EEG test. Ann Neurol 1982; 11:391–395.
Desai BT, Porter RJ, Penry JK. Psychogenic seizures: A study of 42 attacks in six patients, with intensive monitoring. Arch Neurol 1982; 39:202–209.
Gates JR, Ramani V, Whalen S, Loewenson R. Ictal characteristics of pseudoseizures. Arch Neurol 1985; 42:1183–1187.
Leis AA, Ross MA, Summers AK. Psychogenic seizures: Ictal characteristics and diagnostic pitfalls. Neurology 1992; 42:95–99.

Merskey H, Buhrich NA. Hysteria and organic brain disease. Br J Med Psychol 1975; 48:359–366.

Porter RJ. Epilepsy: 100 elementary principles. 2nd ed. Philadelphia: WB Saunders, 1989.

Saygi S, Katz A, Marks DA, Spencer SS. Frontal lobe partial seizures and psychogenic seizures: Comparison of clinical and ictal characteristics. Neurology 1992; 42:1274–1277.

Sperling MR, Pritchard PB, Engel J, et al. Prolactin in partial epilepsy: An indicator of limbic seizures. Ann Neurol 20:716–722.

Williamson PD, Spencer DD, Spencer SS, et al. Complex partial seizures of frontal lobe origin. Ann Neurol 1985; 18:497–504.

TEMPORAL AND EXTRATEMPORAL LOBE SEIZURES

PETER D. WILLIAMSON, M.D.

Specialized epilepsy units offering continuous closed circuit television and electroencephalographic (EEG) monitoring began to be developed in the late 1960s and early 1970s coincident with newly available video technology. At the same time, developments in surgical technique resulted in a renewed interest in surgical intervention for medically refractory epilepsy. The combination of specialized epilepsy units and revitalized epilepsy surgery resulted in the creation of comprehensive epilepsy programs, offering enhanced diagnostic possibilities and modern medical and surgical management of seizures. As the diagnostic power and importance of epilepsy centers was appreciated in the late 1970s and early 1980s, there was a virtual explosion in the number of such centers across the country and throughout the world.

The wealth of clinical data produced by these specialized centers has greatly increased our knowledge and understanding of seizures and epilepsy. Recognition of the enormous potential benefit of resective surgery in selected patients has resulted in improved identification and subclassification of the symptomatic focal, or localization-related epilepsies. This subclassification can take several forms. Because of the long-recognized importance of the temporal lobe as the site of origin for complex partial seizures, an appropriate way to start is to divide the symptomatic localization-related epilepsies into the two broad categories of temporal lobe epilepsy and extratemporal epilepsy. While this separation might seem artificial, it serves an important purpose. Temporal lobe epilepsy is still the single most common type of focal epilepsy associated with successful surgical intervention in adults. However, we also now know that many focal seizures originate in restricted brain regions **outside** of the temporal lobe. How then can these two broad categories be identified and separated?

This can be done by two basic methods, and these are not mutually exclusive. The first involves the identification of a temporal lobe syndrome and then determining whether patients fit the requirements of the syndrome. Using this method, some patients will clearly qualify for the temporal lobe syndrome, while others will have atypical findings, or "red flags." These red flags often suggest that seizures are beginning outside the temporal lobe. The second method involves the identification of extratemporal seizures in different groups of patients, with seizure origin being from a similar region in each group. The overall features of each group of patients are then examined to determine if extratemporal localization-related syndromes can be specified. The identification of both temporal and extratemporal lobe epilepsy syndromes requires that seizure origin be very well documented. The gold standard, of course, is focal cerebral resection that results in cure. Once syndromes have been established, patients can be assigned to one or another group with a fair degree of certainty.

MEDIAL TEMPORAL LOBE EPILEPSY SYNDROME

The temporal lobe syndrome to be described below was derived from a retrospective evaluation of a "pure culture" of temporal lobe epilepsy patients. Patients in this temporal lobe epilepsy syndrome met the following three criteria:

1. Temporal lobe seizure origin determined by intracranial EEG monitoring
2. No space-occupying lesions
3. Seizure elimination following surgery

Since intracranial monitoring demonstrated that all seizures began in the medial temporal structures, the syndrome has been designated the medial temporal lobe epilepsy (MTLE) syndrome. For purposes of convenience, this syndrome has been divided into two components. The first contains the information that would be available after taking an initial detailed history and performing a neurologic examination. The second includes the information that would be available following a comprehensive initial evaluation that included epilepsy unit inpatient monitoring during which seizures were recorded noninvasively.

History and Neurologic Examination

Up to 80 percent of patients with MTLE syndrome have a history of convulsions during infancy or early childhood. In most instances these are complicated febrile convulsions. From 5 to 10 percent of the convulsions are associated with bacterial meningitis, but viral encephalitis or meningoencephalitis is rarely, if ever, documented in these patients. A history of significant head injury or birth trauma is uncommon and probably not related to this syndrome.

Habitual seizures typically begin in the latter part of the first decade or the early part of the second decade of life. Onset of habitual seizures before the age of 2 or after the age of 15 happens uncommonly and should cause concern over the diagnosis of MTLE. If complicated febrile seizures are considered a probable cause of this syndrome, then there is usually a silent period between the presumed cerebral insult and the development of habitual seizures. There is often a second silent period during which seizures appear to come under control with medications. Patients may even remain seizure-free for several years after medications are discontinued, only to have seizures return with a vengeance. Both of these silent periods would suggest that this type of epilepsy is a progressive disease with cerebral changes taking place subclinically.

Almost all patients with the MTLE syndrome have an aura. Auras are so common that their absence is reason for concern about the correct diagnosis. By far the most frequent aura is some type of a visceral sensation. Fear is the second most frequent type of aura, but it is sometimes difficult to determine if the feeling of fear is itself an aura or whether it is a reaction to another symptom associated with seizure onset. Auras that are commonly thought to be associated with temporal lobe epilepsy, such as déjà vu, micropsia, macropsia, depersonalization, and olfactory hallucinations, do occur but are much less common. Some patients have auras that they cannot describe, possibly because the sensations are not part of normal human experience.

All patients with MTLE have partial seizures. One would expect that patients referred to specialized epilepsy centers would all have complex partial seizures (CPS), but occasionally patients are seen who have only auras without alteration of consciousness. Approximately half the patients have secondarily generalized convulsive seizures, either as the initial seizure type or at periodic intervals, but never as the predominant seizure type. These secondarily generalized seizures always occur after the onset of a habitual CPS and never appear to begin de novo.

Neurologic examination is usually entirely normal. A few patients have evidence of a subtle hemiparesis on the side contralateral to seizure origin.

Electroencephalogram, Clinical Seizure Characteristics, and Imaging

Routine or baseline EEGs on patients with the MTLE syndrome are often normal or nonspecific. Long-term monitoring, however, with recording during waking and through all stages of sleep, almost always reveals localized paroxysmal abnormalities. These abnormalities are detectable using the standard 10 to 20 electrodes; special electrodes are seldom required. Paroxysmal abnormalities consisting of spikes or sharp and slow complexes are strictly unilateral in about half the cases, with the other half revealing varying degrees of bilateral, independent paroxysmal activity. Lateralization discordant with the side of seizure origin is very uncommon when the paroxysmal activity is strictly unilateral, but greater paroxysmal activity may be seen in the hemisphere where seizures are *not* originating in as many as 25 percent of patients with bilateral EEG abnormalities. This paroxysmal activity, whether unilateral or bilateral and independent, is almost always located over the anterior temporal regions. Location elsewhere, particularly in the posterior temporal region, is cause for concern regarding the diagnosis of MTLE syndrome. Bilateral, dependent paroxysmal activity (secondary bilateral synchrony) would be unusual with this syndrome.

Scalp EEG changes during an aura or during the initial part of the seizure are very uncommon. Lateralized buildup of sharp theta activity after the seizure has started occurs in over 80 percent of the seizures recorded, and it is usually concordant with the side of seizure origin. Lateralized postictal slowing occurs following about 50 percent of the seizures, and it is a reliable lateralizing sign.

Clinical seizure characteristics are an extremely important part of the evaluation of patients with seizures of any type. This is certainly true for seizures associated with the MTLE syndrome. Some clinical features are more general, while others have the potential to lateralize to the side of seizure origin. As noted previously, almost all these patients have some type of aura, usually a visceral or epigastric sensation. Although some patients have seizures that are quite bland, consisting of loss of contact and staring, most patients have more elaborate seizures. After an aura, there may be a momentary motor arrest followed by semipurposeful coordinated motor activity (automatisms), or the seizure may progress directly to automatic motor activity. Oral alimentary automatisms (lip smacking, chewing, and swallowing) are common and usually occur early in the seizure. Fumbling and picking hand and arm movements are seen frequently. More elaborate motor activity includes repetitive vocalization and semipurposeful reactions to environmental situations. A rich variety of automatic semipurposeful activity can be seen with MTLE, but the repertoire of clinical characteristics for each patient is very stereotyped. Directed aggression and purposeful violence during seizures are exceedingly rare.

Recently, lateralizing features of MTLE seizures have been described. If carefully looked for, they can be detected in seizures in at least 40 to 50 percent of patients. The most common lateralized motor manifestation is dystonic posturing of the arm and hand and sometimes the foot and leg contralateral to the side of seizure origin. This dystonic posturing can be subtle or obvious, but it is constant for a given patient. Often, contralateral dystonic posturing is combined with ipsilateral automatisms of the other hand. Whether or not ipsilateral automatisms in themselves have lateralizing significance is not clear. Head deviation can occur at two different times during MTLE seizures. During the first half of the seizure, head deviation toward the side of seizure origin can occur. This ipsilateral deviation does not have a strongly forced quality, but it is consistent and is not a reaction to the environment. Later in the seizure and sometimes as a prelude to the development of a secondarily generalized seizure, there can be a forced tonic or tonic-clonic head deviation contralateral to the side of seizure origin. When both types of head deviation occur in the same patient, it can be striking, with the head going from one extreme to the other. Finally, postictal aphasia, when it can be clearly demonstrated, is most often due to seizure origin on the language-dominant side. When it occurs, it is often associated with a prolonged period of postictal confusion as well as aphasia. The postictal phase of nonlanguage-dominant seizure origin is significantly shorter.

Neuroimaging has revolutionized the way we practice neurology in general, and it has become an essential part of the presurgical evaluation of patients with epilepsy. Computed tomography scans are generally not helpful in the MTLE syndrome. Magnetic resonance imaging (MRI), however, is proving to be very sensitive in detecting subtle abnormalities in the medial temporal regions. These abnormalities are increased hippocampal signal intensity on T2 weighted coronal views, and relative smallness (atrophy) of the hippocampus on T1 weighted coronal images. Patients in whom these MRI abnormalities are detected and who eventually go to surgery almost always have typical medial temporal (hippocampal) sclerosis demonstrated on pathologic examination. This MRI finding is so important that its absence should cause serious concern about the diagnosis of the MTLE syndrome.

The foregoing sections describe the syndrome of MTLE. If a patient presents with all of the above findings, the diagnosis is virtually assured. If all lateralizing findings are congruent, then medial temporal lobectomy is highly effective in curing the epilepsy. Further studies such as intracranial EEG are unnecessary. How far the clinical findings need to stray from the ideal described above in order to exclude the diagnosis of MTLE is not known, but certain common sense considerations should prevail. For example, a patient with no known risk factors whose seizures begin with an asymmetrical tonic posture, with no preceding aura, followed by rapid secondary generalization into a tonic-clonic seizure does not have the MTLE syndrome, and seizure origin is certainly outside the temporal lobes. Some patients without the MTLE syndrome will fit into one of the categories of extratemporal lobe epilepsy described below. The final diagnosis will depend on careful assessment of all the information for each patient.

EXTRATEMPORAL EPILEPSY SYNDROMES

The term *extratemporal epilepsy* is largely a product of epilepsy surgery programs. Most CPS begin in the temporal lobe, and most temporal lobe seizures are associated with seizure origin in the medial temporal structures. Although a small percentage of temporal lobe seizures begin in the lateral or neocortical temporal structures, surprisingly little well-documented data is available concerning them. Available information suggests that neocortical temporal seizures spread rapidly to medial structures and are therefore clinically indistinguishable from the seizures of MTLE. Elementary auditory hallucinations and possibly vertiginous auras have been associated with temporal neocortical seizure origin. Formed or complex visual and auditory hallucinations, as well as complex memories, have also been considered indications of temporal neocortical seizure origin, but documentation is uneven at best. Risk factors, history, neuroimaging, and possibly EEG findings often do not fit the MTLE syndrome. Since it requires future study, the syndrome of neocortical temporal epilepsy is not examined further here. The remainder of this discussion concentrates on examining the different types of seizures that originate in the frontal, occipital, and parietal lobes.

Frontal Lobe Epilepsy

A variety of frontal lobe seizure types have been described. Most include some type of motor activity: tonic, clonic, prominent motor automatisms, or a combination of all three. All types of status epilepticus, convulsive and nonconvulsive, have been associated with frontal lobe seizure origin, as have seizures that rapidly secondarily generalize into tonic-clonic convulsions. The protean manifestations of frontal lobe seizures make syndromic classification difficult, but there are at least two seizure types that can be identified with some consistency: frontal lobe complex seizures (FLCPS) and supplementary motor area (SMA) epilepsy.

Frontal Lobe Complex Partial Seizures

Frontal lobe seizures with loss of contact and complex clinical manifestations are uncommon attacks that have only recently been recognized and defined. They begin suddenly, often explosively, and end the same way. They are brief, frequent seizures that are followed by little, if any, postictal confusion. Frenetic, fumbling motor automatisms include bimanual or bipedal activity or both. Vocalization is common and varies from simple humming to shouted obscenities. Sexual automatisms with genital manipulation and pelvic thrusting are common. Warnings or auras occur, but they are nonspecific, such as vague cephalic sensations or feelings of muscle tightness. Complex partial status epilepticus occurs in about half of patients with FLCPS. This is manifested by prolonged repetitive or continuous abnormal behavior. This constellation of clinical seizure manifestations often results in very bizarre-appearing attacks. It is not surprising that these patients are frequently considered hysterical or diagnosed as having pseudoseizures. Some patients have histories of prolonged confinement in psychiatric institutions solely because of their clinical seizure manifestations.

The only consistent risk factor, found in a minority of patients with FLCPS, is a history of head trauma. Some patients have small, circumscribed space-occupying lesions in the medial or orbital frontal regions. Unequivocal paroxysmal interictal EEG abnormalities are found in some of these patients. There are, however, patients with very unusual attacks whose ictal and interictal EEGs are normal or nonspecific and whose neuroimaging studies are normal. In these cases, only awareness of and familiarity with these uncommon seizures will prevent diagnostic error.

Intracranial recording shows that when these seizures occur in their typical form, seizure activity remains confined to the frontal lobes even during episodes of complex partial status epilepticus. Spread into the temporal lobe in some patients results in seizures that initially have the characteristics of frontal lobe CPS and subsequently resemble temporal lobe seizures. Although very few documented examples exist, seizure origin has been shown to occur most consistently in the medial or orbital frontal regions. There is some evidence that these seizures may also begin in the lateral frontal convexities. Since these peculiar seizures can begin in various different frontal lobe regions, they do not constitute a single localization-related epilepsy syndrome. They are, however, a unique and identifiable type of frontal lobe epilepsy.

Supplementary Motor Area Epilepsy

Seizures that originate in the SMA are rare. When they present in their typical form, they are recognizable. Again, experience is helpful. Typically, these seizures begin suddenly with the assumption of an asymmetrical tonic posture. The arm contralateral to the side of seizure origin is abducted at the shoulder, flexed at the elbow and externally rotated. The head and eyes turn toward the up-raised hand. Both legs and the other arm may be held in tonic extension. These seizures are brief and consciousness is usually maintained. They may spread to involve the adjacent primary motor area with consequent focal clonic activity. They may also generalize rapidly. Many variations of this posture have been described. The literature, however, contains very few well-documented examples of SMA epilepsy. As with frontal lobe CPS, the EEG is often nonspecific or normal in these patients, a finding that can promote diagnostic error. Furthermore, many seizures originating outside the SMA and, in some cases, outside the frontal lobe can exhibit asymmetrical tonic posturing, thereby mimicking SMA seizures. This is a critical observation because seizures with asymmetrical tonic posturing originating outside the SMA are much more common than true SMA seizures. It has been speculated that seizure spread is responsible for the tonic motor activity. This has been

documented with intracranial recording in some, but not all, patients.

A common risk factor for SMA epilepsy has not been identified. Modern neuroimaging has frequently demonstrated structural abnormalities in the few well-documented patients.

Other Types of Frontal Lobe Seizures

Focal clonic motor activity has long been associated with seizures involving the prerolandic gyrus. However, this can be and often is due to the spread of seizure activity from clinically silent areas in front of or behind the rolandic fissure. Very brief tonic seizures, accompanied often by vocal grunts or snorting noises, have been described as beginning in the frontal convexities. Some frontal seizures can spread very rapidly and can present as generalized convulsive tonic-clonic events. In the absence of structural lesions, frontal lobe seizures can be extremely difficult to localize and, in some instances, may represent diffuse, possibly bilateral disease.

Occipital Lobe Epilepsy

Occipital lobe epilepsy presents with multiple seizure types and, as such, does not constitute a single syndrome. Intracranial recording has conclusively demonstrated that the different types of seizures seen are due to variable spread patterns from the occipital lobe. Seizures can spread medially or laterally and above or below the sylvian fissure. Different seizure types can be seen among different patients but can also occur in the same patient. When multiple clinical seizure types are seen in the same patient, it can also suggest multifocal epilepsy. Most seizures of occipital lobe origin, however, can be identified by virtue of their initial signs or symptoms. These include the well-recognized phenomenon of elementary visual hallucinations, usually consisting of flashing colored lights. When these elementary hallucinations are lateralized, they are always lateralized to the visual field contralateral to the side of origin. A less well-recognized but quite common initial symptom of occipital lobe epilepsy is ictal amaurosis. This is manifested by the sudden dimming or complete loss of vision, either a blackout or a whiteout. While theoretically the ictal blindness could be confined to one visual field, this has never been reported. Eye movement or eye pulling sensations in the absence of detectable movement also occur in patients with occipital lobe seizure origin. Forced blinking or eyelid flutter can occur shortly after seizure origin, as can eye deviation. While eye deviation is usually contralateral to the side of seizure origin, ipsilateral deviation can occur in some patients with occipital lobe seizures.

Occipital lobe epilepsy is often one of the most difficult and complex types of seizure disorder encountered in specialized referral centers. Only recently has this type of epilepsy been well defined. In addition to careful attention to the initial signs and symptoms described above, visual field examination often provides evidence of occipital lobe disease. Field cuts can be very subtle in these patients, detectable only by formal testing. MRI-detectable lesions are present in over half of the adult patients with occipital lobe epilepsy.

Parietal Lobe Epilepsy

Very little has been written about parietal lobe epilepsy. It may be that outside the primary sensory region the parietal lobes are clinically silent in terms of seizure activity. If this were the case, clinical manifestations of parietal lobe epilepsy would not be apparent until after the seizures had spread beyond the confines of the parietal lobe. Recent reports on well-documented parietal lobe epilepsy confirm this possibility and show that parietal lobe epilepsy, like occipital lobe epilepsy, can present with multiple different seizure types, depending on seizure propagation patterns. Unfortunately, somatosensory auras or warnings are the exception rather than the rule in these seizures, so there are often no initial signs or symptoms to help identify the correct region of seizure origin. However, many patients with parietal lobe seizure origin have causative structural lesions demonstrated on MRI.

COMMENTS

Most patients with typical MTLE can be identified on the basis of clinical findings alone. Neuroimaging increases the yield. In a specialized epilepsy referral center, patients with the MTLE syndrome are the single most common type of epilepsy patient seen and constitute 50 to 60 percent of the patients evaluated for surgery. From 20 to 30 percent of the patients referred have extratemporal seizure origin as determined by clinical seizure characteristics, structural lesions, or both. The remaining 20 to 30 percent of patients with partial seizures who are thought to have symptomatic localization-related epilepsy have normal MRIs and do not fit into any particular diagnostic category. Some of these are probably atypical examples of temporal lobe

epilepsy, possibly with seizures originating in the temporal neocortex. Other patients may have one or more epileptogenic foci from such conditions as neural migration disorders. Some patients may have a more diffuse epileptic encephalopathy that presents mainly with partial seizures. It is this last 20 to 30 percent of patients who currently represent the greatest diagnostic challenge in terms of localizing regions of seizure origin.

SUGGESTED READING

Chauvel P, Delgado-Escueta A, Halgren E, Bancaud J. Frontal lobe seizures and epilepsies: Advances in neurology. Vol 57. New York: Raven Press, 1992.

Geier S, Bancaud J, Talairach J, et al. The seizures of frontal lobe epilepsy: A study of clinical manifestations. Neurology 1977; 27:951–958.

Jackson GD, Berkovic SF, Tress BM, et al. Hippocampal sclerosis can be reliably detected by magnetic resonance imaging. Neurology 1990; 40:1869–1875.

Kanner AM, Morris HH, Lüders H, et al. Supplementary motor seizures mimicking pseudoseizures: Some clinical differences. Neurology 1990; 40:1404–1407.

Kotagal P, Lüders H, Morris HH, et al. Dystonic posturing in complex partial seizures of temporal lobe onset: A new lateralizing sign. Neurology 1989; 39:196–201.

Quesney LF. Clinical and EEG features of complex partial seizures of temporal lobe origin. Epilepsia 1986; 27(suppl 2):527–545.

Waterman K, Purves SJ, Kosaka B, et al. An epileptic syndrome caused by mesial frontal lobe foci. Neurology 1987; 37:577–582.

Williamson PD, Boon PA, Thadani VM, et al. Parietal lobe epilepsy: Diagnostic considerations and results of surgery. Ann Neurol 1992; 31:193–201.

Williamson PD, Mattson RH, Spencer DD, Spencer SS. Complex partial status epilepticus: A depth electrode evaluation. Ann Neurol 1983; 18:647–654.

Williamson PD, Spencer DD, Spencer SS, et al. Complex partial seizures of frontal lobe origin. Ann Neurol 1985; 18:497–504.

Williamson PD, Spencer SS. Clinical and EEG features of complex partial seizures of extratemporal origin. Epilepsia 1986; 27(suppl 2):46–63.

Williamson PD, Thadani VM, Darcey TM, et al. Occipital lobe epilepsy: Clinical characteristics, seizure spread patterns and results of surgery. Ann Neurol 1992; 31:3–13.

Williamson PD, Wieser HG, Delgado-Escueta AV. Clinical characteristics of partial seizures. In: Engel J Jr, ed. Surgical treatment of the epilepsies. New York: Raven Press, 1987:101.

GENERALIZED CONVULSIVE, NONCONVULSIVE, AND FOCAL STATUS EPILEPTICUS

DAVID M. TREIMAN, M.D.

Table 1 Classification of Status Epilepticus

Generalized convulsive status epilepticus (includes both primarily and secondarily generalized seizures)
  Overt (GTCS or major motor SE)
  Subtle (most cases of "myoclonic" SE and "electrical" SE)
Nonconvulsive SE (epileptic twilight state)
  Complex partial SE
  Absence SE (spike-wave stupor)
Simple partial SE (no impairment of consciousness)

GTCS = generalized tonic-clonic seizures; SE = status epilepticus.
From Treiman DM. Generalized convulsive status epilepticus in the adult. Epilepsia 1993; 34 (suppl1): S2-S11; with permission.

The term *status epilepticus* (SE) is used whenever a seizure recurs frequently enough or lasts long enough that there is a sustained alteration in the physiologic function of the brain. This may take the form of failure to recover full neurologic function, including normalization of the electroencephalogram (EEG) between successive seizures or of progressive physiologic and neurochemical changes during prolonged continuous seizure activity. Operationally, we make the diagnosis of SE if a patient does not completely recover to baseline neurologic functioning between two or more seizures or if there is more or less continuous seizure activity for at least 30 minutes, whether or not there is an impairment of consciousness or of other neurologic functions.

The implication of this operational definition is that any seizure type that recurs repetitively in a short period of time or persists sufficiently long may be considered SE. Thus, the types of SE can be classified using the same scheme as the International Classification of Epileptic Seizures. However, clinically it is most convenient to divide SE into convulsive and nonconvulsive forms, as outlined in Table 1.

FORMS OF STATUS EPILEPTICUS

Generalized Convulsive Status Epilepticus

The most common type of SE is generalized convulsive status epilepticus (GCSE). In this presentation of SE, the patient has recurrent or continuous convulsions that may be symmetrical or asymmetrical and overt or subtle but are associated with a marked impairment of consciousness (especially at the time of convulsive activity) and bilateral (although at times asymmetrical) ictal discharges on the EEG. Initially the convulsions are discrete seizures that usually progress through a tonic and then clonic phase before the motor activity stops. Interictally, there may be some recovery of consciousness, but if recovery is not complete before another seizure occurs, we make the diagnosis of SE. If GCSE is allowed to continue without treatment adequate to stop all clinical and electrical seizure activity, there is a progressive decline in the intensity of the convulsive activity, though ictal discharges persist on the EEG. Ultimately, in prolonged untreated or undertreated SE, the patient exhibits characteristics of what I have called subtle GCSE. In this presentation of GCSE the patient is in profound stupor or coma and exhibits ictal discharges on the EEG. However, the convulsive activity at this stage is subtle and may consist of no more than small twitches of the fingers or abdominal or facial muscles, or nystagmoid jerks of the eyes. Sometimes, when the episode of GCSE is caused by a severe encephalopathy, there may only be one or two generalized convulsions before the patient undergoes an electromechanical dissociation and exhibits only subtle convulsive activity despite persisting ictal discharges on the EEG.

Just as there is a conversion of motor activity from overt to increasingly subtle convulsive movements during untreated or undertreated GCSE, there is also a predictable sequence of progressive EEG changes during GCSE (Figs. 1 to 5).

Initially the EEG exhibits discrete electrographic seizures associated with overt generalized convulsions. If GCSE is allowed to progress without adequate treatment, the discrete seizures begin to merge to form a waxing and waning pattern of rhythmic ictal discharges that ultimately become monomorphic and continuous. The continuous seizure activity then begins to be punctuated by periods of relative flattening that become progressively longer as the ictal discharges shorten, until finally the patient exhibits periodic epileptiform discharges on a relatively flat background.

It is important to recognize that GCSE is a diagnosis of a dynamic epileptic phenomenon. The clinical and electrographic characteristics of GCSE are different in early SE and late SE, but there is a continuum between early, usually overt, GCSE and late, usually subtle, GCSE. Furthermore, in my opinion, what others have called *myoclonic SE* (in patients with anoxic or other severe encephalopathies) is really subtle GCSE and part of the continuum described above. Sometimes late GCSE progresses still further, from subtle convulsive activity to a complete cessation of motor movements, though electrical seizure activity persists on the EEG. Other physicians have called this electrical presentation of GCSE *nonconvulsive SE*. This, I think, is also a mistake. Electrical GCSE is part of the progressive decrease in the extent and intensity of convulsive activity that may be seen as GCSE progresses from early to late stages and should be treated as vigorously as overt or subtle GCSE.

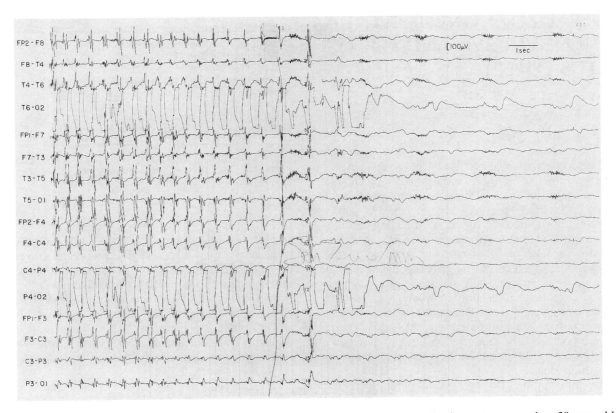

Figure 1 Discrete generalized tonic-clonic seizures with interictal slowing, recorded prior to treatment in a 39-year-old man. Example shows end of clonic phase of the seizure and appearance of postictal slowing. (From Treiman DM, Walton NY, Kendrick C. A progressive sequence of electroencephalographic changes during generalized convulsive status epilepticus. Epilepsy Res 1990; 5:49–60; with permission.)

Nonconvulsive Status Epilepticus

The term *nonconvulsive SE* should, I think, be reserved for the epileptic twilight state that is caused by either continuous spike-wave stupor or complex partial SE. Both forms of SE are manifested clinically by a partial impairment of contact with the environment that may, under some circumstances, be extremely subtle. Spike-wave stupor usually presents as continuous alteration of contact with the environment and at times may be so subtle that the patient simply appears more quiet and withdrawn than usual but otherwise can participate in organized behavior. Complex partial SE characteristically presents as a distinct cycling of behavior, and the patient exhibits a continuous epileptic twilight state during which he or she can respond to environmental stimuli in a limited way. This continuous behavior is punctuated periodically by brief periods of cessation of movement and of response to environmental cues that are frequently accompanied by stereotyped automatisms.

Simple Partial Status Epilepticus

Simple partial SE is operationally defined as continuous or recurrent seizure activity that, like any simple partial seizure, is not associated with any impairment of

contact with the environment. The most common type of simple partial SE is focal motor status, sometime known as epilepsia partialis continuans. But any focal impairment of neurologic function due to continuous or recurrent seizure activity that remains sufficiently localized that there is no impairment of consciousness is considered simple partial SE. Examples of simple partial SE include simple partial sensory SE and epileptic aphasia.

CAUSES

SE may occur in a variety of situations. SE may be the initial seizure presentation in a patient who is going to develop chronic epilepsy. Patients with existing epilepsy may develop SE if antiepileptic drug concentrations drop because of poor compliance or because of increased metabolism during an intercurrent infection. Abuse or withdrawal of alcohol or other drugs also may precipitate SE in epileptic patients with previously controlled seizures. SE also may be a presentation or complication of cerebral infarction of an intracranial mass lesion. SE associated with these conditions is most often overt in its presentation. However, GCSE also may occur as a complication of a variety of toxic, metabolic,

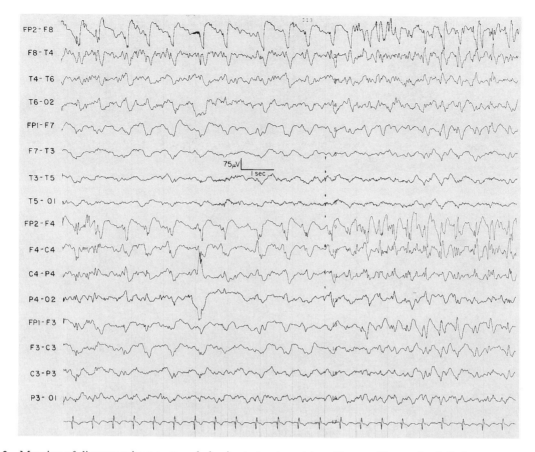

Figure 2 Merging of discrete seizures, recorded prior to treatment in a 64-year-old man. Ictal discharges are continuous but with waxing and waning of frequency and amplitude. An increase in frequency and amplitude can be seen beginning on the right side of the recording. (From Treiman DM, Walton NY, Kendrick C. A progressive sequence of electroencephalographic changes during generalized convulsive status epilepticus. Epilepsy Res 1990; 5:49–60; with permission.)

and infectious encephalopathies. Such patients most often present with subtle GCSE and are frequently seen in hospital intensive care units. In any patient with unexplained coma, the diagnosis of subtle GCSE should be considered.

DIAGNOSIS

Generalized Convulsive Status Epilepticus

The diagnosis of overt GCSE is not difficult when it is based on the observation of two or more generalized convulsions without full recovery of consciousness between seizures. However, there are several potential pitfalls to be avoided when considering this diagnosis. The first is to be sure that the observed seizures are epileptic rather than nonepileptic seizures. Some patients who exhibit psychogenic seizures, whether due to malingering or true conversion reactions, can be extremely convincing. I find three characteristics of genuine epileptic seizures helpful: (1) evolution of behavior during the seizure, (2) stereo-

typed seizures, and (3) sustained convulsive activity without pauses.

Most generalized convulsive seizures evolve through a sequence of tonic and then clonic or clonic-tonic-clonic movements. The clonic jerks tend to slow but increase in amplitude toward the end of the seizure. When generalized convulsions start with focal motor activity and then exhibit Jacksonian spread, the spread is anatomically consistent with the organization of the homunculus on the motor cortex. If a seizure does not evolve in a typical pattern, this raises the question of a possible nonepileptic seizure. However, it is important to recognize that some seizures, particularly complex partial and secondarily generalized convulsive seizures of frontal lobe origin, may exhibit bizarre behavioral characteristics, including strange vocalizations, flailing of the arms, head jerking from side to side, and sexually suggestive pelvic thrusting. If such seizures are stereotyped—that is, exhibit essentially the same pattern of behavior from seizure to seizure—then it is most likely they are true epileptic seizures despite their bizarre presentation. Bizarreness alone is not sufficient to make the diagnosis of psychogenic seizures. In addition to variability of the

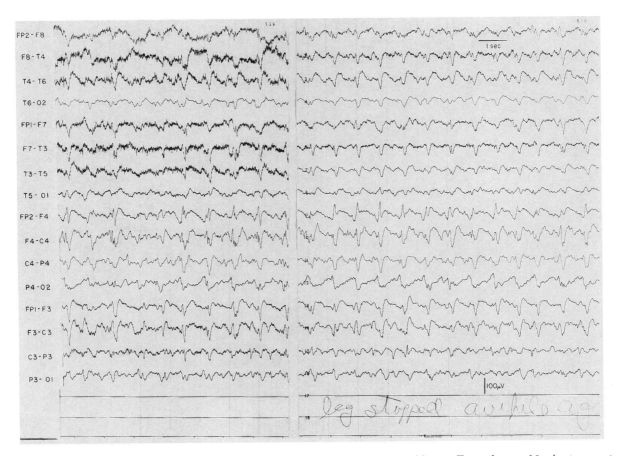

Figure 3 Continuous ictal discharges recorded prior to treatment in a 68-year-old man. Examples are 16 minutes apart. Continuous ictal activity persisted 101 minutes, stopping only after phenytoin infusion was completed and 4 minutes after the end of lorazepam infusion. (From Treiman DM, Walton NY, Kendrick C. A progressive sequence of electroencephalographic changes during generalized convulsive status epilepticus. Epilepsy Res 1990; 5:49–60; with permission.)

behavioral characteristics of psychogenic seizures from event to event, an important clue is the occurrence of pauses during convulsive activity. During true epileptic convulsions the tonic and/or clonic activity is usually sustained without pause until the end of the seizure. However, a conscious patient undergoing a psychogenic seizure cannot sustain continuous intense clonic or even tonic muscle contractions without at least brief periods of rest.

Ultimately, of course, the EEG recording is the most definitive way to differentiate between epileptic seizures and psychogenic seizures. If the EEG recorded during a generalized convulsion has the appearance of a normal resting awake record with good background alpha activity in the posterior derivations (at least in the part that is not obscured by muscle artefact), this is good evidence for a psychogenic seizure. After a true convulsion there should be postictal slowing, at least initially, although patients with seizures of frontal lobe origin rapidly recover consciousness and their EEGs rapidly normalize.

As indicated above, one operational definition of SE is that the patient has repeated seizures without full recovery of consciousness between seizures. A common error is failure to diagnose SE because the patient appears to be recovering consciousness before the next seizure occurs. Because SE refers to a state where the frequency or duration of epileptic activity has caused an alteration in the physiologic functioning of the brain in addition to the seizure activity, any residual impairment of consciousness short of full alertness when the next seizure occurs is an indicator of SE and of sustained pathophysiologic changes. The diagnosis of SE must be made under these circumstances.

GCSE may be asymmetrical in its clinical presentation and in the ictal patterns observed on the EEG. The essential criteria for the diagnosis of GCSE are: (1) impairment of consciousness, (2) convulsive activity during the episode (at least initially), and (3) bilateral abnormalities on the EEG, with ictal discharges apparent from at least one hemisphere. Physicians may erroneously make the diagnosis of focal motor (simple partial) SE when a comatose patient exhibits only unilateral convulsive movements. Such a patient should be considered to have GCSE with an asymmetrical or unilateral presentation.

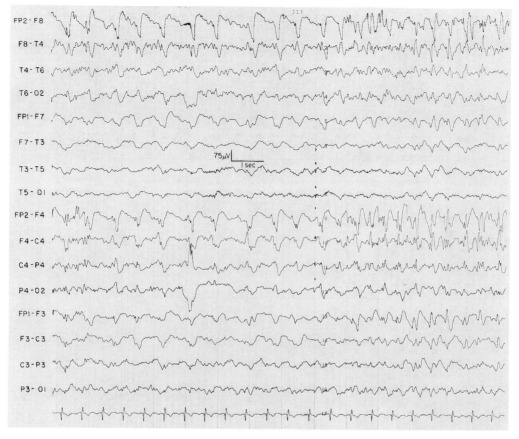

Figure 2 Merging of discrete seizures, recorded prior to treatment in a 64-year-old man. Ictal discharges are continuous but with waxing and waning of frequency and amplitude. An increase in frequency and amplitude can be seen beginning on the right side of the recording. (From Treiman DM, Walton NY, Kendrick C. A progressive sequence of electroencephalographic changes during generalized convulsive status epilepticus. Epilepsy Res 1990; 5:49–60; with permission.)

and infectious encephalopathies. Such patients most often present with subtle GCSE and are frequently seen in hospital intensive care units. In any patient with unexplained coma, the diagnosis of subtle GCSE should be considered.

DIAGNOSIS

Generalized Convulsive Status Epilepticus

The diagnosis of overt GCSE is not difficult when it is based on the observation of two or more generalized convulsions without full recovery of consciousness between seizures. However, there are several potential pitfalls to be avoided when considering this diagnosis. The first is to be sure that the observed seizures are epileptic rather than nonepileptic seizures. Some patients who exhibit psychogenic seizures, whether due to malingering or true conversion reactions, can be extremely convincing. I find three characteristics of genuine epileptic seizures helpful: (1) evolution of behavior during the seizure, (2) stereo-

typed seizures, and (3) sustained convulsive activity without pauses.

Most generalized convulsive seizures evolve through a sequence of tonic and then clonic or clonic-tonic-clonic movements. The clonic jerks tend to slow but increase in amplitude toward the end of the seizure. When generalized convulsions start with focal motor activity and then exhibit Jacksonian spread, the spread is anatomically consistent with the organization of the homunculus on the motor cortex. If a seizure does not evolve in a typical pattern, this raises the question of a possible nonepileptic seizure. However, it is important to recognize that some seizures, particularly complex partial and secondarily generalized convulsive seizures of frontal lobe origin, may exhibit bizarre behavioral characteristics, including strange vocalizations, flailing of the arms, head jerking from side to side, and sexually suggestive pelvic thrusting. If such seizures are stereotyped—that is, exhibit essentially the same pattern of behavior from seizure to seizure—then it is most likely they are true epileptic seizures despite their bizarre presentation. Bizarreness alone is not sufficient to make the diagnosis of psychogenic seizures. In addition to variability of the

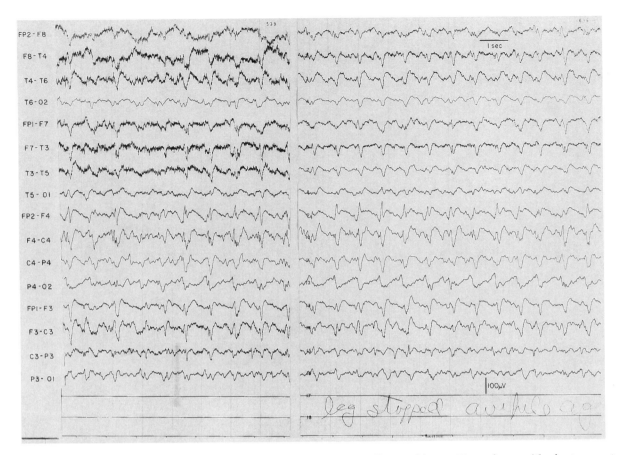

Figure 3 Continuous ictal discharges recorded prior to treatment in a 68-year-old man. Examples are 16 minutes apart. Continuous ictal activity persisted 101 minutes, stopping only after phenytoin infusion was completed and 4 minutes after the end of lorazepam infusion. (From Treiman DM, Walton NY, Kendrick C. A progressive sequence of electroencephalographic changes during generalized convulsive status epilepticus. Epilepsy Res 1990; 5:49–60; with permission.)

behavioral characteristics of psychogenic seizures from event to event, an important clue is the occurrence of pauses during convulsive activity. During true epileptic convulsions the tonic and/or clonic activity is usually sustained without pause until the end of the seizure. However, a conscious patient undergoing a psychogenic seizure cannot sustain continuous intense clonic or even tonic muscle contractions without at least brief periods of rest.

Ultimately, of course, the EEG recording is the most definitive way to differentiate between epileptic seizures and psychogenic seizures. If the EEG recorded during a generalized convulsion has the appearance of a normal resting awake record with good background alpha activity in the posterior derivations (at least in the part that is not obscured by muscle artefact), this is good evidence for a psychogenic seizure. After a true convulsion there should be postictal slowing, at least initially, although patients with seizures of frontal lobe origin rapidly recover consciousness and their EEGs rapidly normalize.

As indicated above, one operational definition of SE is that the patient has repeated seizures without full recovery of consciousness between seizures. A common error is failure to diagnose SE because the patient appears to be recovering consciousness before the next seizure occurs. Because SE refers to a state where the frequency or duration of epileptic activity has caused an alteration in the physiologic functioning of the brain in addition to the seizure activity, any residual impairment of consciousness short of full alertness when the next seizure occurs is an indicator of SE and of sustained pathophysiologic changes. The diagnosis of SE must be made under these circumstances.

GCSE may be asymmetrical in its clinical presentation and in the ictal patterns observed on the EEG. The essential criteria for the diagnosis of GCSE are: (1) impairment of consciousness, (2) convulsive activity during the episode (at least initially), and (3) bilateral abnormalities on the EEG, with ictal discharges apparent from at least one hemisphere. Physicians may erroneously make the diagnosis of focal motor (simple partial) SE when a comatose patient exhibits only unilateral convulsive movements. Such a patient should be considered to have GCSE with an asymmetrical or unilateral presentation.

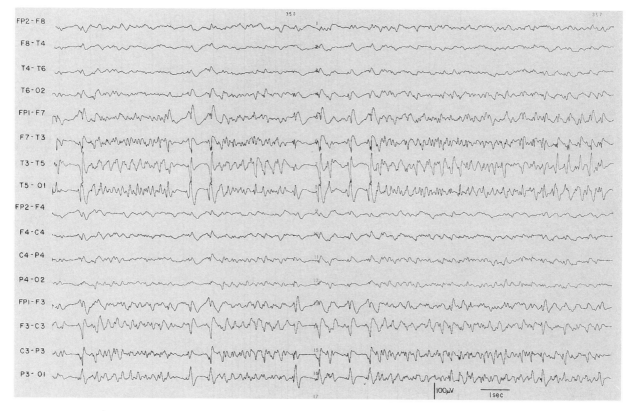

Figure 4 Continuous ictal discharges with flat periods recorded prior to treatment in a 68-year-old man. The seizure focus is clearly in the left hemisphere, but spread of ictal activity to the right hemisphere can be seen as well. (From Treiman DM, Walton NY, Kendrick C. A progressive sequence of electroencephalographic changes during generalized convulsive status epilepticus. Epilepsy Res 1990; 5:49–60; with permission.)

Role of the EEG

I believe all cases of SE should be managed using simultaneous EEG recording. However, initiation of treatment should never be delayed while waiting for the EEG, since emergency EEG recording is difficult to arrange in some hospitals. Although highly desirable, EEG monitoring during management of SE is not absolutely necessary if all convulsive activity stops with treatment and the patient is obviously recovering consciousness. However, if after convulsive movements have been stopped the patient does not rapidly regain consciousness, then cessation of all electrical seizure activity must be verified by EEG. Furthermore, if a patient has a single convulsion but fails to recover consciousness, emergency EEG recording is essential. Such a patient is likely to be in subtle GCSE following the single convulsion.

The diagnosis of subtle GCSE must be made by EEG. This is because subtle GCSE is operationally defined as a condition characterized by profound coma and convulsive motor activity so subtle that the diagnosis cannot be made with confidence without observing ictal discharges on the EEG. By ictal discharges I mean any of the patterns discussed above and illustrated in Figures 1 to 5.

Nonconvulsive Status Epilepticus

The diagnosis of nonconvulsive SE may be difficult at times. In general, the diagnosis of any type of SE is suggested by a sudden or rapid alteration of neurologic function. This, of course, is also true of individual seizures, but such seizures are isolated events from which the patient rapidly recovers. Nonconvulsive SE is manifested by a partial depression of consciousness and/or contact with the environment that may take a variety of forms. These may include repeated typical complex partial seizures with impaired consciousness and automatic behavior, withdrawn behavior, decreased responsiveness only, confusion, or psychiatric symptoms such as paranoia, mania, or depression. The clue that such symptomatology may be epileptic is that it appears abruptly and independently of the psychological environment. The diagnosis is confirmed by the demonstration of ictal activity on the EEG. However, some patients with CPSE may have nonspecific EEG changes, such as rhythmic theta activity or diffuse slowing without the characteristic rhythmic, sharp activity usually thought of as ictal. Under these circumstances, normalization of the EEG accompanied by improvement of contact with the environment after intravenous benzodiazepine or phenytoin admininstration supports the diagnosis.

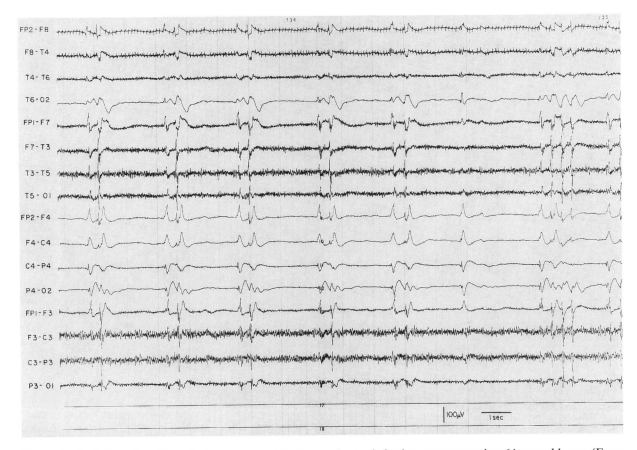

Figure 5 Periodic epileptiform discharges on a flat background recorded prior to treatment in a 64-year-old man. (From Treiman DM, Walton NY, Kendrick C. A progressive sequence of electroencephalographic changes during generalized convulsive status epilepticus. Epilepsy Res 1990; 5:49–60; with permission.)

Nonconvulsive SE must be differentiated from a variety of psychiatric conditions, including fugue states, bipolar affective disorder, schizophrenia, and other psychoses. Some movement disorders, particularly those that occur as a complication of drug therapy or other toxic exposures, may be confused with nonconvulsive SE. Oculogyric crisis or other acute dystonic reactions, because of the abruptness of onset, may be confused with nonconvulsive SE if the practitioner is not familiar with these conditions. Occasionally other movement disorders such as buccal-lingual dyskinesias, hemiballismus, or various presentations of choreoathetosis, if presenting abruptly in a patient without a known neurologic disorder, may suggest nonconvulsive status. A variety of metabolic disorders, especially hypoglycemia, may produce a rapidly developing depression of consciousness and be confused with nonconvulsive SE.

Simple Partial Status Epilepticus

The diagnosis of simple partial SE is made by observing more or less continuous focal seizure activity in a completely conscious and alert patient. Such activity must persist for at least 30 minutes to be considered SE by most physicians, and I think this is a reasonable,

though arbitrary, criterion. Focal ictal activity on the EEG anatomically consistent with the nature and location of the behavioral seizure activity makes the diagnosis of simple partial SE easy. However, frequently the cortical seizure discharges in simple partial SE are so focal that no ictal activity is apparent on the EEG. The EEG may be completely normal. Under these circumstances the diagnosis of simple partial SE is supported by the observation of repetitive stereotyped movements that are not significantly modified by environmental changes, suggestion, or efforts to distract the patient. Sometimes the only way to make a definitive diagnosis of simple partial SE is a therapeutic trial of intravenous antiepileptic drugs.

DIAGNOSTIC ALGORITHM

Ultimately, the diagnosis of SE depends on intelligent observation of a patient, careful assessment of the history, and critical reading of the EEG. Because there is no "serum seizure factor" that has been identified, the diagnosis of seizures, including SE, is a clinical one that calls for superb clinical skills and excellent medical judgement. Diagnosis of SE must be approached logi-

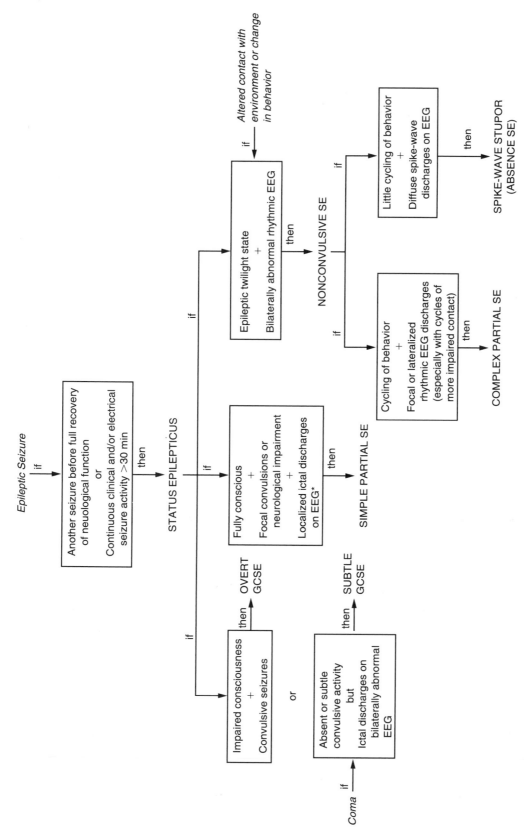

Figure 6 Algorithm for the diagnosis of various types of status epilepticus. Clinical presentations that start the diagnostic process are in italics. Decision parameters are in boxes. Specific types of status epilepticus are capitalized. SE = status epilepticus; GCSE = generalized convulsive status epilepticus. *Scalp EEG may be normal during a simple partial seizure if the seizure activity remains sufficiently localized.

cally and systematically. The algorithm in Figure 6 presents in schematic form the approach to the diagnosis of SE that has been discussed in this chapter.

SUBSEQUENT EVALUATION

Because one-third of the cases of SE occur as a complication of an underlying encephalopathy and another one-third as the first presentation of chronic epilepsy, it is important to determine the cause of the episode. Once SE has been controlled, the underlying cause can be considered. A blood sample should have been drawn for serum chemistry determinations, hematology, and toxic substance screening even before treatment is initiated. Once the seizures are controlled, most patients without a previous history of epilepsy or recurrent SE should have a cerebral imaging study, preferably a magnetic resonance scan. If there is any suspicion of central nervous system infection, the cerebrospinal fluid should be examined. Even if the management of the episode of SE included simultaneous EEG recording, a follow-up routine awake and sleep EEG, perhaps with nasopharyngeal electrodes, may provide useful information regarding the presence of structural abnormalities (perhaps not visible on the cerebral imaging study) or of an epileptic focus.

SUGGESTED READING

Delgado-Escueta AV, Treiman DM. Focal status epilepticus: Modern concepts. In: Luders H, Lesser RP, eds. Epilepsy: Electroclinical syndromes. Berlin: Springer-Verlag, 1987:347.
Delgado-Escueta AV, Wasterlain GC, Treiman DM, Porter RJ, eds. Advances in neurology, Vol 34, Status epilepticus: Mechanisms of brain damage and treatment. New York: Raven Press, 1983.
Porter RJ, Penry JK. Petit mal status. In: Delgado-Escueta AV, Wasterlain CG, Treiman DM, Porter RJ, eds. Advances in neurology, Vol 34, Status epilepticus: Mechanisms of brain damage and treatment. New York: Raven Press, 1983:61.
Treiman DM. Status epilepticus. In: Resor J, Kutt H, eds. The medical treatment of epilepsy. New York: Marcel Dekker, 1992:183.
Treiman DM. Status epilepticus. In: Laidlaw J, Richens A, Chadwick D, eds. A textbook of epilepsy. Edinburgh: Churchill Livingstone, 1993:205.
Treiman DM. Generalized convulsive status epilepticus in the adult. Epilepsia 1993;34 (suppl1): S2-S11.
Treiman DM, Delgado-Escueta AV. Complex partial status epilepticus. In: Delgado-Escueta AV, Wasterlain CG, Treiman DM, Porter RJ, eds. Advances in neurology, Vol 34, Status epilepticus: Mechanisms of brain damage and treatment. New York: Raven Press, 1983:69.
Treiman DM, Walton NY, Kendrick C. A progressive sequence of electroencephalographic changes during generalized convulsive status epilepticus. Epilepsy Res 1990; 5:49–60.

INTERICTAL BEHAVIORAL CHANGES IN EPILEPSY

ORRIN DEVINSKY, MD.
KENNETH PERRINE, Ph.D.

Behavioral changes in epilepsy were debated more than 2,000 years ago. Controversy continues. Most of the controversy arises from the poor methodology and selection bias in many early studies, which showed that psychopathology was frequent and severe among people with epilepsy. Few disorders have been or are associated with the stigma and discrimination of epilepsy. As recently as 1982, the state of Missouri finally repealed legislation that made it illegal for persons with epilepsy to marry, and in 1986 women with epilepsy in South Carolina could still be involuntarily sterilized. Some of the greatest advancements in the care of people with epilepsy have consisted in erasing misconceptions that pervade medical and public opinion. People with epilepsy have been depicted as having stereotypical personality styles, mental retardation, psychosis, aggression, and various other behaviors that are not characteristic of people with epilepsy. However, certain cognitive, affective, and other behavioral changes may be associated

with epilepsy. These changes impair function and quality of life and may require medical intervention. The desire to protect people with epilepsy from degrading and stigmatizing labels must be respected. However, people with epilepsy who are suffering from major depression or other serious behavioral disorders must be diagnosed and treated.

In considering behavioral changes in epilepsy, we must not be locked into a purely psychiatric framework that pigeonholes patients into specific diagnostic categories. Epilepsy has been associated with a wide variety of behavioral changes (Table 1), some of which may be considered positive or neutral, while others are pathologic. The extensive list of famous religious, political, and

Table 1 Reported Interictal Behavioral Changes

Obsessiveness
Viscosity
Emotionality
Hypergraphia
Circumstantiality
Paranoia
Depression
Aggression
Anger
Dependence
Increased religious concerns
Increased philosophical and moral concerns
Altered sexual interests

artistic figures alleged to have had epilepsy has led to the concept that epilepsy is associated with genius. Nietzsche wrote that "four men most thirsty for action of all time were epileptics (Alexander, Caesar, Mohammed, and Napoleon)."

DIAGNOSIS OF BEHAVIORAL CHANGES IN EPILEPSY: CAVEATS

The pendulum on interictal behavioral changes swings back and forth over time: such changes are there, then they aren't; they are related to epilepsy, then they are related to other factors; they are specific for epilepsy, then they aren't. It may be hard to diagnose what some feel strongly does not exist — that is, interictal behavioral changes. Such changes do exist. The key questions are: What are these changes? How often do they occur? What are the pathogenetic factors responsible? Which ones should be treated? How should they be treated?

To identify interictal behavioral changes, one needs to look for them. As with many phenomena such as myoclonic jerks, reflex epilepsy, and ictal autoscopy, the patient will not spontaneously offer the complaint or diagnosis. You must specifically inquire about it. The comment is occasionally made,"I have cared for hundreds of patients with temporal lobe epilepsy and I have never seen one with hypergraphia or hyperreligiosity." (No one makes that comment about viscosity!) Norman Geschwind once examined a patient with temporal lobe epilepsy and asked the man if he had deep convictions or interest in religion. He responded "No, I have no interest in religion." Dr. Geschwind inquired further, "Why not? Were you ever religious?" The man responded, "God, he is the one who gave me the epilepsy" and then proceeded into a long discussion of his very strong personal views on this matter.

Depression is one of the most common and debilitating behavioral disorders in patients with epilepsy. Yet neurologists routinely ask about seizures and medication side effects such as double vision or unsteadiness but do not routinely ask patients how their spirits have been.

Cognitive changes are common in people with epilepsy. Cognition, including attention, language, arithmetic skills, memory, planning and organization and abstract thought, is often affected in epilepsy. While the cause of congitive changes varies from the underlying lesion, to epilepsy, to antiepileptic drugs (AEDs), the disability related to these problems deserves recognition. In some patients, the effects of chronic AED therapy are impossible to measure since they have been on medications for the majority of their childhood and adult life. They do not know what they would be like off, or on lower doses, of AEDs. Some people deny, while others exaggerate, the severity of cognitive dysfunction. Cognitive functions may be improved by better seizure control or reduction or discontinuation of sedating AEDs such as phenobarbital and primidone.

The presence of certain behavioral changes provides only weak support for a diagnosis of epilepsy. None of the personality traits or psychopathologic disorders are pathognomonic of epilepsy. Certain constellations of behavioral features may suggest the possibility of epilepsy, but these features cannot be used to establish the diagnosis. If the person does not have characteristic paroxysmal symptoms, such as staring with impairment of consciousness and automatisms (complex partial seizures [CPS]), tonic-clonic (grand mal) seizures, or simple partial seizures (SPS), the diagnosis of epilepsy should not be made. Further, among patients who present with primary psychiatric or behavioral phenomena, the presence of paroxysmal autonomic, somatosensory, cognitive, or affective symptoms does not establish the diagnosis of epilepsy. These symptoms also occur in psychiatric disorders such as major depression, bipolar disorder, schizophrenia, generalized anxiety, panic, and somatization disorders. Also, other psychiatric disorders are commonly confused with epilepsy. For example, episodes of staring and impaired consciousness or abnormal movements manifesting as psychogenic or nonepileptic seizures are a very common presentation of conversion disorder. Dissociative disorders are also confused with epilepsy because numerous neurologic complaints together with periods of amnesia may suggest epilepsy.

PERSONALITY

Subtle as well as more prominent personality traits and changes occur in some people after they develop epilepsy. Following Bear and Fedio's study of patients with temporal lobe epilepsy (TLE), the concept of a characteristic personality profile emerged but was soon under siege. Of the 18 self-rated traits they studied, the most significant differences were an increased prevalence of humorlessness, circumstantiality, dependence, and sense of personal destiny in patients with TLE. Raters identified TLE patients as significantly different from controls in 14 traits, most strongly circumstantiality, obsessionalism, and dependence. Right-sided TLE patients displayed more emotional traits and exhibited "denial" or "polished" their self-images, while left-sided TLE patients displayed more ideational traits and "tarnished" their self-images. These laterality effects on self-image are consistent with other investigations of lateralized brain disorders. Right hemisphere lesions are associated with denial and neglect. Left hemisphere lesions are associated with depression.

However, all of these personality traits are also reported in patients with other brain or psychiatric disorders. The controversy surrounding the TLE personality syndrome is largely a product of methodologies, such as comparison groups or selection bias, and conceptions. How one defines a syndrome is central to the conceptual issue. A syndrome is a constellation of signs and symptoms that are not usually associated with each other. Thus, the combination of hypergraphia, religiosity, hyposexuality, and viscosity is an unusual constellation, not typical of psychiatric or neurologic disorders. However, such a constellation is also quite uncommon among patients with epilepsy, or more specifically, TLE.

There is no characteristic personality among people with TLE or other forms of epilepsy. Most people with epilepsy have a normal personality structure. However, there are certain traits that are more commonly found among people with epilepsy, some of which may be more common in those with temporal lobe seizure foci. In some cases these traits coexist and can create a striking and relatively distinct behavioral syndrome.

Altered Sexuality

Interictal hyposexuality in temporal lobe and other forms of epilepsy is well documented. Hyposexuality, including decreased libido and impotence, occurs in approximately half of TLE patients, without sex bias. Many patients, especially those whose seizures began before puberty, do not marry or regard their hyposexuality as a problem. Complaints usually come from the spouse or the parent who observes lack of interest in the opposite sex. Impotence may result from AEDs, especially barbiturates. The pathogenetic role of TLE in hyposexuality is supported by observations that sexual activity may increase following successful seizure control with AEDs and temporal lobectomy. Rarely, postlobectomy subjects develop marked hypersexuality, similar to that observed in the Kluver-Bucy syndrome.

Interictal hypersexuality is rare but may respond to AED therapy with insight into the inappropriateness of sexual thoughts and actions. Deviant sexual behavior during the interictal period has also been reported in TLE, including exhibitionism, transvestism, transsexualism, and fetishism.

Religiosity

Religiosity is not a consistent personality feature among patients with epilepsy or TLE. Although a small subgroup may have unusually strong religious beliefs, and an even smaller fraction have ecstatic seizures, the evidence for pronounced hyper-religiosity in epilepsy patients as a group is weak. Detailed questionnaires on the subject do not reveal any differences between patients with right versus left TLE, TLE versus generalized epilepsy, or epilepsy subjects and controls. There are some well-documented cases of sudden religious conversions occurring in close temporal proximity to seizures, however.

Viscosity

Viscosity refers to a sticky and cohesive interpersonal style with a tendency for prolonged verbal contacts, talking repetitively, circumstantially, and in some cases, pedantically. Viscosity is more common among patients with TLE, with the highest scores in those with left-sided foci. However, patients with primary generalized epilepsy may be more viscous than normal controls.

Viscosity may result from some combination of linguistic impairment, mental slowness, psychological dependence, and a tendency for social cohesion. In some patients there may be an emotional need to seek and maintain the company of others. Animal studies demonstrate that discrete limbic lesions, in the septum for example, alter social awareness and the desire to maintain contacts with other animals within or between species

Hypergraphia

This trait, first described in relation to TLE, is characterized by a tendency toward extensive and, in some cases, compulsive writing. There is a striking preoccupation with detail. Words are defined and redefined and underlined, and parentheses are used to make word meaning absolutely clear. The writers accord great importance to their material, which often focusses on moral and religious concerns. Hypergraphia occurs in approximately 8 percent of TLE patients. Duration of epilepsy, hypomania, and number of significant life events during the past year correlate positively with hypergraphia.

PSYCHOPATHOLOGY

General Aspects

Patients with epilepsy have significantly increased mental pathology when compared with normal controls. When compared to patients with chronic medical or neurologic illnesses, however, psychopathology measures are only slightly increased, most often for psychosis, depression, and anxiety, or unchanged (Table 2). The higher rate of psychiatric hospitalization in patients with epilepsy compared to those with other chronic illnesses largely reflects the increased risk of psychosis in epilepsy. Comparisons of psychopathology between TLE and non-TLE groups (primary generalized epilepsy or focal, non-TLE) are inconclusive. In general, group differences on the MMPI, other psychopathology scales, and psychiatric diagnoses (none using DSM-IIIR) do not demonstrate robust intergroup differences.

The prevalence of psychopathology among patients with epilepsy is high, even though group differences are slight (see Table 2). Increased psychopathology is associated with other variables, including the seizure phenomenology, brain pathology, AEDs, and psychosocial factors (Table 3). Factors associated in some studies with increased psychopathology include medial-limbic temporal foci (in contrast to neocortical-lateral), early seizure onset, left-handedness, left temporal or bilateral temporal foci, multiple seizure types, total lifetime

Table 2 Reported Interictal Psychopathologic Disorders

Mood disorders
  Depression
    Major depression
    Dysthymia
  Mania

Psychosis
  Schizophrenic-like
  Forced normalization

Anxiety disorders
  Panic disorder
  Generalized anxiety disorder

Personality disorders

Dissociative disorders
  Depersonalization
  Poriomania (fugue)
  Multiple personality

Disorders of impulse control
  Intermittent explosive disorder
  Conduct disorders

Table 3 Factors Contributing to Psychopathology in Epilepsy

Genetic predisposition

Gender

Epilepsy-related factors
  Anatomic focus
  Lateralization
    Temporal
    Frontal
    Multifocal
    Primary generalized seizures
  Seizure type
    Simple partial
    Complex partial
    Generalized tonic-clonic
    Myoclonic
  Prolonged seizures
  Status epilepticus
  Low seizure frequency
  Age of onset

Brain pathology
  Known cause
  Diffuse brain dysfunction
  Early brain injury
  Temporal lobe pathology
  Lateralized cerebral injury
  Cognitive impairment

Antiepileptic drugs
  Polytherapy
  Withdrawal
  Acute or chronic toxicity

Psychosocial factors
  Low socioeconomic status
  Low educational level
  Vocational problems
  Premorbid personality
  Stigmatization
  Discrimination
  Fear of seizures
  Deprivation

number of convulsions, presence of focal atrophic lesion, and history of ictal fear.

Depression

Depression occurs during the prodromal, ictal, postictal, and interictal periods in patients with epilepsy. Prodromal symptoms precede seizures by hours or days, and among affective prodromata, depression is common. Depression is the second most common ictal affect after fear-anxiety. In some cases, feelings of sadness can persist hours or days after the seizure has ended. In rare cases, simple partial or absence status cause prolonged depressive affect.

Depression is the most common interictal psychiatric disorder in patients with epilepsy. Up to 80 percent of patients with epilepsy report feelings of depression, and endogenous depression occurs in up to a third of patients. The rate of suicide is elevated two- to five-fold in patients with epilepsy. When added to the complex behavioral web of medication side effects, neurologic and cognitive impairment, and psychosocial disability, depression can devastate these patients. Given the high prevalence and the associated morbidity and mortality, recognition and treatment of depression in patients with epilepsy must be prime concerns of neurologists.

The phenomenology of depression in epilepsy is consistent with both endogenous and reactive mechanisms. The psychosocial problems that accompany epilepsy include (1) neurologic impairment in patients with structural pathology or frequent seizures, (2) social bias and stigma leading to restrictions on employment, living situations, and companionship, and (3) disturbed family relations (e.g., dependency, overprotection, rejection, negative self-image), all of which act to reduce an individual's capacity to enjoy life and grow.

Depression in epilepsy is more than a reaction to chronic illness. Biological factors also contribute. These factors include a family history of depression, left-sided seizure focus, and use of barbiturates. Left hemisphere lesions and left carotid amobarbital injections induce greater depressive reactions than right-sided ones. The interictal hypometabolism in patients with CPS is ipsilateral to the seizure focus, suggesting that hypometabolism may represent the physiologic correlate of a left hemisphere "lesion."

Depression often remains unrecognized or untreated in epilepsy patients, which is unfortunate because there are effective treatments for depression. Epilepsy is not an absolute contraindication for use of antidepressants. Although antidepressants may lower the seizure threshold, most patients tolerate these medications without an increase in seizure frequency.

Psychosis

The relationship between epilepsy and psychosis, especially persistent interictal psychoses, remains controversial. Is there an increased prevalence of psychosis among patients with epilepsy? Are seizures antagonistic to the development of psychosis, or is there a pathogenetic affinity between epilepsy and psychosis?

Peri-ictal Psychosis

Differentiation of peri-ictal delirium from psychosis is critical. Delirium is a transient mental disorder with impaired attention, disorientation, global disturbance of cognitive function, autonomic dysfunction (usually sympathetic hyperactivity), and alterations of the sleep-wake cycle and psychomotor activity. Delirium may begin acutely or subacutely. Symptoms usually fluctuate. In contrast, postictal psychosis occurs with relative preservation of attention and with delusions or hallucinations that are typically more systematized and structured than the fragmentary phantasms of delirium. Despite the clear textbook distinction between delirium and psychosis, as one carefully reviews cases of peri-ictal psychosis, features of delirium are often superimposed.

Nonconvulsive status epilepticus rarely mimics psychosis but more often causes delirium. During absence and atypical absence status, there is confusion, prominent inattention, and partial reduction in the level of consciousness. Complex partial status of temporal or frontal lobe origin typically present as a series of discrete seizures rather than a continuous ictal state. However, invasive recordings may document continuous but localized ictal discharges between seizures. These patients are often confused and lethargic, although agitation may be present, especially if the person is restrained. Simple partial status is rare but can be easily confused with primary psychiatric disorders. These patients report hallucinations, affective symptoms, and dissociative phenomena with preserved consciousness. Psychosis developed in over 10 percent of cases of simple partial status in one series. Periodic lateralized epileptiform discharges have been associated with delirium in elderly patients. Electroencephalography is essential to identify atypical cases of nonconvulsive status but may be normal during simple partial and frontal lobe CPS.

Approximately 25 percent of all psychoses in epilepsy are postictal. There is typically an increase in seizure frequency, cessation of seizures with a lucid interval of 1 to 2 days, followed by psychosis. Psychosis most often follows a series of generalized tonic-clonic seizures, which may be primary or secondary generalized. Prominent mood alterations are common with postictal psychosis. Spontaneous recovery is usual, but episodes of psychosis often recur if seizure control lapses. In high-risk patients, we have successfully used a combination of oral lorazepam and molindone for 1 to 4 days after seizures.

Interictal Psychosis

Poorly derived epidemiologic data and anecdotal observations of an antagonistic relationship between epilepsy and psychosis formed part of the theoretical basis for electroconvulsive therapy in psychiatry. Subsequently, an increased prevalence of psychosis among patients with epilepsy has been stressed. Despite a vast literature, we remain uncertain whether people with epilepsy are at greater than usual risk to develop psychosis. The answer appears to be yes, but the risk has probably been overestimated because of selection bias.

Interictal psychosis differs from schizophrenia. The psychoses of epilepsy are characterized by a preservation of warm affect and personality with a predominance of visual rather than auditory hallucinations. Formal thought disorder, incoherent thought, emotional withdrawal, catatonia, and negative symptoms are less common in interictal psychosis than in schizophrenia. Outcome is more favorable in epileptic compared to schizophrenic psychoses, and there is less need for neuroleptics and institutionalization. However, there can be extensive overlap between the phenomenology of epileptic and schizophrenic psychoses. Further, in some cases, there is a coincidental occurrence of epilepsy and schizophrenia.

Possible risk factors for psychosis in patients with epilepsy are listed in Table 4. In the only prospective study of psychosis and epilepsy, children with temporal lobe seizure foci had a 10 percent chance of developing interictal psychosis during a follow-up that lasted up to 30 years. Although a significant relation between temporal lobe seizure foci and psychosis has frequently been reported, this relation remains unproven. Among the nine studies that compared rates of psychosis among patients with different epilepsy types, two found significantly higher rates and most others found nonsignificant increases among those with temporal lobe foci.

Landolt introduced the term *forced normalization* to describe the paradoxical emergence of an acute psychosis following achievement of seizure control or resolution of epileptiform discharges. The phenomenon is considered extremely rare by some, while others report that up to 8 percent of psychoses associated with epilepsy result from forced normalization. These psychoses may be more clinically pleomorphic than other interictal psychoses. Most patients respond to therapy with antipsychotic medications. Forced normalization has been postulated as a mechanism of other acute behavioral changes in epilepsy, including conversion symptoms, depression, and mania.

Identification of risk factors for psychosis may permit effective preventive measures. Social deteriora-

Table 4 Possible Risk Factors for Interictal Psychosis

Onset of epilepsy before age 20
Duration of epilepsy greater than 10 years
Social deterioration
Antiepileptic drug polytherapy
High-dose antiepileptic drug therapy
Female sex
History of complex partial seizures
Temporal > frontal lobe seizure focus
Left-sided seizure focus
Glial tumors and hamartomas

tion and development of new behavioral complaints should lead to careful assessment of psychiatric status. Social services and psychiatric treatment may prevent further behavioral decline.

Anxiety Disorders

Anxiety is commonly reported by patients with epilepsy. Anxiety and related feelings of fear and paranoia may occur as (1) SPS (auras), (2) psychological reactions to other warning symptoms that alert the patient that a seizure is imminent, (3) postictal states, (4) interictal behavior, or (5) panic attacks. The boundaries between these pathologic processes are usually clear but may be blurred. Further, medical causes of increased anxiety and fear reactions must be considered, including mitral valve prolapse, hyperthyroidism, hypoglycemia, pheochromocytoma, Cushing's syndrome, acute asthma, hypo- or hypercalcemia, alcohol or sedative drug withdrawal, and use of central nervous system stimulants such as cocaine or amphetamines.

Ictal Fear

Fear and anxiety are the most common affective symptoms in spontaneous and electrically induced SPS. Among partial seizure patients, fear is reported as an aura by 10 to 15 percent. Fear and anxiety usually occur with anteromedial temporal seizures, although mesial frontal seizures may also cause fear. The quality and intensity of ictal anxiety-fear varies tremendously. Some patients report a slight uneasy and nervous feeling. Others describe an intense emotion of fear and horror. As with other SPS symptoms, the onset of ictal fear is paroxysmal and the duration is brief (30 to 180 seconds). In contrast, panic attacks often build up over minutes and last more than 5 minutes. However, simple partial status rarely causes fear that lasts longer than 10 minutes.

Ictal fear is associated with psychopathologic features in some patients. These features include increased rate of psychiatric hospitalization, interictal anxiety, and increased scores on MMPI scales of psychaesthenia, psychopathic deviancy, paranoia, schizophrenia, and social introversion. Whether behavioral effects of recurrent ictal fear or pathophysiologic changes associated with specific anatomic abnormalities contribute to the psychopathology is unknown.

Differentiation between spontaneous and reactive fear is often difficult, and the forms may coexist. Spontaneous fear is a sudden emotion not evoked by a frightening thought or stimulus. Ictal reactive fear is the patient's response to the realization that a seizure may occur. It is an appropriate reaction, not an SPS. A subgroup of patients experience prolonged (hours or days) postictal fear and anxiety. It has been our experience that most of these patients have fear or anxiety as their aura and that postictal anxiety follows a cluster of CPS. Ictal and postictal anxiety are treated

with AEDs. In some postictal cases, benzodiazepine for several days may be helpful.

Interictal Fear and Anxiety

There is an increased rate of generalized anxiety and panic disorders among patients with epilepsy. Interictal anxiety symptoms are reported by as many as 66 percent of patients with epilepsy. The prevalence of generalized anxiety or panic disorders in epilepsy is unknown. Although interictal anxiety and panic has been reported most commonly among patients with partial seizures arising from limbic foci, we have also observed an increased rate of these disorders among patients with primary generalized epilepsy such as juvenile myoclonic epilepsy.

Dissociative Disorders

Psychiatric dissociative disorders are characterized by disturbances in the sense of self and in memory. The disturbances of self include loss of memory for self-referential information (psychogenic amnesia), elaboration of secondary identities (psychogenic fugue, multiple personality), or depersonalization (loss of personal reality, feeling detached from one's mind, like an automaton). Memory changes usually consist of amnesia (complete or partial) for events during a dissociative state. Psychogenic amnesia and fugue states are often associated with amnesia for important personal data, such as, home address and spouse's name. Dissociative disorders can occur suddenly or gradually. They can be brief or persistent.

Ictal dissociative phenomena include depersonalization, derealization (loss or impairment of environmental reality; feeling as if the world is unreal), autoscopy (seeing one's double or out-of-body experiences), and, rarely, personality alteration (dual or multiple personalities). In a structured interview of patients with partial epilepsy, the frequencies of ictal dissociative phenomena were: depersonalization (15 percent), derealization (18 percent), and autoscopy (6 percent). Cases of dual or multiple personality states temporally associated with seizures are rare. Further, when studied with video-EEG monitoring, six consecutive patients who had been diagnosed as having multiple personality disorder and epilepsy were found to have psychogenic seizures.

Poriomania refers to prolonged periods of confusion in which the patient may travel and subsequently have no memory of events during this period (that is, a fugue state). These episodes have been only occasionally reported in epilepsy patients, and there is no documentation during these attacks. Their pathophysiology remains poorly defined. These episodes are probably postictal states such as delirium or psychosis after prolonged seizures or seizure clusters.

It is uncertain whether dissociative states occur between seizures. Dual personalities and the Capgras syndrome, a dissociative disorder in which patients make only approximate answers to questions, have been reported in association with control of seizures and normalization of interictal epileptiform activity. In a standardized questionnaire concerning dissociative phenomena, patients with partial seizures scored significantly lower than those with multiple personality disorder. However, there was a 20 percent overlap of scores between these groups. In patients with psychogenic dissociative disorders such as multiple personalities, there is often a history of major emotional trauma, especially repetitive physical or sexual abuse in childhood.

COMMENTS

Epilepsy can be accompanied by changes in cognition, personality, affect, and other elements of behavior. There is no single "epileptic constitution" or personality complex. The main characteristic of behavior encountered in epilepsy is diversity. As one looks at the behavioral traits reported in epilepsy, a specific and consistent pattern is lacking. Rather, extremes of behavior are accentuated, sometimes in one direction, often in both directions. Changes in emotional state are prominent in epilepsy. Some authors describe a prominent deepening or increase in emotionality, while others identify a global decrease in emotional life and content. Emotional lability is also reported. Sexuality and libido are typically decreased, but fetishism, transvestism, exhibitionism, and hypersexual episodes also occur. Concerns over morality may be lacking or exaggerated. Patients may be irritable and aggressive or timid and apathetic. The impressive list of people with epilepsy in politics, religion, the arts, and the sciences suggests a potentially positive expression of this behavioral spectrum. Psychosis, depression, paranoia, and personality disorders may represent the negative pole of epilepsy-related behavioral changes.

The most important aspect of behavioral changes in epilepsy, for physicians, is the need to recognize and treat dysfunctional behavior. Depression is a common problem that is often unrecognized and untreated. Other treatable problems include impotence, anxiety, panic attacks, and psychosis. Identifying risk factors should assist in developing methods to prevent these disorders.

SUGGESTED READING

Altschuler LL, Devinsky O, Post RM, Theodore WH. Depression, anxiety and temporal lobe epilepsy: Laterality of focus and symptomatology. Arch Neurol 1990; 47:284–288.

Bear DM. Temporal lobe epilepsy: A syndrome of sensory-limbic hyperconnection. Cortex 1979; 15:357–384.

Bear DM, Fedio P. Quantitative analysis of interictal behavior in temporal lobe epilepsy. Arch Neurol 1977; 34:454–467.

Bromfield EB, Altshuler L, Leiderman DB, et al. Cerebral metabolism and depression in patients with complex partial seizures. Arch Neurol 1992.

Devinsky O, Bear D. Varieties of aggressive behavior in temporal lobe epilepsy. Am J Psychiatry 1984; 141:651–656.

Dewhurst K, Beard AW. Sudden religious conversions in temporal lobe epilepsy. Br J Psychiatry 1970; 117:497–507.

Falconer MA. Reversibility by temporal-lobe resection of the behavioral abnormalities of temporal-lobe epilepsy. N Engl J Med 1973; 289:451–455.

Fenwick PBC, Toone BK, Wheeler MJ, et al. Sexual behavior in a centre for epilepsy. Acta Neurol Scand 1985; 71:428–435.

Flor-Henry P. Psychosis and temporal lobe epilepsy: A controlled investigation. Epilepsia 1969; 10:363–395.

Hermann BP, Schwartz MS, Karnes WE, Vahdat P. Psychopathology in epilepsy: Relationship of seizure type to age at onset. Epilepsia 1980; 21:15–23.

Landolt H. Serial encephalographic investigations during psychotic episodes in epileptic patients and during schizophrenic attacks. In: de Hass L, ed. Lectures on epilepsy. Amsterdam: Elsevier, 1958:91.

Ounstead C. Aggression and epilepsy: Rage in children with temporal lobe epilepsy. J Psychosom Res 1969; 13:237–242.

Reynolds EH. Mental effects of antiepileptic medication: A review. Epilepsia 1983; 24 (suppl 2):S85–S95.

Robertson MM, Trimble MR, Townsend HRA. The phenomenology of depression in epilepsy. Epilepsia 1987; 28:364–372.

Taylor DC. Aggression and epilepsy. J Psychosom Res 1969; 13: 229–236.

Taylor DC. Sexual behavior and temporal lobe epilepsy. Arch Neurol 1979; 21:510–516.

Trimble MR, Thompson PJ. Anticonvulsant drugs, cognitive function, and behavior. Epilepsia 1983; 24 (suppl 1):S55–S63.

Tucker DM, Novelly RA, Walker PJ. Hyperreligiosity in temporal lobe epilepsy: Redefining the relationship. J Nerv Ment Dis 1987; 175:181–184.

Waxman SG, Geschwind N. Hypergraphia in temporal lobe epilepsy. Neurology 1974; 24:629–631.

Waxman SG, Geschwind N. The interictal behavior syndrome in temporal lobe epilepsy. Arch Gen Psychiatry 1975; 32:1580–1586.

Whitman S, Hermann BP, Gordon A. Psychopathology in epilepsy: How great is the risk? Biol Psychiatry 1984; 19:213–236.

Williams D. The structure of emotions reflected in epileptic experiences. Brain 1956; 79:29–67.

NEONATAL SEIZURES

GREGORY L. HOLMES, M.D.

Seizures are one of the most common, and frequently ominous, neurologic signs occurring in neonates and require prompt evaluation. One of the first steps when facing the child with suspected neonatal seizures is to determine whether the events have an epileptic basis. The electroencephalogram (EEG) can be of enormous value in differentiating seizures from nonepileptic events and providing prognostic information. Following the diagnosis, the clinician must search vigorously for a cause of the seizures since cause will be the most important factor in determining outcome. In deciding how vigorously to treat the seizures, the clinician must weigh the risks of seizure-induced brain damage against the potential risk of antiepileptic therapy.

There is little question that neonatal seizures are associated with a high morbidity and mortality rate. Even with recent advances in the areas of obstetrics and perinatal care, seizures continue to be a significant predictor of poor neurologic outcome. Their recognition is very important since they may be the first and, occasionally, only sign of a central nervous system (CNS) disorder.

Neonatal seizures differ markedly from those occurring in older subjects in their clinical manifestations, causes, and short- and long-term prognosis. The clinician evaluating a neonate with seizures is faced with a striking dichotomy: roughly half of the affected newborns are destined to poor outcomes, the others escaping with little or no sequelae. Many seizures are epiphenomena of insults occurring before, during, or after birth or of transient metabolic, systemic disorders. Causative factors are more readily identifiable at this age, and idiopathic seizures are quite uncommon. As noted, cause is the most important determinant of outcome.

CLINICAL MANIFESTATIONS

Because neonatal seizures can be covert, because their expression can be erratic or fragmentary, and because some of the vast and peculiar repertoire manifested by normal and especially encephalopathic infants can mimic seizure manifestations, careful observation and monitoring are helpful in distinguishing between seizure and nonseizure activities. As will be discussed, the EEG may be of major assistance to the clinician.

Neonatal seizures were separated by Volpe into five types based solely on clinical manifestations: subtle,

Supported in part by grants from the National Institutes of Neurological Disorders and Stroke (RO1-NS27984) and the Stephen Linn Fund.

tonic, focal clonic, multifocal clonic, and myoclonic. While the classification of neonatal seizures continues to evolve, Volpe's classification system remains important.

The manifestations of subtle seizures include repetitive sucking and other oral-buccal-lingual movements, assumption of a fixed or immobile posture, pedaling movements of the legs or paddling movements of the arms, blinking, momentary fixation of gaze with or without eye deviation, nystagmus, and apnea. Although clinically unimpressive, subtle seizures are commonly associated with severe CNS insults.

Tonic seizures resemble decerebrate or opisthotonic posturing and consist of intermittent tonic extension of the arms, legs, or all four extremities. Without EEG confirmation, it is very difficult to differentiate these activities from nonepileptic abnormal motor activity. They are usually associated with severe brain lesions and occur most frequently in preterm infants.

Clonic seizures consist of rhythmic jerking of groups of muscles and occur in either a focal or multifocal pattern. In multifocal clonic seizures, movements may migrate from one part of the body to another. Although focal seizures may be seen with localized brain insults, they may also be seen in disorders that diffusely affect the brain such as asphyxia, subarachnoid hemorrhage, hypoglycemia, or infection.

Myoclonic seizures are similar to those seen in older children, consisting of rapid, isolated jerks. The myoclonic seizures usually consist of bilateral jerks, although occasionally unilateral or focal jerks can occur.

Using this classification system, it became clear to clinicians that clonic seizures were frequently associated with EEG ictal discharges, usually contralateral to the side of clinical involvement. Subtle and tonic seizures were less frequently associated with EEG ictal discharges. It was also observed that while clonic seizures frequently responded to antiepileptic drugs (AEDs), subtle and tonic seizures were less likely to cease with drug therapy. This raised the question of whether subtle and tonic seizures were in fact epileptic events or some other paroxysmal disorder of the ill neonate.

This issue was addressed by Mizrahi and colleagues, who, by utilizing EEG with simultaneous video monitoring techniques, demonstrated that many events previously thought to be epileptic seizures had no EEG correlate. Focal clonic and tonic seizures and some myoclonic seizures had a close correlation with ictal EEG discharges, while generalized symmetrical tonic posturing, some myoclonic jerking, and most behaviors considered to be subtle seizures (oral-buccal-lingual movements, irregular, random, eye movements, nystagmus, pedaling movements, stepping movements, and rotary arm movements) were not associated with EEG activity.

A few comments about terminology are necessary. A seizure is a sudden electrical discharge of brain gray matter that results in an alteration of functioning. Epilepsy is defined as two or more *unprovoked* seizures. Unfortunately, Mizrahi and colleagues used the term *seizure* to describe any stereotyped, repetitive behavior, and differentiated epileptic from nonepileptic seizures by whether there was an accompanying EEG discharge. This terminology is unfortunate because in older children and adults all seizures are considered to be secondary to CNS discharges. In addition, many infants have recurrent seizures provoked by acute CNS events that are self-limited. Calling these seizures epileptic is inappropriate. In this review I will use the term *seizure* to describe paroxysmal events secondary to brain electrical discharges.

One other caution is necessary. There are problems in depending solely upon consistent EEG correlates as the sine qua non for diagnosing epileptic seizures. As in older children and adults, EEG discharges may not always be recorded from the scalp in infants that clearly have seizures. When faced by the child with stereotyped repetitive behaviors, the clinician should attempt some simple maneuvers. Tonic movements and motor automatisms that can be arrested by restraint or repositioning are unlikely to be seizures. Likewise, jitteriness may be confused with neonatal seizures. Jitteriness is usually stimulus-sensitive; exhibits a rapid to-and-fro, symmetrical movement of the extremities; and ceases with passive flexion of the extremity. One additional condition that may mimic a neonatal seizure is *benign neonatal sleep myoclonus*. In this disorder there is bilateral, synchronous, repetitive jerking of the upper and/or lower extremities. The myoclonus may be quite dramatic but only occurs during sleep.

CAUSES

Although an extensive array of disorders may be associated with neonatal seizures, only a few disorders account for the majority of cases. Idiopathic or cryptogenic seizures are rare in the neonate. Determining cause is critical because this dictates therapy and is highly correlated with outcome. Therapy with AEDs will be of no value to the infant with unrecognized hypoglycemia or meningitis. Unfortunately, the ill neonate may present with a constellation of disturbances, each of

Table 1 Causes Commonly Associated with Neonatal Seizures

Cause	Comments
Hypoxia-ischemia	While often diagnosed inappropriately, hypoxia-ischemia remains a major cause of neonatal seizures.
Hypocalcemia	Hypocalcemia was formerly among the most frequent causes of neonatal seizures. In more recent studies, however, hypocalcemia as a primary cause is rare. Hypocalcemia is often seen in infants that have had other insults.
Hypoglycemia	Like hypocalcemia, hypoglycemia is often associated with other neonatal disorders such as trauma, hemolytic disease, or asphyxia. Infants of diabetic and toxemic mothers, small for gestational age infants, and twins are at risk. Neurologic signs include jitteriness, hypotonia, lethargy, and apena, in addition to seizures.
Hyponatremia/ hypernatremia	Hyponatremia, like hypocalcemia, usually occurs in association with other disorders, such as intracranial hemorrhage or meningitis, and is secondary to inappropriate antidiuretic hormone. Hypernatremia is usually iatrogenic, most frequently secondary to improper mixing of formula.
Intracranial hemorrhages	Primary subarachnoid hemorrhage occurs in both term and preterm infants. Bleeding is from venous structures and is often associated with asphyxia or trauma. Although many subarachnoid hemorrhages are mild and inconsequential except for causing transient seizures, some result in a stormy course with hydrocephalus and brain parenchymal damage. Intraventricular hemorrhage is the most common type of intracranial hemorrhage and accounts for a large percentage of morbidity and mortality primarily, but not exclusively, in preterm infants. While intraventricular hemorrhage is an unusual cause of neonatal seizures, many of these infants have hypoxic-ischemic encephalopathies.
Infection	Intrauterine or postnatal CNS infections may lead to seizures. Intrauterine causes include rubella, toxoplasmosis, cytomegalovirus, herpes simplex, and coxsackievirus B. Intrauterine infections are usually associated with other systemic signs: microcephaly, jaundice, rash, hepatomegaly, and chorioretinitis. Common postnatal infections include E. coli and group B beta-streptococcus. Any infant without a clear cause for seizures requires prompt lumbar puncture. Sepsis without meningitis may also lead to seizures.
Congenital malformation	Virtually all disorders of neuronal migration and organization (i.e., polymicrogyria, neuronal heterotopias, lissencephaly, holoprosencephaly, and hydranencephaly) may lead to severe neonatal seizures.
Metabolic disorders	Although the differential diagnosis of neonatal seizures includes inherited metabolic disorders, these are fortunately rare and usually produce other significant symptoms such as peculiar odors, protein intolerance, acidosis, alkalosis, lethargy, or stupor. In most cases of metabolic disease, pregnancy, labor, and delivery are normal. While food intolerance may be the earliest indication of a systemic abnormality, seizures are commonly the first specific clue to CNS involvement. If untreated, metabolic disorders commonly lead to lethargy, coma, and death. In surviving infants, weight loss, poor growth, and failure to thrive are common.
Drug withdrawal	A significant cause of neonatal seizures in urban hospitals is withdrawal from narcotic-analgesics, sedative-hypnotics, and alcohol. Infants born to heroin- or methadone-addicted mothers have an increased risk of seizures, although the most common neurologic findings are jitteriness and irritability. Infants of methadone-addicted mothers may have late withdrawal symptoms, with seizures occurring as long as 4 weeks after birth.
Toxins	Although rare, seizures may be a prominent feature in infants poisoned with local anesthetics. Inadvertent fetal anesthetic injection usually occurs in deliveries at the time of local anesthesia administered for episiotomy. The infant presents at birth with bradycardia, apnea, and hypotonia. Seizures usually occur within the first 6 hours and are generally tonic in type. The infants may have mydriasis and loss of lateral eye movements and pupillary light reflexes.

which may contribute to the development of seizures. For example, hypoxic-ischemic encephalopathies, hypoglycemia, hypocalcemia, and intracranial hemorrhages, all sufficient to cause seizures on their own, may occur together in the same infant. Table 1 lists common causes of neonatal seizures.

EVALUATION

Determining the cause of neonatal seizures is more urgent than beginning AED treatment. Neonates do not have generalized tonic-clonic seizures, and the systemic abnormalities seen with prolonged seizures in older patients rarely occur in neonates.

The first step in the evaluation should be a careful history and physical examination. A family history of neonatal seizures is suggestive of benign familial neonatal seizures, while a history of maternal drug ingestion may implicate drug withdrawal as a cause. The clinician should ask about maternal infections or drug ingestion and review the delivery record for clues to cause. While Apgar scores provide the physician with information about the child's condition at birth, they do not indicate causation. Many infants with neuromuscular disease or encephalopathic processes occurring well before birth have low APGAR scores. A tense fontanel may suggest an infection or hypoxic-ischemic injury. If the child has microcephaly, a congenital infection or cerebral malformation should be considered. Congenital malformations may be associated with dysmorphic facial features. Chorioretinitis, hepatosplenomegaly, or skin rashes suggest a con-

Table 2 Diagnostic Tests in the Evaluation of Neonatal Seizures

Test	Disorder
Recommended in All Infants with Unexplained Seizures	
Complete blood count	Infection, subarachnoid hemorrhage
Glucose	Hypoglycemia
Calcium/magnesium	Hypocalcemia/hypomagnesemia
Electrolytes	Hyponatremia/hypernatremia
Cerebral spinal fluid	Meningitis/encephalitis
Ammonia	Urea cycle abnormalities
TORCH titers	Toxoplasmosis, cytomegalovirus disease, rubella, herpes congenital infections
Head ultrasound	Congenital malformations, intraventricular hemorrhage
Recommended if Clinically Indicated	
CAT scan	Strokes, hypoxic-ischemic injuries
Amino acids	Disorders of amino acid metabolism
Organic acids	Disorders of organic acid metabolism
Long-chain fatty acids, lactate, pyruvate, chromosomes, lysosomal enzymes	Obtain if clinically suspected (i.e., peroxisomal disorders, mitochondrial diseases, storage disorders, chromosome abnormalities)

genital infection such as toxoplasmosis, while needle marks in the scalp raise the possibility of inadvertent injection of a local anesthetic such as lidocaine during delivery.

Following the history and physical examination, the appropriate diagnostic studies should be performed and treatment for the seizures begun. Table 2 lists recommended diagnostic studies for a neonate with a seizure. A "shotgun" approach to the evaluation of a patient should be avoided. However, all infants with unexplained seizures should have a spinal fluid examination. Neonates can have meningitis without fever, a bulging fontanel, or nuchal rigidity.

All infants with suspected seizures should have an EEG. The EEG is an important tool in diagnosing seizures that might be clinically unsuspected, and, conversely, it may eliminate the need for AEDs. While the EEG alone generally fails in revealing specific diagnostic conditions, it may be the first test to guide the clinician in reaching an unsuspected diagnosis. For example, an interhemispheric or regional asymmetry of background patterns may suggest an underlying lesion, such as an intrauterine vascular accident. The EEG may suggest dysgenetic brain anomalies, inborn errors of metabolism (like nonketotic hyperglycinemia or pyridoxine dependency), or infection, such as herpes simplex encephalitis. Another important value of the neonatal EEG is its powerful contribution to the assessment of short- and long-term prognosis. This noninvasive test is singularly more valuable in this respect during the neonatal period than at other ages.

For prognostic purposes, the background EEG patterns are more significant than the patterns of EEG epileptiform discharges, though some of these may also be revealing. Infants with isoelectric, burst-suppression, or low-voltage EEGs, especially if persistent on serial studies, have a high risk of neurologic sequelae regardless of seizure cause. Rowe et al, in a prospective study of 74 neonates with clinical seizures, found that in both preterm and full-term infants the EEG background patterns correlated highly with outcome. The EEG discharges interictally were not as highly significant. However, ictal discharges, when evaluated independently of interictal discharges, were clearly correlated with generally poor outcomes.

As mentioned above, the EEG has few specific patterns to indicate precise causes. One pattern has been proposed as diagnostic for neonatal herpes simplex encephalitis by several authors. A multifocal, periodic, or quasi-periodic pattern is an EEG paroxysmal feature that in itself is nonspecific, but when associated with the proper clinical and cerebrospinal fluid findings should strongly suggest neonatal herpes simplex encephalitis. Another instance in which the EEG is useful for specific diagnosis is the very rare condition of pyridoxine dependency. However, the diagnosis is empirically confirmed by administration of pyridoxal, which causes cessation of the intractable clinical and electrographic seizures.

SUGGESTED READING

Hill A, Volpe JJ. Seizures, hypoxic-ischemic brain injury, and intraventricular hemorrhage in the newborn. Ann Neurol 1981; 10:109–121.

Holden KR, Mellitis ED, Freeman JM. Neonatal seizures: I. Correlation of prenatal and perinatal events with outcomes. Pediatrics 1982; 70:165–176.

Holmes GL. Neonatal seizures. In: Pedley TA, Meldrum BS, eds. Recent advances in epilepsy. Number 2. New York: Churchill Livingstone, 1985:207.

Mikati MA, Feraru E, Krishnamoorthy K, Lombroso CT. Neonatal herpes simplex meningoencephalitis: EEG investigations and clinical correlates. Neurology 1990; 40:1433–1437.

Mizrahi EM, Tharp BR. A characteristic EEG pattern in neonatal herpes simplex encephalitis. Neurology 1982; 32:1215–1220.

Painter MJ, Bergman I, Crumrine P. Neonatal seizures. Pediatr Clin North Am 1986; 33:91–109.

Rowe JC, Holmes GL, Hafford J, et al. Prognostic value of the electroencephalogram in term and preterm infants following neonatal seizures. Electroencephalogr Clin Neurophysiol 1985; 60: 183–196.

Scher MS, Painter MJ. Controversies concerning neonatal seizures. Pediatr Clin North Am 1989; 36:281–310.

Shewmon DA. What is a neonatal seizure? Problems in definition and quantification for investigative and clinical purposes. J Clin Neurophysiol 1990; 7:315–368.

Volpe JJ. Neonatal seizures: Current concepts and revised classification. Pediatrics 1989; 84:422–428.

VASCULAR DISORDERS

SYMPTOMATIC CAROTID STENOSIS

ERNESTO FERNÁNDEZ-BEER, M.D.
JEFFREY L. SAVER, M.D.

When referring to symptomatic carotid stenosis we are practically speaking of atherosclerotic occlusive disease, since all other causes of symptomatic carotid stenosis (e.g., fibromuscular dysplasia, arterial dissection, endarteritis) are so rare and distinctive in their clinical presentation as to be considered altogether different diseases. The results obtained thus far from the North American Symptomatic Carotid Endarterectomy Trial (NASCET) and the European Carotid Surgery Trial (ECST) have conclusively demonstrated that carotid endarterectomy is superior to aspirin alone in the management of symptomatic patients with severe (more than 70 percent) stenosis of the extracranial internal carotid artery. Additionally, the European trial found that symptomatic patients with mild (0 to 29 percent) stenoses derive insufficient benefit from carotid endarterectomy to outweigh the risks of the operation. This information was much needed. However, its usefulness will be appreciated if the selection process for the endarterectomy is made on solid clinical and laboratory information. This means being able to objectively conclude that a patient's symptoms and signs are caused by carotid stenosis and not some other frequently associated condition. We still do not know whether medical or surgical treatment is best for asymptomatic (moderate to severe) or for symptomatic moderate (30 to 69 percent) carotid stenosis. Ongoing prospective randomized trials may soon give us an answer. Given the current state of information, we cannot overemphasize the importance of developing the necessary clinical skills to plan an efficient, cost-effective, low-risk investigation of patients with carotid disease and to distinguish symptomatic from asymptomatic carotid stenoses.

CLINICAL EVALUATION

History

At the first encounter, the physician should be willing to sit calmly with the patient and family and obtain a detailed history of the complaints. The time invested at this point is crucial. We suspect that diagnostic errors most commonly occur at this stage, probably because it is the most time-consuming. If subsequent investigation of the patient yields evidence of occlusive carotid disease, but vague, nonfocal symptoms or focal symptoms outside the distribution of the carotid artery in question are being attributed to the stenosed vessel, the patient may be referred for an unnecessary operation, or medical treatment may be instituted that is not directed at the source of symptoms.

Background historical data that are helpful in predicting the presence of extracranial carotid atherosclerosis include white race, male sex, and age. The presence of associated risk factors such as hypertension, diabetes, coronary disease, peripheral vascular disease, hyperlipidemia, and tobacco use all correlate with the presence of carotid disease.

The symptoms caused by carotid artery stenosis, regardless of the mechanism (hemodynamic versus embolic), are either transient or permanent. Transient symptoms pose a particular diagnostic challenge. The spells are brief and often alarming. Only one in ten is witnessed by a physician, and, when examined during an attack, patients complaining of only one symptom will often exhibit additional signs. Empathic but pointed questioning regarding differential features is critical. The temporal course and distribution of a symptom and any subtle accompanying secondary symptoms should be determined as precisely as possible: Were hand paresthesias accompanied by minor perioral paresthesias? Was unilateral visual disturbance due to problems in one eye or in one hemifield (did the patient close one eye at a time during the attack)? Was there a march?

The arbitrary temporal definition of a transient ischemic attack (TIA) has been challenged in recent years. We agree with the caveats incorporated in the recent Classification of Cerebrovascular Diseases from the National Institute of Neurological Disorders and Stroke (NINDS), which defines a TIA as follows:

A brief episode of focal loss of brain function, thought to be due to ischemia, that can usually be localized to that portion of the brain supplied by one vascular system (left or right carotid or vertebrobasilar system) and for which no other cause can be found. Arbitrarily, by convention, episodes lasting <24 hours are classified as TIAs although the longer the episode the greater the likelihood of finding a cerebral infarct by computed tomography (CT) or magnetic resonance imaging (MRI). TIAs commonly last 2-15 minutes and are rapid in onset (no symptoms to maximal symptoms in <5 minutes and usually in <2 minutes). Fleeting episodes lasting only a few seconds are not likely to be TIAs. Each TIA leaves no persistent deficit, and there are often multiple attacks. There are unusual instances that fall outside this definition.

Transient ischemic events lasting less than 24 hours but associated with radiologic evidence of infarction might more accurately be labeled *cerebral infarction with transient signs.* This is a distinction without an important therapeutic difference: both spells without and spells with associated infarcts represent symptomatic carotid stenosis.

The symptoms common to left and right carotid TIAs include motor, sensory, and visual features (Table 1). Among motor symptoms are dysarthria, and weakness, paralysis, or clumsiness of the contralateral extremities or face. Sensory symptoms encompass numbness or paresthesias of the contralateral extremities or face. Visual symptoms include loss or distortion of vision in the ipsilateral eye or, rarely, the contralateral hemifield. Sensory and motor symptoms commonly occur together, but occasionally the patient will report pure motor or pure sensory disturbance. All degrees of weakness may be seen. If patients are examined during an attack, they will exhibit the reported signs of motor and speech dysfunction, but sensory symptoms will usually not be accompanied by objective sensory loss. Of cognitive symptoms, only aphasia is recognized commonly, and only a history of comprehension difficulties allows a clear differentiation from dysarthria. Transient aphasia is a symptom of a dominant hemisphere TIA, casting suspicion on the left carotid in 99 percent of right-handers and 60 percent of left-handers.

Transient monocular blindness (amaurosis fugax) should always suggest ipsilateral carotid stenosis, although less than half of patients with transient monocular visual loss will demonstrate more than 50 percent carotid stenosis on angiography. Close attention should be paid to the pattern of visual loss reported. An altitudinal or lateralized visual loss, often described as a descending shadow or closing curtain, is most strongly predictive of ipsilateral carotid disease. Other patterns, such as diffuse loss of vision simultaneously involving the entire monocular visual field or concentric constriction of vision inward from the periphery, less frequently reflect carotid lesions. The duration of the typical attack

Table 1 Recognition of Carotid Transient Ischemic Attacks (TIAs)

Symptoms suggestive of carotid TIAs
  Unilateral weakness
  Unilateral sensory loss
  Dysarthria (not in isolation)
  Transient monocular blindness
  Rarely, homonymous hemianopia
  Dysphasia

Symptoms not suggestive of carotid TIAs
  Symptoms suggesting vertebrobasilar TIAs
    Weakness, bilateral or shifting
    Sensory loss, bilateral or shifting
    Blindness, bilateral or homonymous
    Vertigo, diplopia, dysphagia, dysarthria, ataxia – only if two or more symptoms occur together
  Symptoms not acceptable as evidence of TIA
    Nonfocal symptoms
      Syncope
      Dizziness
      Confusion
      Incontinence of urine or feces
      Generalized weakness
    Isolated symptoms
      Vertigo, diplopia, dysphagia, ataxia, tinnitus, amnesia, drop attacks, dysarthria

is measured in seconds to minutes, and recurrent spells tend to be stereotyped. Episodes in the same patient of transient monocular blindness and ipsilateral hemispheral TIAs are highly suggestive of carotid disease.

A less common manifestation of carotid distribution TIA includes loss of vision precipitated by exposure to sunlight. These episodes have been associated with severe obstructive carotid disease ipsilateral to the affected eye. The visual loss is diffuse rather than altitudinal or sectorial. Recovery occurs when the patient returns to a darker environment over minutes to hours. The mechanism is not well understood but is felt to be related to slow regeneration of retinal pigment due to ischemia.

Rarely, positive transient symptoms may be attributed to ischemia in the distribution of the carotid arteries. A well-known event is that of limb shaking episodes, which commonly are confused with simple partial seizures. They are precipitated by postural changes, walking, or neck hyperextension but also occur independent of precipitating factors. The movements are involuntary, coarse, nonrhythmic, often unilateral, and tend to involve the distal portions of the extremity more than the proximal. Their duration is measured in seconds to minutes, and their frequency varies between 3 and 12 Hz. During the episode there is no alteration of consciousness. They are not associated with spike-wave discharges on electroencephalograms and do not respond to anticonvulsant treatment, but rather to optimization of cerebral blood flow through adjustment of antihypertensive medication or endarterectomy. The pathogenesis of positive limb shaking during ischemia is poorly understood but may involve release of subcortical motor circuitry.

Table 2 TIAs in the Carotid Territories: Features Distinguishing Different Vascular Mechanisms

Mechanism	Duration	Multiplicity	Symptom Distribution and Type	Precipitants
Cardioembolic	>1 hour	Single or only a few episodes	Limb symptoms restricted to one body part or distal portions of two body parts; aphasia; different vascular distributions in different episodes	Palpitations; chest pain
Lacunar	Minutes	Variable	Pure motor or pure sensory limb symptoms affecting three body parts or entire portion of two body parts; no cortical signs	
Large vessel stenosis				
Hemodynamic	Brief, seconds to minutes	Multiple, may occur in clusters	Highly stereotyped episodes; limb shaking TIAs; monocular visual loss on exposure to bright light	Orthostatic changes; exertion
Artery to artery embolic	<25 minutes	Multiple	Less strictly stereotyped; limb symptoms restricted to one body part or distal portions of two body parts; aphasia; TMB and ipsilateral hemispheral symptoms	

Recognizing symptoms that are not due to carotid stenosis is perhaps as important as recognizing those that are. Nonfocal symptoms occurring in isolation do not reliably reflect focal brain ischemia in either the anterior or posterior circulation. Isolated lightheadedness, wooziness, vertigo, or syncope are not manifestations of carotid disease. Vertebrobasilar TIAs may be characterized by bilateral motor or sensory symptoms, vertigo, diplopia, dysphagia, or unilateral or bilateral homonymous visual field loss. Posterior circulation ischemia should not be attributed to disease in anterior circulation vessels. Alternating neurologic symptoms, such as left then right hemiparesis, suggest vertebrobasilar disease, cardiac embolism, or diffuse vascular disease.

An attempt should be made to distinguish TIAs in the carotid territory due to large artery disease from those due to vascular mechanisms unrelated to carotid stenosis (Table 2). TIAs caused by carotid occlusive disease are generally believed to occur through either of two mechanisms: artery to artery embolism (most commonly), and intermittent hemodynamic reduction of blood flow across a tightly obstructed vessel. Flow-related TIAs are characteristically short in duration and highly stereotyped, often occurring in clusters. They may be precipitated by changes in posture or exertion. Artery-to-artery embolic TIAs may be more long-lived. Cardioembolic TIAs tend to be quite long lasting (from one to several hours), do not recur frequently, and may produce symptoms in different vascular distributions during different episodes. Recent studies have suggested that lacunar TIAs may be recognized by the absence of cortical signs and the distribution of motor and sensory symptoms. Pure motor or pure sensory symptoms affecting face, arm, and leg simultaneously, or both proximal and distal portions of two limbs, are probably of small vessel origin. Monopareses, sensory symptoms confined to a single limb, and restricted, distal faciobrachial or brachiocrural symptoms are more characteristic of large vessel TIAs.

Focal ischemia is not the only cause of transient or permanent focal neurologic deficits. High in the differential diagnosis are migraine with aura and epilepsy. Both present with a march of neurologic symptoms, in a leisurely 5 to 20 minute fashion in migrainic spells, a rapid few second pace in seizures. TIAs have an all-at-once or, less commonly, a stuttering onset. Additionally, ischemia usually produces negative symptoms, implying loss of function of the responsible neuronal networks, while both migraine and seizures may usually be distinguished by the presence of positive symptoms, implying excess of function, such as paresthesiae rather than numbness, clonic activity rather than weakness, photopsias rather than blindness. With migraine the presence of a headache and a past personal or family history of similar stereotyped neurologic symptoms strongly support the diagnosis. However, from 25 to 35 percent of ischemic neurologic events may be associated with a headache, and therefore we always consider migraine a diagnosis of exclusion. In the case of epilepsy, the physician needs to be familiar with the rare inhibitory or "negative" type of focal seizure, which presents with transient symptoms identical to those of an ischemic nature, such as monoparesis or hemiparesis, hemisensory symptoms, and any degree of language or speech disturbance. The most common underlying structural lesions in these cases are tumor and infarct. Occasionally, primary or metastatic brain tumors produce "transient tumor attacks," which may be clinically indistinguishable from the ischemic occlusive variety. Supratentorial meningiomas and arteriovenous malformations are well known to mimic TIAs. Rarely, especially in elderly patients, a subacute subdural hematoma may produce transient neurologic symptoms suggestive of carotid occlusive disease. Helpful differentiating clinical features in these cases are the associated fluctuation in level of consciousness (lethargy or stupor) and cognitive function. Amyloid angiopathy, which more commonly causes lobar hemorrhages, has been reported to cause recurrent episodes of sensory symptoms as well as ischemic infarctions. Multiple sclerosis may produce TIA-like symptoms during exacerbations, but these usually last several hours in contrast to the briefer duration of most TIAs. Finally, other systemic derangements that may give rise to carotid distribution symptoms are hypertensive encephalopathy, symptomatic hypoglycemia, and hyperventilation.

In contrast to transient ischemic attacks, recognition of minor or major stroke in the carotid territories is generally not difficult. The patient exhibits persistent symptoms that correlate with CT or MRI demonstrated infarction in the deep or superficial territories of the middle cerebral artery, anterior cerebral artery, or both. A diagnostic dilemma arises when patients evidence more than one potential vascular mechanism for their stroke, such as coexistent cardiac source of embolism or small vessel disease and carotid stenosis. Historical features suggestive of symptomatic carotid stroke rather than cardioembolism are preceding TIAs (present in 40 to 50 percent of cases), stuttering course, and onset during sleep. Penetrating artery disease is the more likely, though not invariable, cause of small, deep strokes less than 1.5 cm in diameter. Large subcortical strokes greater than 1.5 cm in diameter more frequently reflect large artery disease.

Physical Examination

In addition to a detailed neurologic examination, particular attention should be devoted to the cardiovascular and neurovascular exams. Blood pressure and pulse recordings and cardiac auscultation are geared at detecting cardiac dysfunction in the forms of congestive heart failure, rhythm abnormalities, and murmurs. Signs of peripheral vascular disease may suggest the presence of diffuse atherosclerosis. The neck and head are auscultated for bruits, bearing in mind their shortcoming as specific and sensitive indicators of carotid disease. Many patients without bruits harbor significant extracranial stenosing lesions. Conversely, only 50 to 60 percent of cervical bruits are associated with high-grade internal carotid artery stenosis. Bruits that extend into diastole and are well localized near the angle of the jaw are most likely to correlate with underlying carotid disease. The presence of an ocular bruit may signify ipsilateral intracranial carotid siphon stenosis. Hemodynamically significant extracranial stenosis with collateral flow through the orbit or an intracranial vascular malformation may also produce a cranial bruit.

Palpation of neck and facial pulses may be helpful, but findings again must be interpreted with caution. Patients with severe internal carotid stenosis or occlusion may have normal neck pulses originating in patent common and external carotid arteries. An absent or markedly diminished carotid artery pulse suggests severe occlusive disease. When the external carotid circulation serves as a source of collateral supply for a markedly stenosed internal carotid artery, the ipsilateral superficial temporal artery may dilate and have a bounding pulse, and the supraorbital pulse may be obliterated by compression of the superficial temporal artery (frontal artery sign).

The ophthalmologic examination may yield rewarding findings, such as cholesterol or platelet retinal emboli, or a milder degree of hypertensive retinopathy ipsilateral to a high-grade carotid stenosis in a patient with systemic hypertension. Rarely, signs of chronic orbital ischemia may be seen, such as pupillary dilation with poor light reaction, neovascularization of the iris (rubeosis iridis), elevated intraocular pressure with secondary glaucoma, and proliferative retinopathy.

LABORATORY INVESTIGATION

The laboratory investigation of a patient with carotid TIAs or stroke can be divided into three phases: the basic, the noninvasive vascular, and the invasive vascular. The basic evaluation includes screening and atherosclerotic risk factor labs performed on all patients. These include complete blood count, serum electrolytes, blood urea nitrogen, serum creatinine, lipid profile, erythrocyte sedimentation rate, syphilis serology, prothrombin and partial thromboplastin times, liver function tests, a chest radiograph, and electrocardiogram (ECG). In addition, a neuroimaging study is obtained to document the presence and extent of infarction and rule out hemorrhage, tumor, or other structural lesion with a strokelike presentation. An MRI is preferable to CT: Its greater sensitivity is especially helpful in detecting small infarctions in patients with transient neurologic deficits. When evaluating a patient within a few hours of symptom onset, an initial CT should be obtained because it more reliably identifies acute hemorrhage. We routinely admit to the hospital patients with newly developed symptoms, or stroke or TIA episodes within the preceding 7 days, and proceed with investigations to disclose the pathophysiology as swiftly as possible, thus decreasing the possibility of stroke progression or recurrence.

The objective of the noninvasive vascular workup is the detection of carotid atherosclerotic disease, a cardiac source of embolism, or both. We customarily obtain carotid duplex studies, an echocardiogram, and, when rhythm abnormalities are suspected, a 24 hour Holter ECG. Advantages of carotid ultrasonography are wide availability and sensitivity and specificity exceeding 90 percent in the detection of moderate to severe carotid stenosis. When employed judiciously it is an excellent screening instrument for determining whether a patient should proceed to the third, invasive or risky, phase of the evaluation, which is carotid angiography.

However, several limitations of ultrasound must be borne in mind. Carotid duplex studies are operator dependent. If one is not confident of the reliability of a noninvasive laboratory, it is better to proceed directly to angiography in a patient with suspected symptomatic carotid stenosis than be deterred by a false-negative ultrasound finding. Even in the best of hands, duplex instruments, including those with color flow imaging, cannot reliably distinguish hairline residual lumina from total occlusions. The former are operable, the latter are not. Duplex studies suggesting occlusion should be confirmed by angiography, including an injection with delayed exposures to detect late, trickle flow.

Carotid ultrasound and angiographic measurements correlate more precisely at higher than at lower grades of stenosis. Consequently, angiography is indicated not only for most patients with carotid symptoms and 70 percent or more stenosis by ultrasound, but also for those with moderate (30 to 70 percent) stenosis on duplex study who should go on to arteriography to rule out a higher grade obstruction.

If the patient has minimal (less than 30 percent) stenosis by ultrasonography, angiography may initially be deferred, and further investigations should address whether the patient's symptoms are due to more distal stenosis (e.g., in the carotid siphon or middle cerebral artery) as well as the possibility of cardioembolism.

Lastly, the clinician should be aware that ultrasound laboratories differ widely in the algorithms employed to translate ultrasound velocity measures that reflect the cross-sectional *area* of stenotic lumen to angiographic measures of lumen *diameter*. In other words, a 75 percent stenosis means different things in different settings. Many of these conversion formulas predate the reporting of the results of the NASCET and ECST, and these two trials themselves used different measurement methods to determine angiographic stenosis. It is of paramount importance that the physician elucidate what formula the local neurosonology laboratory is relying upon, whether it pre- or postdates the NASCET and ECST trials, and with which of these or other angiographic measurement techniques the reported percentage stenoses are intended to correlate.

The recent availability of transcranial Doppler ultrasound and magnetic resonance angiography (MRA) allows noninvasive investigation of intracranial anterior circulation stenosis. Surgical therapy is no longer at issue in these patients. Since both intracranial atherosclerotic occlusive disease and nonhemodynamically significant extracranial carotid stenosis will be managed medically, the risks of angiography are generally not justified. An exception to this rule may be the patient with suspected internal carotid artery dissection.

If carotid duplex scanning reveals moderate stenosis, severe stenosis, or occlusion in the symptomatic carotid artery, the clinician is faced with the decision of whether to perform a carotid angiogram to define more precisely the true extent of stenosis, exclude tandem extracranial and intracranial stenoses, and determine the degree of stenosis of the opposite carotid. We believe that at present, carotid angiography remains a mandatory assessment before carotid endarterectomy. Overall, this procedure is associated with a 4 percent risk of neurologic complications and a 1 percent risk of permanent stroke, though recent studies suggest that intra-arterial digital subtraction arteriography may have lower morbidity than conventional arteriography. Before consigning a patient to angiography, the physician needs to determine if the patient is medically fit for the procedure and for a subsequent endarterectomy, and whether he or she would consent to surgery if recommended (Table 3).

An interesting recent British study suggests that the optimal strategy of carotid artery imaging depends on the degree of stenosis considered critical to detect. To

Table 3 Selection Criteria for Carotid Angiography

TIA likely, or small to medium-sized infarction definitely, in distribution of carotid artery.*

CT/MR excludes primary hemorrhage or nonvascular structural lesion.

Carotid duplex suggests moderate or severe stenosis or occlusion of carotid artery on side appropriate to symptoms.

Patient has no medical contraindications to carotid endarterectomy.

Patient is willing to undergo endarterectomy if angiogram is abnormal.

---

*A massive infarction, leaving little further territory at risk, would preclude any benefit from endarterectomy.

detect only patients with more severe stenosis (more than 50 to 75 percent) it is safer and more cost-effective to screen all patients with duplex ultrasonography, reducing the number of angiograms required and the number of strokes after angiography. To detect stenosis of more than 25 percent, it is more cost-effective to take into account the presence or absence of a carotid bruit, proceeding directly to angiography in symptomatic patients harboring a bruit, and screening patients without a bruit with duplex ultrasonography.

Magnetic resonance angiography (MRA) is a most promising development in the diagnostic investigation of symptomatic carotid stenosis. Using time-of-flight and black blood techniques, MRA has emerged as a useful noninvasive procedure to image the extracranial and intracranial vasculature of patients who are medically too ill for carotid endarterectomy and can be spared the risks of conventional cerebral angiography. At present, we do not recommend MRA in lieu of angiography to assess patients for endarterectomy. MRA techniques often overestimate the degree of stenosis and are insensitive in the detection of plaque ulceration. However, both MRA and sonographic techniques are evolving rapidly, and it is entirely possible that over the lifetime of this text, endarterectomy based on noninvasive testing alone may become a justifiable and standard practice.

SUGGESTED READING

Calanchini PR, Swanson PD, Gotshall RA, et al. Cooperative study of hospital frequency and character of transient ischemic attacks IV: The reliability of diagnosis. JAMA 1977; 238:2029–2033.

Feldmann E, Wilterdink J. The symptoms of transient cerebral ischemic attacks. Semin Neurol 1991; 11:135–145.

Furlan AJ. Transient ischemic attacks: Recognition and management. Heart Dis & Stroke 1992; 1:33–38.

Hankey GJ, Warlow CP. Symptomatic carotid ischemic events: Safest and most cost effective way of selecting patients for angiography, before carotid endarterectomy. BMJ 1990; 300:1485–1491.

Huston J, Lewis BD, Wiebers DO, et al. Carotid artery: Prospective blinded comparison of two-dimensional time-of-flight MR angiography with conventional angiography and duplex US. Radiology 1993; 186:339–344.

Mohr JP, Gautier JC, Pessin MS. Internal carotid artery disease. In: Barnett HJM, Mohr JP, Stein BM, Yatsu FM, eds. Stroke: Pathophysiology, diagnosis, and management. 2nd ed. New York: Churchill Livingstone, 1992: 285.

Moore WS, Mohr JP, Najafi H, et al. Carotid endarterectomy: Practice guidelines. J Vasc Surg 1992; 15:469–479.

Sandercock PAG. Recent developments in the diagnosis and management of patients with transient ischemic attacks and minor ischemic strokes. Q J Med 1991; 78:101–112.

Wolpert SM, Caplan LR. Current role of cerebral angiography in the diagnosis of cerebrovascular diseases. AJR Am J Roentgenol 1992; 159:191–197.

STROKE IN THE YOUNG

BARNEY J. STERN, M.D.
ROBERT J. WITYK, M.D.

Diagnosing the cause of a stroke in a 15- to 45-year-old patient is often challenging because of the diverse causes to be considered. Fortunately, the diagnosis can be secured in most individuals if the patient is approached in a systematic fashion. Information gleaned from the patient's history and physical examination, together with easily obtainable ancillary studies, can help direct further evaluation.

Inquiry should be made as to whether the patient has had any prior strokes or transient neurologic symptoms. One should always consider the possibility of multiple sclerosis or malignancy mimicking stroke. Historical information may provide clues to the cause of the stroke (Table 1). Some caveats need to be mentioned: (1) in a young patient, the presence of risk factors for a particular disease does not mean that the disease is present or is the cause of the patient's stroke; (2) a particular disorder can cause a stroke by a variety of mechanisms; and (3) a stroke can occur in the presence of several risk factors or diseases, making it difficult to assign a single cause.

The physical examination should be directed not only at a neurologic assessment, but also to the cardiovascular system. In addition, important information can be obtained by a formal ophthalmologic evaluation and careful survey of the skin (Table 2).

Table 1 Selected Historical Information

May suggest a vascular cause:
  Atherosclerosis
    Smoking
    Hypertension
    Hyperlipidemia
    Diabetes mellitus
    Radiation therapy
  Dissection
    Trauma
    Chiropractic manipulation

May suggest a cardiac cause:
  Intravenous drug abuse
  Association of stroke with exercise or straining
  Deep venous thrombosis
  Murmur
  Valve replacement
  Cancer
  Bone marrow transplantation

May suggest a hematologic cause:
  Sickle cell disease
  Deep venous thrombosis
  Livedo reticularis
  Bone marrow transplantation

Other clues:
  Recurrent headaches
  Use of oral contraceptives
  Alcohol use
  Recent febrile illness
  Pregnancy
  Human immunodeficiency virus infection/acquired immunodeficiency syndrome
  Family history of stroke or premature myocardial infarction
  Known systemic disorders

Table 2 Clues from Examination of the Eyes and Skin

Ocular examination
  Corneal arcus: hypercholesterolemia
  Corneal opacity: Fabry's disease
  Lisch nodules: neurofibromatosis
  Lens subluxation: Marfan's syndrome, homocystinuria
  Retinal perivasculitis: sickle cell disease, syphilis, connective tissue diseases, sarcoidosis, inflammatory bowel disease, Behçet's disease, Eales' disease
  Retinal arteriolar occlusions: emboli, angiopathic syndrome with sensorineural hearing loss and multiple small strokes
  Retinal angioma: cavernous malformation, von Hippel-Lindau disease
  Optic atrophy: neurofibromatosis
  Retinal hamartoma: tuberous sclerosis
  Angioid streaks: pseudoxanthoma elasticum

Skin Examination
  Osler nodes, splinter hemorrhages, needle tracks: endocarditis
  Xanthoma, xanthalasma: hyperlipidemia
  Café-au-lait spots, axillary freckles, neurofibromas: neurofibromatosis
  Excessive laxity: Ehlers-Danlos syndrome
  Telangiectasia: Osler-Weber-Rendu disease, scleroderma
  Purpura: coagulopathy, Henoch-Schönlein purpura, cryoglobulinemia
  Capillary angioma: cavernous malformation
  Aphthous ulcers: Behçet's disease
  Angiokeratosis: Fabry's disease
  Livedo reticularis: Sneddon's disease
  Facial angiofibromas, ash leaf spot, ungual fibroma, shagreen patch: tuberous sclerosis
  Papules, atrophic lesions: Degos' disease (malignant atrophic papulosis)

CATEGORIZING THE TYPE OF STROKE

It is critical to define whether the patient has a primarily ischemic or hemorrhagic neurologic disorder since this will help direct further investigation. Ischemic infarctions can be broadly categorized as being caused by vascular disease, cardiac emboli, hematologic disorders, substance abuse, oral contraceptives, migraine, and an array of miscellaneous conditions, many of them rare. Hemorrhagic processes include subarachnoid, intra-parenchymal, and intraventricular bleeding.

Ischemic Stroke

Vascular diseases involving large arteries can be classified as being caused by atherosclerosis (3 to 48 percent of patients) and nonatherosclerotic disorders (3 to 33 percent of patients). We believe it is important not to attribute a young patient's stroke to atherosclerosis just because risk factors for atherosclerosis are present. Risk factors such as duration of smoking, diabetes mellitus, hypertension, and certain lipoprotein abnormalities are correlated with atherosclerosis, but unless significant arterial disease, such as over 70 percent diameter internal carotid stenosis, can be demonstrated by imaging studies, a continuing search for the cause of the patient's stroke is indicated. If atherosclerotic-type lesions are present in the absence of common risk factors, disorders of homocysteine metabolism and prior radiation therapy should be considered.

Nonatherosclerotic arterial disorders include dissection, Takayasu's disease, fibromuscular dysplasia, idiopathic or secondary forms of moya moya disease, peripartum angiopathy, and arteritis. Dissection can occur spontaneously or following mild trauma, chiropractic manipulation, or neck hyperextension. Dissection is also associated with fibromuscular dysplasia and possibly migraine. If arteritis is present, evaluation is necessary to determine if the process is limited to the central nervous system (CNS) (isolated angiitis of the CNS, "primary" and "benign" forms) or a manifestation of a systemic disorder.

Some 4 to 18 percent of young stroke patients have small, deep infarctions and a "classic lacunar syndrome" such as a pure motor or sensory stroke, a sensorimotor stroke, or ataxic-hemiparesis. If a young patient does not have a history of severe hypertension, other causes of small, deep infarctions such as inflammatory or infectious disorders or cardiogenic emboli should be considered.

Cardiac embolism is the cause of stroke in 8 to 35 percent of young stroke patients. As outlined in Table 3, some conditions are a more probable source of emboli than others, an important consideration when deciding upon the extent of further evaluation in a patient in whom there is a finding only *possibly* associated with stroke. This is especially true for mitral valve prolapse, which commonly occurs in the general population. Another example would be the presence of a right to left shunt such as a patent foramen ovale,

which is more common in stroke patients than in controls. In the absence of a right-sided (venous) source of emboli to traverse the shunt, the presence of a patent foramen ovale should be considered only a possible cause for the stroke and further evaluation would be appropriate.

A hematologic cause of stroke is implicated in 3 to 18 percent of young patients. The spectrum includes primary hypercoagulable syndromes, abnormalities of coagulation-fibrinolysis associated with systemic conditions or drugs, platelet abnormalities, and disordered blood rheology or vascular surfaces. Ischemic stroke can be the presenting feature of a hematologic disorder (Table 4). A hypercoagulable state is of greater concern with any of the following: a personal or family history of recurrent thromboses, clots in atypical sites such as the

Table 3 Conditions Associated with Cardiac Emboli

Probable Source
Endocarditis
Atrial fibrillation
Recent myocardial infarction
Akinetic segment
Dilated cardiomyopathy
Intracardiac thrombus or tumor
Valvular vegetations including nonbacterial thrombotic endocarditis
Prosthetic valve
Right-to-left shunt with associated venous thrombosis
Spontaneous atrial contrast echo
Atrial septal aneurysm

Possible Source
Mitral valve prolapse
Atrial flutter
Remote myocardial infarction
Left ventricular hypertrophy
Hypokinetic segment
Isolated atrial septal defect or patent foramen ovale (without associated venous thrombosis)
Mitral annular calcification
Calcific aortic stenosis

Table 4 Selected Hematologic Disorders Associated with Stroke

Sickle cell disease
Hemoglobin SC disease
Polycythemia
Dysglobulinemia
Leukoagglutination
Thrombocytosis
Thrombotic thrombocytopenic purpura
Disseminated intravascular coagulation
Antiphospholipid
  Lupus anticoagulant
  Anticardiolipin
Antithrombin III deficiency
Protein C deficiency
(Free) protein S deficiency
Disorders of fibrinolysis

arms and neck, simultaneous bilateral leg thromboses, and continued clotting in spite of therapeutic anticoagulation.

Many conditions cause hematologic changes that can lead to stroke. Examples include pregnancy, cancer, nephrotic syndrome, leukemia, ulcerative colitis, paroxysmal nocturnal hemoglobinuria, and Behçet's syndrome. The hematologic changes are typically complex, and arterial or venous thrombosis can occur. Paradoxically, a hemorrhagic component can also be present, as in venous infarction or eclampsia. The primary and secondary antiphospholipid syndromes are another example of the complex manner in which hematologic disorders lead to stroke. Large or small artery or venous thrombosis can occur, as well as cardiac valvular lesions presumably leading to emboli. Associated deep venous thrombosis can predispose to paradoxical emboli if there is a right to left cardiac shunt.

Substance abuse is an important consideration in young stroke patients. Alcohol abuse seems to confer a modest excess risk of ischemic and hemorrhagic stroke. "Crack" cocaine is associated with both ischemic and hemorrhagic stroke, whereas cocaine more commonly causes hemorrhagic events. An associated aneurysm or arteriovenous malformation may be present in patients who have bled, especially if cocaine has been used. Other drugs associated with stroke include heroin, sympathomimetics, phencyclidine, and LSD. As for how drugs cause stroke, multiple mechanisms have been hypothesized. The possibility of septic endocarditis should always be considered. Since patients may not be forthcoming about their drug history, acquaintances should be questioned and blood and urine toxicology surveys obtained expeditiously. The presence of needle marks, hypertension, and cardiac arrhythmias, especially tachycardia, should raise the suspicion of drug use.

Oral contraceptives are implicated as a cause of stroke in 4 to 16 percent of patients. However, there are no adequate data correlating the risk of stroke for women using the currently available low-dose estrogen and progestin preparations. The potential relationship between oral contraceptives and migraine is especially relevant to the pathogenesis of stroke in young women. There may also be an increased risk of intracranial occlusive disease in smokers using oral contraceptives. We are hesitant to attribute an ischemic stroke to oral contraceptive use without first evaluating the patient for other causes.

Although migraine is considered a cause of stroke in only 2 to 18 percent of patients, it is quite often a consideration. Because there is no diagnostic marker for migraine, the clinician must rely on the patient's history. The 1988 International Headache Society definition of migrainous cerebral infarction is as follows:

One or more migrainous aura symptoms not fully reversible within seven days and/or associated with neuroimaging confirmation of ischemic infarction. Diagnostic criteria: (1) Patient has previously fulfilled criteria for migraine with neurologic aura. (2) The present attack is typical of previous attacks, but neurologic deficits are not completely reversible within seven days and/or neuroimaging demonstrates ischemic infarction in the relevant area. (3) Other causes of infarction ruled out by appropriate investigations.

Some controversial issues include: (1) Can a migrainous stroke occur within the context of a typical episode of migraine without aura (common migraine)? (2) Can a patient with a history of migraine who awakens without a headache but with a neurologic deficit have had a migrainous stroke? (3) What is the relationship of migrainous stroke to other conditions that may predispose to stroke such as pregnancy or oral contraceptive use and mitral valve prolapse? Until the pathophysiology of migraine is better understood or there is a readily available diagnostic marker, it will be difficult to resolve these controversies. Our current bias is to allow a diagnosis of migrainous stroke in migraine patients both with and without aura who have a stroke within the context of their typical headache and have no other readily identifiable stroke cause. In some patients, angiography at the time of the event can show segmental narrowing of cranial arteries suggestive of vasospasm. Subsequent angiography is typically normal, confirming the reversible nature of the lesion. It is important not to assign a diagnosis of migrainous stroke until after a thorough evaluation. For instance, patients with an arteriovenous malformation, arterial dissection, antiphospholipid syndrome, or MELAS (mitochondrial encephalomyopathy, lactic acidosis, and strokelike episodes) can have a history of migraine-like headaches.

Many other disorders have been associated with stroke in the young. A detailed discussion of each of these entities is beyond the scope of this chapter, but many not otherwise mentioned here are listed in Table 5. Several other conditions, however, warrant brief comment.

Only a small proportion of patients with acquired immunodeficiency syndrome (AIDS) have a strokelike

Table 5 Other Conditions Associated with Stroke

Inflammatory diseases: rheumatoid arthritis, systemic lupus erythematosus, scleroderma, Sjögren's syndrome, polymyositis, Henoch-Schönlein purpura, polyarteritis nodosa, Churg-Strauss syndrome, Wegener's granulomatosis, lymphomatoid granulomatosis, sarcoidosis, isolated angiitis of the central nervous system (primary and benign variants)

Infectious diseases: neuroborreliosis, cysticercosis, herpes zoster

Cancer: tumor emboli, L-asparaginase treatment, malignant angioendotheliomatosis

Hereditary disorders: Marfan's syndrome, epidermal nevus syndrome, autosomal dominant leukoencephalopathy with multiple small, deep infarctions

Ovarian hyperstimulation syndrome

illness. Diagnostic considerations in this setting include meningovascular syphilis, cardiogenic embolism from nonbacterial thrombotic endocarditis, vasculopathies associated with cryptococcal, tuberculous, and lymphomatous meningitis and herpes zoster, and human immunodeficiency virus (HIV)–associated vasculitis. Patients can also have transient neurologic events, especially with toxoplasmosis.

MELAS, which is most often associated with a point mutation in a mitochondrial DNA-encoded transfer RNA for leucine, is now recognized as a cause of "stroke" in young adults. The pathophysiology of the neurologic deficits is not known, and angiograms are unremarkable. The spectrum of clinical manifestations, including the abrupt onset of focal neurologic deficits, headaches, vomiting, seizures, lactic acidosis, and ragged red fibers on muscle biopsy, is well known.

Table 6 Selected Causes of Central Nervous System Hemorrhage

Trauma
　Delayed "spat" apoplexy
Aneurysm
　"Berry," mycotic
Vascular malformation
　Arteriovenous, cavernous, venous
Hypertension
Coagulopathy
Arteritis
　Sterile
　Infectious
Sympathomimetic drugs
　Cocaine and "crack" cocaine
Hemorrhage into a tumor
Moya moya disease or syndrome
Cold exposure
Migraine

However, we have diagnosed MELAS in patients who were otherwise asymptomatic or had only sensorineural hearing loss. With the recent availability of a rapid screening test for MELAS utilizing a polymerase chain reaction assay on leukocytes or urinary epithelial cells, it will be interesting to see if the prevalence of atypical MELAS in the young stroke population is higher than previously suspected.

The cause of ischemic stroke remains unknown in 4 to 36 percent of young patients. This wide range reflects referral biases of published surveys and the dates of patient accrual. Furthermore, there are many challenges inherent both in clinically evaluating young stroke patients, as has been discussed, and in categorizing their diagnoses for scientific publication. No doubt the broad ranges reported in this chapter for the various diagnostic groups also reflect these issues. There is an ever expanding list of diagnostic considerations in young stroke patients. An extensive multidisciplinary evaluation is indicated for patients with stroke of indeterminate cause. The use of computerized literature surveys is also critical to comprehensive, up-to-date evaluation of these patients.

Hemorrhagic Stroke

Selected causes of hemorrhagic events are listed in Table 6. Patients with cavernous malformations occasionally have a familial history, as do rare individuals with an aneurysm. Disorders associated with aneurysms include polycystic renal disease, pseudoxanthoma elasticum, Ehlers-Danlos and Marfan's syndromes, coarctation of the aorta, arteriovenous malformations, moya moya disease or syndrome, and endocarditis. The relationship of bleeding with sympathomimetic drugs and cocaine and "crack" cocaine is again worthy of mention. Normotensive individuals with a lobar he-

Table 7 Major Risk Periods for Selected Syndromes During Pregnancy and the Puerperium

	Trimester				
	1	*2*	*3*	*Labor/Delivery*	*Postpartum*
Eclampsia			*	*	*
Intracranial hemorrhage					
Subarachnoid bleed					
Aneurysm			*	*	*
Arteriovenous malformation		*		*	*
Takayasu's disease				*	
Moya moya disease		*	*		*
Venous thrombosis					*
Cardiogenic embolus					
Peripartum cardiomyopathy			*		*
Nonbacterial thrombotic endocarditis					*
Fat embolus				*	
Trophoblastic disease					*
Arterial occlusions		*	*		*

Adapted from Stern BJ: Cerebrovascular disease and pregnancy. In: Goldstein PJ, Stern BJ, eds. Neurological disorders of pregnancy. 2nd rev ed. Mount Kisco, NY: Futura, 1992; with permission.

Table 8   Diagnostic Testing for Ischemic Infarction

Laboratory	Neurodiagnostics	Cardiovascular
Phase One		
CBC	CT −/+ contrast	ECG
Differential		
Erythrocyte sedimentation rate		
Electrolytes		
Glucose		
Blood urea nitrogen, creatinine		
Liver function tests		
Platelets		
PT, aPTT		
Blood, urine toxicology		
RPR/VDRL		
Sickle prep		
Blood cultures		
Pregnancy test		
Cholesterol		
Triglycerides		
HDL-C		
Phase Two		
	CSF (include as indicated): cryptococcal antigen, cytology, VDRL, IgG index, Oligoclonal bands, *Borrelia burgdorferi* titer	Echocardiogram: transthoracic; transesophageal; air contrast; Holter monitor
	Brain MRI	
Phase Three		
	Angiography	
	(Carotid duplex)	
	(Transcranial Doppler)	
	(MR angiography)	
Phase Four		
FTA-ABS		DVT evaluation
HIV assay		
Hemoglobin electrophoresis		
Antinuclear antibody		
Serum protein electrophoresis		
Cryoglobulins		
Lupus anticoagulant		
Anticardiolipin		
D-dimer		
Clotting factor assays (antithrombin III, Proteins S and C, etc.)		
Thrombin time (dysfibrinogenemia)		
Serum homocyste(i)ne		

CBC = complete blood count; BUN = blood urea nitrogen; PT = prothrombin time; aPTT = activated partial thromboplastin time; RPR/VDRL = rapid plasmin reagin/Venereal Disease Research Laboratory; HDL-C = high-density lipoprotein cholesterol; CSF = cerebrospinal fluid; MRI = magnetic resonance imaging; FTA-ABS = fluorescent treponemal antibody; HIV = human immunodeficiency virus; DVT = deep venous thrombosis.

Adapted from Stern BJ, Kittner S, Sloan M, et al. Stroke in the young: Parts I and II. Md Med J 1991; 40:453–462, 565–571; with permission.

matoma are especially likely to harbor an identifiable vascular lesion predisposing to hemorrhage.

Pregnancy and the puerperium can set the stage for an assortment of ischemic and hemorrhagic processes. As illustrated in Table 7, the time at which an event occurs can help narrow diagnostic considerations. Furthermore, hemorrhagic events can sometimes be caused by processes unique to pregnancy such as eclampsia and trophoblastic carcinoma. Needless to say, any of the many causes of stroke in the young can precipitate a stroke during pregnancy.

APPROACH TO THE PATIENT

The diagnostic approach to the young stroke patient is influenced by the individual's history and physical examination. A brain computed tomography (CT) scan will help determine whether the patient has had a primarily ischemic or hemorrhagic event. If an ischemic stroke is suspected, the information provided by readily available Phase I studies (Table 8), integrated with the already available data, can guide the clinician to initially favor cardiogenic embolism, large artery disease, a

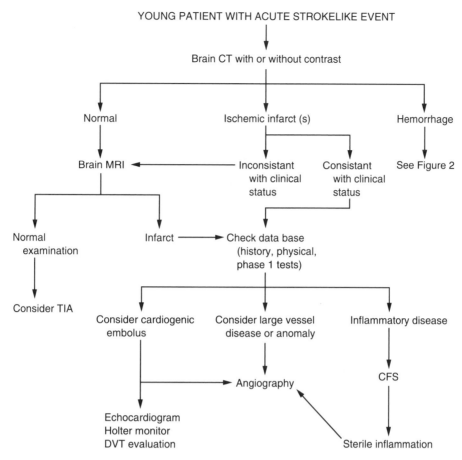

Figure 1 Algorithm for the evaluation of a young person who has experienced an acute strokelike event. CT = computed tomography; MRI = magnetic resonance imaging; TIA = transient ischemic attack; CSF = cerebrospinal fluid; DVT = deep venous thrombosis. (Adapted from Stern BJ, Kittner S, Sloan M, et al. Stroke in the young: Parts I and II. Md Med J 1991; 40:453–462, 565–571; with permission.)

vascular anomaly, or an inflammatory disorder. The algorithm outlined in Figure 1 can be followed, and appropriate Phase 2 and 3 studies (Table 8) obtained within a day or so.

A brain magnetic resonance imaging (MRI) can yield additional information if the CT scan is normal or provides inconclusive information. An MRI is especially useful when evaluating a woman early in pregnancy when radiation exposure should be avoided. A cerebrospinal fluid sample should be obtained emergently if infection is suspected and there is no contraindication to lumbar puncture.

We believe that early cerebral angiography can provide extremely valuable information and should be considered an integral part of the evaluation of a young stroke patient. Angiography can document cerebral emboli and characterize large artery disease and vascular anomalies. Though the angiographic appearance of small artery "beading" is relatively nonspecific, this finding can guide further investigation. If the patient has a systemic or cardiac condition closely linked to ischemic stroke, angiography may not be indicated. Furthermore,

some conditions such as sickle cell disease and homocystinuria may make angiography risky. Therefore, angiography should not be performed indiscriminately. Lastly, unless atherosclerotic disease is strongly suspected, carotid duplex imaging, transcranial Doppler, and magnetic resonance angiography may not provide adequate information about vascular anatomy, especially small artery disease. Obtaining these noninvasive studies should not be a cause for delay in performing intra-arterial angiography.

Phase 4 studies (Table 8) should be considered if the diagnosis remains elusive. Most of these tests are not obtainable in a timely fashion, and patient management will need to proceed empirically pending test results. We expect the items in Phase 4 to grow as new causes of stroke are defined.

If the patient has had a hemorrhagic event, the evaluation is usually more straightforward (Fig. 2). The algorithm emphasizes the need for angiography to fully evaluate normotensive patients with a lobar or intraventricular hemorrhage.

In summary, the evaluation of the young stroke

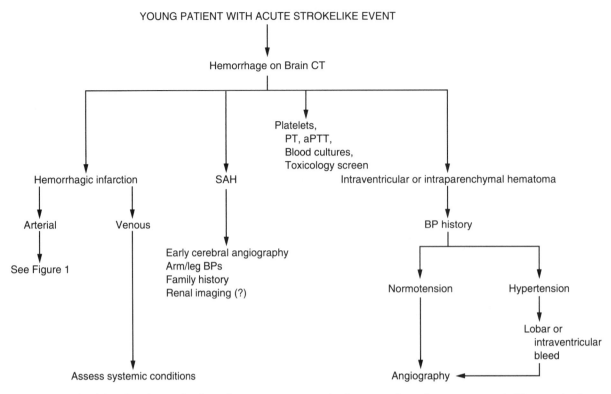

Figure 2 Algorithm for the evaluation of a young person who has experienced an acute strokelike event when hemorrhage is found on brain CT scanning. (Adapted from Stern BJ, Kittner S, Sloan M, et al. Stroke in the young: Parts I and II. Md Med J 1991; 40:453–462, 565–571; with permission.)

patient is a challenge. However, if the patient is approached in a systematic fashion and advantage is taken of an interdisciplinary assessment, the mystery can often be deciphered.

Acknowledgment. The authors wish to thank their fellow members of the Young Stroke Study Group (Baltimore, Maryland) for the insightful discussions that helped mold this chapter: Doctors David Buchholz, Constance Meyd, Christopher Earley, Steven Kittner, Thomas Price, and Michael Sloan.

SUGGESTED READING

Bogousslavsky J, Pierre P. Ischemic stroke in patients under age 45. Neurol Clin 1992; 10:113–124.

Calabrese LH, Furlan AJ, Gragg LA, Ropos TJ. Primary angiitis of the central nervous system: Diagnostic criteria and clinical approach. Cleve Clin J Med 1992; 59:293–306.

Hart RG, Kanter MC: Hematologic disorders and ischemic stroke: A selective review. Stroke 1990; 21:1111–1121.

Natowicz M, Kelly RI. Mendelian etiologies of stroke. Ann Neurol 1987; 22:175–192.

Stern BJ: Cerebrovascular disease and pregnancy. In: Goldstein PJ, Stern BJ, eds. Neurological disorders of pregnancy. 2nd rev ed. Mount Kisco, NY: Futura, 1992.

Stern BJ, Kittner S, Sloan M, et al. Stroke in the young: Parts I and II. MMJ 1991; 40:453–462, 565–571.

Welch KMA, Levine SR: Migraine-related stroke in the context of the International Headache Society classification of head pain. Arch Neurol 1990; 47:458–462.

CARDIAC SOURCES OF EMBOLISM

CHARLES H. TEGELER, M.D.

In recent years interest in cardiac and aortic sources of brain embolism has increased dramatically. Epidemiologic and clinical studies suggest that 15 to 20 percent of all strokes have a cardioembolic mechanism. Nonvalvular atrial fibrillation is now recognized as the most frequent cause of cardioembolism, accounting for about 45 percent of all cardioembolic strokes. At least two-thirds of the strokes associated with atrial fibrillation are due to cardioembolic mechanisms, with most attributed to thrombi formed within the left atrium (LA) or left atrial appendage (LAA). Ischemic heart disease is the second most common cause of cardioembolism, due to either acute myocardial infarction with left ventricular dysfunction or chronic left ventricular aneurysm. Recent reports suggest that aortic atherosclerosis is a frequent unsuspected source for cardioembolism. Despite the increased interest, understanding the pathophysiology of cardioembolism has been limited by several factors, including the absence of diagnostic methods capable of sensitively evaluating the LA and LAA, the heterogeneity of potential cardioembolic mechanisms, and the necessity of having to infer stroke mechanism based merely on identification of a potential source of embolism in the heart (the "smoking gun" approach).

Accurate identification of the ischemic mechanism has assumed a pivotal role in the clinical management of patients with, or at risk for, stroke. Recent clinical trials have confirmed that for patients with nonvalvular atrial fibrillation, antithrombotic therapy can safely reduce the risk of a first stroke by up to 80 percent. Although lacking confirmation with clinical trials, long-term anticoagulation with warfarin is now the accepted therapy for secondary prevention following cardioembolism. Clinical trials have confirmed that carotid endarterectomy effectively reduces the risk of stroke in patients with symptomatic tight carotid stenosis. In addition, new therapies for acute stroke, currently in clinical trials, such as thrombolytic therapy, are generally mechanism-specific. However, for an individual patient, understanding and documenting the stroke mechanism often remain problematic.

APPROACH TO DEFINING THE ISCHEMIC MECHANISM

Identification of the ischemic mechanism is particularly important in cardioembolism since confirmation of the diagnosis will probably result in the use of long-term anticoagulation, a potentially risky therapy. Given this clinical imperative to document cardioembolic mechanisms, all available diagnostic tools must be utilized, in a logical and cost-effective manner. When faced with patients manifesting acute focal neurologic deficits, I follow the same initial approach for identification of the stroke mechanism, including cardioembolism, in all. The first objective is to determine whether the event is vascular as opposed to nonvascular (brain tumor, hypo- or hyperglycemia, seizure with persisting Todd's paralysis, psychiatric conversion reaction, or metabolic encephalopathy) (Fig. 1). For those events that appear vascular, the next step is to decide if the stroke is hemorrhagic (intracerebral hemorrhage, subarachnoid hemorrhage, subdural hematoma, epidural hematoma) or an ischemic infarction. Beyond this, the goal is to determine whether the mechanism was large vessel atherothromboembolism, due to either hemodynamic effects or artery-to-artery embolism, small vessel intracranial disease (lacunar infarction), cardioembolism, or a variety of less common causes.

I approach the acute decision regarding vascular causation by starting with a detailed history and physical examination, screening laboratory studies (Table 1), a chest roentgenogram, and an electrocardiogram (ECG). This allows quick identification of hypo- or hyperglycemia, acute myocardial infarction, significant cardiac arrhythmia, history of a seizure disorder, or other nonvascular conditions that may require alternative approaches. Additional laboratory studies may ultimately be needed to understand the stroke mechanism in some patients, especially young patients or those without the usual risk factors for cerebrovascular disease. Key historical elements to help identify the vascular nature of the event include the temporal profile of the onset (acute versus chronic, hours versus days), the pattern of progression, any resolution of symptoms (Table 2), a history of prior similar episodes, and the nature of any accompanying symptoms such as headache, nausea or vomiting, visual loss, vertigo, aphasia, dysphagia, and the like. The neurologic examination will also help to identify an event as vascular and may suggest a cause (Table 3).

Although I may have a high index of suspicion regarding the vascular nature of an event based on the history and physical examination, I routinely obtain an unenhanced computed tomography (CT) scan of the brain, or a magnetic resonance imaging (MRI) scan if available, to identify nonvascular causes such as hydrocephalus, tumor, or abscess, and to identify hemorrhagic stroke. If no hemorrhage is seen, but there are well-developed low-density lesions acutely, the CT scan is repeated with contrast, or an MRI obtained, to rule out tumor or abscess. Hemorrhagic infarction offers important clues to the mechanism, since it frequently accompanies cardioembolism. Some hemorrhagic changes are seen on CT scan in up to 20 to 25 percent of cardioembolic strokes by 48 to 72 hours after the event, but they are uncommon with atherothrombotic events.

Once the vascular nature of the event is confirmed and primary brain hemorrhage is ruled out, the task is to identify the ischemic mechanism. The history and

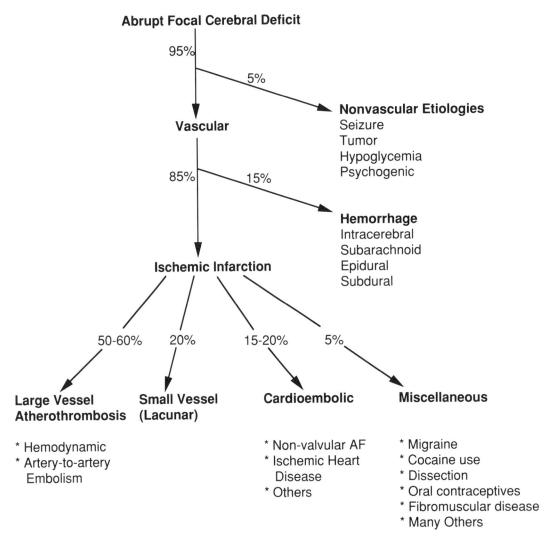

Figure 1 Causes of the stroke syndrome. AF = Atrial fibrillation.

Table 1 Laboratory Studies for Acute Stroke Syndrome

Initial	Later or as Indicated
Complete blood count	Lipid profile
Platelet count	Syphilis serology
Chemistry profile:	Erythrocyte sedimentation rate
Glucose	Serum protein electrophoresis
Electrolytes	Hemoglobin electrophoresis
Blood urea nitrogen	Serum viscosity
Creatinine	Platelet aggregation studies
Prothrombin time	Antiphospholipid antibodies
Partial thromboplastin time	Fibrinogen level
Urinalysis	Antinuclear antibodies

Table 2 Temporal Profile of Ischemic Events

Event	Time Course
Transient ischemic attack	Focal neurologic deficit that resolves by 24 hours (usually < 20 minutes)
Stroke-in-evolution	Definite progression of focal deficits over the preceding minutes to hours
Completed stroke	Focal neurologic deficit that persists for at least 24 hours

physical examination still form the foundation for this endeavor. An abrupt onset while the patient is awake or active, with early maximal severity of deficit, suggests embolism. A sudden or stuttering onset often present on awakening, progression over minutes to hours, or preceding transient ischemic attacks (TIA) suggest atherothrombosis. The history can be crucial in providing a profile of associated risks and can point to an ischemic mechanism. A history of atrial fibrillation, myocardial infarction, congestive heart failure or congestive cardiomyopathy, or prosthetic heart valve points to a cardiac source. Recent neck trauma, hypertension, hyperlipidemia, tobacco use, cervical bruits, or migraine identify risks for other ischemic mechanisms.

The physical examination can also identify patients

Table 3 Key Clinical Features of Vascular Causes of Stroke Syndrome

Type	Onset	Location and Deficits
Atherothrombosis	Abrupt or stuttering onset, often present on awakening, may show progression, half preceded by TIA	Cortical or subcortical, hemiparesis, hemisensory deficit, aphasia, visual field deficits
Embolism	Abrupt onset when awake or active, maximal deficit at onset, prior TIA uncommon	Cortical lesions, MCA branch lesions, hemiparesis, aphasia, cortical sensory loss, visual field deficit, hemorrhagic transformation common, seizures at onset more frequent
Hemorrhage	Gradual, progressive course over minutes to hours, often with headache, vomiting	Cortical or subcortical, progressive, focal deficits, often decreasing level of consciousness

TIA = transient ischemic attack; MCA = middle cerebral artery.

at high risk for cardioembolism. The examination must include assessment for atrial fibrillation (irregularly irregular rhythm, radial pulse deficit), congestive heart failure, cardiac murmurs, or abnormal pulse waves, such as slow upstroke and prolonged impulse with aortic stenosis, or water-hammer pulse of aortic insufficiency. Findings on the general examination suggestive of atherothrombosis might include cervical bruits, retinal emboli, or blood pressure asymmetry.

The pattern of neurologic deficits can help localize the brain area affected, often providing clues to the mechanism. Cardioembolism most commonly results in cortical infarction. Thus, it is important to look for signs of focal cortical dysfunction such as visual field deficits, gaze preference, aphasia, cortical sensory loss, neglect, or anosognosia. An isolated Wernicke's aphasia is most often due to cerebral embolism.

DIAGNOSTIC STUDIES TO RULE IN CARDIOEMBOLISM

The physician's index of suspicion for cardioembolism depends on the features of the clinical presentation and the profile of cardiac risk factors. If the index of suspicion is very high, a cardiac evaluation should be considered, irrespective of the results of other diagnostic studies. Otherwise, the decision to pursue specific cardiac evaluation should be made based on both the clinical features and results of other diagnostic studies. For example, the absence of severe carotid stenosis in a patient with a large stroke suggests the need for cardiac evaluation. In every patient, the physician must decide prior to additional workup whether the information gathered will affect management or outcome. Even if the clinical features and other test results suggest the need for a cardiac workup, the patient must also be a candidate for treatment options; that is, the deficits must not be so severe as to preclude preventive therapy, and there must be no bleeding diathesis that precludes the use of antithrombotic or anticoagulant therapy. Otherwise, no further cardiac testing should be performed.

Bedside clinical features can generate a high index of suspicion but cannot by themselves reliably identify the stroke mechanism. I use additional diagnostic evaluation to help identify specific and even unsuspected causes, including cardioembolism. CT or MRI scans most often show cortical infarction patterns in cardioembolism. A pattern of branch infarctions in the middle cerebral artery territory is most often due to cerebral embolism. Infarction in multiple vascular territories provides evidence of a source proximal to the extracranial carotid artery. Silent infarction, which occurs in up to 40 percent of those with "asymptomatic" atrial fibrillation, may also be an important clue. Cardioembolism may cause large (1.5 cm diameter), deep infarcts (lagoons) by occluding the ostia for several penetrating arteries. While experimental evidence is mounting that cardioembolism may cause small, deep infarcts (lacunes), such infarcts are more often due to associated hypertension or diabetes mellitus. In virtually all patients with stroke in whom a diagnostic workup is appropriate, I obtain carotid duplex sonography, with or without color-flow imaging, to identify carotid stenosis as a potential cause of the event. Although the presence of carotid stenosis does not prove causality, the identification of severe carotid stenosis has direct management implications. Transcranial Doppler (TCD) sonography should also be performed to evaluate the intracranial circulation for stenosis, define collateral flow patterns, and document the cerebral hemodynamics of both the anterior and posterior circulations. TCD also allows detection of cerebral microembolism (see later).

CARDIAC DIAGNOSTIC EVALUATION

Specific cardiac diagnostic evaluation should include an ECG and a chest roentgenogram, as well as some form of long-term assessment for arrhythmia. The latter might be accomplished with cardiac monitoring via telemetry in an intensive care unit or by 24 hour Holter monitoring. Again, the decision regarding additional cardiac diagnostic testing depends on whether such additional information will affect clinical management. If so, I proceed with the highest yield, least risky techniques. Evaluation of cardiac structure and function is best accomplished with echocardiography. Transthoracic, or surface, two-dimensional echocardiography (TTE) revolutionized the field of cardiac diagnostic testing. This method is noninvasive, relatively low in cost, and widely available. A surface echocardiogram can

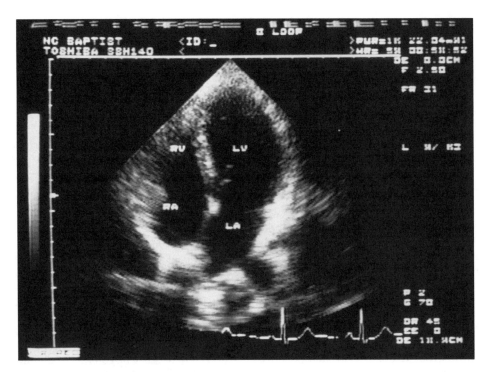

Figure 2 Transthoracic echocardiogram. The left atrium (LA) is deep and farthest from the transducer on the skin surface. RA = right atrium; RV = right ventricle; LV = left ventricle. (From Tegeler CH, Downes TR. Thrombosis and the heart. Semin Neurol 1991; 11:339–352; with permission.)

accurately evaluate chamber size and performance, valvular structure and function, intracardiac masses or thrombi, especially those in the ventricles, and pericardial structures. The addition of Doppler methods (duplex Doppler, continuous-wave Doppler, or color-flow imaging) allows evaluation of cardiac hemodynamics. However, due primarily to location of the heart, and specifically the LA, LAA, and interatrial septum, deep and posterior within the chest, TTE is often unable to adequately assess these key structures (Fig. 2). Elderly patients are frequently more difficult to image with TTE, as are those with pulmonary disease. Thus, when used to evaluate the general population of stroke patients for intracardiac thrombosis or source of embolism, TTE has a low yield. The diagnostic yield is improved by selecting patients with higher risk of cardioembolism based on the history and physical examination or the results of the ECG, chest radiograph, or Holter.

Transesophageal echocardiography (TEE) overcomes many of the limitations of TTE and provides high resolution cardiac images and functional data, particularly of the LA, LAA, and interatrial septum. This method is semi-invasive but has proven to be safe and well tolerated in stroke patients. It has at least a fivefold higher yield for identification of potential cardiac sources of embolism in stroke patients (Fig. 3), even in those with a normal TTE study. The use of biplane or omniplane TEE transducers allows interrogation of virtually all areas within the heart and surrounding structures. This includes the arch of the aorta, a frequent

site of atherosclerosis, which was previously hidden to monoplane TEE. The yield of TEE is increased further with the use of ultrasound bubble contrast agents, particularly when administered in conjunction with a Valsalva's maneuver, to identify right to left intracardiac shunts. TEE frequently reveals a variety of potential cardiac sources of embolism (Table 4), many of which are of uncertain clinical significance. The higher yield of potential cardiac sources of embolism may be especially important in the young patient, who rarely has another identifiable cause of stroke. Other cardiac imaging modalities such as cardiac CT, MRI, or positron emission tomography have potential to provide important information but to date have no proven utility or advantage over echocardiographic methods.

When it is clear that greater understanding of the ischemic mechanism will affect clinical management, I proceed with specific cardiac testing using echocardiography (Fig. 4). Both TTE and TEE have unique strengths and limitations and are complementary. Because of the semi-invasive nature of TEE, its higher cost, and the continued uncertainty regarding the clinical importance of many potential cardiac sources of embolism, I recommend starting with TTE. A TTE study is indicated for stroke patients in whom no other obvious cause has been established or when there is an increased risk of cardioembolism. Patients included in the group with an increased risk are those having evidence of cardiac disease by history, physical examination, ECG, Holter, or chest roentgenogram, those with atrial fibril-

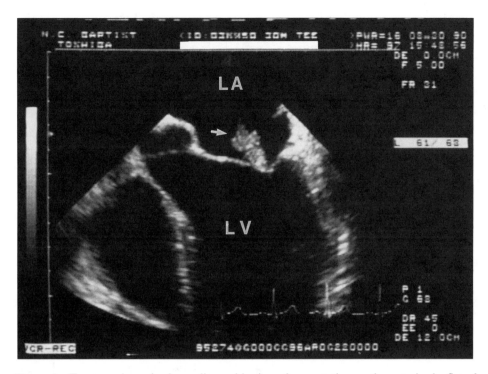

Figure 3 Transesophageal echocardiographic view of a vegetation on the anterior leaflet of the mitral valve (*arrow*). LA = left atrium; LV = left ventricle. (From Tegeler CH, Downes TR. Thrombosis and the heart. Semin Neurol 1991; 11:339–352; with permission.)

Table 4 Potential Sources of Cardioembolism Identified by Echocardiography

Aortic atherothrombosis or dissection
Atrial septal defect or atrial septal aneurysm
Patent foramen ovale
Cardiomyopathy
Thrombus or mass in the left ventricle, left atrium, or appendage
Left atrial enlargement
Left ventricular dysfunction (dyskinesis, akinesis, or aneurysm)
Mitral or aortic valvular stenosis, strands, vegetations, or prolapse
Spontaneous echo contrast

lation, patients less than 45 years of age, and those in whom there is any clinical suspicion of cardioembolism. Because cerebral ischemia is associated with an increased risk of cardiac or coronary artery disease, the presence of which might significantly affect management, TTE could be considered in all stroke patients.

If the TTE study is negative or technically inadequate, especially in those without clinical cardiac disease or those less than 45 years old, I usually obtain a TEE examination. The TEE study is best performed in the echocardiography laboratory in awake or mildly sedated patients. Monitoring devices used during the study should include ECG and pulse oximeter. Topical anesthesia should be applied to the posterior pharynx, and mild intravenous sedation is usually desirable (diazepam or midazolam). An intravenous agent, glycopyrrolate, is frequently used to dry secretions. Usually with a bite-block in place, the scope is introduced and advanced

to a position behind the heart, in the mid-esophagus. The scope is advanced or withdrawn, flexed or extended, to interrogate the heart from a variety of standardized views. The rate of unsuccessful insertion should be 1 to 2 percent, and a typical clinical study should take 10 to 20 minutes. The only clear contraindication to TEE is a history of dysphagia or known esophageal disease. Use of anticoagulation is considered a relatively minor contraindication and does not preclude a TEE examination. However, in anticoagulated patients, elective TEE should be performed after ensuring that the patient is not overanticoagulated. Bubble contrast assessment should be a routine part of TEE studies performed to identify a source of embolism.

EMBOLUS DETECTION

Doppler ultrasound is able to detect the passage of microembolic material through the cerebral arteries. The difference in acoustic impedance between embolic material and the surrounding blood causes an increase in the intensity of the returning signal when embolic material passes through the Doppler beam. This is displayed as an increased intensity in a trace of the total spectral intensity, or a focal area of increased intensity within the Doppler spectrum. This method has been successfully used in the setting of ischemic stroke, TIA, postmyocardial infarction, prosthetic heart valves, cardiopulmonary bypass, and carotid endarterectomy. The technique can be applied to virtually any accessible

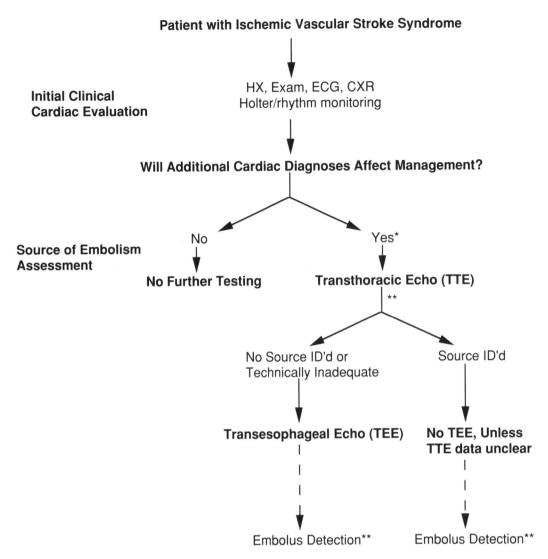

Figure 4 Algorithm of evaluation for cardiac source of embolism.
* If no clear etiology and < 45, no clinical evidence of cardiac disease, or atrial fibrillation, consider going directly to TEE.
** Embolus detection projected for use to confirm cardioembolism in vivo, follow natural history, and assess effect of therapy. May ultimately prove useful to identify high-risk patients who should have additional cardiac testing.

artery but has most frequently been used in the common carotid arteries, middle cerebral arteries, and vertebrobasilar vessels. Embolism detection offers an opportunity to move beyond the "smoking gun" approach, to actually identify and document the occurrence of embolism in patients. Such information could increase our understanding of stroke mechanism in specific patients, help localize the source of embolism, identify high-risk patients either before or after stroke, and provide objective evaluation of the effect of preventive therapies. In our institution, embolism detection is often used to evaluate patients for an embolic mechanism and to help localize an embolic source to a position either proximal or distal to the common carotid artery. Application in patients with all types of ischemic infarction suggests that this may be a more precise method than any other clinical approach to identify stroke mechanism. It can not only confirm embolism when suspected clinically, but

can also identify unsuspected cardioembolism. Embolus detection might even allow initial identification of patients at high risk (evidence of active cerebral embolization) that require additional cardiac diagnostic studies. The prevalence and natural history of these embolic signals, and their clinical importance as regards management, require further study. However, this promises to become a standard part of the diagnostic evaluation for ischemic stroke, particularly cardioembolism.

COEXISTENT DISEASE

The presence of both carotid stenosis and potential cardiac or aortic sources of embolism presents a difficult management dilemma. Clinical features and test results may suggest which problem caused the acute event and guide initial therapy. More often, it remains unclear which lesion was the culprit, and treatment must address both. This may mean choosing a preventive medication to try to affect both the heart and the carotid stenosis, such as aspirin, ticlopidine, or warfarin, or performing a carotid endarterectomy prior to placing the patient on long-term anticoagulation. The ability of Doppler embolus detection to localize an embolic source may prove quite helpful in patients having both carotid disease and cardiac sources of embolism, by documenting which is the active process requiring specific therapy.

If all studies are negative and no clear cause is found in the cerebral circulation or in the heart, I usually use antithrombotic therapy (aspirin or ticlopidine) rather than anticoagulation (warfarin). If the studies are negative but there is a high clinical index of suspicion regarding cardioembolism, I often treat patients for at least a few months with warfarin, then consider switching to antithrombotic therapy. There are few data to provide guidance in this area.

SUGGESTED READING

Amarenco P, Cohen A, Baudrimont M, Bousser MG. Transesophageal echocardiographic detection of aortic arch disease in patients with cerebral infarction. Stroke 1992; 23:1005–1009.

Bogousslavsky J, Van Melle G, Regli F. Middle cerebral artery pial territory infarcts: A study of the Lausanne Stroke Registry. Ann Neurol 1989; 25:555–560.

Caplan LR. Brain embolism revisited. Neurology 1993; 43:1281–1287.

Cerebral Embolism Task Force. Cardiogenic brain embolism: Second report of the Cerebral Embolism Task Force. Arch Neurol 1989; 46:727–743.

DeRook FA, Comess KA, Albers GW, Popp RL. Transesophageal echocardiography in the evaluation of stroke. Ann Intern Med 1992; 117:922–932.

Markus H. Transcranial Doppler detection of circulating cerebral emboli: A review. Stroke 1993; 24:1246–1250.

Pearson AC, Labovitz AJ, Tatineni S, Gomez CR. Superiority of transesophageal echocardiography in detecting cardiac source of embolism in patients with cerebral ischemia of uncertain etiology. J Am Coll Cardiol 1991; 17:66–72.

Ringelstein EB, Koschorke S, Holling A, et al. Computed tomographic patterns of proven embolic brain infarctions. Ann Neurol 1989; 26:759–765.

Rothrock JF, Hart RG. Antithrombotic therapy in cerebrovascular disease. Ann Intern Med 1991; 115:885–895.

Sherman DG, Dyken ML, Fisher M, et al. Antithrombotic therapy for cerebrovascular disorders. Chest 1992; 102(Suppl):529S–537S.

Sirna S, Biller J, Skorton DJ, Seabold JE. Cardiac evaluation of the patient with stroke. Stroke 1990; 21:14–23.

Stroke Prevention in Atrial Fibrillation Investigators. Stroke prevention in atrial fibrillation study: Final results. Circulation 1991; 84:527–539.

Stump DA, Stein CS, Tegeler CH, et al. Validity and reliability of an ultrasound device for detecting carotid emboli. J Neuroimag 1991; 1:18–22.

Tegeler CH, Downes TR. Cardiac imaging in stroke. Curr Concepts Cerebrovasc Dis Stroke 1991; 26:13–18.

Tegeler CH, Downes TR. Thrombosis and the heart. Semin Neurol 1991; 11:339–352.

Tegeler CH, Kitzman DW. Clinical utility of echocardiography in neurologic disorders. Neurol Clin 1993; 11:353–374.

Tegeler CH, Sherman DG. Ischemic cerebrovascular disease: Diagnosis and management. J Intensive Care Med 1986; 1:184–196.

Toole JF, Tegeler CH. Atherogenic embolism causing cerebral infarction (editorial). J Stroke Cerebrovasc Dis 1992; 2:65–66.

REVERSIBLE VASOSPASM OF INTRACEREBRAL VESSELS

GREGORY K. CALL, M.D.

Reversible vasospasm of intracerebral arteries refers to the phenomenon of one or more cerebral arteriograms showing multiple arterial narrowings that resolve on a later arteriogram. It is a purely descriptive diagnosis based on the pattern of cerebral arterial narrowing. In certain clinical circumstances the same phenomenon may be called vasculitis. We have also called it reversible vasoconstriction. This chapter focuses on the arterial patterns seen at arteriography, the clinical circumstances under which these studies are done, and what I believe they mean diagnostically.

One point of caution before starting. The word *spasm* may be inferred by some to mean an involuntary convulsive muscle contraction *without* a structural change within the arterial wall. In at least some conditions discussed in this chapter, this is not the case.

Likewise, the term *vasculitis* implies an inflammatory infiltrate as a defining characteristic, but not all cases of reversible arterial narrowing involve an inflammatory process. Clinically, the terms *vasospasm* and *vasculitis* are strongly tied to an arteriographic pattern and should be interpreted as descriptive only. We should keep an open mind about underlying pathophysiology in most instances. Such terms as *narrowing, constriction,* or *vasculopathy* may be preferable because they are more neutral.

CASE EXAMPLE

A 70-year-old woman was admitted to the hospital with a severe occipital headache, nausea, and vomiting. She first developed a severe headache 5 days prior to admission. It had lessened though never resolved in the intervening 4 days. Past medical history was remarkable for 5 years of frequent, probably daily, use of a cough preparation containing pseudoephedrine. Her general and neurologic examinations were normal. A cranial computed tomography (CT) scan was normal. The cerebrospinal fluid (CSF) contained 2 white cells and 2,080 red blood cells. The protein was 36 mg per

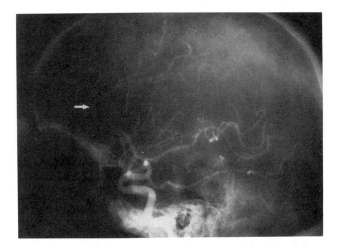

Figure 1 Initial right carotid artery injection was thought to show tapering of the distal anterior cerebral artery (*arrow*) and mild irregularity of distal branches but was not diagnostic.

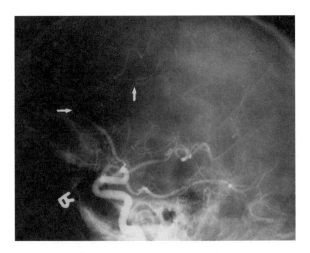

Figure 3 Subsequent right carotid artery injection 11 days after the first study shows definite tapered narrowing of the distal anterior cerebral artery and irregularities of pericallosal branches.

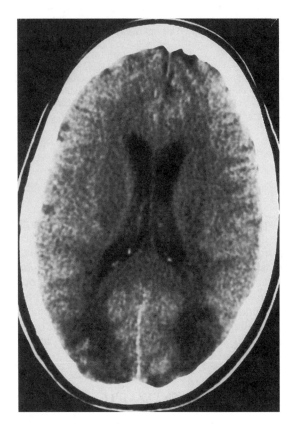

Figure 2 Plain cranial computed tomography shows bilateral parietal-occipital low density lesions in the border zone.

deciliter, and the glucose was 63 mg per deciliter. A cerebral arteriogram (Fig. 1) showed slight tapering and mild irregularities of some vessels but was not considered diagnostic. There was no aneurysm. Her headache resolved almost completely, and she was sent home 4

days later. The headaches recurred while the patient was at home, and 5 days after discharge she was readmitted with severe headache, nausea, vomiting, and complaints that she could not see. The patient and family were certain she had not used more of the cough preparation. During the first 24 hours in the hospital she was intermittently delirious, displayed visual-spatial disorientation, and experienced alternating bilateral motor and sensory deficits that varied from mild to severe. At times she was nearly normal. On the second hospital day a repeat CT scan showed bilateral parietal-occipital infarcts in a border zone pattern (Fig. 2). The CSF contained 1 white cell, 550 red cells, and normal protein and glucose. A repeat arteriogram (Fig. 3) showed arterial narrowings that were much more definite than those on the original study.

CLINICAL CHARACTERISTICS

This case illustrates the typical characteristics of reversible cerebral vasospasm, regardless of specific underlying pathology. Characteristically, the clinical onset is with a severe headache, approaching if not equaling the severity seen in subarachnoid hemorrhage (SAH). Sometimes, of course, SAH is the clinical circumstance in which reversible vasospasm occurs. The emphasis of this chapter is on those cases not associated with SAH. The point here is that those cases not associated with SAH also present with a SAH-like headache. In fact, most of my cases are initially thought to be SAH, so that brain imaging, CSF studies, and frequently arteriography are promptly performed. This is a common circumstance in which I am consulted: the arteriogram shows "spasm," but there is no SAH.

When the brain image and CSF study fail to show blood after a severe headache, arteriography may not immediately follow. In these instances the patient's condition dictates when the study will be performed. Sooner or later the clinical circumstances inevitably lead to arteriography.

The headache may wax and wane. The neck remains supple. Frequently the patient is to some degree encephalopathic. Initially, focal neurologic deficits suggesting stroke are mild or transient. Visual symptoms implicating the eye or brain are common. Days to weeks later, a definite stroke will usually occur. It is the occurrence of such strokelike events that finally leads to arteriography, if not already performed.

The stroke syndromes associated with reversible vasospasm often seem unusual. First, there is the severe head pain, far beyond that commonly seen in stroke. Second, the initial symptoms are often fleeting and multifocal. One is often not certain that the condition is a stroke syndrome at all, at least initially. Though arterial occlusive disease is usually thought of early, other conditions frequently considered are venous sinus thrombosis and encephalitis. It is in these circumstances that arteriography is performed. Other than CSF analysis, most laboratory studies are usually of no help. The study of the CSF will eliminate SAH and meningoencephalitis. In reversible vasospasm the CSF is usually nonspecifically abnormal, with an elevated protein or a mild pleocytosis or both. A normal CSF is, however, not uncommon.

Arteriography shows a variety of arterial narrowings, sometimes alternating with dilatations (Fig. 4). The narrowings are multifocal and involve multiple vessels, though the severity can vary greatly. The length of a narrowing may be very short (1 mm), and several may be closely grouped, or they may be long (cm) and cylindrical. Sometimes segments of apparent or definite dilatation are interspersed with areas of short or long narrowings. This latter pattern of apparent dilatation is rarely if ever seen in the spasm of SAH, where long segments of variable narrowing beginning at the circle of Willis is the predominant pattern. A variety of patterns are often seen in the same patient. Furthermore, the patterns change with time in the same patient, as in the case example. Hence "reversible" vasospasm could also be called "changing" vasospasm.

The narrowings do not resemble the irregular, crescentic indentations of atherosclerosis, which are virtually never present in such great numbers intracranially, except perhaps following previous whole head irradiation. The number and severity of the narrowings may be obvious or subtle. They are usually present only distal to the circle of Willis, but I have seen involvement of the basilar artery and the distal internal carotid artery.

In addition to SAH, the conditions most frequently associated with the arteriographic pattern I have described are primary (granulomatous) vasculitis of the central nervous system (CNS) involving vessels within the resolution of imaging techniques (1 mm or greater in diameter), and sympathomimetic amine use or abuse. Much less frequently the pattern is seen with

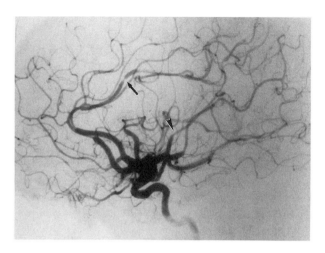

Figure 4 This intracranial left carotid study shows multiple abnormalities. There are short, severe narrowings (*arrow*), which are sometimes adjacent to apparent dilatations (*segment distal to arrow*). There are multiple segments of long, cylindrical narrowings or taperings; a severe one is indicated by the arrowhead.

one of the systemic vasculitides, following craniotomy, closed head injury, with unruptured aneurysm and eclampsia. I have also wondered if it might occur as part of migraine, but this is very uncertain and difficult to prove or disprove.

Primary vasculitis of the CNS often involves vessels less than 1 mm in diameter and hence is not seen on arteriography. In other words, a normal arteriogram is entirely consistent with this form of vasculitis. However, primary vasculitis of the CNS can involve larger vessels, in which case the arteriogram will show the narrowings as described here. The vasculitis is convincingly diagnosed by leptomeningeal biopsy, which is reported to be positive 60 to 70 percent of the time. Unlike the systemic vasculitides, the sedimentation rate is usually normal and various serologic studies including antinuclear antibodies are negative. The systemic vasculitides rarely involve the CNS. Treatment with immunosuppressive agents will result in reversal of the narrowings in weeks to months.

Sympathomimetic drug use has been associated with SAH and intracerebral hemorrhage most frequently, but also with reversible vasospasm, or vasculitis. I have seen spasm and brain parenchymal hemorrhage together. The amines implicated include illicit cocaine and amphetamine, as well as over-the-counter preparations of ephedrine, pseudoephedrine, and phenylpropanolamine. Other sympathomimetics should also be suspect. The strength of this association is increased by animal studies in which monkeys given methamphetamine developed characteristic angiographic changes and a necrotizing angiitis on histologic examination. The animals developed infarctions and hemorrhages. Hence the mechanism of action of these agents appears not to be pharmacologic, since these agents taken systemically have little or no effect on the cerebrovasculature (unlike their potent topical effect), and because pathologically a true vasculitis is present, at least in animals. The necrotizing, largely polymorphonuclear infiltrate can explain why both arterial narrowings and rupture with hemorrhage are seen. By contrast, the infiltrate of primary vasculitis of the CNS is primarily round cell and granulomatous.

In cases associated with sympathomimetic drug use, repeat arteriography days, weeks, or months later will show different locations of the narrowings and ultimately resolution, with or without treatment.

Since sympathomimetic induced vasculitis may be a true inflammatory process, it may be related to primary vasculitis of the CNS. Is the granulomatous vasculitis a more chronic form of sympathomimetic or other drug or antigen-induced acute vasculitis? I do not know the answer to this question, but we are seeing more sympathomimetic-associated stroke, sometimes with the characteristic arteriographic pattern, so the question should be answerable.

A similar pattern of narrowings may on occasion be seen following head trauma and craniotomy and has been reported with unruptured aneurysm, though this latter association may be coincidental. It has also been suggested that vasospasm might in some cases be migrainous in nature. This seems unlikely. Recent research in migraine has developed other models for the pain, making the classic model of vasoconstriction and dilatation less tenable. I have also induced migraine in migraneurs undergoing arteriography for other reasons and have yet to see the development of arterial narrowings of the type I have described.

DIAGNOSIS

The diagnostic problem usually begins when spasm or a "vasculitic" pattern is found unexpectedly on the arteriogram. The problem can begin earlier if arteriography is performed in a person with a severe SAH-like headache and encephalopathy, but arteriography is often not performed until a transient neurologic deficit or stroke appears. Arteriography is better performed sooner than later, however, before serious or multiple strokes occur. It is my impression that the initial injury is usually not severe and there is a window of opportunity to make the diagnosis and begin therapy.

Once the arteriographic pattern is recognized, we know we are dealing with a reversible vasculopathy associated with the processes and situations listed in Table 1. SAH is ruled out by CT and CSF study. Unruptured aneurysm will be seen on arteriogram but may be incidental. Preceding head trauma is obvious. Hence the diagnostic problem is to distinguish between primary vasculitis of the CNS or a sympathomimetic amine-induced vasculitis. Leptomeningeal biopsy can settle the issue if positive, but 30 to 40 percent of the time it is negative. I think this nondiagnostic rate is unacceptably high, and therefore pursue an alternative diagnostic and therapeutic pathway. This path is empir-

Table 1 Clinical Conditions Associated with Reversible Vasospasm

Subarachnoid hemorrhage
Primary (granulomatous) vasculitis of the CNS
Sympathomimetic amine use
Closed head injury
Craniotomy
Unruptured aneurysm
Systemic vasculitis
Eclampsia

ical, but a definitive course of action has yet to be established.

Once I encounter the characteristic arteriographic features, I vigorously pursue the possibility of sympathomimetic use by history and toxicology screening, if timely. The history of drug use must be energetically and repeatedly tracked. Illicit drug use is often denied and over-the-counter sympathomimetic use ignored. At my hospital, the arteriographic pattern of reversible spasm is usually associated with sympathomimetic use. Hence, when I see this pattern in patients who use these agents I assume they are the cause. So far, use of the sympathomimetics has generally been concurrent with the onset of symptoms, though this is sometimes not classified immediately. For example, a cocaine user assured me that he had not used cocaine for "more than a year." I later learned from his wife that he continued to use cocaine regularly.

Aside from the historical difficulties of establishing the use of sympathomimetics, we also do not know how recent such use must have been to be considered causative. If these agents do induce a vasculitis in humans, as they do in monkeys, it is conceivable that many days or even weeks may pass between last use and the onset of symptomatic arterial narrowing or hemorrhage. I consider this an unresolved clinical question.

If I am confident that sympathomimetic use is not present, I assume as an initial working hypothesis that the condition is primary vasculitis of the CNS. I do not pursue evidence for a systemic vasculitis with laboratory tests if the history and physical examination do not suggest such a process.

If the arteriographic findings are not definite, I proceed with a second arteriogram in 1 week. In cases of both sympathomimetic use and primary vasculitis, the process seems to be dynamic, the arteriographic abnormalities evolving with time. If the process still remains in doubt or therapy seems to be ineffective, I proceed with biopsy. It can be argued that all cases should be biopsied. If this course is pursued, it should be remembered that a negative biopsy does not disprove either diagnosis. Furthermore, since we still have much to learn about the natural history of the inflammatory process in these conditions, a biopsy that does show an inflammatory infiltrate may not be specific. In either event, I repeat the arteriogram in 6 to 12 weeks to demonstrate resolution of the arteriographic abnormalities. I repeat the study sooner if clinical improvement does not occur. Therapy need not be delayed until the diagnosis is certain. However, if biopsy is contemplated, I presume it is most likely to be diagnostic if performed before or very soon after immunosuppressive therapy is started. Resolution of the arteriographic abnormalities while on therapy demonstrates the reversible nature of the vasculopathy.

DISCUSSION

Reversible vasospasm of cerebral arteries refers to a changing pattern of multiple arterial narrowings seen by arteriography. It is associated with a variety of medical conditions, most commonly subarachnoid hemorrhage from a saccular aneurysm. Less frequently, changing and reversible narrowings are associated with sympathomimetic amine use, a circumstance of increasing frequency

at my hospital. Much less frequently it is due to primary vasculitis of the CNS. All three conditions result in similar dramatic clinical presentations, with severe headache, encephalopathy, and ultimately a stroke syndrome, often multifocal. Early recognition and prompt therapy can improve prognosis.

SUGGESTED READING

Calabrese LH, Mallek JA. Primary angiitis of the central nervous system. Medicine 1987; 67:20–39.
Call GK, Fleming MC, Sealfon S, et al. Reversible cerebral segmental vasoconstriction. Stroke 1988; 19:1159–1170.
Glick RP, Anson JA. Vasculitis related to substance abuse. In: Churg A, Churg J, eds. Systemic vasculitides. New York: Igaku-Shoin, 1991; 315.
Moore PM. Diagnosis and management of isolated angiitis of the central nervous system. Neurology 1989; 39:167–173.

SPINAL CORD ISCHEMIA

DAVID R. LYNCH, M.D., Ph.D.
STEVEN L. GALETTA, M.D.

Though less common than cerebral ischemia, spinal cord infarction may have devastating neurologic consequences. The relative lack of redundancy of spinal cord neurons makes ischemia of this area among the most serious of neurologic events. However, because of the rarity of spinal cord ischemia, fewer clinicians are familiar with its characteristics and logical evaluation. Though spinal cord ischemia and cerebral ischemia share many features, spinal cord ischemia requires a different evaluation. The diagnostic approach to spinal cord ischemia rests upon several prioritized requirements: (1) the need to exclude other processes that may resemble spinal cord ischemia; (2) the need to define the causes of ischemia, particularly those such as aortic dissection that require immediate attention, and (3) the need to understand spinal cord ischemia associated with aortic surgery, because this represents perhaps the most common cause of spinal cord infarction.

SPINAL CORD BLOOD SUPPLY

The unusual characteristics of spinal cord ischemia result from the intricacy and variability of spinal cord blood supply. There are two components to spinal cord blood supply: the radicular arteries, which reinforce spinal blood supply at a given level, and the anterior and

posterior spinal arteries, which run longitudinally along the spinal cord (Fig. 1).

Although 31 pairs of radicular arteries penetrate each level of the spinal canal, usually only seven or eight contribute to the spinal cord blood supply. Those radicular arteries that supply the spinal cord are commonly unilateral and are best termed medullary or radiculomedullary arteries (see Fig. 1). Radiculomedullary arteries course obliquely as they enter the spinal canal to supply the cord more rostrally than at their point of entry. The cervical cord is supplied by the descending anterior spinal artery arising from both vertebrals, as well as by radiculomedullary arteries derived from the costocervical and thyrocervical trunks. The upper thoracic cord receives supply from 2 to 4 radiculomedullary arteries arising from intercostal branches of the aorta (more commonly on the left). The lower thoracic and lumbar regions receive supply from 1 or 2 radiculomedullary arteries. The larger of these, called the artery of Adamkiewicz, or the artery radicularis magnus (ARM), typically arises from the aorta at levels from T9 to T12. It is left-sided in 85 percent of patients and may be accompanied by an artery supplying the cauda equina when it arises in the high thoracic region. There is considerable variability in this pattern of blood supply because the ARM arises from T9 to T12 in 75 percent of patients, T5 to T8 in 15 percent of patients, and from lumbar levels in 10 percent of patients.

The anterior spinal and posterior spinal arteries comprise the longitudinal supply of the spinal cord. These arteries receive contributions from the radiculomedullary arteries and are connected by pial anastomoses. The anterior spinal artery supplies the ventral two-thirds of the spinal cord, including most of the gray matter along with the corticospinal and spinothalamic

A

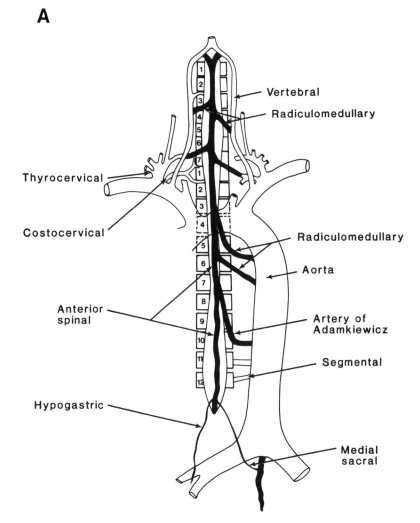

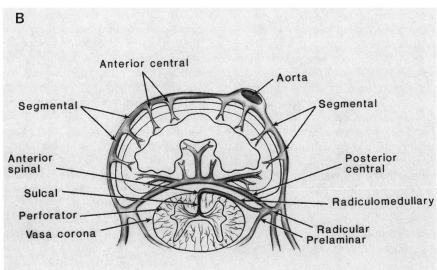

Figure 1 *A,* Anterior view of spinal cord blood supply. The anterior spinal artery and its radiculomedullary feeders are shown in black. The large trunks that these vessels arise from (such as the aorta) are in white. As demonstrated, radiculomedullary arteries are frequently unilateral and have an ascending course. *B,* Axial view of spinal cord blood supply demonstrating segmental anatomy. Radicular arteries arise from the aorta and supply the vertebrae through posterior central and prelaminar vessels. At selected levels, a unilateral radiculomedullary artery derived from the radicular artery reinforces the spinal cord blood supply. (Modified from Yuh WTC, Marsh EE, Wang AK, et al. MR imaging of spinal cord and vertebral body infarction. AJNR Am J Neuroradiol 1992; 13:145–154. © by American Society of Neuroradiology; with permission.)

tracts, while the posterior spinal artery supplies posterior circumferential white matter including the posterior columns. Penetrating branches known as sulcal arteries arise from the anterior spinal artery to enter the spinal cord at each level. In contrast, penetrating arteries arising from the posterior spinal arteries are more diffuse. Several vessels supplying the lateral and superficial aspects of the cord are derived from the plexus between the anterior and posterior spinal arteries. Though the anterior and posterior arteries run longitudinally down the spinal cord, they are not truly continuous. Longitudinal anastomoses are usually most limited in the thoracic area so that blood entering from the ARM runs rostrally to supply the higher thoracic levels. The area most vulnerable to watershed infarction is the upper thoracic cord, especially in the anterior spinal artery distribution. The posterior spinal arteries are frequently reinforced by segmental radiculomedullary arteries and have more anastomoses, particularly at the level of the conus medullaris. Thus, the portion of the spinal cord supplied by the posterior spinal arteries is less vulnerable to ischemia following the occlusion of a single radiculomedullary artery or to watershed events.

Venous return parallels the arterial system by draining blood from the spinal cord through two systems: (1) penetrating veins running in tandem with penetrating arteries and (2) radial veins that drain the lateral aspects of the cord into a posterior venous plexus. Anterior venous return starts with the ventral penetrating veins that eventually drain into the anterior spinal vein. Venous connections are then made to anterior radicular veins to reach the intervertebral plexus. Posteriorly, the large pial plexus of veins connects with two posterior spinal veins. They drain every two to three segments into radicular veins and then eventually to the vena cava or azygos venous systems.

CLINICAL FEATURES

Spinal cord ischemia may manifest as a transient ischemic attack or as an infarction. The symptoms usually include bilateral weakness, sensory loss, and bladder dysfunction. These symptoms may be asymmetric and are less commonly unilateral. Back pain is a complaint of many patients, particularly when associated with aortic dissection. The pain of aortic dissection may also begin in the chest and radiate into the lower extremities. The course of spinal cord ischemia is usually rapid, typically advancing over minutes to several hours, but a chronic presentation may occasionally occur. Venous infarctions in particular may manifest acutely or evolve as a progressive myelopathy. It is also important to realize that an acute course does not exclude a compressive lesion or even a demyelinative process.

Other historical features may be useful in determining the cause of acute spinal cord injury. Information should be sought about the usual and unusual vascular risk factors. Illicit drug use or pre-existing conditions such as sickle cell disease or lupus may narrow the differential diagnosis. Ischemia may be distinguished from compressive spinal cord lesions or transverse myelitis by a history of previous neoplasm or prior neurologic dysfunction such as optic neuritis. The presence of skin lesions or constitutional symptoms suggests an infectious myelitis such as herpes zoster or Lyme disease. Although a history of trauma precedes traumatic spinal cord injury, it must be remembered that trauma may also lead to an aortic dissection and resultant spinal cord ischemia.

Neurologic findings depend on the specific vessel and cord level involved. In occlusions of the anterior spinal artery, the patient develops weakness of all extremities below the level of the lesion with loss of bowel and bladder function. Pinprick and temperature sensation below the level of infarction are also decreased or lost. In severe infarctions, the legs may be flaccid initially, but with time upper motor neuron signs such as extensor plantar reflexes, increased tone, and hyperreflexia develop. Vibration and proprioceptive sensations are spared in a pure anterior spinal artery infarct. If the lesion is in the cervical area, the patient may develop quadriparesis with upper motor neuron signs in the legs. In the arms, lower motor neuron signs (decreased tone, decreased reflexes, and later atrophy and fasciculations) predominate from ischemic injury to the anterior horn cells at that level. Occasionally, patients will have the features of a Brown-Séquard's syndrome with weakness on one side of the body and pain and temperature loss on the opposite side. Sparing of sacral sensation may also characterize cervical cord ischemia since the sacral sensory fibers are peripherally located within the cord and therefore receive a component of their blood supply from superficial vessels. Infarction of the conus medullaris will produce lower motor neuron weakness of the legs associated with sexual and bladder dysfunction. Because of the rich blood supply at the level of the conus, infarcts in this region are less common.

Posterior spinal artery infarcts should affect the posterior columns selectively, leading to loss of proprioceptive and vibratory sensation. However, because the posterior spinal artery has more extensive collaterals, posterior spinal infarcts rarely occur in a pure form. Frequently, posterior spinal artery infarcts are associated with anterior spinal infarction leading to a complete spinal cord infarct.

Venous infarcts of the spinal cord occur less frequently than arterial events. As the venous distribution is similar to the arterial distribution, venous infarcts typically present with the same signs as arterial infarcts and may be either hemorrhagic or nonhemorrhagic. Hemorrhagic infarcts usually affect the spinal cord gray matter, and nonhemorrhagic venous infarcts tend to affect the white matter. Venous infarcts are usually large because of the extensive venous anastomoses around the spinal cord. It is this anastomotic network that allows a small proximal venous occlusion to obstruct many tributaries from a large segment of the cord.

The combination of bilateral weakness, a sensory level, bowel and bladder dysfunction, with preservation

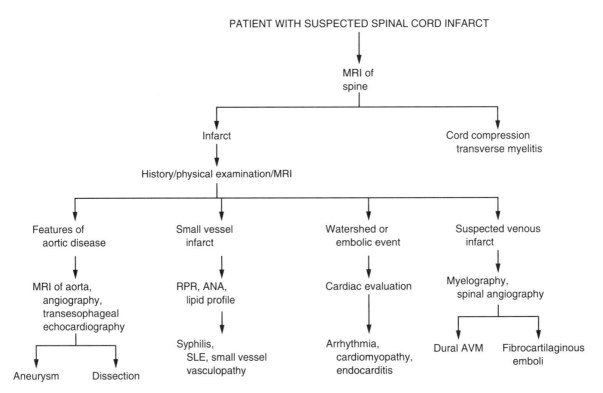

Figure 2 Algorithm for the evaluation of suspected spinal cord infarct (ANA = antinuclear antibody test, AVM = arteriovenous malformation, RPR = rapid plasma reagin test, SLE = systemic lupus erythematosus).

of mental status and cranial nerve function always suggests spinal cord dysfunction. However, when this syndrome is incomplete or when the underlying process involves other levels of the nervous system, the anatomic localization may be unclear. For example, bilateral watershed cerebral infarcts can produce a syndrome of quadriparesis involving the legs more than the arms. Apart from an alteration of mental status, this may resemble the quadriparesis of a cervical spinal cord infarct. In certain cases, such as infarction following hypotension, both cerebral and spinal cord dysfunction may exist. Similarly, aortic aneurysm and dissection may produce sudden bilateral lower extremity peripheral nerve dysfunction that clinically simulates acute cord ischemia.

When the examination clearly demonstrates a spinal cord syndrome, the clinician must separate infarcts from other causes of rapidly evolving spinal cord dysfunction (Fig. 2). The most important of these are compressive lesions from neoplastic disease, disc herniation, or degenerative joint disease. Trauma and transverse myelitis are occasionally diagnostic considerations. When the spinal cord infarct involves the lower thoracic and lumbar region such that weakness and lower extremity sensory loss are present, a rapidly progressive peripheral neuropathy such as the Guillain-Barré syndrome should be considered.

Once the diagnosis of spinal cord ischemia is established, the cause must be sought. The causes of spinal cord infarction include the usual causes of cerebral ischemia such as hypertension and diabetes as well as special causes arising from the unique anatomy of the spinal cord. Embolism from the heart may lead to spinal ischemia but is relatively uncommon. The unusual causes of cerebral ischemia, including systemic lupus erythematosus, syphilis, vasculitis, sickle cell disease, and cocaine abuse, may also involve the spinal cord. There are several causes that are unique to the spinal cord, including disk embolism, cervical spondylosis, air embolism (particularly in diving accidents), and aortic vascular diseases. Spinal cord venous infarcts most commonly arise in association with a dural arteriovenous malformation and venous hypertension. The condition of spinal venous hypertension in association with an arteriovenous malformation and progressive myelopathy is also known as the Foix Alajouanine syndrome. In rare instances, venous infarcts may be caused by embolism of fibrocartilaginous disk to the venous plexus.

RADIOLOGIC AND LABORATORY EVALUATION

Magnetic resonance imaging (MRI) is now the method of choice for the evaluation of the patient with a suspected spinal cord infarct. A myelogram will show compressive lesions but is usually normal in spinal cord infarction. MRI studies can exclude structural lesions that compress the spinal cord and demonstrate the signal characteristics of an evolving infarct. Typically, the MRI will reveal an enlarged cord with decreased signal

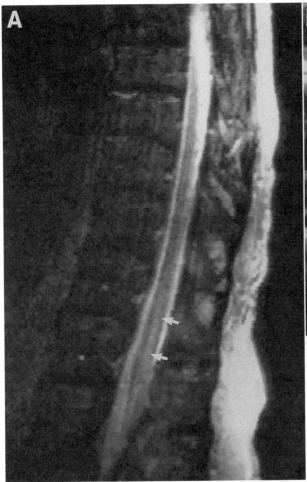

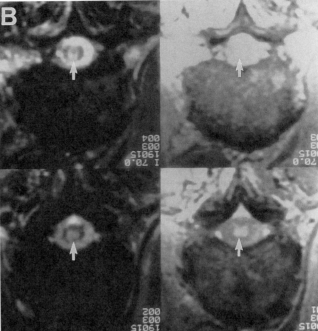

Figure 3 Anterior spinal artery infarct. *A,* Sagittal magnetic resonance study of an anterior spinal artery infarction demonstrating high signal abnormality on a T2 weighted image (*arrow*). *B,* Axial view of an anterior spinal artery infarct demonstrated on spin echo (*left*) and proton density (*right*) magnetic resonance images. Abnormal high signal is seen in the grey matter and the ventral white matter (*arrows*).

intensity on T1 weighted sequences and increased signal on T2 weighted images (Fig. 3). Similar to cerebral infarcts, these lesions show no initial contrast enhancement on T1 weighted images but may enhance 5 days to several weeks after the onset of the ischemia. The longitudinal extent of the infarct may vary from one to several segments. Infarction of a single level is more commonly found in small vessel vasculopathies or watershed infarctions, while aortic disease or dissection infarcts multiple levels.

Spinal cord infarction may be associated with vertebral abnormalities on MRI. Occlusion of a radicular artery may produce high signal change in the endplate and medullary portion of the vertebral body. However, because blood in the radiculomedullary artery runs obliquely as it enters the spinal canal, the spinal cord segment involved is usually located rostral to the ischemic vertebral body. This noncontiguous involvement of the spinal cord and vertebral body differs from the neuroimaging findings observed in compressive lesions and infectious processes.

Venous infarcts resemble arterial infarcts on MRI scan in spite of their different clinical course (Fig. 4). Venous infarcts may have unusual causes such as fibrocartilaginous emboli or a dural arteriovenous mal-

formation (AVM). MRI may demonstrate abnormal signal associated with an AVM, but myelography is occasionally needed to demonstrate the abnormal draining veins. Selective angiography is required to define the arterial feeders, which may even arise from branches of the vertebral or external carotid distributions.

Occasionally, examination of the cerebrospinal fluid (CSF) may be of value. Bloody or xanthochromic fluid suggests an AVM rupture or a venous infarct. CSF also may be used to support other diagnostic possibilities such as demyelinating disease or infection.

The intimate anatomic relationship of the spinal cord and the aorta puts it at particular risk in aortic vascular disease. Spinal cord infarction is among the most dreaded complications of aortic dissection, aortic aneurysms, and aortic surgery. Such patients must be recognized because they require immediate intervention. Spinal MRI and transesophageal echocardiography (TEE) may be helpful by demonstrating an unsuspected dissection or aneurysm. TEE may also detect artherosclerotic plaques in the thoracic aorta. Angiography still remains the test of choice for these aortic abnormalities, but MRI and TEE can provide substantial information and are less invasive.

The evaluation of patients with arterial spinal

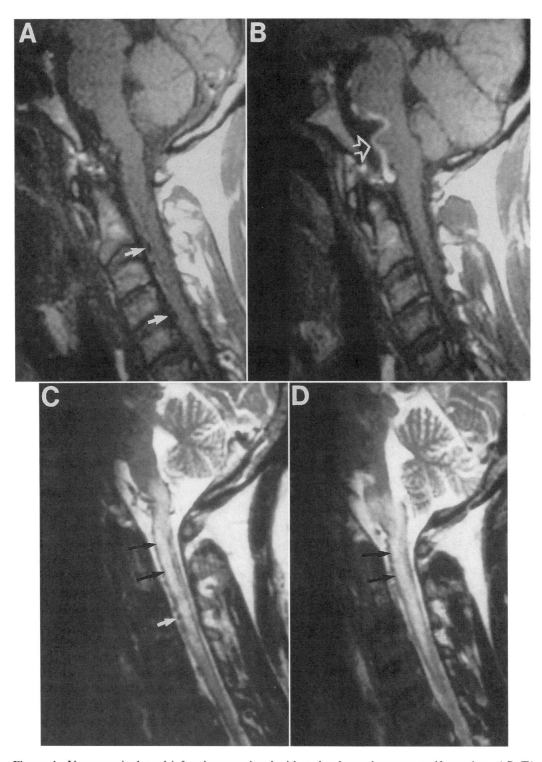

Figure 4 Venous spinal cord infarction associated with a dural arteriovenous malformation. *A,B,* T1 weighted MR images showing thrombosed median ponto-mesencephalic vein (*open arrow*) and prominent vessels over ventral surface of cord (*white arrows*). *C,D,* T2 weighted MR images showing infarct throughout cervical spinal cord (*black arrows*) and abnormal vessels over surface (*white arrow*).

infarcts without aortic disease should include the usual vascular testing. A lipid profile, a vasculitis screen, noninvasive vascular studies, and a cardiac evaluation should be pursued as necessary (see Fig. 2).

SPINAL CORD ISCHEMIA IN AORTIC SURGERY

Perhaps the most common cause of spinal cord infarction is aortic surgery. Evaluation of the patient who has undergone aortic surgery is clearly different from that for other spinal cord infarcts and requires an understanding of the pathophysiology of the surgical procedure.

Operations on the aorta require disruption of blood supply to the spinal cord by cross-clamping of the aorta. With clamping of the aorta, there is an increase in blood pressure proximal to the clamp with hypoperfusion distal to the clamp. Following release of the clamp, there is a period of hypotension and hypoperfusion associated with vasodilatation. Any of these events may affect the blood supply to the spinal cord.

The location of the aneurysm to be resected determines the risk of spinal cord infarct. It is highest in patients with thoracoabdominal aneurysms because the ARM most frequently arises from the region included in the cross-clamp. Spinal cord infarction occasionally occurs in resection of thoracic aneurysms, but infrequently in surgery of the abdominal aorta. Those patients with spinal cord infarcts following abdominal aneurysm repair are presumed to have an ARM that arises very low in the lumbar region.

The location of the ARM is not the only risk factor for spinal cord ischemia. Other factors include the cross-clamp time, aneurysm size, and the presence of rupture. A variety of techniques have been attempted to improve spinal cord blood supply. Shunts to supply blood around the cross-clamp have been ineffective in most series. Such shunts do not account for ARM location and may disrupt normal anastomoses. Many vascular surgeons stress the need to reattach as many intercostal arteries as possible so that the ARM is not disrupted. Unfortunately, this can require increased cross-clamp time.

The complex physiologic changes that occur during cross-clamping suggest that other mechanisms besides simple decrease in blood flow through the ARM are involved in perioperative ischemia. The hypotension following release of the cross-clamp may make the spinal cord susceptible to watershed infarction. So-called spinal cord tamponade may also play a role. When the aorta is proximally clamped, cerebral blood flow increases and consequently intracranial pressure rises. This increased pressure is transmitted to the spinal cord venous system. Since spinal cord arterial pressure is already reduced, cord perfusion pressure may be greatly affected.

The appropriate neurologic preoperative evalua-

tion of a candidate for aortic surgery is yet unclear. If the location of the ARM could be determined perioperatively, the need for intercostal repair and its location would be known. Spinal angiography has proven useful in selective circumstances but is unsuccessful in a relatively high number of patients and is not entirely without risk (2 percent morbidity). Another recently developed technique is the intraoperative injection of hydrogen into the aorta to determine the site of the ARM. The location is ascertained by monitoring spinal cord motor potentials. This approach has been successful in animals but is not yet well tested in humans.

Intraoperatively, attempts have been made to alter the frequency of spinal cord infarction in several ways. One method involves decreasing the spinal cord tamponade. In animals, removal of CSF to lower intraspinal pressure has proven effective. However, a double blind study in humans showed no improvement in postoperative paraplegia with spinal fluid drainage. Another approach for reducing morbidity involves evoked potential monitoring of spinal cord ischemia as an index of damage. Somatosensory evoked potentials (SSEP) monitoring has been attempted but has many limitations. Theoretically it measures only posterior column function, so it would not reflect the more important anterior spinal artery distribution. Motor evoked potentials, which reflect anterior horn cell and corticospinal tract function, show more promise for monitoring ischemic spinal cord damage.

It is hoped that the improved characterization of patients at risk in aortic surgery will decrease the incidence of neurologic complications. At this time, no method of preoperative or intraoperative evaluation can precisely define the outcome.

SUGGESTED READING

Anderson NE, Willoughby EW. Infarction of the conus medullaris. Ann Neurol 1987; 21:470–474.

Case records of the Massachusetts General Hospital: Case 5 – 1991. N Engl J Med 1991; 324:322–332.

Crawford ES, Mizrah EM, Hess KR, et al. The impact of distal aortic perfusion and somatosensory monitoring on prevention of paraplegia after aortic aneurysm operation. J Thorac Cardiovasc Surg 1988; 95:357–367.

Dawson DM, Potts F. Acute nontraumatic myelopathies. Neurol Clin North Am 1991; 9:585–598.

Henson RA, Parsons M. Ischemic lesions of the spinal cord: An illustrated review. Q J Med 1967; 36:205–222.

Lynch DR, Dawson TM, Raps EC, Galetta SL. Risk factors in the neurologic complications of aortic aneurysms. Arch Neurol 1992; 49:284–288.

Roos RT. Spinal cord infarct in disease and surgery of the aorta. Can J Neurol Sci 1985; 12:289–295.

Weisman AD, Adams RD. Neurologic complications of dissecting aortic aneurysms. Brain 1944; 67:69–92.

Yuh WTC, Marsh EE, Wang AK, et al. MR imaging of spinal cord and vertebral body infarction. AJNR Am J Neuroradiol 1992; 13: 145–154.

CEREBRAL AMYLOID ANGIOPATHY

CARLOS S. KASE, M.D.

Cerebral amyloid angiopathy (CAA), or "congophilic" angiopathy, affects the cerebral vasculature selectively, with no amyloid deposited elsewhere in the body. The amyloid is deposited in the walls of small and medium-sized arteries and veins of the cerebral cortex and leptomeninges. The angiopathy is virtually nonexistent in the deep portions of the hemispheres, brain stem, and cerebellum. The presence of amyloid in the vessel wall is recognized by a salmon-pink color on Congo-red stain, with a typical apple-green birefringence under polarized light. These abnormal deposits tend to be more extensive in areas of vascular bifurcations. The involved blood vessels often have intramural clefts in areas of extensive amyloid deposition, resulting in the appearance of a "double-barreled" lumen. Amyloid can also be stained with thioflavin T and S, producing fluorescence under ultraviolet light. The amyloid-laden blood vessels in CAA are superficially located in the cerebral hemispheres, involving all lobes with similar frequency, although a heavier concentration of affected vessels in the parieto-occipital areas has been suggested.

CAA characteristically increases in frequency with advancing age. In an autopsy study, CAA was documented in only 5 percent of individuals in the seventh decade of life, but the frequency rose steadily in subsequent decades, reaching values close to 50 percent in persons older than 90 years, without differences between men and women (Table 1). The rarity of CAA in middle-aged persons results in a virtual absence of its clinical consequences before age 50.

CAA is associated with several clinical and histologic correlates, some of which are causally related to the angiopathy, while others are probably merely coincidental. Among the former, intracerebral hemorrhage (ICH) is the most consistent consequence of CAA, whereas Alzheimer's disease, cerebral infarcts, and leukoencephalopathy occur less commonly.

Table 1 Frequency of Cerebral Amyloid Angiopathy in Relation to Age

Age Group (yr)	Men (%)	Women (%)
60–69	9.3	13.6
70–79	18.3	23.3
80–89	38.0	36.1
90+	42.8	45.8

From Masuda J, Tanaka K, Ueda K, Omae T. Autopsy study of incidence and distribution of cerebral amyloid angiopathy in Hisayama, Japan. Stroke 1988; 19:205–210; with permission.

INTRACEREBRAL HEMORRHAGE

CAA as a histologic entity has been known to pathologists since the nineteenth century, but its clinical significance was not fully appreciated until the 1970s, when a number of authors independently reported the association of CAA with ICH. Early reports on the condition stressed its importance as a cause of ICH in the elderly, its potential association with head trauma and neurosurgical interventions, and the recognition of a familial form of the disease in Iceland. It is now well established that CAA-related ICH presents in two forms, one as a frequent sporadic and age-related condition, the other as a rare familial and geographically distinct form of the disease.

Sporadic Form

The sporadic form of CAA-related ICH is thought to account for about 2 to 9 percent of the cases of ICH, the variation reflecting in part the age groups under consideration. When the analysis is limited to the elderly (60 to 90 years of age), the frequency of CAA as the mechanism of ICH approaches 15 percent.

The most consistent anatomic feature of these hemorrhages is their lobar location, which results from the cortical and leptomeningeal distribution of the angiopathy. Hypertension may or may not be present. As a result, these hemorrhages occur in the white matter of the cerebral lobes, at a distance from the deep hemispheric structures that are most commonly the site of hypertensive ICH. The superficially located angiopathy rarely leads to instances of pure subarachnoid or subdural hemorrhage. More commonly, local subarachnoid hemorrhage (SAH) occurs next to a superficial lobar ICH, giving at times an irregular and variegated character to the hemorrhage. This is a typical aspect of CAA, clearly distinct from hypertensive ICH, which occurs as a single homogeneous focus of parenchymal hemorrhage that almost never communicates with the subarachnoid space of the cerebral convexity or base. CAA-related hemorrhages are evenly distributed among the cerebral lobes, with a slight predominance in the frontoparietal areas.

The other distinctive feature of CAA-related ICH is its tendency toward recurrence, another feature that separates it from hypertensive ICH, which usually occurs as a single event. Recurrent ICHs can be at times separated by periods of 2 or more years. These ICHs appear on gross pathologic examination as lobar hematomas of different ages or as simultaneous ICHs in both cerebral hemispheres. The latter is also a rare occurrence in hypertensive ICH, which generally presents as an isolated focus of hemorrhage. These features stress the need for strongly considering the diagnosis of CAA-related ICH in patients with multiple, recurrent lobar ICHs, especially in those older than 60 years.

The mechanism of bleeding in CAA-related ICH has not been established. Although occasional examples have followed head trauma or a neurosurgical procedure, in the majority of patients the event is spontaneous, without a clear precipitating event. Because of this, attention has been directed at the angiopathy itself, with attempts to elucidate the features that may relate to hemorrhage. The vascular infiltration with amyloid is thought to render the vessels mechanically "brittle" and prone to rupture. Another possible mechanism of rupture of these vessels is the association of CAA with other vasculopathies, either related to hypertension or coincidental with CAA. Among these, formation of microaneurysms and fibrinoid degeneration of the vessel wall are thought to relate to arterial rupture. Microaneurysms are commonly found in amyloid-laden vessels, but their presence at the rupture site has not been consistently documented, raising questions about their ultimate role in vascular rupture and hemorrhage. Fibrinoid necrosis of vessel walls, on the other hand, has been found in up to 70 percent of brains with CAA and ICH, whereas such change is generally absent in brains with CAA but without ICH. The presence of fibrinoid necrosis at sites of arterial rupture suggests that this vasculopathy plays an essential role in producing hemorrhage. Other vascular changes, such as a form of inflammation resembling rheumatoid vasculitis, have a less clear correlation with bleeding. Finally, a possible role for iatrogenic factors in promoting ICH in elderly patients with CAA is suggested by the occurrence of hemorrhage in patients treated with thrombolytic agents for acute myocardial infarction. Since these agents are being used with increasing frequency, generally in combination with aspirin and intravenous heparin, concern exists about their potential for causing ICH in elderly or demented patients at risk of harboring CAA.

These issues of the pathogenesis of CAA-related ICH have an impact on the selection of conservative versus surgical treatment of this condition. Several authors have argued that surgical drainage of large ICHs related to CAA is unsafe because the fragile amyloid-laden vessels are thought to be prone to bleed throughout and after the surgery, resulting in reaccumulation of the hematoma. Others have a different view, based on the rarity of postoperative hematoma accumulation. Surgery is often followed by progressive neurologic improvement, at times with return to independence in activities of daily living. Furthermore, these data have suggested a vital prognosis in patients with surgically treated ICHs that is less dismal than previously quoted figures of 75 percent mortality. My own experience with over a dozen operated patients with CAA-related ICH is similarly reassuring, since I have not observed a single instance of intraoperative bleeding or postoperative recurrence of the hematoma. As a result, my approach is to recommend surgical evacuation of hematomas in patients with medium-sized or large lobar ICHs that are causing mass effect, regardless of the potential for CAA as their underlying mechanism. Surgery also affords the opportunity to confirm the diagnosis by providing tissue for histologic analysis.

Familial Form

The familial form of CAA-related ICH was first recognized in Iceland, where 23 patients within a family of 117 individuals in three generations had ICH. Postmortem examination of five of these patients showed recent ICHs and widespread cerebrovascular amyloidosis without systemic amyloidosis. The distribution of the vascular amyloid deposits was more extensive than in the sporadic variety of CAA, with involvement of cortical and leptomeningeal vessels, as well as those of the basal ganglia, brain stem, and cerebellum. The ICHs in these Icelandic patients occurred early in life, affecting individuals in the third, fourth, and fifth decades of life. This condition is now referred to as "hereditary cerebral hemorrhage with amyloidosis—Icelandic type." The pattern of inheritance of the condition is autosomal dominant.

The biochemical composition of the amyloid fibrils from the Icelandic familial cases is similar to the microprotein gamma-trace, or cystatin C, which is present in abnormally low concentrations in the CSF. The same CSF abnormality has been documented in asymptomatic family members who subsequently go on to develop ICH.

A second form of hereditary CAA-related ICH has been reported in the Netherlands and is known as "hereditary cerebral hemorrhage with amyloidosis—Dutch type." These patients present with ICH between the ages of 45 and 65 years. About two-thirds of the patients have died as a result of the first episode of ICH, and the survivors have had recurrent hemorrhages between 3 weeks and 14 years later. The mode of

Table 2 Familial Forms of Cerebral Amyloid Angiopathy–Related Intracerebral Hemorrhage

	Icelandic	*Dutch*
Mode of inheritance	Autosomal dominant	Autosomal dominant
Age of onset of intracerebral hemorrhage	Early (mean: 30 yr)	Later (mean: 55 yr)
Distribution of amyloid angiopathy	Extensive (cerebral, cerebellar, brain stem arteries)	More limited (cerebral cortex, leptomeninges)
Type of amyloid protein, molecular weight	Cystatin C (gamma-trace), 11,000–12,000 Da	Beta-peptide, 4,200 Da

Da = Dalton

inheritance is also autosomal dominant. The intracerebral hematomas are of lobar location, predominating in the parietal subcortical white matter. In a recent series, one-half of the acute hematomas were multiple, and the mortality for the group of 24 patients was 33 percent. Microscopically, vascular amyloidosis is present in the cerebral cortex and leptomeninges, being absent from the basal ganglia, brain stem, and spinal cord, following a pattern of distribution similar to the sporadic rather than the Icelandic familial form of CAA.

The biochemical characterization of the amyloid protein in the Dutch cases has shown a further difference from the Icelandic cases, since it is not related to cystatin C, but rather to the amyloid beta-protein (Alzheimer A4 or beta-peptide) of Alzheimer's disease and Down's syndrome. The main features of the Icelandic and Dutch forms of hereditary CAA-related ICH are shown in Table 2. Recent studies have indicated that the likely genetic defect in the Dutch form of CAA is in the amyloid beta-protein precursor (APP) gene located in chromosome 21.

OTHER CAA-RELATED CONDITIONS

Several conditions have been reported in association with CAA, some in high enough frequency to suggest a pathogenic link to the angiopathy, while others are rare, probably coincidental, occurrences. Among those possibly related to the angiopathy are Alzheimer's disease, cerebral infarcts, and leukoencephalopathy.

Alzheimer's Disease

In patients with sporadic CAA, histologic brain examination shows neuritic plaques and neurofibrillary tangles with a frequency that is higher than that of the age-matched general population. About 40 percent of patients with sporadic CAA-related ICH show Alzheimer's histologic changes at postmortem examination, and similar figures (30 to 40 percent) for clinically documented cases of dementia preceding the ICH have been reported. However, the correlation between the two processes is poor, since neuritic plaques can occur in the absence of CAA, and CAA can be present without coexistent neuritic plaques. The same lack of close correlation applies to the presence of Alzheimer's histologic changes in patients with CAA and the presence and severity of clinically documented dementia.

The familial forms of CAA with ICH are also different in this regard from the sporadic form. No histologic features of Alzheimer's disease have been documented in the young Icelandic patients who died as a result of ICH. Those with the Dutch variety have shown "primitive" neuritic plaques without the typical amyloid core seen in Alzheimer's disease, and neurofibrillary tangles have not been observed.

The coexistence of CAA with histologic features of Alzheimer's disease has suggested a common metabolic origin for both conditions. This has been supported by the biochemical similarity of the abnormal protein (Alzheimer A4 or beta-peptide) of the sporadic form of CAA and the Dutch variety of familial CAA, with that of Alzheimer's disease and Down's syndrome. However, the origin and mechanism of deposition of the amyloid are still unknown. It has been suggested that the amyloid beta-proteins originate from a common circulating precursor that penetrates the central nervous system (CNS) via injured capillaries with abnormal permeability, with deposition of amyloid in vessel walls and in the core of neuritic plaques. This hypothesis, however, does not fully explain the fact that CAA and neuritic plaques do not always coexist.

Cerebral Infarcts

Since its early pathologic descriptions, CAA has been known to be associated with ICH, as well as small cortical infarcts. These occur where the vascular amyloid deposits are severe, at times with marked thickening of the vessel walls and luminal occlusions. However, some authors have found infarcts with equal frequency in patients with and without CAA. These authors have commented on the generally patent lumens of affected arteries, regardless of the severity of involvement of the wall by CAA.

Small and superficial CAA-related cerebral infarcts do not typically result in stroke syndromes related to the distribution of single large cerebral arteries. It is more likely that the clinical effect of multiple small cortical infarcts in CAA is mediated by their coexistence with other causes of neurologic dysfunction, such as Alzheimer's changes, the effects of repeated episodes of ICH, and a progressive leukoencephalopathy, all contributing to a progressive dementia.

Leukoencephalopathy

A leukoencephalopathy is recognized as another radiologic and histologic concomitant of CAA. It is characterized pathologically by diffuse or patchy pallor of the white matter, with maximal involvement of the centrum semiovale, sparing the subcortical U fibers, corpus callosum, internal capsule, optic radiation, and temporal lobe white matter. Histologically, the white matter shows vacuolation leading to a spongy aspect, with swelling of oligodendrocytes, dilatation of perivascular spaces, astrocytic proliferation, and occasional Rosenthal fibers. No areas of infarction or amyloid angiopathy are present in the affected white matter itself.

Computed tomography (CT) scans show bilateral hypodensity of the hemispheric white matter. Magnetic resonance imaging scans show white matter hyperintensities on T2-weighted sequences, in a distribution that parallels pathologic descriptions. It has been suggested that the leukoencephalopathy develops as a result of chronic ischemia secondary to hypoperfusion by amyloid-laden cortical penetrating arteries. The presence of spongiosis, swollen oligodendrocytes, and enlarged perivascular spaces is thought to correlate with subacute edema, which eventually leads to loss of myelin and astrocytosis.

Miscellaneous Conditions

A number of conditions have been described in association with CAA (Table 3). Some of these are rare in patients with CAA and are probably coincidental, whereas others may have a common pathogenesis. In patients with Down's syndrome, Alzheimer's changes have coexisted with CAA. CAA is more likely to occur in older patients with Down's syndrome. The link between CAA, Alzheimer's disease changes, and Down's syndrome is the common biochemical origin of the abnormal amyloid protein (beta-protein) in the three conditions.

The association of giant-cell arteritis with CAA may not represent the combination of two different types of angiopathy, but rather a giant-cell reaction to vascular amyloid deposits. However, one report documented the association of both forms of vascular disease with chronic inflammatory changes in cortical and subarachnoid vessels and multinucleated giant cells in areas of disrupted elastic membranes. The report of CAA in vessels affected by an inflammatory reaction akin to that of rheumatoid vasculitis suggests that, in some instances, the pathogenesis of CAA may relate to chronic local vascular inflammation. The same applies to the reported instances of CAA associated with granulomatous angiitis of the CNS. A close topographic association between the two types of angiopathy suggests a pathogenic relationship between them rather than a coincidental occurrence. Immunosuppressive treatment with prednisone and cyclophosphamide has resulted in resolution of the granulomatous angiitis as well as a reduction in the severity of CAA. This suggests that the treatment may have resulted in both suppression of vascular inflammation and amyloid formation.

A familial condition characterized by the association of CAA with progressive dementia, spasticity, and ataxia has been described. Despite the presence of profuse CAA in the CNS, and the description of strokelike episodes in several members of the families, no cases of ICH have been recorded in this condition. Its pattern of inheritance is autosomal dominant.

In postirradiation brain necrosis, abundant amyloid deposits, both as irregular masses within the necrotic brain parenchyma and in the walls of blood vessels, have been described. These patients have presented with signs of a focal brain lesion with mass effect 3 or 4 years after cranial radiation therapy. Histologic examination has documented postirradiation demyelination, angionecrosis, thrombosis, and ischemic necrosis.

Vascular malformations of the brain rarely develop amyloid deposits. In some instances, episodes of ICH have been thought to relate to "weakening" of blood vessels by the amyloid deposits. At other times, dense amyloid deposits within vessels of an arteriovenous malformation have been described in the absence of episodes of bleeding.

The presence of CAA in the spongiform encephalopathies has been rarely reported, but parenchymal amyloid deposits in plaque form are frequent in Creutzfeldt-Jakob disease and kuru. CAA is occasionally present in the brains of patients with the Gerstmann-Sträussler form of slowly progressive, predominantly cerebellar spongiform encephalopathy. However, no case of ICH has been reported in this condition.

A single autopsy report documented widespread CAA and a fatal right hemispheric hemorrhage in a boxer with "dementia pugilistica," characterized by symptoms of parkinsonism and progressive dementia. In addition to CAA, histologic examination showed abundant neuritic plaques and neurofibrillary degeneration. Rarely, CAA can present as a mass lesion or amyloidoma, with focal seizures and an expanding hypodense lesion on CT scan. Histologic examination has showed prominent CAA in leptomeningeal and cortical vessels, as well as masses of amyloid free in the parenchyma. CAA in association with a demyelinating disorder has been rarely reported. The demyelinating white matter lesions were consistent with plaques of multiple sclerosis, and blood vessels in their vicinity had profuse vascular and perivascular amyloid deposits. None of the cases reported showed evidence of ICH related to the deposits of vascular amyloid.

A rare familial disorder with oculoleptomeningeal amyloidosis leads to episodes of cerebral infarction as a result of occlusion of large intracerebral arteries by a process of intimal proliferation coincident with heavy adventitial amyloid deposits. No instances of ICH have been recorded in any of the affected families.

Table 3 Conditions Reported in Association with Cerebral Amyloid Angiopathy

Down's syndrome
Vasculitis
    Giant-cell arteritis
    Rheumatoid vasculitis
    Granulomatous angiitis of the CNS
Familial ataxia with dementia
Postcerebral irradiation
Vascular malformations
Spongiform encephalopathy
"Dementia pugilistica"
Mass lesion
Demyelinating disorder
Oculoleptomeningeal amyloidosis

CNS = Central nervous system.
Modified from Vinters HV. Cerebral amyloid angiopathy: A critical review. Stroke 1987; 18:311–324; with permission.

SUGGESTED READING

DeWitt LD, Louis DN. Case records of the Massachusetts General Hospital: Case 27-1991. N Engl J Med 1991; 325:42–54.
Feldmann R, Tornabene J. Diagnosis and treatment of cerebral amyloid angiopathy. Clin Geriatr Med 1991; 7:617–630.

Finelli PF, Kessimian N, Bernstein PW. Cerebral amyloid angiopathy manifesting as recurrent intracerebral hemorrhage. Arch Neurol 1984; 41:330–333.

Gilles C, Brucher JM, Khoubesserian P, Vanderhaeghen JJ. Cerebral amyloid angiopathy as a cause of multiple intracerebral hemorrhages. Neurology 1984; 34:730–735.

Greene GM, Godersky JC, Biller J, et al. Surgical experience with cerebral amyloid angiopathy. Stroke 1990; 21:1545–1549.

Gudmundsson G, Hallgrimsson J, Jonasson TA, Bjarnason O. Hereditary cerebral haemorrhage with amyloidosis. Brain 1972; 95: 387–404.

Masuda J, Tanaka K, Ueda K, Omae T. Autopsy study of incidence and distribution of cerebral amyloid angiopathy in Hisayama, Japan. Stroke 1988; 19:205–210.

Pendlebury WW, Iole ED, Tracy RP, Dill BA. Intracerebral hemorrhage related to cerebral amyloid angiopathy and t-PA treatment. Ann Neurol 1991; 29:210–213.

Vinters HV. Cerebral amyloid angiopathy: A critical review. Stroke 1987; 18:311–324.

Vonsattel JP, Myers RH, Hedley-Whyte ET, et al. Cerebral amyloid angiopathy without and with cerebral hemorrhages: A comparative histological study. Ann Neurol 1991; 30:637–649.

SENTINEL HEADACHES AND ANEURYSMAL SUBARACHNOID HEMORRHAGE

JANET L. WILTERDINK, M.D.

Intracranial aneurysms cause the majority (80 percent) of nontraumatic subarachnoid hemorrhages (SAH). Aneurysms are acquired defects in the arterial wall, although the propensity to form an aneurysm may be congenital and, in some cases, inherited. They most commonly occur at the bifurcations of the large arteries at the base of the brain and are usually asymptomatic until they rupture into the subarachnoid space surrounding the brain. Occasionally the hemorrhage extends into the intracerebral or subdural space. Untreated, 30 to 50 percent of ruptured aneurysms will rehemorrhage in the next days or weeks. Aneurysmal SAH is very uncommon in persons under 20 years; the incidence increases with age, peaking at age 50 to 60.

SAH has a morbidity and mortality of 50 to 70 percent. Most deaths occur in the first 1 to 2 months following SAH. Early mortality, in the first hours and days, correlates with the patient's neurologic condition and is due to increased intracranial pressure and focal and generalized ischemia. Subsequent morbidity and mortality also occur in patients who present in good neurologic condition with the development of complications such as vasospasm, hydrocephalus, and, especially, rehemorrhage.

Early surgical intervention in patients who present in good clinical condition is believed to significantly improve their prognosis by decreasing the risk of rehemorrhage. However, the overall impact of this change in practice on SAH mortality has been disappointing because a significant number of patients die before arriving at the hospital or soon thereafter.

Sentinel headache is a retrospective diagnosis of headache symptoms occurring in the days to weeks preceding a recognized SAH. Because the symptoms are similar although sometimes less severe than those of the recognized SAH, the majority of sentinel headaches are believed to represent a "warning leak" or a minor SAH. Some clinicians feel, however, that some sentinel headaches represent a different pathophysiology, such as acute enlargement or thrombosis of the aneurysm, or isolated hemorrhage into the aneurysm wall.

Between 20 and 50 percent of patients have had a sentinel headache or warning leak prior to their major aneurysmal SAH. This suggests that improved recognition of minor SAH will provide an opportunity for early surgical intervention and possibly improve prognosis in a significant number of patients. Because of the retrospective nature of the diagnosis, it is not always possible to determine why these apparent minor SAHs were misdiagnosed. One-quarter to one-half of these patients do not seek medical attention. Those who are medically evaluated are given alternate diagnoses such as migraine, viral illness, hypertensive crisis, brain tumor, meningitis, sinusitis, alcohol and other intoxications, and cerebral and myocardial infarction, or are simply treated symptomatically. In the overwhelming majority of cases, a failure to diagnose SAH occurs because the diagnosis is not considered and the appropriate workup is not initiated. A failure to diagnose correctly following appropriately ordered diagnostic testing is very rare.

CLINICAL PRESENTATION

History

Headache is virtually a sine qua non of aneurysmal SAH. Even when other symptoms and signs are present, it is usually the major and often the only complaint. Common descriptors of the headache include exploding, bursting, crushing, agonizing, tremendous, awful, terrible, terrific, tearing, excruciating, and unbearable. These emphasize its two most distinctive features: sudden onset and unusual severity. The symptoms may be less severe or stereotyped in the smaller hemorrhages or "warning leaks." Chronic migraine and other headache sufferers with SAH usually note that the headache associated with minor SAH is very different from their previous headaches. When evaluating a patient with an acute headache, suddenness of onset and unusual severity should alert the clinician to the possibility of SAH.

Other features of the headaches are less distinctive. There is no typical location for the headache of SAH. Virtually every type of headache pattern has been reported with SAH, including generalized, retro-orbital, occipital, hemicranial, and bitemporal. These do not accurately predict hemorrhage or aneurysm location. The headache associated with SAH is occasionally fleeting but usually persists for several hours or days.

Rarely, in 1 to 2 percent of SAH patients, headache does not occur, requiring a high index of suspicion for the diagnosis. It is also important to remember that a history of headache may not be obtainable in the obtunded or comatose patient.

Meningitis-like symptoms, such as a painful stiff neck, vomiting, photophobia, and a low-grade fever, accompany headache in SAH in about 20 to 60 percent of patients. Occasionally the neck discomfort may be more prominent than the headache. These symptoms may shift attention to infectious causes. However, the precipitous onset of these symptoms in SAH would be unusual for meningitis and should alert the clinician to the correct diagnosis.

Loss of consciousness, brief or prolonged, may be an associated or presenting feature of aneurysmal rupture. Often the patient will complain of headache seconds before losing consciousness or will awaken shortly afterward complaining of severe headache. Some patients awaken with a clouded sensorium, and some present in coma. Therefore, SAH should be considered in the differential diagnosis of patients in coma or metabolic encephalopathy, especially if accompanied by headache or physical distress.

The clinical setting in which the headache occurs may suggest its cause. Classically SAH occurs in the setting of physical exertion such as sexual intercourse, presumably due to acute blood pressure elevation. However, the absence of this history should not dissuade the clinician from this diagnosis. Many SAHs occur during normal activity or rest, and some occur during sleep.

Because a history of warning symptoms is not uncommon, patients should be questioned about unusual symptoms in the days or weeks prior to presentation. Sentinel headache from a warning leak is the most common of these and is usually similar, but perhaps less severe, than the current presentation. Enlargement of the aneurysm prior to rupture may also produce symptoms such as facial or eye pain, visual field deficits, diplopia, and other visual symptoms.

The patient's past medical and family history may reveal medical conditions known to be associated with intracranial aneurysms. These include polycystic kidney disease, coarctation of the aorta, and, less commonly, moyamoya disease, Ehler-Danlos disease, fibromuscular dysplasia, and other connective tissue diseases. Pregnancy may also increase the risk of aneurysmal rupture. Some intracranial aneurysms are familial. However, most aneurysmal SAHs do not occur in association with any one of these conditions or with a family history of SAH.

Physical Examination

Features of the physical examination are less specific for the diagnosis of SAH than the clinical history. Patients are often ill-appearing and in physical distress. Meningismus with Kernig's or Brudzinski's signs or a low-grade fever may be present. High temperatures, more suggestive of bacterial meningitis, are not associated with SAH. The neurologic examination, while of prognostic value, is usually not helpful in the diagnosis of SAH per se, as it may fall anywhere along the spectrum from normal, to isolated cranial nerve deficits, to hemiparesis, to coma.

The exception to this rule is a third cranial nerve palsy associated with an enlarging posterior communicating artery aneurysm. Unlike the ischemic third nerve palsy associated with diabetes, which affects the central nerve fibers and spares the peripherally located pupillary fibers, compression of the nerve by an enlarging aneurysm usually affects sympathetic fibers first, producing a large unreactive pupil with ptosis and oculomotor paresis. When this develops acutely, it is a very specific finding that requires the diagnosis of intracranial aneurysm be pursued.

Other clinical syndromes may suggest the aneurysm location in patients with SAH. Middle cerebral and internal carotid artery aneurysms may rupture into the temporal lobe producing aphasia and hemisensory or hemimotor deficits. Aneurysms arising from the anterior communicating artery may be associated with abulia and lower extremity weakness.

Funduscopic examination may reveal subhyaloid or preretinal hemorrhages, dark red globular swellings around the optic disc secondary to rapid venous engorgement. While these are present in only 20 percent of patients with SAH, when seen in the setting of acute headache they are virtually pathognomonic for SAH. Papilledema is seen rarely in acute SAH.

Acute elevation of blood pressure is common after SAH, secondary either to increased intracranial pressure (Cushing's response) or to acute catecholamine release.

Table 1 Clinical Features Suggesting the Diagnosis of Subarachnoid Hemorrhage

History
  Headache: any location, severe, sudden onset, persistent
  Meningitis-like symptoms: neck stiffness, nausea, vomiting, photophobia
  Loss of consciousness: brief or prolonged
  Warning symptoms: headache or diplopia, days to weeks before presentation
  Setting of symptom onset: physical exertion, sexual intercourse
  Past medical history: coarctation of the aorta, Ehler-Danlos, other (see text)
  Family history of SAH

Examination
  Physical distress
  Meningismus, low-grade fever
  Elevated blood pressure
  Subhyaloid or preretinal hemorrhages
  Neurologic deficits, especially nonpupillary sparing oculomotor palsy

This may suggest the diagnosis of hypertensive encephalopathy rather than SAH. However, the presence of headache or other neurologic symptoms should alert the clinician to perform further investigation.

The signs and symptoms of aneurysmal SAH are summarized in Table 1.

DIAGNOSTIC TESTING

An outline of the diagnostic workup is presented in Figure 1. Diagnostic testing should proceed without delay once the diagnosis of SAH is considered. The high mortality rate of untreated aneurysmal rupture mandates diagnostic evaluation even when the clinical suspicion for the diagnosis is not very high.

Noncontrast *computed tomography* (CT) of the head should be the first test performed in a patient with suspected SAH. Because most aneurysms are located at the base of the brain, most of the blood appears as a hyperdense outline of the basal cisterns. Depending on the amount of blood and the location of the aneurysm, SAH also appears as a blush over the cerebellar

tentorium, in the cortical sulci, and in the ventricles (Fig. 2A). As subarachnoid blood is absorbed over the first few days, the density of the signal decreases, becoming isodense with brain tissue (Fig. 2B). A CT scan at this stage may appear as effacement of the cisterns or sulci. Gradually the signal becomes more hypodense, resembling normal spinal fluid.

The sensitivity of CT for the detection of SAH depends on its temporal relationship to aneurysm rupture, and the amount of blood in the subarachnoid space. Because blood becomes diluted by cerebral spinal fluid (CSF), minor amounts of SAH may not be detected by CT. The earlier the CT is performed after aneurysm rupture, before blood is hemolyzed and cleared, the greater its sensitivity. The sensitivity of CT in SAH is over 90 percent in the first 24 hours and remains high for the first 72 hours.

Specific patterns of hemorrhage on CT may suggest the location of the ruptured aneurysm. Blood in the basal cisterns is the most common and least specific location. A large amount of blood in the sylvian fissure suggests middle cerebral artery aneurysm. Blood in a cavum septum pellucidum or in the interhemispheric

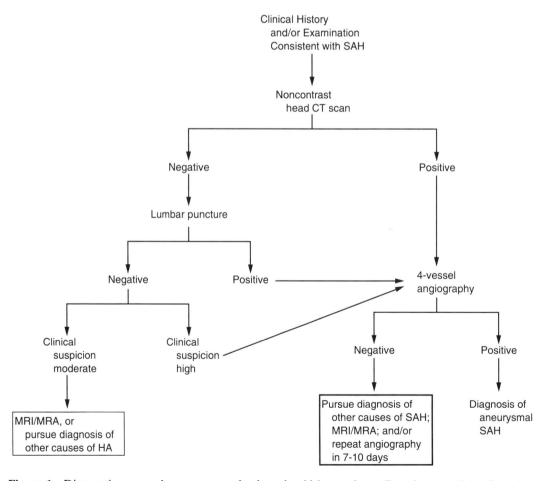

Figure 1 Diagnostic approach to aneurysmal subarachnoid hemorrhage. Boxed areas of the flow chart require case-by-case consideration as outlined in the text. (HA = headache.)

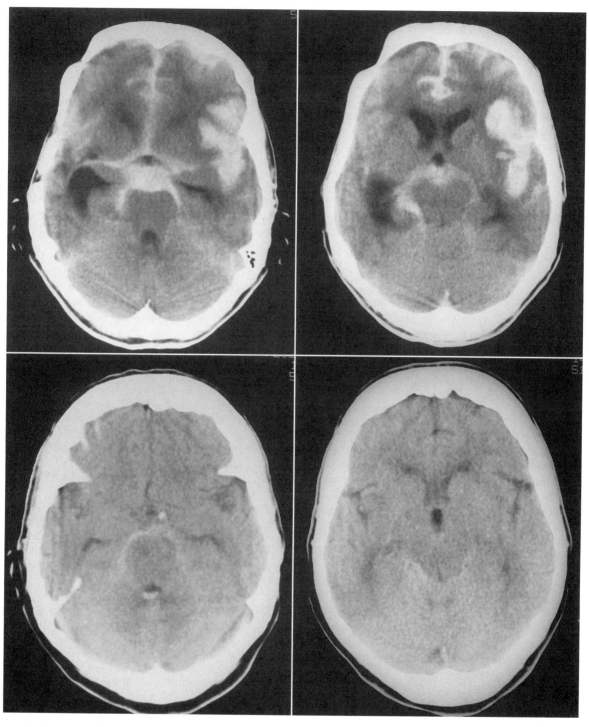

Figure 2 Spectrum of computed tomography (CT) appearance in SAH. *(Top, left and right)* This 60-year-old woman presented within hours after acute left middle cerebral artery aneurysm rupture. There is a large quantity of blood in basal cisterns and cortical sulci, especially in left sylvian fissure, where there is some intracerebral extension into the temporal lobe. *(Bottom, left and right)* This 35-year-old male presented 36 hours after a left posterior communicating artery aneurysm rupture. The extent of subarachnoid hemorrhage is less than in the top left and right panels. Also, partial resorption of the blood decreases its density on CT such that it is approaching the density of normal gray matter.

fissure is typical of anterior communicating aneurysms. Isolated intraventricular hemorrhage is more common with anterior communicating and basilar artery aneurysms. Because the pattern of hemorrhage depends not only on aneurysm location but also on size and orientation, these patterns are not always reliable. They are most useful in patients with multiple aneurysms, to identify which aneurysm is most likely to have ruptured.

Intracerebral hemorrhage (ICH) into the temporal lobe and basal ganglia is associated with middle cerebral or internal carotid artery aneurysm rupture. Anterior cerebral artery aneurysms may rupture into the frontal lobe. The presence of ICH on CT may obscure the diagnosis of SAH by drawing attention away from the presence of subarachnoid blood. Also, because intracerebral blood is cleared more slowly than subarachnoid blood, a CT performed several days after aneurysm rupture may reveal only intracerebral blood. Aneurysmal rupture should be considered in the differential diagnosis of "primary" ICH in the frontal or temporal lobes or deep white matter when imaging studies are performed late and there is no clear cause for ICH.

Recent data suggest that subarachnoid hemorrhage isolated to the basal cisterns around the midbrain is highly associated with nonaneurysmal SAH. While this pattern of bleeding does not preclude the need for angiography to rule out an aneurysm, it may allow more confidence in the diagnosis of nonaneurysmal SAH when angiography is negative.

While *magnetic resonance imaging* (MRI) may also detect SAH, there are many reasons why CT is usually the test of choice. The sensitivity of MRI is less well defined than CT but appears to be lower than CT in the hyperacute setting. MRI is perhaps equally or more sensitive in the subacute period (4 to 14 days). However, at this late stage neither test has a very high sensitivity. CT is also less expensive, more readily available, and can be reliably performed in the ventilated or unstable patient. While MRI is more likely than CT to detect the underlying structural cause of SAH, it only rarely obviates the need for conventional angiography.

Lumbar puncture (LP) and CSF analysis must be performed in a patient with suspected SAH if the CT is negative. The CT should precede LP, however, because of the possibility of mass effect from subarachnoid hemorrhage or ICH, which would contraindicate LP. CSF findings depend on the temporal relationship of the LP to the rupture. Red blood cells appear almost immediately. Over the first day and next few weeks, the number of red blood cells decreases as they are hemolyzed, producing a pigment in the CSF known as xanthochromia. Depending on the amount of blood, xanthochromia generally peaks at about 7 days and persists for about 2 weeks. A mild reactive meningitis may develop, with an elevated protein, a minimally decreased or normal glucose, and a moderate leukocytosis with lymphocyte predominance.

Occasionally it is difficult to distinguish bloody CSF following traumatic LP from that of a SAH. In a traumatic tap, the number of red blood cells usually decreases between the first and last tubes of CSF collected, but remains constant in SAH. This is not always a reliable means of distinguishing the two problems. A tube of CSF should be centrifuged and the supernatant examined for xanthochromia, which suggests that the blood is due to SAH rather than a traumatic tap. However, xanthochromia requires at least 2 to 4 hours, sometimes up to 12 hours, to appear. Therefore, false-negatives (absent xanthochromia with true SAH) may occur if the LP is performed too soon. False positive xanthochromia may occur if the CSF from a traumatic tap is not examined immediately or if previous traumatic attempts at LP have occurred. The presence of xanthochromia is unreliable if the red blood cell count is very high, greater than 100,000 cells per cubic millimeter.

Prospective studies suggest that the presence of red blood cells or xanthochromia in the CSF has a 100 percent sensitivity for SAH when CSF is obtained between 12 hours and 2 weeks after hemorrhage and remains as high as 70 percent for the first 3 weeks. It is important that the fluid be examined for xanthochromia by spectrophotometry because the naked eye can miss up to one-half of xanthochromic samples in patients with SAH.

Cerebral angiography to look for an intracranial aneurysm is necessary when CT or CSF analysis reveals subarachnoid hemorrhage not produced by trauma. Four vessels must be injected because of the occurrence of multiple aneurysms in 20 percent of patients. The angiogram must be filmed in at least two projections to avoid concealment of the aneurysm by other vascular structures.

Occasionally angiography will fail to reveal the aneurysm in patients with aneurysmal SAH. Thrombosis of the aneurysm or compression of the aneurysm by subarachnoid clot may preclude contrast filling of the aneurysm. Vasospasm in the proximal artery may also prevent adequate contrast filling of the aneurysm. Other vascular structures may overlie and conceal the aneurysm in certain projections. Rarely, the aneurysm is obliterated after it ruptures.

When angiography is negative in the patient with nontraumatic SAH, other causes such as cerebral or spinal arteriovenous malformation are considered. However, many neurologists and neurosurgeons would consider repeating angiography 7 to 10 days later, especially if the angiography was incomplete or of poor quality or if vasospasm was present. If the initial angiogram is well performed with no vasospasm present, the yield of a second angiogram is very low. However, because of the high mortality associated with an untreated aneurysm and the low morbidity and mortality of angiography in our institution, it is our policy to repeat angiography in such patients if they are in good clinical condition.

While *magnetic resonance angiography* (MRA) has obvious appeal because it is noninvasive, it currently has a limited role in the diagnosis of aneurysmal SAH. At the present time, MRA can detect aneurysms greater than 4 mm in diameter, but its sensitivity remains undefined, particularly in the setting of SAH. The size of the aneurysm is frequently underestimated by MRA. Even if an aneurysm were to be detected by MRA, angiography would still be required to better define its anatomy and size and to rule out the presence of other aneurysms. Surgeons require adequate visualization of the aneurysm and its arterial attachment in order to plan specific surgical strategy.

THE PATIENT WITH ACUTE HEADACHE AND NEGATIVE CT AND LP

There are a number of benign headache syndromes that can mimic SAH. These go by such names as crash migraine and benign exertional and coital headache. Because of their similarity to the headache of SAH, most of these patients are examined on at least one occasion with CT and LP. When these are negative, the patients have an overwhelmingly benign outcome on follow-up.

However, there are a handful of reported cases in the literature of patients with "thunderclap headache" suggestive of SAH, whose CT and LP did not reveal SAH but whose angiography revealed an intracranial aneurysm. When specific details of testing are lacking, such as timing after symptom onset, incomplete or delayed investigation are possible explanations for testing failure. However, there are a few well-documented cases in which appropriately performed CT and LP were negative and angiography revealed an aneurysm and diffuse cerebral vasospasm. At surgery these patients had no evidence of SAH or had minimal bleeding into the vessel wall. The explanation of such cases is controversial. Some suggest that the aneurysm was responsible for the symptoms by a different mechanism than bleeding. Others suggest that the aneurysm was an incidental finding and that the headache or vasospasm were due to another cause, such as migraine.

This situation requires considerable clinical judgment. The consequences of failing to diagnose a symptomatic aneurysm are severe but must be weighed against subjecting a patient to the risk of angiography when the prior probability of a positive result is low. If the CT and LP are performed late after symptom onset, so that negative results are unreliable, and if there are suggestive clinical features and the angiographer is experienced, such patients should probably undergo four-vessel angiography. Suggestive clinical features include a family history or a past medical history suggesting the patient is at risk, a classic history of SAH-like symptoms, or the presence of neurologic signs, in particular a third cranial nerve palsy affecting the pupil. In patients with negative studies in whom we feel the diagnosis of aneurysmal SAH is possible but very unlikely, we use MRI and MRA as screening tests and follow the patient clinically if these are negative.

SUGGESTED READING

Bassi P, Bandera R, Loiero M, et al. Warning signs in subarachnoid hemorrhage: A cooperative study. Acta Neurol Scand 1991; 84: 277–281.

Day JW, Raskin NH. Thunderclap headache: Symptom of unruptured cerebral aneurysm. Lancet 1986; ii:1247–1248.

Iwanaga H, Wakai S, Ochiai C, et al. Ruptured cerebral aneurysms missed by initial angiographic study. Neurosurgery 1990; 27:45–51.

Ogawa T, Inugami A, Shimosegawa E, et al. Subarachnoid hemorrhage: Evaluation with MR imaging. Radiology 1993; 186: 345–351.

Rinkel GJE, Wijdicks EFM, Hasan D, et al. Outcome in patients with subarachnoid haemorrhage and negative angiography according to pattern of haemorrhage on computed tomography. Lancet 1991; 338:964–968.

Vermeulen M, Hasan D, Blijenberg BG, et al. Xanthochromia after subarachnoid haemorrhage needs no revisitation. J Neurol Neurosurg Psychiatry 1989; 52:826–828.

Vermeulen M, Lindsay KW, Van Gijn J. Subarachnoid haemorrhage. London: WB Saunders, 1992.

Wijdicks EFM, Kerkhoff H, van Gijn J. Cerebral vasospasm and unruptured aneurysm in thunderclap headache. Lancet 1988; ii:1020.

Wolpert SM, Caplan LR. Current role of cerebral angiography in the diagnosis of cerebral vascular disease. AJR Am J Roentgenol 1992; 159:191–197.

PERIMESENCEPHALIC SUBARACHNOID HEMORRHAGE

JAN van GIJN, M.D., F.R.C.P.E.
GABRIËL J.E. RINKEL, M.D.

Perimesencephalic hemorrhage constitutes 10 percent of all subarachnoid hemorrhages and two-thirds of all subarachnoid hemorrhages with a normal angiogram. In these particular cases the hemorrhage probably originates from a ruptured vein, although this remains to be proved, and the prognosis is invariably excellent. Therefore the management is completely different from that of patients with aneurysmal subarachnoid hemorrhage. The diagnosis can be clinched only when the physician recognizes the typical pattern of hemorrhage on an early computed tomography (CT) scan, and should be subsequently confirmed by a normal angiogram. Unfortunately, the clinical features are usually indistinguishable from those of aneurysmal subarachnoid hemorrhage.

CLINICAL FEATURES

It is not possible to infer the perimesencephalic origin of subarachnoid hemorrhage in a given patient from the clinical symptoms and signs. The features are those of subarachnoid hemorrhage in general. The patient is an adult of any age but typically over 40 years. Sudden headache is the cardinal feature, often described as a blow on the head or an explosion inside. Physical exercise or straining may have precipitated the attack, but other patients are struck while reading the newspaper or turning over in bed. Neurologic examination is normal except for neck stiffness, but even this sign may be absent if the patient is examined soon after the onset of the headache. Neck stiffness from subarachnoid hemorrhage takes hours to develop, a fact that many medical teachers fail to impress on future family practitioners and emergency officers.

In retrospect, patients in whom this diagnosis is eventually confirmed are less ill than patients with ruptured aneurysms, their headache has more often developed in minutes rather than seconds, and initial loss of consciousness does not occur. However, the predictive value of these clinical characteristics in distinguishing perimesencephalic (nonaneurysmal) from aneurysmal subarachnoid hemorrhage is very limited, for two reasons. First, patients with perimesencephalic hemorrhage are a minority (10 percent) of all patients with subarachnoid hemorrhage, whereas patients with a ruptured aneurysm are the vast majority (85 percent). Second, the divisions are far from absolute: in patients with perimesencephalic hemorrhage the headache may come on in seconds, and many patients with a ruptured

aneurysm do not lose consciousness during the ictus and are not seriously ill on first examination.

COMPUTED TOMOGRAPHY

CT scanning is the first-line investigation for patients with suspected subarachnoid hemorrhage, of any type. The sensitivity depends mainly on the interval after the event, but also on the quality of the equipment and the radiologist. Under optimum conditions, evidence of blood after aneurysmal hemorrhage can be detected in at least 95 percent of cases within a day versus only 50 percent after a week. If the initial CT scan is performed later than 3 days after the hemorrhage, much of the extravasated blood will have disappeared. Also, in patients with aneurysmal subarachnoid hemorrhage the remaining blood may be mainly confined to the cisterns around the midbrain. This might lead to the erroneous conclusion of a nonaneurysmal origin of the hemorrhage (see next paragraph). Therefore, the diagnosis of perimesencephalic subarachnoid hemorrhage can be made with confidence only if the first CT scan is performed within 3 days of the onset of the symptoms.

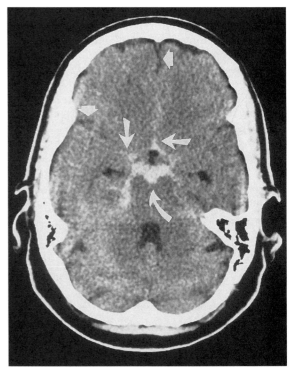

Figure 1 Computed tomography scan of a patient with perimesencephalic subarachnoid hemorrhage. Center of bleeding is in interpeduncular cistern (*curved arrow*). There is some extension to medial-horizontal part of one sylvian fissure and to posterior part of frontal interhemispheric fissure (*straight arrows*). No blood is seen in lateral parts of sylvian fissure or in anterior part of frontal interhemispheric fissure (*arrowheads*), and there is no intraventricular hemorrhage.

In perimesencephalic subarachnoid hemorrhage the extravasated blood is confined to, or at least predominantly located in, the cisterns around the midbrain (Fig. 1). The center of the hemorrhage is most often in the interpeduncular cistern, sometimes in the prepontine cistern. The ambient cistern is involved in more than half of the cases, the quadrigeminal cistern less commonly, depending on the overall severity of the hemorrhage. From the interpeduncular fossa the blood may extend anteriorly to the chiasmatic cistern and to the medial-horizontal part of the sylvian fissure, but never to the anterior interhemispheric fissure or to the lateral sylvian fissures. An intraparenchymal hematoma rules out the diagnosis, as does frank intraventricular hemorrhage (other than some sedimentation of red blood cells in the posterior horns).

Aneurysms at the bifurcation of the basilar artery give rise to hemorrhages that are also centered around the interpeduncular fossa, but as a rule in those cases the jet resulting from a tear in an artery propels the blood much farther forward and laterally, as far as the anterior interhemispheric and lateral sylvian cisterns. Nevertheless, occasionally a basilar artery aneurysm bleeds locally rather than in a diffuse fashion. Angiography discloses such an aneurysm in about one in 20 patients with a perimesencephalic pattern of hemorrhage.

OTHER INVESTIGATIONS

Magnetic resonance imaging (MRI) may be used to indicate the source of bleeding if CT scanning is performed after too long an interval. In some patients with a ruptured aneurysm this technique can still detect subpial depositions of hemosiderin near the aneurysm, but in patients with perimesencephalic subarachnoid hemorrhage, no such traces can be detected by MRI.

Lumbar puncture should be reserved for patients in whom no blood is detected by CT or MRI. At best, this helps to establish the diagnosis of subarachnoid hemorrhage in general. It provides no information about its origin. It is essential to distinguish between a traumatic tap and a true hemorrhage. A widely held but erroneous belief is that this distinction can be reliably made by collecting the cerebrospinal fluid (CSF) in three consecutive test tubes and by comparing the degree to which these are bloodstained. The only sound method is to centrifuge the CSF and to examine the supernatant for xanthochromia. The CSF cannot be declared normal unless spectrophotometry has been used. The yellow color stems from xanthochromic pigments released from disintegrating red cells in the CSF. These pigments can invariably be found between 12 hours and 2 weeks after subarachnoid hemorrhage. Lumbar puncture should therefore be deferred until at least 12 hours after the onset of the headache. The only legitimate exception is the rare patient with such an incomplete history that meningitis cannot be ruled out. If lumbar puncture is done too soon and the CSF is bloodstained, perhaps due to a traumatic tap, the patient cannot escape an angiogram and may suffer unnecessary anxiety even if this is normal.

Angiography cannot be omitted, because of the rather remote possibility of a ruptured basilar artery aneurysm. However, when angiography is normal there is no need to repeat it. Given that a basilar artery aneurysm underlies at most one in 20 hemorrhages with a perimesencephalic distribution on CT, and that at most one in 20 angiograms fails to demonstrate the expected aneurysm in patients with an "aneurysmal" type of subarachnoid hemorrhage on CT, the chance that a repeated angiogram will reveal an aneurysm in a patient with perimesencephalic subarachnoid hemorrhage is one in 400. It is clear that the complications of 399 unnecessary angiograms (an estimated four to six deaths or strokes) far outweigh the benefits of finding this single aneurysm.

Our admonition not to repeat cerebral angiography in patients with perimesencephalic subarachnoid hemorrhage and a normal angiogram by no means applies to patients with negative angiograms in general. When the pattern of hemorrhage on CT suggests a ruptured aneurysm the search for an occult aneurysm should be relentlessly pursued, not only by repeated angiograms but in some circumstances (such as rebleeding) even by exploratory craniotomy.

MANAGEMENT IN HOSPITAL

As soon as a negative angiogram has confirmed the initial impression gained from the CT scan that the source of the hemorrhage in the cisterns around the midbrain is not an aneurysm or any other detectable anomaly of the cerebral vasculature, management should be tailored to that of an innocuous disorder. Such a policy is backed up by experience gained from a prospective series of more than 100 patients with perimesencephalic subarachnoid hemorrhage. In these patients, not a single episode of rebleeding or of delayed cerebral infarction has ever occurred. The only possible complication is the development of hydrocephalus in the acute phase by blockage of the CSF circulation because the perimesencephalic cisterns form a narrow passage at the level of the tentorial hiatus. But even then the disorder is usually self-limiting, and only in exceptional cases does drainage of CSF have to be considered. In those rare cases lumbar puncture should be tried first, and insertion of a ventricular catheter only as a last resort. In general, the practical consequences of the diagnosis of nonaneurysmal perimesencephalic hemorrhage are several.

First, the patient should be told the good news that his or her hemorrhage is not one of the dangerous kind, with many possible complications and usually the need for intracranial surgery, but rather a harmless variety that is not known to recur and that does not interfere with future life-style.

Second, special drugs and measures that were initially given with a view to the possibility of an aneurysm should be discontinued. This applies, for instance, to nimodipine, continuous supervision by nursing staff, an intravenous drip and a total fluid intake of at least 3 L a day, electrocardiographic monitoring, and limitation of visitors and other stimuli.

Third, even continued bed rest is no longer necessary, at least when the patient is no longer troubled by headache. Apart from the patient's symptoms, there are no obstacles to being up and about and subsequently to resuming a normal life.

LONG-TERM PROGNOSIS

The outcome in the long term is, as far as we know, as good as in the short term. More than 80 patients have now been followed up for an average period of 4 years, and not a single patient reported a rebleed or a sudden bout of headache reminiscent of their hemorrhage. Only a few patients had not resumed their previous activities, because of unrelated diseases or because unnecessary fears of rebleeding induced their employers' medical advisers to declare them unfit for work. Thus, the alleviation of worries should be directed not only to the patients and their relatives, but also to general practitioners and to doctors on whose advice employers and insurance companies base their assessment of risks.

PATHOGENESIS

The excellent prognosis is the very reason that no autopsy study of this condition has been performed to unveil the source of nonaneurysmal perimesencephalic hemorrhage. Yet some compelling arguments lead us to assume that this source is not an artery, and most probably a vein.

The local nature of the hemorrhage is one of its main characteristics. In perimesencephalic hemorrhage it is not rare to find evidence of extravasated blood in the interpeduncular fossa but not in the chiasmatic cistern, although these two adjoining CSF spaces are either continuous or separated by nothing more than a flimsy arachnoid membrane. Furthermore, the hemorrhage never extends into the ventricular system or into the brain parenchyma. This restricted pattern of extravasation differs in a striking fashion from that of arterial hemorrhage, in particular with a ruptured aneurysm of the basilar artery, which is also located in the interpeduncular fossa.

That delayed cerebral ischemia does not occur after perimesencephalic subarachnoid hemorrhage cannot be attributed only to lesser degrees of cisternal blood on the initial CT scan, because we found in a separate study that ischemic complications did occur after aneurysmal hemorrhages with similar amounts of blood. The proportions of other well-known predictors of delayed cerebral ischemia were also similar in the two groups. In other words, only a different origin of the hemorrhage, other than a ruptured artery, can explain the absence of delayed cerebral ischemia in perimesencephalic subarachnoid hemorrhage.

Finally, the mild clinical features differ in at least some patients from those of ruptured aneurysms: loss of consciousness does not occur (against 50 percent in aneurysmal hemorrhage), and a gradual onset of the headache is more common with perimesencephalic hemorrhage.

ANGIOGRAM-NEGATIVE SUBARACHNOID HEMORRHAGE: A MIXED BAG

Two-thirds of all patients with subarachnoid hemorrhage and a negative angiogram have a nonaneurysmal perimesencephalic hemorrhage. Most of the remaining one-third have aneurysms that for some reason do not show up on angiography, perhaps because of vasospasm or compression from an adjoining hematoma. The remainder consists of a collection of rarities: vertebral artery dissection, dural arterial malformation, spinal arterial malformation, and pituitary apoplexy. Given this heterogeneity of causes, the blanket term *angiogram-negative subarachnoid hemorrhage* is meaningless, in individual patients as well as in scientific communications.

SUGGESTED READING

Ferbert A, Hubo I, Biniek R. Non-traumatic subarachnoid hemorrhage with normal angiogram: Long term follow-up and CT predictors of complications. J Neurol Sci 1992; 107:14–18.

Rinkel GJE, Wijdicks EFM, Hasan D, et al. Outcome in patients with subarachnoid haemorrhage and negative angiography according to pattern of haemorrhage on computed tomography. Lancet 1991; 338:964–968.

Rinkel GJE, Wijdicks EFM, Ramos L, van Gijn J. Progression of acute hydrocephalus in subarachnoid haemorrhage: A case report documented by serial CT-scanning. J Neurol Neurosurg Psychiatry 1990; 53:354–355.

Rinkel GJE, Wijdicks EFM, Vermeulen M, et al. Outcome in perimesencephalic (nonaneurysmal) subarachnoid hemorrhage: A follow-up study in 37 patients. Neurology 1990; 40:1130–1132.

Rinkel GJE, Wijdicks EFM, Vermeulen M, et al. The clinical course of perimesencephalic nonaneurysmal subarachnoid hemorrhage. Ann Neurol 1991; 29:463–468.

Rinkel GJE, Wijdicks EFM, Vermeulen M, et al. Nonaneurysmal perimesencephalic subarachnoid hemorrhage: CT and MR patterns that differ from aneurysmal rupture. AJNR Am J Neuroradiol 1991; 12:829–834, AJR Am J Roentgenol 1991; 157:1325–1330.

Rinkel GJE, Wijdicks EFM, Vermeulen M, et al. Acute hydrocephalus in nonaneurysmal perimesencephalic hemorrhage: evidence of CSF block at the tentorial hiatus. Neurology 1992; 42:1805–1807.

Van Gijn J. Subarachnoid haemorrhage. Lancet 1992; 339:653–655.

Van Gijn J, van Dongen KJ, Vermeulen M, Hijdra A. Perimesencephalic hemorrhage: A nonaneurysmal and benign form of subarachnoid hemorrhage. Neurology 1985; 35:493–497.

Vermeulen M, Lindsay KW, van Gijn J. Subarachnoid haemorrhage. London: WB Saunders, 1992.

ECLAMPSIA

JAMES O. DONALDSON, M.D.

Toxemia of pregnancy is an idiopathic hypertensive disease peculiar to gravid women, commonly nulliparas beyond the twentieth week of gestation. I prefer toxemia to the term currently in vogue, *pregnancy-induced hypertension* (PIH), because toxemia encompasses the entire spectrum of the disease and its manifestations in multiple organs, sometimes, as in the liver and kidney, in manners unique to this disorder.

The death rate for eclampsia was 30 percent as recently as 1930 and remains 7 percent. The mortality associated with eclampsia is much greater than the 1 to 2 percent mortality of severe preeclampsia, in part because other organs are more seriously involved. Cerebral pathology causes 30 to 60 percent of eclamptic deaths. The hypoxia and lactic acidosis that accompany a tonic-clonic seizure can precipitously worsen an already sick woman. Additionally, fetal bradycardia lasts for 20 minutes following the convulsion.

The basic criteria for the diagnosis of preeclampsia in a pregnant woman are hypertension and proteinuria. Edema has been included by some authorities. However, leg edema is commonplace and has many other causes. Edematous hands and face are more suggestive of toxemia. In mild preeclampsia, proteinuria is best determined by analysis of a 24 hour urine collection, but in more quickly evolving situations this is supplanted by a dipstick. In this instance, determinations at two different times are usually required, mainly because it can be difficult to collect an uncontaminated urine specimen unless the patient's bladder is catheterized.

Obstetricians still argue about blood pressure criteria for toxemia. In the United States, many obstetricians require a blood pressure of 140/90 mm Hg for a diagnosis of mild preeclampsia. However, in the second trimester, when blood pressure typically dips, a diastolic blood pressure of over 75 mm Hg may warrant monitoring. Systolic blood pressures between 160 and 180 mm Hg and diastolic pressures between 100 and 110 mm Hg are commonly used as criteria for severe preeclampsia. More recently, the incremental rise in blood pressure has been incorporated into standard definitions of severe preeclampsia. Heavy proteinuria, thrombocytopenia, and involvement of the liver, lungs, and heart also suggest a patient with severe preeclampsia.

ECLAMPTIC CONVULSIONS

Soon after invention of the blood pressure cuff, eclamptic seizures were found to occur in the presence of arterial hypertension, often following an added rise in an already elevated blood pressure. The blood pressure at which eclamptic convulsions occur varies and is often below levels at which some obstetricians begin to treat hypertension. To internists and neurologists accustomed to evaluating older patients, blood pressures such as 150/95 mm Hg seem commonplace, and acceptable for some patients with chronic hypertension. However, that is significant hypertension for a teenager whose customary blood pressure is 95/60 mm Hg. In the autopsy-proven series collected by Sheehan and Lynch, 26 percent of cases convulsed at systolic blood pressures less than 160 mm Hg. In Nigeria, Lawson considered 125/85 mm Hg to be worrisome and found convulsions to occur at 140/90 mm Hg.

Eclampsia is toxemia severe enough to cause a convulsion. Seizures are often preceded by visual hallucinations, headache, and brisk reflexes. As described by Sir William Gowers in 1888, eclamptic convulsions are generalized tonic-clonic seizures, sometimes with superimposed clinical features of multiple foci activated in succession. For instance, aversive eye movements due to a focus in one hemisphere and isolated limb jerking due to a focus in the other hemisphere can irregularly punctuate successive seizures or a prolonged eclamptic convulsion. In 1928, Oppenheimer and Fishberg understood that the classic form of the eclamptic attack consisted of epileptiform seizures in every way analogous to those occurring in acute glomerulonephritis. They included eclampsia and glomerulonephritis as causes of hypertensive encephalopathy in usually normotensive young patients.

Although a seizure is an important, time-honored criterion for eclampsia, it should be understood that the onset of brain lesions sometimes precedes the first eclamptic convulsion. The traditional definition excludes both visual hallucinations and cortical blindness, even though these are manifestations of lesions in the occipital cortex that are identical to lesions which elsewhere could cause convulsions. Visual hallucinations, usually streaks of light, often precede eclamptic convulsions. More recently, computed tomography (CT) and magnetic resonance imaging (MRI) have demonstrated changes in the brain in toxemic women who have not convulsed. The traditional diagnostic criteria for eclampsia also exclude toxemic women who suddenly become comatose due to a large intracerebral hematoma without convulsing.

PATHOGENESIS

Hypertensive encephalopathy results from the failure of arteriolar vasoconstriction at relatively high blood pressures to limit both perfusion through the capillary bed and the pressure exerted upon capillary endothelial cells. In pathophysiologic terms, the upper limit of the autoregulation of cerebral blood flow is exceeded in hypertensive encephalopathy. The breakthrough occurs first in the occipital lobes and in the watersheds between territories of major cerebral arteries. At higher pressures the process operates throughout the brain, and generalized vasogenic cerebral edema results. The upper limit of autoregulation of cerebral perfusion is directly dependent upon an individual's customary blood pressure. Currently the only method to predict the upper limit of autoregulation for a particular patient is an estimate based on the patient's customary blood pressure. However, this can be unknown for the many women who do not participate in prenatal care.

THE CONSULTATION

In most instances, obstetricians diagnose toxemia and treat eclamptic convulsions without the input of neurologists. The earlier toxemia develops during pregnancy, the more likely it is to be superimposed on another disease, especially vascular diseases such as chronic essential hypertension, diabetes mellitus, and lupus erythematosus. The occurrence of eclampsia in the second trimester in association with a hydatidiform mole has suggested to generations of obstetricians that toxemia is a disease requiring a placenta or placentation onto the uterus and not the presence of a fetus.

Neurologists are usually consulted if the patient has atypical features, focal deficits, impaired consciousness, or convulses more than 24 hours after childbirth. We may have plenty of time to ruminate, or we may be plunged into a desperate situation requiring immediate action. Most neurologists need not be reminded to examine the eye grounds.

Chart Review

When circumstances permit, review the chart with attention to blood pressure, medications, especially magnesium sulfate, level of responsiveness, and evidence of disseminated intravascular coagulopathy (DIC). Tracking the patient's blood pressure can be frustrating because blood pressures are usually recorded in several sites: prenatal record, labor flow sheets, anesthesia record if a cesarean section was done, recovery room record, and postpartum floor notes.

Ventilation is important because CO_2 retention lowers the upper limit of autoregulation. Tachypnea should not be taken as evidence of adequate ventilation, as anyone who takes care of patients with myasthenia gravis knows. Arterial blood gases need to be checked if ventilation is impaired by hypermagnesemia or if respiratory drive is diminished by drugs or disease. Thus, women with severe preeclampsia can convulse in the recovery room following general anesthesia for a cesarean section, with a blood pressure that before anesthesia was evidently within their zone of autoregulation.

Approximately 15 percent of eclamptic women develop DIC, which predisposes a woman whose capillary blood-brain barrier has been damaged by hypertensive encephalopathy to develop intracerebral hemorrhages. Coma due to intracerebral bleeding has occurred hours after eclamptic seizures. Uterine hemorrhage and oozing from venous punctures is uncommon. A platelet count below 150,000 per cubic millimeter is suggestive of

DIC. Remember that baseline plasma fibrinogen levels are increased by 50 percent during pregnancy.

Neurodiagnostic Studies

Usually if a neurologist has been summoned, CT or MRI has been arranged or already performed. CT has the advantage of a faster scanning, and it is an excellent method of detecting major acute hemorrhages. In eclampsia, CT can be normal, show diffuse cerebral edema with slitlike ventricles, or show regions with decreased density denoting increased brain water, sometimes in arcuate bands through the internal and external capsules. CT may not visualize petechial hemorrhages or detect some areas of edema in the cortex. MRI is superior to CT in detecting edema in the cortical mantle and elsewhere in the brain. Single-photon emission computed tomography shows increased perfusion adjacent to abnormal regions on CT and MRI.

The timing of the appearance of cerebral edema is important. Unlike the delay of several days in the CT appearance of cytotoxic cerebral edema following a common ischemic stroke, vasogenic cerebral edema in hypertensive encephalopathy can be apparent on CT immediately after the crisis and often disappears in a few days. This distinction escapes many radiologists, who interpret hypodense areas as cerebral infarctions without considering timing.

The electroencephalogram (EEG) reflects the status of the patient, ranging from mild slowing of the background activity in patients just having difficulty thinking to delta activity in stuporous patients, often prominently in the posterior regions in patients with cortical blindness.

Cerebrospinal fluid (CSF) pressure is normal or increased. The concentration of protein in CSF is typically 50 to 150 mg/dl. A few red cells or pink-tinged fluid is not unusual. A grossly bloody CSF is a poor prognostic sign.

Angiography is discussed at the end of this chapter.

DIFFERENTIAL DIAGNOSIS

The antepartum presentation of toxemia is well known to obstetricians and obstetric nurses. Sometimes the course of mild preeclampsia can suddenly accelerate. Neurologists should understand that postpartum eclampsia, with the first eclamptic convulsions beginning within 24 hours following childbirth, makes up about one-fourth of all cases of eclampsia. In addition to eclampsia, the differential diagnosis of intrapartum convulsions and hypertension includes pheochromocytoma, thrombotic thrombocytopenic purpura, porphyric crisis, and autonomic hyperreflexia in quadriplegics and paraplegics with a cord level above T5 to T6. The differential diagnosis of intrapartum convulsions without hypertension includes:

1. The inadvertent intravenous injection of local

anesthetics in the course of a paracervical or pudendal nerve block

2. Water intoxication—usually large amounts of a dilute oxytocin solution have been administered after fetal death.

3. Epilepsy—1 percent of epileptics convulse during labor, perhaps due to hyperventilation.

Late Postpartum Toxemic Encephalopathy

The diagnosis of toxemic hypertensive encephalopathy is more complicated when it occurs more than 24 hours after childbirth or termination of a molar pregnancy. Almost all of these rare cases have occurred within 10 to 14 days postpartum. Once again, seizures need not occur, but if convulsions do occur the diagnosis can be more specifically called late postpartum eclampsia. Once again the presence of hypertension is important. Causes of postpartum hypertension include cocaine abuse, diet pills with phenylpropanolamine, and bromocriptine for suppression of lactation. Most cases of late postpartum eclampsia in the antiquarian literature were instances of postpartum cerebral venous thrombosis. In Europe and North America, most cases of postpartum cerebral venous thrombosis occur from 4 days to 4 weeks after childbirth. The condition can sputter for days. Headache is common to both conditions. In both situations the severity and nature of the condition may not be appreciated until a seizure demands a diagnosis. The CSF profile and neuroimaging studies may not distinguish between these two possibilities.

If CT and MRI can not establish a diagnosis of cerebral venous thrombosis, arteriography can help to establish the diagnosis. In late postpartum eclampsia, vasospasm is found in large and medium-caliber cerebral arteries, which resembles spasm following rupture of a berry aneurysm. In Europe, this entity is called postpartum angiopathy. Transcranial Doppler studies have shown a marked increase in the velocity of flow in the middle cerebral arteries of women who developed postpartum eclampsia.

PROGNOSIS

Most signs and symptoms of toxemia abate within 48 hours. Hypertension takes longer to resolve but is usually back to customary levels in 2 weeks. Although most women recover following eclampsia and seemingly have no cerebral sequelae, including epilepsy, a few have focal deficits and epileptic foci. A persistent vegetative state is rare.

SUGGESTED READING

Aguglia U, Tinuper P, Farnarier G, et al. Electroencephalographic and anatomo-clinical evidences of posterior cerebral damage in hypertensive encephalopathy. Clin Electroencephalogy 1984; 15:53–60.

Bogousslavsky J, Despland PA, Regli F, et al. Postpartum cerebral angiopathy: Reversible vasoconstriction assessed by transcranial Doppler ultrasounds. Eur Neurol 1989; 29:102–105.

Cunningham FG, Lindheimer MD. Hypertension in pregnancy. N Engl J Med 1992; 326:927–932.

Donaldson JO. Neurology of pregnancy. 2nd ed. London: WB Saunders, 1989.

Fish SA, Morrison JC, Bucovaz ET, et al. Cerebral spinal fluid studies in eclampsia. Am J Obstet Gynecol 1972; 112:502–512.

Lewis LK, Hinshaw DB, Will AD, et al. CT and angiographic correlation of severe neurological disease in toxemia of pregnancy. Neuroradiology 1988; 30:59–64.

Raroque HG, Orrison WW, Rosenberg GA. Neurologic involvement in toxemia of pregnancy: Reversible MRI lesions. Neurology 1990; 40:167–169.

Redman CWG, Jefferies M. Revised definition of pre-eclampsia. Lancet 1988; 1:809–812.

Richards A, Graham D, Bullock R. Clinicopathological study of neurological complications due to hypertensive disorders of pregnancy. J Neurol Neurosurg Psychiatry 1988; 51:416–421.

Schwartz RB, Jones KM, Kalina P, et al. Hypertensive encephalopathy: Findings on CT, MR imaging, and SPECT imaging in 14 cases. AJR Am J Roentgenol 1992; 159:379–383.

CEREBRAL VENOUS THROMBOSIS

JOSEPH P. BRODERICK, M.D.

Cerebral angiography, computed tomography (CT), and, most recently, magnetic resonance imaging (MRI) have revolutionized the diagnosis and treatment of cerebral venous thrombosis. Prior to cerebral angiography, the diagnosis of cerebral venous thrombosis was usually made at autopsy after a progressive history of headache, papilledema, seizures, focal deficits, coma, and death. At autopsy, it was commonly found that hemorrhagic infarction had accompanied thrombosis of the major cerebral venous sinuses. Treatment with anticoagulation was considered controversial because of the risk of exacerbating brain hemorrhage.

This classical clinical and pathologic scenario is now recognized as an uncommon sequelae of cerebral venous thrombosis. Instead, the syndrome of isolated increased intracranial pressure has become the most frequent presentation of cerebral venous thrombosis, and anticoagulation has become the standard treatment for most patients. This chapter outlines the common presentations of and diagnostic approach to cerebral venous thrombosis.

CLINICAL PRESENTATION BY LOCATION OF THROMBUS

The clinical presentation of cerebral venous thrombosis depends on the location and extent of the thrombus within the cerebral venous system. The superior sagittal sinus (Fig. 1), which is involved in more than 70 percent of cases of cerebral venous thrombosis, drains the major part of the cerebral cortices and plays a major role in the reabsorption of cerebrospinal fluid. Obstruction of this sinus elevates intracranial pressure by increasing both intravenous and cerebrospinal fluid pressure. Not surprisingly, the large majority of patients with sagittal sinus occlusion initially present with signs and symptoms of increased intracranial pressure such as headache and papilledema. If the thrombus extends into the superficial cortical veins, cerebral edema, infarction, and hemorrhage may occur. In this latter setting, patients may experience focal or generalized seizures, focal weakness, sensory or visual loss, aphasia, or a change in the level of consciousness.

The lateral sinus (see Fig. 1), which is involved in 70 percent of cases, drains blood from the cerebellum, brain stem, and posterior part of the cerebral hemispheres. As with sagittal sinus occlusion, most patients present with signs and symptoms of increased intracranial pressure. Isolated occlusion of either the lateral or sagittal sinuses is uncommon. Patients often have thrombosis of multiple sinuses or cerebral veins.

The deep cerebral veins and sinuses (see Fig. 1), which are involved in more than 10 percent of cases, drain the deep white matter of the cerebral hemispheres and the basal ganglia. Extensive involvement of this system is almost always associated with headache and changes in the level of consciousness. More severe presentations may include the focal findings of aphasia and hemiparesis accompanied by bilateral or unilateral edema or hemorrhagic infarction of the thalami and basal ganglia on brain imaging. At first glance, the CT or MRI findings may resemble those of bilateral infarction seen with occlusion of the thalamoperforating arteries. However, in cases of deep cerebral sinus thrombosis, abnormalities of the deep sinuses are usually evident on CT or MRI (see below).

The cavernous sinuses, which are involved in less than 5 percent of cases, are located on each side of the sella turcica. They drain blood from the orbits through the ophthalmic veins and from the anterior part of the base of the brain by the sphenoparietal sinus and middle cerebral veins. Cavernous sinus thrombosis usually presents with headache, chemosis, proptosis, and painful ophthalmoplegia, which is initially unilateral but frequently becomes bilateral. Cavernous thrombosis can also present more insidiously as an isolated sixth nerve palsy with mild chemosis and proptosis.

CAUSES OF CEREBRAL VENOUS THROMBOSIS

The known causes of cerebral venous thrombosis can be placed into one of six general categories: infection, inflammatory disorders, structural damage to venous sinuses from local trauma or adjacent lesions, blood disorders (disorders of coagulation and thrombolytic proteins, red blood cells, or platelets), miscellaneous, and idiopathic. The incidence of cerebral venous thrombosis due to bacterial sepsis or localized infection, such as otitis media, has dramatically declined in developed countries with the use of antibiotics. In Ameri and Bousser's series, only nine (8 percent) of 110 cases of venous thrombosis were attributed to infection (see Suggested Reading). However, the skin overlying the face and scalp, the oropharynx, the nose, and the ear should be examined carefully in a patient with cerebral venous thrombosis to rule out a local infectious cause. Spread of local infection from facial cellulitis or sphenoid sinusitis is still the most common cause of cavernous sinus thrombosis.

Inflammatory causes of cerebral venous thrombosis include connective tissue diseases such as lupus erythematosus, Behçet's disease, and sarcoidosis. Although the sinus thrombosis usually occurs in the setting of a previously diagnosed inflammatory disease, it may be a disease's first manifestation, particularly in Behçet's disease.

Head trauma and intracranial operations are two of

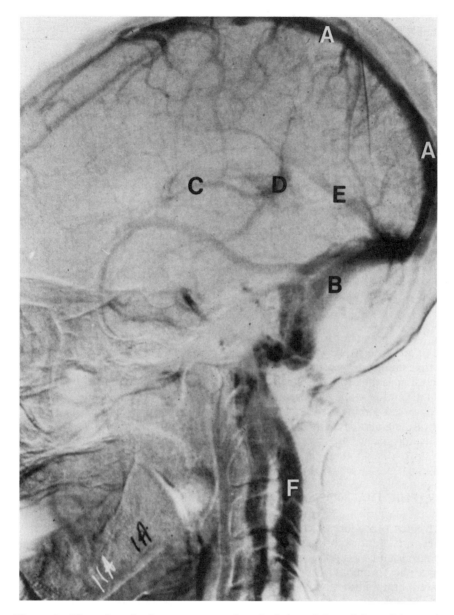

Figure 1 Normal cerebral venous system: *A,* sagittal sinus; *B,* lateral sinus; *C,* internal cerebral vein; *D,* vein of Galen; *E,* straight sinus; *F,* jugular vein.

the most common structural causes of cerebral venous thrombosis. Other structural causes include tumors, carcinomatous meningitis, arachnoid cysts, and local or surgical trauma to the jugular vein.

Hypercoagulability associated with the immediate postpartum period, pregnancy, or oral contraceptives is the most common cause of cerebral venous thrombosis in women of childbearing age. According to Srinivasan, the incidence of cerebral venous thrombosis in the peripartum period in India is about 4.5 cases per 1,000 obstetric admissions, compared to the Western incidence of less than one in 3,000. In Ameri and Bousser's series of 100 patients, nine women (8 percent) had no risk factor for cerebral venous thrombosis other than the use of oral contraceptives. Other disorders of the hemostatic control system that may lead to cerebral venous thrombosis include acquired or inherited protein C deficiency, antithrombin III deficiency, protein S deficiency, sickle cell disease, polycythemia vera, paroxysmal nocturnal hemoglobinuria, thrombocythemia, antiphospholipid antibody syndrome, the nephrotic syndrome, and hypercoagulability associated with malignancy.

Miscellaneous causes include severe dehydration, neonatal asphyxia in infants, and severe heart failure in adults. However, despite extensive diagnostic workups, the cause of cerebral venous sinus thrombosis remains unknown in 20 to 35 percent of cases.

DIFFERENTIAL DIAGNOSIS OF COMMON PRESENTATIONS

Isolated increased intracranial pressure, which occurs in over 40 percent of all patients, is the most common clinical syndrome of cerebral venous thrombosis. Many of these patients receive an initial diagnosis of benign intracranial hypertension or pseudotumor cerebri, but this latter diagnosis should only be made after cerebral venous thrombosis is excluded by an appropriate imaging study. More severe elevation of intracranial pressure, which may be associated with subacute changes in the level of consciousness, can mimic encephalitis or meningitis. Cerebrospinal fluid (CSF) examination can help exclude these conditions.

Focal symptoms and signs indicating unilateral or bilateral cerebral hemisphere involvement is another common presentation, and it may be preceded by signs and symptoms of increased intracranial pressure. Focal presentations include acute stroke syndromes, focal or generalized seizures, or a combination of focal neurologic deficits, change in level of consciousness, and seizures. Determining whether an arterial or venous occlusion is the cause of an acute stroke syndrome may be difficult. Features that should suggest the possibility of cerebral venous occlusion as the cause of a stroke are listed in Table 1. Whatever the clinical presentation, identification of a thrombosed cerebral venous sinus by brain imaging, cerebral angiography, or autopsy is necessary for a definitive diagnosis.

RADIOGRAPHIC DIAGNOSIS

High-quality MRI is the procedure of choice for a patient suspected of cerebral venous thrombosis. MRI noninvasively detects absence of blood flow in cerebral venous sinuses, images the thrombus itself (Fig. 2), demonstrates associated brain infarction, edema, or hemorrhage, detects structural causes of the thrombosed sinus such as tumor, and rules out other conditions such as arterial stroke or abscess. Most importantly, it can be repeated to evaluate resolution or progression of thrombosis.

Selection of the correct MRI protocol is critical, and images in multiple planes and sequences must be evaluated by an experienced physician. For example, on some conventional T1 and T2 weighted MR images, flowing blood can be of high or low signal intensity as well as isointense. These characteristics may also be shared by clots. More recent advances in two-dimensional time-of-flight MRI, phase-contrast MRI, and contrast-enhanced three-dimensional time-of-flight MR angiography (Fig. 3) allow for an accurate picture of the presence or absence of flow within the major venous sinuses. MR angiography may become the gold standard for imaging cerebral venous thrombosis in the near future.

Table 1 Features Suggesting Cerebral Venous Thrombosis as a Cause of Stroke

Papilledema
Bilateral edema, infarction, or hemorrhage in the upper part of the cerebral hemispheres or thalami
Hemorrhagic infarction not conforming to a typical arterial vascular distribution or with surrounding feathered edema
Prominent and persistent seizure activity
Clinical setting, such as the postpartum period
Prominent headache for days prior to the stroke

MRI is not available in some institutions and is usually unobtainable for patients who are intubated or uncooperative. Until the recent developments in MRI, CT of the brain was the initial test of choice in the diagnosis of cerebral venous thrombosis. Like MRI it rules out other conditions such as arterial strokes or tumors and visualizes cerebral edema, infarction, or hemorrhage associated with cerebral venous thrombosis (Fig. 4). With contrast administration, an "empty delta sign" (Fig. 5) may be seen, which represents the opacification of collateral veins in the wall of the sagittal sinus surrounding the nonenhancing clot within the sinus. However, the usefulness of this sign is limited since it is present in only 30 percent of reported cases. In addition, the posterior sagittal sinus divides into two channels in nearly a quarter of normal persons, which can appear as a false delta sign on CT imaging. Other CT findings include contrast enhancement of the falx, tentorium, and small cerebral ventricles. Thus, CT is insufficient in most cases to definitively diagnose cerebral venous thrombosis, and subsequent cerebral angiography is usually indicated.

Cerebral angiography has been the gold standard in the diagnosis of cerebral venous thrombosis for many years. Four-vessel digital or conventional angiography with visualization of the entire venous phase on at least two projections is necessary. Partial or complete lack of filling of a sinus is the classic angiographic sign of cerebral venous thrombosis. However, the anterior part of the sagittal sinus may be absent in normal persons, and nearly a fifth of normal persons have partial or total agenesis of one lateral sinus. Nonfilling of the posterior portion of the sagittal sinus (Fig. 6) or the deep venous sinuses, or multiple sinus occlusions are the most specific radiographic markers of thrombosis. MRI is superior to cerebral angiography in that it not only visualizes the absence of blood flow but also the clot itself. Angiography also carries some risk that the dehydrating effects of the contrast agent may result in progression of the thrombosis.

In summary, MRI is the test of choice for suspected cerebral venous thrombosis. CT, followed by cerebral angiography, is another excellent diagnostic option. If MRI is inconclusive, cerebral angiography should be done.

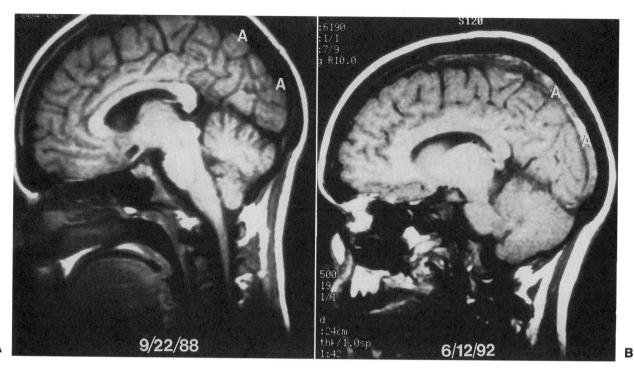

Figure 2 A 22-year-old woman with a normal MRI scan in 1988 presented with sagittal and lateral sinus occlusions in 1992. Sagittal T1 weighted MR images from 1988 show a normal sagittal sinus (*A*), while images from 1992 show a clot within the sagittal sinus (*B*). Patient had marked and progressive increase in intracranial pressure with loss of vision, despite heparin, and was subsequently treated with multiple doses of intravenous tissue plasminogen activator. Patient's condition and thrombus formation stabilized, but the thrombus did not resolve despite thrombolytic therapy. Optic nerve fenestrations and finally a lumbar-peritoneal shunt successfully relieved the patient's symptoms of increased intracranial pressure.

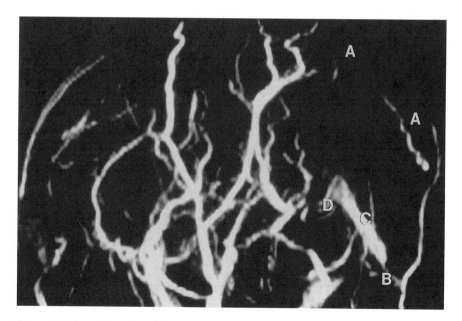

Figure 3 Two-dimensional time-of-flight angiography in patient described in Figure 2. *A,* occluded sagittal sinus; *B,* occluded lateral sinus; *C,* patent straight sinus; *D,* patent vein of Galen.

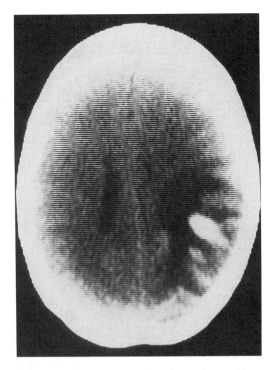

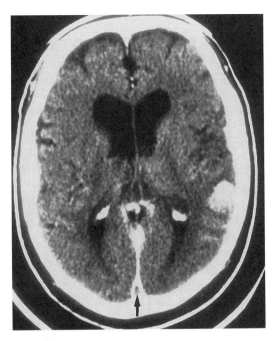

Figure 5 Appearance of delta sign (*black arrow*) in patient with sagittal sinus occlusion.

Figure 4 Hemorrhagic infarction in patient with sagittal sinus thrombosis. Note feathered pattern of edema surrounding hemorrhage, which is atypical for arterial infarction and more typical of edema surrounding a hemorrhagic tumor.

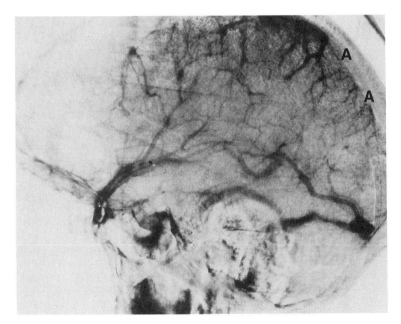

Figure 6 Angiographic appearance of sagittal sinus occlusion (*A*). Note patent deep cerebral veins and sinuses.

OTHER DIAGNOSTIC TESTS

CSF examination is a useful diagnostic, and sometimes therapeutic, procedure. Evaluation of the CSF can exclude infection or leptomeningeal cancer as a cause of the sinus thrombosis. Repeated lumbar drainage of CSF may also relieve the symptoms of increased intracranial pressure. CSF examination should be avoided, if possible, in the setting of an intracranial mass lesion such as a large cerebral infarction or hemorrhage. CSF findings in cerebral venous thrombosis include mild to moderate elevation of CSF protein in two-thirds of patients, more than 20 red cells in two-thirds of patients, and a mild pleocytosis in one-third of patients. Increased CSF pressure is seen in almost all patients with signs and symptoms of increased pressure.

Electroencephalography (EEG) should be obtained in patients with cerebral venous thrombosis who are in coma or have recurrent seizures. Nonconvulsive status epilepticus, periodic epileptiform discharges, or frequent electrographic seizures on an EEG may point to causes of unresponsiveness other than increased intracranial pressure or stroke, and may respond to changes in anticonvulsant therapy.

Other investigations include complete blood count, sedimentation rate, renal and liver panels, prothrombin time, partial thromboplastin time, antinuclear antibody, rheumatoid factor, serum protein electrophoresis, antiphospholipid antibodies, and chest radiography. If an obvious cause of venous thrombosis is not initially found, a more extensive evaluation of the hemostatic and thrombolytic systems should be performed. If hemostatic abnormalities are detected, long-term anticoagulation will likely be needed.

OUTCOME

In recent series of cerebral sinus thrombosis, the reported mortality was between 6 and 30 percent. Factors related to poor prognosis include involvement of deep cerebral sinuses, coma, a large intracerebral hemorrhage or cerebral infarction, patient age (infants and the very elderly), and the underlying cause. For example, septic cerebral venous thrombosis still has a mortality of at least 30 percent. For those patients who do survive, the outcome is usually good with full recovery in more than three-quarters of patients. Persistent deficits in some patients can include optic nerve atrophy, hemiparesis, or epilepsy.

SUGGESTED READING

Ameri A, Bousser MG. Cerebral venous thrombosis. Neurol Clin 1992; 10(1):87–111.

Barnwell S, Higashida R, Halbach V, et al. Direct endovascular thrombolytic therapy for dural sinus thrombosis. Neurosurg 1991; 28:135–142.

Bousser MG, Chiras J, Bories J, Castaigne P. Cerebral venous thrombosis: A review of 38 cases. Stroke 1985; 16:199–213.

Einhaupl K, Villringer A, Meister W, et al. Heparin treatment in sinus venous thrombosis. Lancet 1991; 338:597–600.

Enevoldson TP, Russell RW. Cerebral venous thrombosis: New causes for an old syndrome? Q J Med 1990; New Series 77 (284):1255–1275.

Erbguth F, Brenner P, Schuierer G, et al. Diagnosis and treatment of deep cerebral vein thrombosis. Neurosurgery 1991; Rev. 14: 145–148.

Gates PC. Cerebral venous thrombosis: A retrospective review. Aust N Z J Med 1986; 16:766–770.

Hanley D, Feldman E, Borel C, et al. Treatment of sagittal sinus thrombosis associated with cerebral hemorrhage and intracranial hypertension. Stroke 1988; 19:903–909.

Levine SR, Twyman RE, Gilman S. The role of anticoagulation in cavernous sinus thrombosis. Neurol 1988; 38:517–522.

Srinivasan K. Cerebral venous and arterial thrombosis in pregnancy and puerperium: A study of 135 patients. Angiology 1983; 731–746.

CEREBRAL VASCULAR ANOMALIES

CAMILO R. GOMEZ, M.D.
ROEKCHAI TULYAPRONCHOTE, M.D.

Congenital vascular anomalies result from faulty development of blood vessels in utero. Various types of anomalies have been identified in the brain, their specific morphology depending on the aberrant stage of cerebrovascular embryogenesis. *Arteriovenous malformations* (AVMs) represent direct communications between arterial and venous systems, without the interposition of arteriolar and capillary beds. *Venous angiomas* consist of anomalous veins, usually arranged in a radial pattern, which empty into a central draining vein. *Cavernous angiomas* (or malformations) are composed of thin-walled vascular channels without smooth muscle or brain tissue in their interstices. Finally, *capillary telangiectasias* are small dilated capillary blood vessels separated by normal neural parenchyma, sometimes drained by enlarged tortuous veins.

CLINICAL PRESENTATION

The natural history of any congenital vascular anomaly varies according to its type. In general, an asymptomatic period of variable length is followed by the development of acute symptoms determined by propensity to bleed or to induce dysfunction of the neighboring neurologic tissue (Table 1). Some vascular anomalies are often found coincidentally during the evaluation of patients for unrelated reasons.

Arteriovenous Malformations

The symptoms produced by an AVM are quite variable and depend upon its size and location. The overwhelming majority of cerebral AVMs are located above the tentorium. With the exception of children younger than 2 years of age, in whom congestive heart failure or hydrocephalus may dominate the clinical picture, the majority of patients afflicted by AVMs will present with symptoms of subarachnoid or intraparenchymal hemorrhage. The specific deficit will directly reflect the area of the brain in which the hemorrhage occurs, and the presentation is commonly highlighted by headache, nausea, vomiting, and alteration of consciousness. Less commonly, seizures of the partial motor or

Table 1 Morbidity and Mortality Associated with Various Congenital Vascular Anomalies

Anomaly	Rupture Rate	Morbidity	Death Rate
Arteriovenous malformation	3–4%/year	2%	1%/year
Venous angioma	Unknown	Unknown	Unknown
Cavernous angioma	1%/lesion/year	Unknown	Unknown

partial complex type, often with secondary generalization, are the initial manifestation of an AVM. The seizure focus can typically be traced to the area adjacent to the AVM, reflecting perhaps the local metabolic disturbance caused by the malformation. Other symptoms of AVMs include headaches, usually resembling migraine and often associated with exercise.

Venous Angiomas

Although venous angiomas were traditionally considered rare, recent data suggest that they are more frequent than previously suspected. In fact, some authorities consider them the most common type of congenital vascular anomaly affecting the brain, with an incidence approximately four times greater than that of AVMs. The more frequent identification of venous angiomas is due to advances in diagnostic imaging and, consequently, has allowed the recognition of the benign nature of these malformations. The true incidence of hemorrhage related to venous angiomas is not known (see Table 1), but based upon their common coincidental finding, it is estimated to be low. Recently we have also found that patients harboring venous angiomas may present with exercise-induced headaches.

Cavernous Angiomas

Cavernous angiomas represent 10 to 15 percent of all congenital cerebrovascular anomalies. Their clinical presentation most often includes seizures (35 to 50 percent) or hemorrhage (15 to 25 percent). Two distinct types, isolated and familial, have been described. Although they can be asymptomatic, they can produce hemorrhages with an incidence somewhat less than that of AVMs. Familial cavernous angiomas or the presence of multiple lesions increases the risk of intracranial hemorrhage. Patients may present with seizures refractory to treatment with antiepileptic medications and may require surgical removal of the malformation in order to achieve seizure control.

Capillary Telangiectasias

The overwhelming majority of capillary telangiectasias are small and clinically silent, being found inciden-

tally during autopsy of middle-aged and elderly persons. They have a predilection to be located in the pons, cerebral cortex, and white matter. Their clinical importance is limited, with the exception of a rare familial condition in which they can be found in multiple locations within the nervous system: hereditary hemorrhagic telangiectasia (Rendu-Osler-Weber disease).

DIAGNOSTIC PROCEDURES

The diagnosis of congenital vascular anomalies depends on their identification with imaging techniques capable of studying the anatomic or physiologic characteristics of the cerebral blood vessels. In general, the diagnostic procedures available for the evaluation of these patients can be classified as invasive or noninvasive. The former category comprises cerebral angiography only, but the latter includes radiologic (computed tomography), ultrasonic (transcranial Doppler), and magnetic (magnetic resonance imaging and magnetic resonance angiography) techniques. The proper utilization of these diagnostic procedures depends on the specific patient, his or her clinical presentation and general health status, the type of malformation suspected, and the proposed therapeutic strategy.

Computed Tomography

Computed tomography (CT) is a radiographic technique that measures of the density of tissue and displays it in highly detailed two-dimensional images. The administration of intravenous contrast agents also permits the assessment of vascular structures and their anomalies and the identification of abnormalities of the blood-brain barrier. The great majority of AVMs (approximately 85 percent) can be diagnosed by CT, particularly when the test is performed following the administration of intravenous contrast. If the CT is performed without contrast, only very large AVMs or the hemorrhages that they produce will be readily identified (Fig. 1). In addition, the CT may show areas of calcification within the anomaly and, in patients who have had previous hemorrhages, areas of hypodensity corresponding to encephalomalacia. Some patients may also present with hydrocephalus, which is easily diagnosed by unenhanced CT. Characteristically, the CT performed with contrast shows an enhancing lesion of irregular margins with serpentine vascular channels (Fig. 2A). Even in patients who have suffered intracerebral hemorrhages from the AVM, enhancement of the lesion may reveal its presence within the hematoma.

Venous angiomas are usually only identified if the CT is performed with contrast. The draining vein typically appears as a discrete rectilinear or slightly curved vascular structure, sometimes close to the cortical surface, sometimes located deep within the cerebral hemispheres (Fig. 3A). Cavernous angiomas may be shown as small areas of calcification that develop extensive contrast enhancement, often involving the cortex and resem-

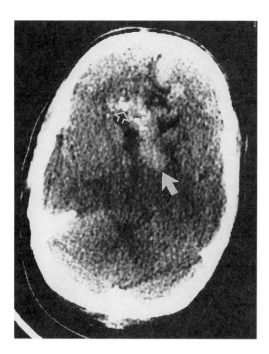

Figure 1 Computed tomography (CT) without contrast of a patient with a large arteriovenous malformation (AVM) located deep in the brain parenchyma. Dilated blood vessels are readily apparent (*white arrow*) and so are calcifications (*open arrow*).

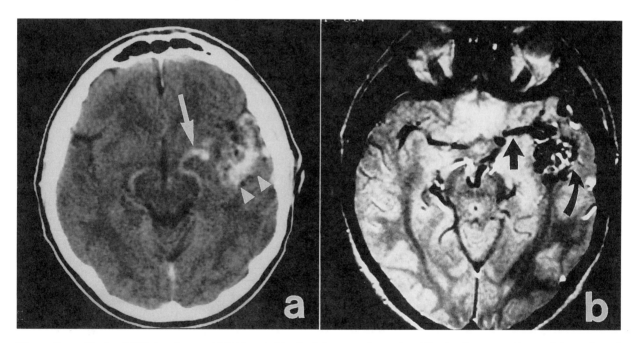

Figure 2 *a,* Contrast CT showing an AVM located in the left opercular region. The feeding artery is noted (*arrow*), and the nidus is well delineated (*arrowheads*). *b,* Spin-density magnetic resonance imaging (MRI) of an opercular AVM showing the feeding artery (*straight arrow*) and the nidus (*curved arrow*).

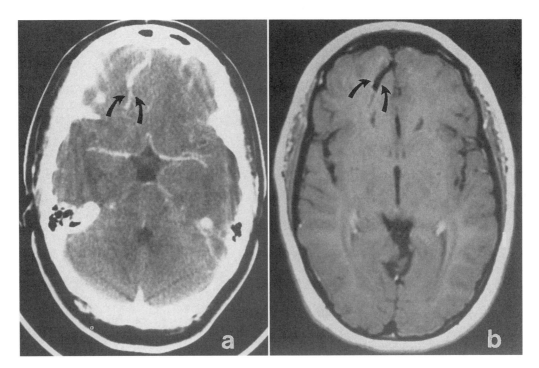

Figure 3   *a,* Contrast CT showing a right frontal venous angioma (*arrows*). *b,* T1 weighted MRI showing the venous angioma as an area of signal void (*arrows*).

bling a tumor (Fig. 4). For the most part, capillary telangiectasias are not readily identified using CT.

Magnetic Resonance Imaging

Magnetic resonance imaging (MRI) is based on the effect radiofrequency waves have on the magnetic behavior of protons located within the human body. Typically, the MRI study of patients harboring AVMs yields images of the brain parenchyma surrounding an area of "signal void" corresponding to the vessels that compose the AVM (Fig. 2B). This picture results from the fast flowing blood within the AVM's vascular channels (see the section on transcranial Doppler), the velocity of which impedes acquisition of the time-dependent echo signals necessary to construct the images. The appearance is almost unequivocal in large AVMs, but in the very small ones, distinction from other vascular anomalies becomes somewhat difficult. The addition of the MRI-specific contrast agent gadolinium does not seem to influence the reliability of MRI in detecting this type of vascular anomaly.

Venous angiomas, when studied using MRI, are displayed as single rectilinear, signal-void vascular structures without the convoluted appearance of AVMs (Fig. 3B). The MRI appearance of cavernous angiomas is quite characteristic: a small or moderate-sized rounded lesion with a core of mixed signal intensity, surrounded by a rim of low signal intensity (Fig. 5). The former corresponds to the cavernous vascular channels in which blood flows slowly and which may be thrombosed,

producing mixed signal intensity. The rim is considered to represent hemosiderin-laden macrophages resulting from previous low-pressure hemorrhages, which may have never caused any symptoms.

Magnetic Resonance Angiography

The advent of fast-scanning MRI pulse sequencing, particularly gradient-echo and bipolar flow-encoding echo gradient, has allowed direct vascular imaging, resulting in the development of magnetic resonance angiography (MRA). Essentially, this technique is the antithesis of conventional MRI since it provides images of the flowing blood only, disregarding the stationary structures that surround it. The study of cerebrovascular pathology using MRA is still in its early stages. However, it is already possible to see how AVMs can be identified and displayed in three dimensions using this technique (Fig. 6A). Less information exists regarding the potential utilization of MRA for the diagnosis of venous angiomas, and it is unlikely that it will be of significant assistance in the evaluation of patients with cavernous angiomas or capillary telangiectasias.

Transcranial Doppler

Until now, and perhaps with the relative exception of MRA, the techniques described provide only an anatomic account of the vascular anomaly and its localization with respect to other cerebral structures, an issue of special interest in planning treatment. The

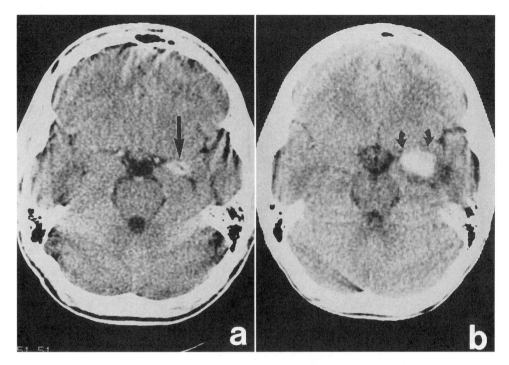

Figure 4 CT of a patient with a cavernous angioma. Before contrast administration (*a*), the lesion is displayed as a round, somewhat calcified structure (*straight arrow*). Following intravenous contrast (*b*), there is diffuse enhancement, resembling a tumor (*curved arrows*).

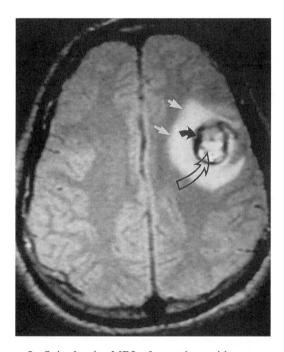

Figure 5 Spin-density MRI of a patient with a cavernous angioma. A reticulated core of mixed signal intensity (*open arrow*) is surrounded by a rim of low intensity (*black arrow*). Some degree of edema also surrounds the anomaly (*white arrows*).

anomalous development of cerebral blood vessels, however, gives rise to aberrant hemodynamics within the malformation. This is particularly true in AVMs, where the direct communication between arteries and veins implies a bypass of the vasomotor arterioles, which provide the resistance of the cerebral circulation. This peculiar arrangement results in drastic changes in the flow dynamics of the arteries that feed the AVM and makes these anomalies detectable by physiologic vascular tests such as transcranial Doppler (TCD). Characteristically, examination of an AVM-feeding vessel using TCD leads to the identification of greatly elevated blood flow velocities, concurrent with a decrease in pulsatility reflective of the decreased resistance secondary to the absence of vasomotor arterioles (Fig. 7). In addition, changes in the partial pressure of carbon dioxide will have little or no effect upon the TCD-measured blood flow velocities of AVM feeders, also because of the absence of vasomotor vessels. It is important to note that if the AVM is of very small size, the changes incurred by the feeding vessels may not be detectable with conventional TCD. In general, other types of vascular anomalies do not display any significant hemodynamic changes that would make them readily apparent to TCD examination.

Cerebral Angiography

In spite of advances in noninvasive imaging, cerebral angiography remains the definitive test for the evalua-

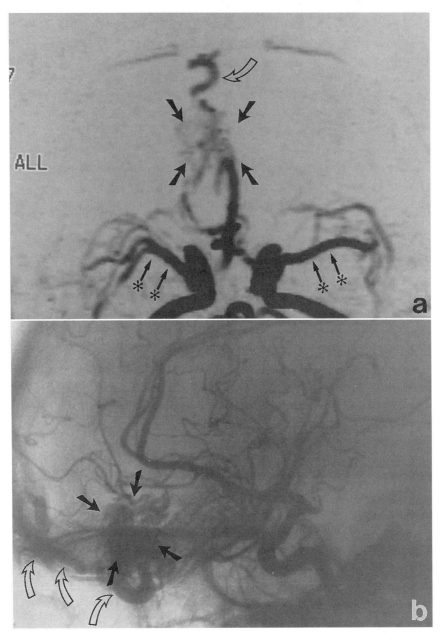

Figure 6 Magnetic resonance angiography (MRA) (*a*) and angiogram (*b*) of a patient with a frontal AVM are shown. Note how both tests display the AVM nidus (*confluent black arrows*), as well as a large draining vein (*open arrows*). The middle cerebral arteries are noted (**).

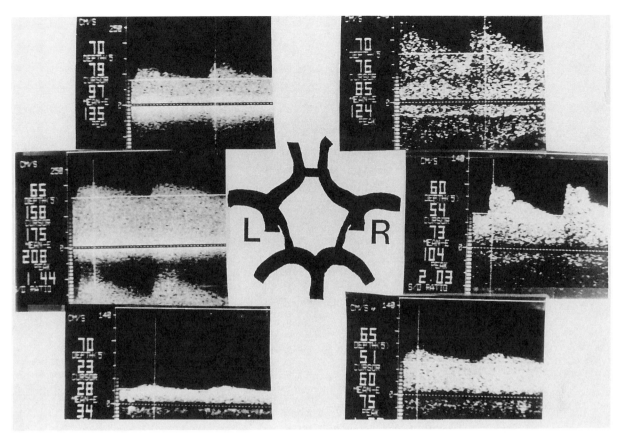

Figure 7 Transcranial Doppler (TCD) of a patient with an AVM in the left sylvian fissure. Note the high velocities and low pulsatility found in the left middle cerebral artery (*left, center panel*), the main feeding vessel.

tion of vascular anomalies. The techniques utilized include subtraction film screen angiography and intra-arterial digital subtraction angiography (DSA). The latter provides a good survey but does not give sufficient detail, and we prefer to make decisions regarding care based upon the subtraction "cut" films. Angiography carries a relatively low morbidity and mortality in expert hands and provides extremely detailed information about the vessels that constitute the anomaly. In patients with AVMs, angiography will show the main feeding and draining vessels (Fig. 6B). The absence of resistance vasomotor arterioles leads to the angiographic picture of early draining veins. Whenever performed, cerebral angiography should include as selective a series of injections as possible, not only of the internal carotid artery and its branches but also of the external carotid artery, in order to identify dural feeding arteries. Finally, since the association between AVMs and aneurysms is well established, a comprehensive four vessel angiogram should be carried out whenever possible. When studying patients suspected of having venous angiomas, high-volume contrast injection and delayed venous images are indispensable. It is very unlikely, on the other hand, for

cavernous angiomas to be revealed by any type of angiographic technique.

DIAGNOSTIC STRATEGIES

The presence of congenital vascular anomalies of the brain should be suspected in any patient (particularly of young age) presenting with intracranial hemorrhage or partial seizures. They should also be considered in the differential diagnosis of patients with atypical headaches that follow a vascular pattern or are induced by exercise. The choice of which diagnostic procedure to use for any specific patient depends on many factors, including the mode of presentation, the type of vascular anomaly suspected, the neurologic status and general health of the patient, and the projected plans for treatment. In general, the least invasive tests should be performed first. This not only allows screening of all patients suspected of having a vascular anomaly, but also guides the more focused undertaking of cerebral angiography. An important consideration is the clinical picture that brought the

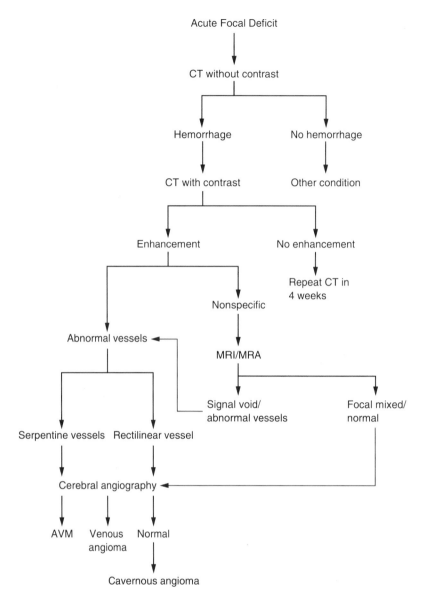

Figure 8 Diagnostic algorithm for patients presenting with acute focal deficits.

patient for evaluation, which appears to us to be the best method for approaching the problem of diagnosing cerebral vascular anomalies.

Patients Presenting with Sudden Focal Deficit

The majority of individuals harboring an undiagnosed vascular anomaly who present with a focal neurologic deficit of sudden onset will be found to have an intracerebral hemorrhage resulting from rupture of the vessels that comprise the malformation. The diagnostic strategy we follow is outlined in Figure 8. Since the majority of these patients are seen as emergencies, the immediate diagnostic procedure of choice is the unen-

hanced CT. If the CT fails to show a hemorrhage, conditions other than a vascular anomaly should be suspected and alternative diagnostic algorithms are recommended. If a hemorrhage is found, and this appears to indicate an underlying vascular anomaly, we recommend a repeat CT following the administration of intravenous contrast. If no enhancement is present, we usually repeat the CT with and without contrast after 4 weeks. The rationale is that the hematoma may have obscured a small anomaly that will be apparent only after resorption of the blood clot has taken place. If repeat CT is negative, patients strongly suspected of harboring a malformation will be tested with MRI or MRA. If enhancement is seen in the original CT, its pattern will

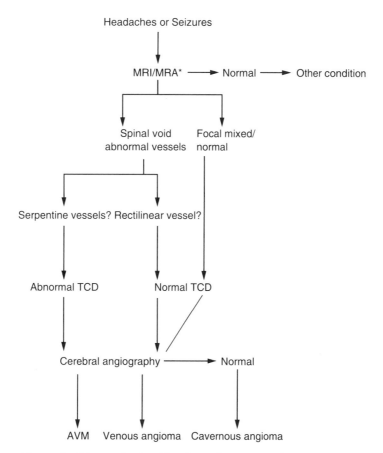

Figure 9 Diagnostic algorithm for patients presenting with headache or seizures.

determine the course to follow. If the enhancement is unspecific (i.e., "blush") we proceed with a combination of MRI and MRA. In some instances, especially if pathology other than a vascular anomaly is a consideration, administration of gadolinium may be helpful. If the CT enhancement or the MRI/MRA results suggest the presence of a malformation, subtraction angiography is the best course to follow. It must be remembered that angiography will be normal in the majority of patients with cavernous angiomas.

Patients with Headaches or Seizures

In contrast to the patients considered above, individuals who present with headaches or seizures are often seen in outpatient clinics, and the diagnosis can be easily made following algorithms similar to that shown in Figure 9. When assessing patients with seizures or headaches, if any feature of the history or physical examination suggests the presence of a vascular anomaly, we start the evaluation with an MRI/MRA. This has the advantage of addressing not only the possibility of vascular anomalies, but also other common conditions that cause seizures and headaches. Again, if the MRI/MRA is completely normal, other conditions should be considered. If, on the other hand, there are abnormalities suggestive of vascular anomalies, we recommend performing a TCD. This not only confirms the diagnosis of AVM in many cases, but it may be of assistance in the follow-up of the patient. As with other patients, however, the definitive test will be subtraction angiography.

SUGGESTED READING

Barrow DL, ed. Intracranial vascular malformations. Park Ridge, Ill.: American Association of Neurological Surgeons, 1990.

Gomez CR, Gomez SM, Rosenfeld WE, Selhorst JB. Cavernous angiomas: Magnetic resonance imaging, transcranial Doppler, and angiographic correlates. J Neuroimag 1992; 2:91–96.

Gomez CR, Malik MM. Exercise-induced headaches and cerebral venous angiomas. J Neuroimag 1992; 2:139–142.

Rigamonti D, Spetzler RF, Medina M, et al. Cerebral venous malformations. J Neurosurg 1990; 73:560–564.

Spetzler RF, Martin NA. A proposed grading system for arteriovenous malformations. J Neurosurg 1986; 65:476–483.

Wilson CB, Stein BM, eds. Intracranial arteriovenous malformations. Baltimore:Williams & Wilkins, 1984.

INFECTIOUS DISEASES

HERPES SIMPLEX ENCEPHALITIS

GREGORY M. BLUME, M.D.
KENNETH L. TYLER, M.D.

EPIDEMIOLOGY AND PATHOGENESIS

Herpes simplex encephalitis (HSE) is the most important cause of fatal sporadic encephalitis in the United States. In the United States and western Europe, the disease affects approximately one in 300,000 individuals per year, accounting for about 10 to 20 percent of all cases of viral encephalitis. Males and females are affected with equal frequency. HSE shows a bimodal age distribution, with nearly half the cases occurring in patients above the age of 50 and one-third in those below the age of 20. Unlike arboviral infections, which are typically clustered in the summer months, cases of HSE are equally distributed throughout the year and show no seasonal or particular geographic preferences. Herpes simplex virus (HSV) 1, which is responsible for the majority of nongenital infections with HSV, is also responsible for the vast majority of cases of HSE and is the focus of the subsequent discussion. HSV 2 is responsible for neonatal HSE in infants with disseminated herpes infections.

HSV is a ubiquitous pathogen, with humans serving as the only natural host and source of transmission. Infection is presumed to occur through respiratory droplet aerosols or through direct contact with infectious oropharyngeal secretions. By adolescence, 70 to 90 percent of most populations worldwide have serological evidence of previous HSV 1 infection, which typically presents as gingivostomatitis. Following this primary infection the virus becomes latent, notably in the trigeminal ganglion. It is estimated that one-third of infected individuals will subsequently develop recurrent disease, usually in the form of herpes labialis. It is important to recognize that despite the widespread distribution of HSV, encephalitis is an astonishingly rare complication of infection. About two-thirds of cases appear to result from reactivation of latent infection in seropositive individuals, with the remainder apparently due to de novo primary infection. The events that determine why only occasional individuals develop central nervous system (CNS) infection remain unknown. The process by which HSV gets from sites of latency or primary infection to the CNS has not been definitively established. It is generally accepted that the virus reaches the brain through the nerves rather than through the bloodstream. The virus may spread either from the olfactory mucosa along the olfactory bulbs to the brain or via tentorial branches from the trigeminal nerve innervating the dura of the middle and anterior fossae. Either of these pathways would explain the predilection of HSV for the temporal and orbitofrontal lobes.

CLINICAL FEATURES

Untreated, the mortality of HSE can exceed 80 percent, leaving many of the survivors with severe residual neurologic sequelae. The untreated disease classically follows a relentless course of neurologic deterioration proceeding toward coma and death. Because of the high morbidity and mortality of this disease, as well as the advent of effective antiviral therapy with acyclovir (ACV), HSE is thought of almost immediately when clinicians are faced with certain clinical presentations. HSE is invariably considered whenever a patient presents with fever, headache, altered consciousness, and focal seizures, or any acute focal findings suggesting pathology in the frontal or temporal lobes. It may present abruptly or following several days of an influenza-like prodrome. The basic clinical features are summarized in Table 1. The classic clinical presentation, which occurs in the majority of patients, is one of fever, headache, and alteration of consciousness. More than two-thirds of cases will have a history of seizures, personality change, and dysphasia. Other common findings include autonomic dysfunction, ataxia, hemiparesis, cranial nerve deficits, and memory loss. Unfortunately, the majority of these findings are nearly as common in patients with non-HSV encephalitis as in those with HSE (see Table 1). Additional findings suggestive of frontotemporal pathology, which have been reported with HSE but which are not specific for the disease, include olfactory or gustatory hallucinations,

Table 1 Clinical Features of Herpes Simplex Encephalitis

	Number (%) of Patients	
	Brain Biopsy Positive	*Brain Biopsy Negative*
Historical findings		
Alteration of consciousness	109/112 (97)	82/84 (98)
CSF pleocytosis	107/110 (97)	71/82 (87)
Fever	101/112 (90)	66/85 (78)
Headache	89/110 (81)	56/73 (77)
Personality change	62/87 (71)	44/65 (68)
Seizures	73/109 (67)	48/81 (59)
Vomiting	51/111 (46)	38/82 (46)
Hemiparesis	33/100 (33)	19/72 (26)
Memory loss	14/59 (24)	9/47 (19)
Clinical findings at presentation		
Fever	101/110 (92)	64/79 (81)
Personality change	69/81 (85)	43/58 (74)
Dysphasia	58/76 (76)	36/54 (67)
Autonomic dysfunction	53/88 (60)	40/71 (56)
Ataxia	22/55 (40)	18/45 (40)
Hemiparesis	41/107 (38)	24/81 (30)
Seizures	43/112 (38)	40/85 (47)
Focal	28	13
Generalized	10	14
Both	5	13
Cranial nerve defects	34/105 (32)	27/81 (33)
Visual field loss	8/58 (14)	4/33 (12)
Papilledema	16/111 (14)	9/84 (11)

CSF = cerebrospinal fluid.

Modified from Whitley RJ, Soong S-J, Linnemann C Jr, et al. Herpes simplex encephalitis: Clinical assessment. JAMA 1982; 247:317–320; copyright 1982, American Medical Association; with permission.

and anosmia. Although the presence of recurrent herpes labialis is indicative of prior infection with HSV, this finding occurred with equal frequency (22 percent) in both HSE and non-HSE patients and is not helpful in diagnosis.

Atypical presentations of HSE are being more frequently reported. Most reports have been of less fulminant subacute or chronic presentations with varying combinations of lethargy, confusion, and focal findings (particularly those related to the temporal lobe). As newer diagnostic studies, such as polymerase chain reaction (PCR) based assays become more widespread, the clinical spectrum of HSE will probably continue to widen.

LABORATORY DIAGNOSIS

There is no pathognomonic clinical presentation of HSE, and diagnosis therefore depends on the appropriate use of laboratory and radiologic tests. Early diagnosis is of utmost importance because the virus replicates rapidly, and morbidity and mortality are directly related to viral load and the duration and severity of illness prior to instituting definitive antiviral therapy. Traditionally the only definitive method of diagnosing HSE has been through brain biopsy, but recent advances in immunologic and molecular biologic techniques have now provided alternate forms of noninvasive diagnosis that are becoming increasingly available.

Cerebrospinal Fluid

The cerebrospinal fluid (CSF) is almost invariably (in more than 97 percent of cases) abnormal in HSE (Table 2). Typical findings include an elevated pressure, a normal or mildly elevated protein, and a mononuclear pleocytosis with between 50 and 500 lymphocytes per cubic millimeter. In rare cases the initial CSF may be acellular or show a polymorphonuclear predominance. The diagnostic usefulness of red blood cells is probably overemphasized. Although common in HSE, they are also frequently found in cases of non-HSV encephalitis. The glucose is almost always normal, although hypoglycorrhachia has been reported as a late finding in isolated cases. Virus is almost never successfully cultured from CSF. The principal value of cultures and stains is to exclude other potential diagnoses.

CSF can be utilized for a variety of immunodiagnostic tests to detect HSV antibody or antigens. As noted earlier, the majority of patients have pre-existing serum antibodies to HSV. As a result, serum serologies are not of diagnostic value. The presence of CNS HSV infection results in intrathecal synthesis of anti-HSV antibodies. A fourfold rise in CSF HSV-specific antibody titer occurs in the majority of patients, as does an increase in the CSF/serum anti-HSV antibody ratio. The specificity of CSF/serum antibody determination can be increased by adjusting the ratios for nonspecific breakdown of the blood-brain barrier by using CSF/serum ratios of albumin or other antiviral antibodies as correcting factors. Unfortunately, the rate of rise in CSF antibody titers is slow, and nonspecific alterations in the blood-brain barrier result in a significant number of false-positives in patients with non-HSV encephalitis. For these reasons, CSF serologic studies are used primarily to assist in retrospective confirmation of a suspected diagnosis, rather than as an aid in acute diagnosis and management.

A more promising approach is to identify the presence of HSV antigens (typically one or more of the viral envelope glycoproteins) in the CSF. Since the antigens detected are actual structural components of the virus, they would not be expected to be present in cases of non-HSV encephalitis. In preliminary studies, antigen detection has proven to be highly specific, with few false-positives. Tests have detected up to 75 percent of confirmed HSE cases within 5 days of disease onset.

Perhaps the most exciting development in the diagnosis of HSE has been the use of PCR to amplify HSV DNA from the CSF of infected individuals. A number of studies have now indicated that PCR assays turn positive as early as 24 to 48 hours after the onset of neurologic symptoms in most cases. In the largest study to date, 42 of 43 patients with verified HSE (biopsy or intrathecal production of HSV immunoglobulin gamma G) were

Table 2   Cerebrospinal Fluid Findings in Herpes Simplex Encephalitis

	Common in HSE	Uncommon in HSE
Opening pressure	Elevated	Normal
Protein	Normal or mildly elevated (median 80 mg/dl)	Markedly elevated
Cell count	Lymphocytic pleocytosis (10–500 cells/mm^3)	Neutrophilic pleocytosis or fewer than 10 cells/mm^3 (both may be seen early) >500 cells/mm^3 (seen in only 8%)
Red blood cells	<50 cells/mm^3 in 50% >500 cells/mm^3 in 20%	No RBC
Glucose	Normal	Hypoglycorrhachia in <5%
Antibody to HSV	Serum to CSF ratio <20 in 90% of patients by third week of illness (compare to control antiviral antibody ratio)	—
Viral cultures	Negative	Positive <10%

Modified from Whitley RJ, Soong S-J, Linnemann C Jr, et al. Herpes simplex encephalitis: Clinical assessment. JAMA 1982; 247:317-320; copyright 1982 American Medical Association; with permission.

positive by PCR for HSV. There were no false-positive PCR results in a control group of 60 patients with acute febrile focal non-HSV encephalopathies; 47 of the controls were seropositive to HSV. PCR results remain positive even 2 to 5 days after initiating acyclovir therapy. The PCR technique may be difficult to master but can give preliminary results within 8 hours, though confirmation will take longer. Because of uncertainty regarding a possible "window of negativity," it is recommended that serial CSF specimens be sent for PCR early in the course of illness. If these results can be replicated in general diagnostic laboratory practice, this will become the procedure of choice for diagnosis of HSE.

Electroencephalogram

The electroencephalogram (EEG) is a useful test in HSE because it is abnormal in 80 to 90 percent of cases. The abnormality generally takes the form of spikes, sharp waves, or spike and slow wave complexes seen over one or both temporal lobes. These abnormalities often evolve into periodic lateralized epileptiform discharges (PLEDS), which, when seen in the context of an acute encephalopathy, are very suggestive of HSE.

Computed Tomography and Magnetic Resonance Imaging

Radiologic tests are of crucial importance in localization of disease prior to biopsy, but no scanning procedure has proven specific or sensitive enough to be reliably diagnostic. Computed tomography (CT) scans may show focal low density lesions, contrast enhancing lesions, areas of hemorrhage, or areas suggestive of mass effect and edema. However, only about 60 percent of patients with biopsy-proven HSE have abnormal CT scans, and distinctive CT findings are often not present at the onset of illness. Growing experience with magnetic resonance imaging (MRI) indicates that it is more sensitive than CT in defining early lesions and the extent

of tissue abnormalities. When available, MRI should be the diagnostic imaging procedure of choice in suspected cases of HSE.

Brain Biopsy

Brain biopsy has traditionally been considered the gold standard for the diagnosis of HSE because of its high degree of sensitivity and specificity. Biopsy material is used for histopathologic study (e.g., detection of Cowdry type A intranuclear inclusions), HSV antigen detection by immunocytochemistry or immunofluorescence, electron microscopy, and culture. When performed by experienced neurosurgeons in major clinical centers, the risk of the procedure has been surprisingly low, with complications reported in only 0 to 3 percent of patients. Although typically minor, these may include hemorrhage, brain herniation secondary to edema, wound dehiscence, and problems secondary to general anesthesia. False-negative brain biopsies may occur when samples are taken from noninvolved areas. This problem can be minimized by using information obtained from EEG and imaging studies to select an appropriate biopsy site.

The controversy over the use of brain biopsy is based largely on two issues. The first relates to the toxicity of antiviral therapy, and the second to the likelihood that biopsy will reveal previously unsuspected treatable conditions in the patients being biopsied. Current evidence suggests that ACV is a relatively nontoxic antiviral agent (see below). However, data concerning potential long-term adverse effects, if any, are not yet available. Widespread and nonspecific use of ACV may also contribute to the emergence of pathogenic ACV-resistant HSV strains. ACV-resistant HSV isolates have already been the source of clinical problems in immunocompromised individuals, including patients with acquired immunodeficiency syndrome.

Data from the NIAID Collaborative Antiviral Study Group trials indicate that up to 40 percent of patients whose biopsy is negative for HSE will have another diagnosis made as a result of the biopsy. In 25 to 50 percent of this group the alternative diagnosis was a potentially treatable illness. Since only about 45 percent of patients undergoing biopsy for suspected HSE have a positive (HSV+) biopsy, these results suggest that 5 to 10 percent of patients with suspected HSE will instead have an alternative treatable diagnosis made as a result of brain biopsy. Interpretation of these data remains controversial for a variety of reasons. Much of the data was accumulated before the widespread routine use of CT and MRI. The availability of these tests would be expected to significantly reduce the incidence of non-HSE diagnoses made at biopsy. The classification of treatable and nontreatable alternate diagnoses is also subject to differences of opinion (Table 3).

Recent attempts to resolve these issues have involved the use of decision analysis techniques. Although also imperfect, these studies do make some interesting points. Perhaps the most clinically useful conclusion is that the higher the likelihood that a patient has HSE based on clinical and laboratory findings, the less the indication for biopsy. Conversely, the lower the clinical likelihood of HSE (e.g., atypical clinical presentation or absence of abnormalities in CSF, EEG, or imaging studies), the greater the indication for biopsy. A practical rule of thumb might be that patients with a typical CSF profile and abnormalities suggesting orbito-frontal or temporal pathology on EEG and MRI should be treated empirically. Patients with an acellular CSF and without typical EEG or imaging studies are far less likely to have HSE and should be considered for biopsy. Perhaps the best hope for clinicians is that the increasingly widespread availability of CSF PCR will liberate us from this conundrum!

PATHOLOGY

The gross pathology of HSE includes inflammation, congestion, hemorrhage, and softening centered asymmetrically around the temporal lobes. Extension into the inferior frontal, parietal, and occipital lobes is often present. There may be clouding and congestion of the overlying meninges. On cut sections, the involvement of the unci, amygdaloid nuclei, hippocampi, insulae, parahippocampal, posterior orbital, fusiform, and cingulate gyri may be seen. After 2 weeks, the areas of involvement may show necrosis and liquefaction. Evidence of subfalcine or uncal herniation may be seen secondary to edema. Microscopic examination initially shows only nonspecific changes, including congestion of small vessels in the cortex and subcortically, sometimes with petechiae. At about the second week, perivascular cuffing with predominantly lymphocytes becomes prominent. As the disease progresses through the second and third weeks, necrosis (often frankly hemorrhagic) and more intense perivascular inflammation are prominent. Gliosis becomes common late in the course of the disease. Cowdry type A inclusions (eosinophilic intra-

Table 3 Alternate Diagnoses in Patients with Suspected Herpes Simplex Encephalitis

Disease	Number of Patients
Treatable	(n = 38)
Infection	
Abscess/subdural empyema	
Bacterial	5
Listeria	1
Fungal	2
Mycoplasma	2
Tuberculosis	6
Cryptococcal	3
Rickettsial	2
Toxoplasmosis	1
Mucormycosis	1
Meningococcal meningitis	1
Tumor	5
Subdural hematoma	2
Systemic lupus erythematosus	1
Adrenal leukodystrophy	6
Nontreatable	(n = 57)
Nonviral (n = 17)	
Vascular disease	11
Toxic encephalopathy	5
Reye's syndrome	1
Viral (n = 40)	
Togavirus infections	
St Louis encephalitis	7
Western equine encephalitis	3
California enecphalitis	4
Eastern equine encephalitis	2
Other herpes viruses	
Epstein-Barr virus	8
Cytomegalovirus	1
Others	
Echovirus	3
Influenza A	4
Mumps	3
Adenovirus	1
Progressive multifocal leukoencephalopathy	1
Lymphocytic choriomeningitis	1
Subacute sclerosing panencephalitis	2

Modified from Whitely RJ, Cobbs CG, Alford CA. Diseases that mimic herpes simplex encephalitis: Diagnosis, presentation, and outcome. JAMA 1989; 262:23; copyright 1989, American Medical Association; with permission.

nuclear inclusions surrounded by a clear unstained zone with a rim of marginated chromatin) may be present. These inclusions are found during the first week of illness in approximately 50 percent of cases of HSE. Electron microscope and immunocytochemical studies indicate that the inclusions are composed of viral proteins and correspond to masses of viral particles that accumulate during assembly.

DIAGNOSTIC CONSIDERATIONS

Only about 40 percent of patients undergoing brain biopsy for suspected HSE have this diagnosis confirmed. Therefore, there are a large number of patients who are suspected of having HSE but who ultimately prove to have another diagnosis (see Table 3). Perhaps the most important treatable group of diagnoses that should be considered are other forms of infection, in particular those caused by bacteria, mycobacteria, fungi, and parasites. It is unlikely that some of the alternative diagnoses listed in Table 3 would be missed if the patients had undergone CT scanning and/or MRI. Current experience suggests that most tumors and adrenoleukodystrophy are unlikely to be confused with HSE.

Our basic diagnostic strategy can be summarized as follows. Patients in whom HSE is suspected on the basis of an acutely altered mental status associated with focal signs or symptoms on history and neurologic examination undergo emergent MRI. If a diagnostic lesion is not found on MRI, and the results of MRI and neurological examination do not suggest the presence of raised intracranial pressure, CSF is obtained for cell count, glucose, protein, culture, stains, and PCR studies. Patients with an appropriate CSF profile (see Table 2) and clinical or MRI evidence of a focal process consistent with HSE are started empirically on ACV (see below) pending results from PCR. Therapy is discontinued after approximately 5 days in patients with negative PCR results and immediately in patients for whom further workup reveals an alternative diagnosis. Patients with atypical CSF findings, and in whom clinical and diagnostic studies do not indicate the presence of a focal process consistent with HSE, are not started on ACV but are followed closely for the development of focal abnormalities. These patients are candidates for brain biopsy. The decision about whether to empirically treat these atypical cases with ACV remains problematic. If brain biopsy is available, these patients should be strongly considered for this procedure. Since their probability of having HSE is low, the likelihood that biopsy may reveal an unsuspected treatable diagnosis is proportionally increased. Some experts advocate instituting ACV therapy in these cases if there is likely to be a significant delay before biopsy can be performed. A brief course (24 to 48 hours) of ACV does not appear to significantly reduce the sensitivity of brain biopsy in the diagnosis of HSE.

SUGGESTED READING

Aurelius E, Johansson B, Skoldenberg B, et al. Rapid diagnosis of herpes simplex encephalitis by nested polymerase chain reaction assay of cerebrospinal fluid. Lancet 1991; 337:189–192.

Booss J, Esiri MM. Sporadic encephalitis I. In: Booss J, Esiri MM, eds. Viral encephalitis. Oxford: Blackwell, 1986:55.

Fishman RA. No, brain biopsy need not be done in every patient suspected of having herpes simplex encephalitis. Arch Neurol 1987; 44:1291–1292.

Hanley DF, Johnson RT, Whitley RJ. Yes, brain biopsy should be a prerequisite for herpes simplex encephalitis treatment. Arch Neurol 1987; 44:1289–1290.

Johnson RT. Herpes virus infections. In: Johnson RT, ed. Viral infections of the nervous system. New York: Raven Press, 1982:129.

Kahlon J, Chaterjee S, Lakeman FD, et al. Detection of antibodies to herpes simplex virus in the cerebrospinal fluid of patients with herpes simplex encephalitis. J Infect Dis 1987; 155:38–44.

Lakeman FD, Koga J, Whitley RJ. Detection of antigen to herpes simplex virus in cerebrospinal fluid from patients with herpes simplex encephalitis. J Infect Dis 1987; 155:1172–1178.

McKendall RR. Herpes simplex. In: McKendall RR, ed. Viral disease: Handbook of clinical neurology. Vol 56/12. Amsterdam: Elsevier, 1989:207.

Nahmias AJ, Whitley RJ, Visintine AN, et al. Collaborative Antiviral Study Group: Herpes simplex virus encephalitis: Laboratory evaluations and their diagnostic significance. J Infect Dis 1982; 145: 829–836.

Rowley AH, Whitley RJ, Lakeman FD, Wolinsky SM. Rapid detection of herpes-simplex-virus DNA in cerebrospinal fluid of patients with herpes simplex encephalitis. Lancet 1990; 335:440–441.

Schroth G, Gawehn J, Thron A, et al. Early diagnosis of herpes simplex encephalitis by MRI. Neurology 1987; 37:179–183.

Soong S-J, Watson NE, Caddell GR, et al. NIAID Collaborative Antiviral Study Group: Use of brain biopsy for diagnostic evaluation of patients with suspected herpes simplex encephalitis: A statistical model and its clinical implications. J Infect Dis 1991; 163:17–22.

Whitley RJ. Viral encephalitis. N Engl J Med 1990; 323:242–250.

Whitley RJ, Alford CA, Hirsch MS, et al. NIAID Collaborative Antiviral Study Group: Vidarabine versus acyclovir therapy in herpes simplex encephalitis. N Engl J Med 1986; 314:144–149.

Whitley RJ, Cobbs CG, Alford CA. Diseases that mimic herpes simplex encephalitis: Diagnosis, presentation, and outcome. JAMA 1989; 262:234–239.

Whitley RJ, Schlitt M. Encephalitis caused by herpes viruses, including B virus. In: Scheld WM, Whitley RJ, Durack DT, eds. Infections of the central nervous system. New York: Raven Press, 1991:41.

Whitley RJ, Soong S-J, Linnemann C Jr, et al. NIAID Collaborative Antiviral Study Group: Herpes simplex encephalitis: Clinical assessment. JAMA 1982; 247:317–320.

CENTRAL NERVOUS SYSTEM HIV AND RELATED OPPORTUNISTIC INFECTIONS

CHRISTINA M. MARRA, M.D.

Patients infected with the human immunodeficiency virus (HIV) are at risk for a number of central nervous system (CNS) disorders. These can present as diffuse processes, characterized primarily by encephalopathy; focal processes, commonly characterized by hemiparesis or visual field cuts; and meningeal processes, usually characterized by headache, stiff neck, and fever. A bewildering array of diagnostic possibilities exists for each category. However, only a handful of diagnoses are most likely. Clues from the history, physical examination, neuroimaging, and routine laboratory tests can often lead to correct diagnosis and successful treatment, as suggested in Table 1 and Figure 1. This chapter focuses on the most common infections of the CNS: acquired immunodeficiency syndrome (AIDS) dementia, toxoplasmic encephalitis, progressive multifocal leukoencephalopathy (PML), and cryptococcal meningitis.

AIDS DEMENTIA

Although the pathophysiology of AIDS dementia is unknown, it is probably a consequence of direct infection of the brain by HIV. Patients usually present with the subacute onset of difficulty with concentration and memory. The patient, family, and friends may note slowed thinking, social withdrawal, and diminished emotional responses. Neurologic examination may demonstrate disorientation, cognitive impairment, slowing of rapid alternating movements of the upper extremities, increased lower extremity tone, upgoing toes, distal sensory loss consistent with peripheral neuropathy, and tremor.

Patients with AIDS dementia almost always have evidence of significant HIV-related immunosuppression, with a CD4 count lower than 200 per microliter. As many as 50 percent of patients with advanced HIV infection develop dementia. Formal neuropsychological tests show difficulties with motor speed and fine control, attention and concentration, and speed of information processing. Computed tomography (CT) and magnetic resonance imaging (MRI) may show atrophy or nonspecific white matter changes. Cerebrospinal fluid (CSF) analysis usually shows a mild increase in total protein (60 to 80 mg per deciliter) and sometimes a low-grade mononuclear pleocytosis. These abnormalities are nonspecific and can even be seen in asymptomatic HIV infection. Recent data from the Multicenter AIDS Cohort Study suggest that CSF beta 2-microglobulin concentrations greater than 3.8 mg per liter are specific for AIDS dementia. Confirmation of the usefulness of this test in clinical practice awaits further study.

AIDS dementia is a diagnosis of exclusion. With the possible exception of CSF beta 2-microglobulin, no test is able to confirm the diagnosis. Neuroimaging and CSF examination are most valuable in excluding other diagnoses. The practical differential diagnosis of AIDS dementia includes metabolic abnormalities and psychiatric disorders. Progressive multifocal leukoencephalopathy can sometimes present with dementia in the absence of focal findings and may have neuroimaging features similar to those in AIDS dementia. Encephalitis should be considered, especially in the setting of fever and CSF pleocytosis, with the most likely culprits being the encephalitic form of CNS toxoplasmosis, and herpes viruses: herpes simplex virus (HSV) types 1 and 2, human cytomegalovirus (CMV) and varicella.

TOXOPLASMIC ENCEPHALITIS

Symptomatic toxoplasmosis in patients with HIV is caused about 95 percent of the time by reactivation of previous infection by the parasite. Reactivation is almost always associated with one or more brain abscesses or, uncommonly, with a picture of diffuse encephalitis. Patients present acutely or subacutely with fever, headache, cognitive changes, weakness, visual changes, or seizures. Neurologic examination often demonstrates hemiparesis or visual field cuts.

Toxoplasmic encephalitis develops in about 10 percent of HIV-infected individuals, usually affecting those with CD4 counts below 200 per microliter. It rarely develops in patients without serologic evidence of previous infection with *Toxoplasma*. Contrast CT scan shows multiple ring or homogeneously enhancing lesions in the basal ganglia or at the gray-white junction. CT less commonly shows single lesions. Multiple lesions are more readily demonstrated by MRI. Toxoplasmic encephalitis is the cause of 60 percent of all CNS mass lesions of any type in patients with HIV. Cimino and co-workers showed that when a lesion enhances with

Table 1 Peripheral Blood CD4 Count and Susceptibility to Central Nervous System (CNS) Disease

	CD4 Count, Cells/μL			
	>500	500–200	<200	<100
Stroke	X	X		
HIV meningitis	X	X		
Syphilitic meningitis	X	X		
Tuberculous meningitis		X	X	X
AIDS dementia			X	X
Cryptococcal meningitis			X	X
Toxoplasmic encephalitis			X	X
Progressive multifocal leukoencephalopathy				X
Primary CNS lymphoma				X

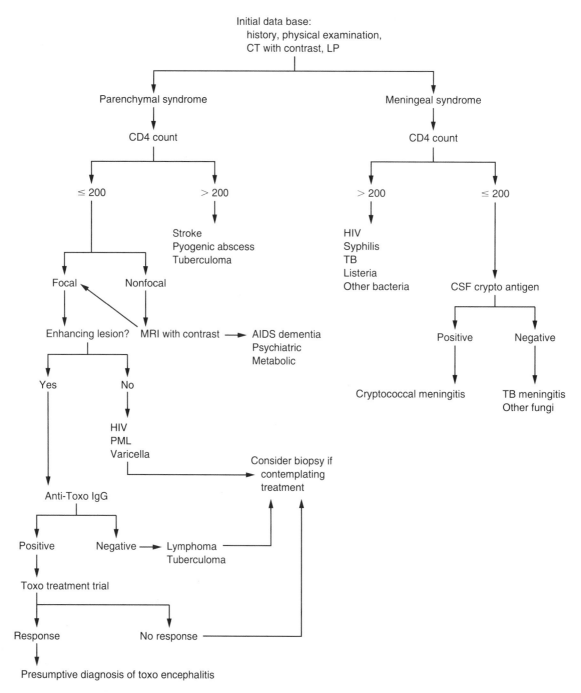

Figure 1 Algorithm for the evaluation of an HIV-infected patient with suspected central nervous system disease. (Crypto = cryptococcal; LP = lumbar puncture; PML = progressive multifocal leukoencephalopathy; Toxo = *toxoplasma*)

contrast on CT in a patient with a high serum anti-*Toxoplasma* IgG titer (greater than 1:64), the probability of toxoplasmic encephalitis goes up to 80 percent. Similarly, when the lesion does not enhance and the serum anti-*Toxoplasma* IgG titer is low, the probability of toxoplasmic encephalitis goes down to 14 percent. Ciricillo and Rosenblum showed that the probability of toxoplasmic encephalitis was only 35 percent when a

single lesion was evident on cranial MRI. Unlike neuroimaging, CSF analysis is not much help in diagnosing toxoplasmic encephalitis. CSF may be normal or show mild increases in cells and protein. Although some authors have demonstrated intrathecal anti-*Toxoplasma* IgG production or identified organisms on cytocentrifuged CSF preparations, these tests are not often useful.

The practical differential diagnosis of toxoplasmic

encephalitis includes primary CNS lymphoma and tuberculoma. The neuroimaging features of primary CNS lymphoma can distinguish it from toxoplasmic encephalitis when an enhancing lesion crosses the midline in the corpus callosum or when a mass lesion is associated with nodular ventricular enhancement. These characteristics have not been reported in toxoplasmic encephalitis. Injection drug users are at particular risk for tuberculoma as are individuals from the developing world and patients with active tuberculosis at other body sites. Less common entities to consider in the differential include metastatic cancer, pyogenic brain abscess, fungal abscesses, herpes viruses (HSV 1, varicella, rarely human CMV), PML, and stroke.

Although definitive diagnosis of toxoplasmic encephalitis can be made by brain biopsy with immunoperoxidase staining for *Toxoplasma,* the diagnosis is usually established by clinical and radiographic response to a 10 to 21 day treatment trial. A major pitfall in using a treatment trial to establish the diagnosis is poor patient selection. Even though toxoplasmic encephalitis is the most common cause of a mass lesion in patients with HIV, it is not the only cause, and precious time can be lost when a patient with a low likelihood of toxoplasmic encephalitis is subjected to an inappropriate trial. Patients appropriate for such an approach are those with multiple enhancing lesions on neuroimaging, detectable serum anti-*Toxoplasma* IgG, and low likelihood of other causes of a CNS mass. Thus a patient with bacteremia or active tuberculosis would be a poor candidate for a treatment trial with anti-*Toxoplasma* medications.

PROGRESSIVE MULTIFOCAL LEUKOENCEPHALOPATHY

PML is caused by a papovavirus that is acquired by about 70 percent of people during childhood. The virus remains latent (in kidney or in brain) and reactivates in the setting of immunosuppression, infecting oligodendrocytes and causing demyelination. PML is seen in about 4 percent of patients with HIV, and most often occurs in patients with CD4 counts below 100 per microliter. Patients complain of cognitive changes, weakness, and visual difficulties. Neurologic examination may identify dementia, hemiparesis, gait disorders, and visual field deficits.

Cranial CT may be normal or may show low-density lesions in the white matter, typically in the parietooccipital regions. MRI more clearly defines one or more white matter lesions that have a characteristic scalloped appearance as the focus of demyelination abuts the gray-white junction. Occasional case reports document involvement of cortical gray matter. Lesions rarely show contrast enhancement, mass effect, or edema. CSF may be normal or show nonspecific abnormalities but does not establish the diagnosis.

The practical differential diagnosis of PML is limited to HIV. AIDS dementia and progressive multifocal leukoencephalopathy can have similar neuroimaging findings. Although focal findings on neurologic examination are common with PML and not with AIDS dementia, the two can be difficult to distinguish clinically when PML presents primarily with cognitive changes. In this setting, biopsy may be required for definitive diagnosis. Rarely, CNS infection with varicella may lead to a subacute, progressive neurologic illness clinically and radiographically similar to PML.

CRYPTOCOCCAL MENINGITIS

Cryptococcus is an encapsulated yeast. It is able to infect many tissues, but lung and meninges are the most important clinically. Cryptococcal meningitis in patients with HIV may represent newly acquired infection or reactivation of a pulmonary source. Cryptococcal meningitis occurs in about 8 percent of patients with HIV, and these patients generally have CD4 counts below 200 per microliter. Patients often complain of headache and fever. Neurologic examination may be entirely normal or show mild meningismus.

Compared to patients without HIV, patients with HIV and cryptococcal meningitis seem to have a higher fungal burden. Blood cultures are frequently positive, and serum cryptococcal antigen is a sensitive test for excluding a diagnosis of cryptococcal meningitis. The number of CSF cells is less than 20 per microliter in 60 percent of HIV-infected patients with cryptococcal meningitis. India ink stain and CSF culture are more frequently positive than in patients not infected with HIV. Cranial CT is usually normal but occasionally shows an enhancing cryptococcoma.

The practical differential diagnosis of cryptococcal meningitis includes HIV, tuberculosis, and syphilis. As discussed above, nonspecific CSF abnormalities due to HIV are common, especially early in the course, with mononuclear cell counts between 10 and 20 and mildly elevated protein. Syphilitic meningitis is probably more common in patients with HIV and syphilis compared to those without HIV and can occur in individuals with relatively normal CD4 counts. CSF abnormalities are similar to those seen with HIV, but the cell count is generally higher and CSF-VDRL may be reactive, especially with longer duration of syphilis infection. Tuberculous meningitis may be seen in those at increased risk for this infection, especially injection drug users. Patients with HIV and tuberculosis are at increased risk for disseminated disease, including meningitis. Unlike cryptococcal meningitis in persons infected with HIV, tuberculous meningitis may occur in HIV-infected individuals with CD4 counts greater than 200 per microliter. Other fungal meningitides, such as those due to *Histoplasma* and *Candida*, CMV, and *Listeria* or other bacteria, should be considered in the differential diagnosis but are uncommon. The diagnosis of *Histoplasma* meningitis can be made by detection of antigen or specific antibody in CSF. CSF culture is positive in 30 to 50 percent of cases. CSF culture is more likely to be positive in *Candida* meningitis. The diagnosis of *Listeria* and other bacterial meningitides in patients infected with HIV is established by culture of CSF or blood. CSF abnormalities in CMV meningitis are similar to those seen with HIV, but ventricular enhancement may be seen on cranial MRI.

A major pitfall in the diagnosis of cryptococcal meningitis is misinterpretation of the cell count or India ink stain. The organism may be so prevalent that yeast is mistaken for red blood cells or white blood cells and the opportunity for rapid diagnosis missed.

COMMENTS

Although the differential diagnosis for processes affecting the CNS in patients with HIV can be extensive, the clues provided by a combination of clinical, neuroimaging, and laboratory data can often lead to a correct diagnosis. An algorithm for evaluation of such patients is shown in Figure 1.

SUGGESTED READING

Berenguer J, Moreno S, Laguna F, et al. Tuberculous meningitis in patients infected with the human immunodeficiency virus. N Engl J Med 1992; 326:668–672.

Berger JR, Kaszovitz B, Donovan-Post MJ, Dickinson G. Progressive multifocal leukoencephalopathy associated with human immunodeficiency virus infection: A review of the literature with a report of sixteen cases. Ann Intern Med 1987; 107:78–87.

Cimino C, Lipton RB, Williams A, et al. The evaluation of patients with human immunodeficiency virus-related disorders and brain mass lesions. Arch Intern Med 1991; 151:1381–1384.

Ciricillo SF, Rosenblum ML. Imaging of solitary lesions in AIDS (letter). J Neurosurg 1991; 74:1029.

Grant IH, Armstrong D. Fungal infections in AIDS: Cryptococcosis. Infect Dis Clin North Am 1988; 2:457–464.

Gray F, Gherardi R, Wingate E, et al. Diffuse "encephalitic" cerebral toxoplasmosis in AIDS: Report of four cases. J Neurol 1989; 236:273–277.

Ho DD, Bredesen DE, Vinters HV, Daar ES. The acquired immunodeficiency syndrome (AIDS) dementia complex. Ann Intern Med 1989; 111:400–410.

Kieburtz KD, Epstein LG, Gelbard HA, Greenamyre JT. Excitotoxicity and dopaminergic dysfunction in the acquired immunodeficiency syndrome dementia complex: Therapeutic implications. Arch Neurol 1991; 48:1281–1284.

Luft BJ, Remington JS. Toxoplasmic encephalitis in AIDS. Clin Infect Dis 1992; 15:211–222.

McArthur JC, Nance-Sproson TE, Griffin DE, et al for the Multicenter AIDS Cohort Study. The diagnostic utility of elevation in cerebrospinal fluid β2-microglobulin in HIV-1 dementia. Neurology 1992; 42:1707–1712.

Powderly WG. Therapy for cryptococcal meningitis in patients with AIDS. Clin Infect Dis 1992; 14(suppl 1):S54–59.

HTLV-I MYELOPATHY

WILLIAM A. SHEREMATA, M.D.
LAWRENCE S. HONIG, M.D., Ph.D.

The human retrovirus, T cell leukemia/lymphoma virus–type I (HTLV-I), is principally associated with two clinical disorders: an acute, rapidly fatal hematologic disease, *adult T cell leukemia/lymphoma* (ATL or ATLL), and a chronic neurologic disorder, *progressive spastic paraparesis*. More common in the tropics, the neurologic disorder is often referred to as *tropical spastic paraparesis* (TSP), or *HTLV-I associated myelopathy* (HAM) since the recognition of its relationship to HTLV-I. Its cardinal clinical features include the insidious development of lower extremity weakness and spasticity with sphincter dysfunction.

HTLV-I, one of the Retroviridae, was originally identified in cells from an ATL patient and belongs to the subfamily Oncoviridae. It is related most closely to another member, HTLV-II, and less to bovine leukemia virus (BLV). It is only distantly related to human immunodeficiency virus (HIV)-I, the agent of acquired immunodeficiency syndrome (AIDS), HIV-II, and to other animal virus members of the subfamily Lenteviridae. Because most patients with HTLV-I associated disease were born or lived in endemic areas, awareness of its worldwide distribution is essential.

HTLV-I endemic areas are largely limited to tropical and subtropical areas of the world (Fig. 1). This geographic distribution generally coincides with the known occurrence of the hematologic disorder but not completely with the neurologic disorder diagnosed as TSP. Most cases of HTLV-I associated nervous system disease have been recognized in the Caribbean, the Pacific coastal area of Colombia, and southern Japan. Although myelopathy is endemic in Africa and India, only in western Zaire is there any substantial number of retrovirus associated cases.

Prior to the identification of the HTLV-I virus, spastic paraparesis occurring in tropical areas was, and still is, usually designated as TSP. In Jamaica, Cruickshank and co-workers described TSP clinically as "Jamaican neuropathy" in 1956 and went on to describe the pathology in 1964. Evidence of an association of TSP and HTLV-I infection was originally reported by Gessain and co-workers in 1985. Within a few months this was confirmed in Japan, and then again in cases from Jamaica and Colombia. A detailed population survey performed in the Seychelles islands by the National Institutes of Health (NIH) team in 1987 further extended knowledge of this disorder. In 1986, Osame and co-workers in Japan originally proposed the term

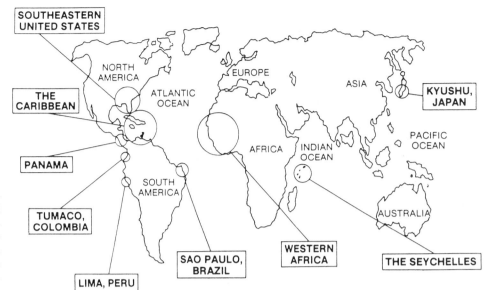

Figure 1 Map showing world-wide distribution of tropical spastic paraparesis (TSP). (From Roman GC. Viral disease. In: McKendall RR, ed. Handbook of clinical neurology. Vol 12(56). New York: Elsevier, 1989; with permission.)

HTLV-I associated myelopathy, or HAM. Following the finding of large numbers in both the Caribbean and Japan, it was agreed that HTLV-I/II seropositive TSP cases and HAM were indeed the same disorder, and a World Health Organization committee accepted the acronym TSP/HAM.

Not all progressive spastic paraparesis patients in the tropics or subtropical areas are HTLV-I positive. Only half of patients show evidence of such infection, and the majority of patients in Africa and the Indian subcontinent are seronegative. Recently, consistent genomic sequence differences between the "cosmopolitan" strain of virus prevalent in the Caribbean and Japan, and the African variant have been shown. However, this finding is unlikely to explain the failure to identify retrovirus infection more often in those populations. Rather, it is likely to reflect different causes within the broad differential diagnosis of myelopathy.

PATIENT CHARACTERISTICS

For practical purposes, we consider the diagnosis of TSP/HAM in all persons who are native to or residing in tropical and subtropical areas and who present with *progressive* gait problems, regardless of any diagnosis previously made. When we began to recognize this disorder almost a decade ago, most patients with HTLV-I infection were either born or had lived in an endemic area, such as the Caribbean islands or Central or South America. With the passage of time, a progressively larger portion of our patient population is American born. However, certain American ethnic groups are known to have a higher HTLV-I/II seroprevalence. These include those of Japanese ancestry in Hawaii, African-Americans in the southeastern United States, and some Native American groups.

TRANSMISSION

As with HIV-I, HTLV-I is transmissible by sexual contact, transfusion, and exposure to blood contaminated objects such as shared drug paraphernalia. Sexual transmission is relatively inefficient, with spouses often being nonseroconcordant. In Japan it has been calculated that about a thousand sexual exposures to an infected male are required for HTLV-I transmission to a female. Study of familial occurrence in Japan has resulted in recognition of mother-to-child transmission by breast-feeding rather than by transplacental or peripartum routes. Infection with HTLV-I probably confers an approximate lifetime risk of myelopathy of about 1 to 4 percent. Evidence of a genetic risk is suggested by human leukocyte antigen studies in Japan, but environmental factors including nutritional status and coexistent infections are likely to be at least as important.

SYMPTOMS

Onset of symptoms may occur at any age, but the initial symptoms typically appear between the ages of 30 and 50 years. Females predominate by a ratio of nearly 3 to 1. Because of the insidious nature of the disease, patients commonly present for medical attention 5 to 10 years after onset of symptoms.

The earliest symptoms of neurologic disease are usually motor in origin. Gait difficulty secondary to slowly progressive bilateral leg weakness and spasticity lead to complaints of leg stiffness, cramps, or pain. Earlier in the course, nocturnal leg cramps may occur in the absence of other complaints. Sensory symptoms are often minimal, but severe back pain may be prominent early in the course of illness. Other symptoms usually consist of numbness and paresthesias in the feet and calves. Urinary symptoms are usually an early feature, with marked frequency and urgency, often rapidly progressing to incontinence. Patients presenting with acute urinary retention often have complicating pyelonephritis or recurrent infections. Bowel complaints consisting primarily of constipation may appear later in the course. In males, sexual dysfunction with erectile difficulties is common.

Less commonly recognized symptoms include tremor, ataxia, and muscle atrophy. Cranial nerve deficits, including visual loss and deafness, have been reported. We have seen retrobulbar neuritis precede the onset of myelopathy by several years, as in multiple sclerosis, but the risk appears to be less than 1 percent. However, visual evoked responses are commonly abnormal, indicating that the disease is more widely disseminated in the central nervous system than is clinically obvious. Cognitive symptoms are rare.

NEUROLOGIC SIGNS

Signs of neurologic disease are predominantly those of a lower cervical and upper thoracic myelopathy, affecting the long white-matter tracts. The mental state is characteristically normal, but the limited educational attainment of many patients and difficulty with English usage may pose important practical limitations in such evaluations. Nevertheless, subtle changes of cognitive function may be detected by neuropsychological examination. Signs of cranial nerve impairment are ordinarily not obvious. However, optic atrophy, nystagmus, and facial palsy have been rarely reported.

Motor examination in the earlier stages of illness usually reveals full strength in the upper extremities contrasting with often prominent hip and knee flexor weakness. These motor findings are often asymmetric initially. Later in the clinical course, foot drop often appears. Tone is increased, often with marked spasticity in the legs. Reflexes are characteristically brisk in all four extremities, although in advanced disease ankle reflexes may be diminished or absent, reflecting either dorsal column or peripheral nervous involvement. Clonus is often present, and Babinski's responses are usually easily demonstrated. The jaw jerk is infrequently exaggerated.

Examination may reveal loss of vibration and proprioception in the feet, although these functions are often spared. Distal loss of pinprick and temperature sensation occur even less often. While a sharp sensory level does not occur, an indistinct thoracolumbar sensory level to pinprick may be demonstrable.

LABORATORY TESTS

HTLV-I/II Antibody

Laboratory examination reveals the presence of HTLV-I/II antibody, or antigen, in both serum and cerebrospinal fluid (CSF). Most ELISA, radioimmunoassay, and even standard Western blot antibody tests cannot distinguish between HTLV-I and HTLV-II with certainty; hence the common reference to "HTLV-I/II" antibody. Recent advances in the use of specific recombinant antigen-antibody tests have provided a less cumbersome and less expensive alternative means of distinguishing HTLV-I from HTLV-II with reasonable certainty.

Polymerase Chain Reaction

Polymerase chain reaction (PCR) detection of proviral DNA in peripheral blood white cells has been considered the gold standard and necessary for certain diagnosis of HTLV-I infection. However, excellent agreement between new recombinant antigen-antibody tests and PCR has recently been established.

Proof of HTLV-I Myelopathy Diagnosis

Virus may be cultured from either blood or CSF, but virus culture is not, and probably never will be, clinically useful. It may be argued that an irrefutable diagnosis requires the detection of antibody or viral antigen by PCR or "antigen capture" in CSF, but this is not necessary in most cases and is beyond the capability of most laboratories at present.

CSF commonly shows a variable, lymphocytic-predominant pleocytosis (5 to 100 cells per cubic millimeter), and mild elevations in protein are frequent. Intrathecal IgG synthesis is often increased, although it may be decreased—indicating the presence of an impaired blood-brain barrier. Some correlation between high levels of intrathecal synthesis of IgG and disease activity is apparent. Oligoclonal bands may be present in both serum and in CSF.

Lobulated lymphocytes of the type seen in ATL have been reported in both CSF and blood, but anything more than the rare cell is unusual. An immunologically stimulated individual will show such cells in very small numbers. The demonstration of significant hematologic abnormality suggests either concomitant ATL or that the myelopathy or other signs are neurologic complications of ATL.

Other Tests

Blood tests for HIV antibody, syphilis (FTA-ABS), and vitamin B_{12} deficiency are especially important and should be performed in all subjects. Some patients with clear laboratory evidence of HTLV-I central nervous system infection may have one of these other conditions concomitantly. Tropical sprue, complicated by intragastrointestinal B_{12} consumption, may be encountered.

Importantly, elevated levels of creatine kinase may identify the occasional case of polymyositis associated with HTLV-I infection. This may be accompanied by myelopathy. Falling or pressure necrosis, which are common, may be the source of such enzyme elevations.

Electrodiagnostic studies usually reveal normal sensory action potentials and nerve conduction velocities, although decreased motor action potential amplitude and abnormal F-responses may be found. Similarly, electromyographic examination is most often normal, although signs of chronic partial denervation may be observed. Somatosensory action potentials are usually abnormally prolonged, malformed, or absent upon lower extremity stimulation and normal upon upper extremity stimulation. Visual evoked potentials are abnormal in a large proportion of cases, but brain stem auditory potentials are less often affected.

Magnetic resonance imaging (MRI) of the spinal cord is usually normal, but cord atrophy may be seen. Rarely, T2 signal abnormalities are seen. Imaging of the brain may show white matter lesions with increased T2 signal, which are often periventricular in location. These are more frequently seen in rapidly progressive cases, such as in our immigrant Haitian population.

Since the manifestations of this illness are neurologic, we will renew the time-honored diagnostic criteria used by the NIH neuroepidemiologic team.

Table 1 Clinical Criteria for Diagnosis of Tropical Spastic Paraparesis

1. Absence of a history of difficulty walking or running during school age
and
2. At least *two* of the following within 2 years of onset
   a. Increasing urinary frequency, nocturia, or retention, with or without penile impotence
   b. Leg cramps or low back pain
   c. Symmetric weakness of the lower extremities within 6 months of onset of the disease
   d. Complaints of numbness or dysesthesias of legs or feet
and
3. A clinical examination revealing
   a. Increased patellar reflexes
   b. Spasticity of both legs (usually manifested by spastic gait)
   c. Absence of a sensory level, pupillary abnormalities, and optic disc changes
and
4. Absence of a history of relapses

Table 2 Workup of HTLV-I Associated Myelopathy

1. History and neurologic examination
2. Magnetic resonance imaging of brain and spinal cord (exclude structural lesion)
3. Lumbar puncture (exclude other meningitides)
4. Determination of HTLV-I infection status
   a. Serologic screening: serum and CSF (ELISA, RIA, Western blot)
   b. Confirmatory testing (recombinant antigen, Western blot, or polymerase chain reaction)
   c. Viral culture (peripheral blood or CSF mononuclear cells)
5. Clinical follow-up

CSF = cerebrospinal fluid, RIA = radioimmunoassay.

DIAGNOSTIC CRITERIA FOR TROPICAL SPASTIC PARAPARESIS

Although the terms HTLV-I associated myelopathy and TSP are often used interchangeably, the association of the clinical disorder and HTLV-I by Gessain and co-workers was made serendipitously when they found viral antibody in 13 of 17 TSP cases included as controls for a study of leukemic patients. TSP is a clinical syndrome and is recognized in many geographically separated parts of the world. Immigrants, visitors, and citizens with gait abnormalities who have resided in these areas are the prime suspects for the diagnosis. There are no obvious signs that immediately distinguish those who will prove to be seropositive from those who are seronegative. The clinical criteria for diagnosis of TSP employed by Roman and co-workers for the NIH neuroepidemiologic studies are outlined in Table 1. Although proposed for a prospective study, they provide helpful guidelines in making a clinical diagnosis. An outline for evaluating the patient is presented in Table 2.

DIFFERENTIAL DIAGNOSIS OF HTLV-I MYELOPATHY

Denny-Brown and Spillane, in presenting their experience with prisoners of war, extensively reviewed the subject of TSP to 1947. More recent surveys of the subject by Roman and co-workers identified a wider variety of problems associated with TSP (Table 3).

Table 3 Differential Diagnosis of HTLV-I Associated Myelopathy

Compressive degenerative disease (spondylosis or disk disease)

Neurodegenerative diseases (amyotrophic lateral sclerosis)

Nutritional
Chronic cyanide intoxication
Cobalamin (vitamin B_{12}) deficiency
Tocopherol (vitamin E) deficiency
Lathyrism

Infectious
Viral (HIV, VZV, HSV)
Bacterial (syphilis, tuberculoma)
Fungal (cryptococcoma, coccidioidomycosis)
Parasitic (strongyloidosis, schistosomiasis)

Inflammatory
Idiopathic transverse myelitis
Multiple sclerosis
Systemic lupus
Sarcoidosis

Neoplastic disease (extramedullary or intramedullary tumors)

Vascular disease (ischemic infarct, arteriovenous malformation)

HIV = human immunodeficiency virus, VZV = varicella zoster virus; HSV = herpes simplex virus.

Myelopathy in HTLV-I endemic regions engenders a broad differential diagnosis, since many conditions may be associated with or confounded with TSP/HAM.

Compressive myelopathy is always a major consideration in the differential diagnosis in patients with progressive myelopathies. The advent of MRI has eased the task of identifying clinically significant intervertebral disk protrusions or spondylolisthesis, and spinal canal tumors can easily be differentiated from syringomyelia and intraparenchymal neoplasms. However, spinal cord lesions having increased T2 signal, with or without contrast enhancement, must not automatically be assumed to represent spinal cord tumors, since they may represent demyelinating lesions associated with edema. Reviewing the history and performing other paraclinical tests in a search for evidence of disseminated disease is most helpful. Follow-up MRI examinations can reveal changes in spinal cord size and signal characteristics. Spinal cord compression secondary to lymphoma must always be considered. The hematologic manifestations of leukemia-lymphoma may be overlooked, particularly in cases presenting with paraplegia. We have also seen seropositive patients with ATL presenting with myelopathy secondary to spinal cord compression.

Nutritional problems have been proposed as causative factors. Malnutrition, once of overriding concern in spastic paraparesis in the tropics and other areas, may be less important. However, pellagra, vitamin B_{12} and vitamin E deficiencies, and possibly other nutritional disorders undoubtedly still occur. *Toxins* in foodstuffs are also factors. Lathyrism, secondary to consumption of flour made from the sweet (chick) pea, has not been seen in North America and disappeared from Europe during the Middle Ages, but it still occurs in India. Aflatoxin, from fungal contamination of nuts, has been described as producing a subacute myelopathy in Thailand. Compelling evidence implicating cyanogenic diets producing chronic cyanide intoxication in some areas has been reported. Conceivably these factors may act as cofactors in HTLV-I infected individuals.

Vitamin B_{12} deficiency may cause subacute combined degeneration of the spinal cord. The symptoms of dorsal column sensory involvement may be less obvious than those due to pyramidal tract involvement. B_{12} deficiency may result from inadequate diet, tropical sprue, or gastric surgery in younger patients. Classic pernicious anemia with atrophic gastritis must also be considered in older patients. B_{12} deficiency should always be ruled out by serum studies.

Vitamin E deficiency is a rare cause of myelopathy, typically found in children with a malabsorption syndrome. Since animal fat is our major source of this essential vitamin, dietary elimination of animal fat has been utilized to produce experimental models in primates. Demyelination as well as motor neuron damage has been demonstrated. Serum tocopherol levels may help in clinical diagnosis.

Infectious causes of myelopathy of several kinds are well established. Treponemal infections, principally syphilis and yaws, are well known and were of overriding concern in the past. Problems with cross-reactive antibodies to *Leptospira* species complicate interpretation of laboratory findings at present. HIV-1 is now a major concern and must always be considered in the diagnosis of any myelopathy. Spinal cord compression still occurs from tuberculous osteomyelitis as well as other granulomatous agents. To cite an unusual case, we have seen an HTLV-I, HIV-1 negative case of coccidioidomycotic abscess compressing the spinal cord in our Florida population. Several viral causes must be considered in the differential diagnosis, including enteroviruses, herpes simplex, and herpes zoster.

An *HTLV-II associated ataxic syndrome* has recently been recognized by our group in Miami and by Appenzeller and co-workers in New Mexico. This ataxic syndrome associated with HTLV-II infection appears to be associated with symptoms of increased urinary frequency and muscle cramps. Increased muscle tone and reflexes may be present, but the finding of severe ataxia on examination distinguishes this syndrome from TSP/HAM. We have suggested that this clinical entity may be the basis of "tropical ataxic neuropathy" (TAN), which was also described in Jamaica when "Jamaican neuropathy" was first recognized. Certain features such as blindness and deafness, described as part of TAN, have not been found in the recently identified cases.

Parasitic infestations are well known. The only infestation occurring in this hemisphere that produces a myelopathy picture is schistosoma (Bilharzia). However, the common clinical picture seen is primarily one of areflexia. While rarely causing neurologic disease, Strongyloides (whipworm) infestation is a serious aggravating factor in accelerating the course of illness in Jamaica, but one which we have not seen in Miami. Malaria may also accelerate the illness.

Transverse myelitis describes a spinal cord disorder apparently involving one or more segments of the spinal cord at a single level. It typically presents with subacute onset of weakness and sensory loss, progressing to paraplegia within days to weeks. Subsequent partial or complete recovery suggests that the process is primarily demyelinative. It is important to note that HTLV-I/II seropositive cases have been recorded in Jamaica and in the Seychelles. Up to a quarter of TSP/HAM cases may present as transverse myelitis. Various other infectious agents, including enteroviruses and other inflammatory diseases such as systemic lupus erythematosus, can cause transverse myelopathy. It may also, rarely, be a manifestation of a paraneoplastic process.

Multiple sclerosis (MS) is frequently a consideration, particularly in the United States where it is a much more common cause of an isolated chronic progressive myelopathy than HTLV-I. Clinically, the presence of prominent brain stem or optic nerve disease suggests MS rather than HTLV-I myelopathy. A fluctuating course with remissions is also more typical of MS, although acute increases in symptoms have been reported occasionally in HTLV-I myelopathy. Serologic studies for HTLV-I should be helpful in doubtful cases, but there will be cases of indeterminant Western blots with nondefinitive clinical pictures leading to uncertainty. The similarity of TSP to the chronic myelopathic presentation of MS has raised the question of whether a virus related to HTLV-I might have a role in the pathogenesis of that illness.

Ischemic spinal cord disease can cause spastic paraplegia and can result from vasculitides or disease of the aorta or the radicular arteries. Acute spinal cord infarction usually has onset over minutes to hours and involves the lower thoracic segments. It may be seen in patients with diabetes, atheromatous vascular disease, or aortic aneurysms, or after aortic surgery. Granulomatous arteritis may also produce spinal cord lesions.

COMMENTS

HTLV-I myelopathy is a chronic progressive spastic paraparesis endemic in many areas of the world. It is seen in the United States primarily in immigrant communities. However, HTLV-I infection is transmissible by blood, sexual contact, and by breast-feeding of infants and is increasingly being recognized among other population groups. Diagnosis of spastic paraparesis is easily made on the basis of the clinical history and examination, with laboratory testing providing evidence of HTLV-I infection. The identification of patients with similar clinical syndromes without HTLV-I/II serum antibody suggests a possible role for other types of retroviral agents.

SUGGESTED READING

Cruickshank JK, Rudge P, Dalgleish AG, et al. Tropical spastic paraparesis and human T cell lymphotropic virus type 1 in the United Kingdom. Brain 1989; 112:1057–1090.
Gout O, Gessain A, Bolgert F, et al. Chronic myelopathies associated with human T-lymphotropic virus type I. Arch Neurol 1989; 46:255–260.
Harrington WJ Jr, Sheremata WA, Snodgrass SR, et al. Tropical spastic paraparesis/HTLV-I associated myelopathy (TSP/HAM): Treatment with an anabolic steroid—danazol. AIDS Res Hum Retroviruses 1991; 7:1031–1034.
Iwasaki Y. Pathology of chronic myelopathy associated with HTLV-I infection (HAM/TSP). J Neurol Sci 1990; 96:103–123.
Janssen RS, Kaplan JE, Khabbas RF, et al. HTLV-I associated myelopathy/tropical spastic paraparesis in the United States.
Osame M, Matsumoto M, Usuku K, et al. Chronic progressive myelopathy associated with elevated antibodies to HTLV-I and adult T-cell leukemia-like cells. Ann Neurol 1987; 21:117–122.
Rodgers-Johnson P, Gajdusek DC, Morgan OStC, et al. HTLV-I and HTLV-III antibodies in tropical spastic paraparesis. Lancet 1985; 2:1247–1248.
Roman GC. Retrovirus-associated myelopathies. Arch Neurol 1987; 44:659–663.
Roman GC, Spencer PS, Schoenberg BS. Tropical myeloneuropathies: The hidden endemias. Neurology 1985; 35:1159–1170.
Sheremata WA, Berger JR, Harrington WJ, et al. Human T lymphotropic virus type I-associated myelopathy: A report of 10 patients born in the United States. Arch Neurol 1992; 29:1113–1118.

CHRONIC MENINGITIS

PATRICIA K. COYLE, M.D.

Chronic meningitis makes up 8 percent of all meningitis cases. It is arbitrarily defined as a meningoencephalitis syndrome with associated cerebrospinal fluid (CSF) abnormalities that persists at least 4 weeks. In reality, the diagnosis is usually raised at the time of initial lumbar puncture in a patient with a suggestive CSF profile who has been symptomatic for less than a month. Clinical features of this syndrome include various combinations of headache, fever, stiff neck, mental status changes, focal deficits, and seizures. CSF abnormalities involve pleocytosis (usually mononuclear), with variable findings of moderately decreased glucose, increased protein, and increased pressure. Many diverse conditions cause chronic meningitis, and it is often not easy to identify the precise cause. Despite extensive investigations, at least a third of patients remain undiagnosed. I find it useful to divide causes into infectious and noninfectious (Table 1). The leading infectious cause is *Mycobacterium tuberculosis* (TB),

followed by *Cryptococcus neoformans*. The leading noninfectious cause is neoplastic meningitis, followed by neurosarcoidosis and vasculitis. Even in modern series, the mortality for this condition ranges from 27 to 35 percent. Among survivors there may be significant morbidity. I feel that it is crucial to have an organized and logical approach to this difficult problem.

HISTORY

I emphasize five major areas when taking a history from chronic meningitis patients (Table 2). Are there pertinent exposures? For example, has there been recent contact with anyone who has active TB? Does the patient's sexual history indicate partners at risk for syphilis or retroviral infection? Has there been exposure to areas infested with deer ticks, the Lyme disease vector? Has the patient consumed snails, raw fish, or contaminated vegetables, which can be infected with the parasite *Angiostrongylus cantonensis?* This worm is endemic in Asia and the Pacific. *Brucella* is a bacterial zoonotic infection. Patients with brucellosis give a history of contact with farm animals, unpasteurized dairy products, or laboratory exposure. *Leptospira interrogans* is a spirochetal zoonotic infection. Patients give a history

Table 1   Causes of the Chronic Meningitis Syndrome

Infectious

Bacterial
   Tuberculosis
   Spirochetal (Lyme disease, syphilis, *Leptospira*)
   Agents that cause sinus tracts (*Actinomyces, Arachnia, Nocardia*)
   Brucella
   Rare causes (*Listeria monocytogenes, Neisseria meningitidis, Francisella tularensis*)

Fungal
   Common (*Candida, Coccidioides, Cryptococcus, Histoplasma*)
   Uncommon (*Aspergillus, Blastomyces, Dematiaceous paracoccidioides, Pseudoallescheria, Sporothrix, Mucormycetes*)

Parasitic
   Cysticercus
   Granulomatous amebic meningoencephalitis (acanthamoeba)
   Eosinophilic meningitis (angiostrongylus)
   Toxoplasma
   Coenurus cerebralis

Viral
   Retrovirus (HIV-1, HTLV-1)
   Enterovirus (in hypogammaglobulinemics)

Noninfectious

Neoplastic

Neurosarcoidosis

Vasculitis
   Primary central nervous system
   Systemic (giant cell arteritis, lymphomatoid granulomatosis, polyarteritis nodosa, Wegener's granulomatosis)

Behçet's disease

Chemical meningitis
   Endogenous
   Exogenous

Chronic benign lymphocytic meningitis

Fabry's disease

Idiopathic hypertrophic pachymeningitis

Systemic lupus erythematosus

Vogt Koyanagi Harada disease

HIV = human immunodeficiency virus; HTLV = human T cell lymphotropic virus.

---

of animal exposure or of swimming in a pond infected with animal urine. *Pseudoallescheria boydii* is an ubiquitous fungi in soil, polluted waters, and sewage. Infection in normal hosts often follows an episode of near drowning. Exposure to IV needles, unsafe sex, or blood transfusion prior to the institution of routine screening raises concerns about retroviruses: human immunodeficiency virus (HIV) 1 and human T cell lymphotropic virus (HTLV) 1.

I probe in the history for evidence of extraneural disease. For example, a history of draining sinuses or abscesses suggests infection with *Actinomyces, Arachnia propionica, Nocardia, Coccidioides,* or *Blastomyces*. Eye complaints consistent with uveitis are seen in sarcoidosis, Behçet's disease, Vogt-Koyanagi-Harada disease, lymphoma, and *Leptospira* or angiostrongylus infection.

Table 2   Key Historical Clues in Chronic Meningitis

Exposures
Extraneural disease
Immunodeficiency
Systemic conditions
Travel

Pulmonary disease is particularly common with TB, *Aspergillus, Blastomyces,* and *Histoplasma* infections and sarcoidosis. Joint involvement is a feature of Lyme disease and Behçet's disease. Skin lesions are associated particularly with Lyme disease (erythema migrans) and Vogt-Koyanagi-Harada disease (alopecia, poliosis, vitiligo).

Specific infections occur in immunocompromised hosts. A variety of congenital and acquired conditions suppress the immune system, including HIV-1 infection, chemotherapy, organ transplant with its concomitant drug treatment, chronic steroid use, and hematologic malignancies. This predisposes to infection with certain fungi (*Aspergillus, Candida, Coccidioides, Cryptococcus, Histoplasma, Mucormycetes, Pseudoallescheria*), bacteria (TB, *Listeria, Nocardia*), parasites (*Acanthamoeba, Toxoplasma*), and viruses (ECHO virus and polio in agammaglobulinemics).

I always check the history for an underlying systemic disorder that can produce meningitis. In patients with known TB, syphilis, brucellosis, acquired immunodeficiency syndrome, extraneural fungal infections, sarcoidosis, or malignancy, the development of a chronic meningitis is likely to reflect extension of their known disease process. Underlying diseases may predispose to certain infections. For example, *Mucormycetes* can infect diabetics in ketoacidosis. *Candida* infection is more likely in patients receiving hyperalimentation and who have chronic indwelling lines.

Finally, certain infections are geographically restricted. Prior travel history in a patient documents potential exposures to *Brucella* (southwest states; Mediterranean region), the Lyme disease agent *Borrelia burgdorferi* (coastal northeast, north central, Pacific states), *Coccidioides* (semiarid southwest states), *Blastomyces* and *Histoplasma* (Ohio, Mississippi, and St. Lawrence river valleys), *Paracoccidioides* (Latin America, Mexico), cysticercus (Mexico, Latin America, India, Africa), angiostrongylus (Southeast Asia, Pacific islands, Cuba), and the HTLV-1 virus (tropics, Caribbean, Japan).

EXAMINATION

My main goals in examining a chronic meningitis patient are: (1) to document concurrent extraneural disease; (2) to identify potential biopsy sites; and (3) to document the type and extent of neurologic involvement. Table 3 outlines some useful examination clues. Any enlarged lymph node or unexplained skin lesion is fair

Table 3 Key Examination Clues in Chronic Meningitis

Adenopathy
Dermatologic lesion
Ophthalmologic features
Organomegaly or organ disease
Associated neurologic features
    Cranial nerve involvement
    Focal lesion
    Hydrocephalus
    Peripheral neuropathy
    Multilevel neuraxis involvement

Table 4 Laboratory Evaluation of the Chronic Meningitis Syndrome

Blood studies

Cerebrospinal fluid (CSF)

Cultures
    At multiple sites
    Multiple (≥ 3) times
    For multiple agents

Antibody studies
    On paired CSF, serum samples

Antigen studies

Skin testing
    Purified protein derivative
    Anergy panel

Imaging
    Chest film
    Contrast magnetic resonance imaging or computed tomography
    Angiography

Biopsy
    Extraneural
    Leptomeningeal/brain

game for biopsy. My patients get a formal neuro-ophthalmologic consultation to look for uveitis, tubercles, or granulomas in the eye. Evidence on my examination for hepatosplenomegaly, pulmonary disease, or bone marrow involvement means that I will pursue organ-specific pathology with additional tests and procedures. Orbit or sinus disease suggests *Aspergillus* or *Mucormycetes* infection or Wegener's disease. Features of the neurologic examination can suggest specific diagnoses. For example, prominent facial nerve involvement is particularly common with meningitis due to Lyme disease or neurosarcoidosis. Focal parenchymal lesions such as abscesses are common with certain fungi as well as *Toxoplasma*, while strokes are seen with vasculitis, TB, and fungi with a predilection to invade blood vessels (*Aspergillus, Histoplasma, Mucormycetes*). Hydrocephalus due to prominent basilar meningeal involvement is particularly seen in TB, fungal meningitis, and cysticercosis. Associated peripheral nerve or root involvement suggests Lyme disease, brucellosis, sarcoidosis, or vasculitis due in particular to polyarteritis nodosa. Neoplastic meningitis can give symptomatic involvement at multiple levels, including spinal nerve roots, cranial nerves, and cerebral cortex.

LABORATORY EVALUATION

My laboratory evaluation for chronic meningitis is outlined in Table 4. Routine blood studies are sometimes helpful. A low sodium or syndrome of inappropriate antidiuretic hormone suggests TB meningitis, while a high sodium or diabetes insipidus syndrome suggests sarcoidosis. Sarcoid patients may also show increased IgG, calcium, and angiotensin converting enzyme (ACE). ACE levels may also be elevated in CSF. I always send collagen vascular and vasculitis blood studies. Antineutrophilic cytoplasmic antibodies can screen for Wegener's, a systemic vasculitis that may involve the meninges.

CSF studies are the most critical in chronic meningitis. My general approach is to plan on performing at least three lumbar punctures at regular intervals in order to send repeat studies and to document changes in CSF parameters. I try to provide large-volume CSF samples (at least 5 to 20 cc) for cultures, stains, and cytologies. When lumbar CSF is unrevealing, and particularly when

there is a prominent basilar process, I proceed to lateral cervical or cisternal puncture, or a ventricular tap. My CSF studies include cell count, differential, glucose, and protein. Certain CSF abnormalities suggest a specific diagnosis (Table 5). I order cytology and request immunocytochemistry with monoclonal antibodies to try to identify abnormal cells. I routinely perform Gram's, acid fast, and india ink stains and will request a wet prep study if amebae are suspected. I order oligoclonal bands and IgG index to rule out a demyelinating process.

I send at least three cultures from multiple sites, including CSF, blood, urine, gastric washes, joint fluid, prostatic secretions, sputum, and stool for ova and parasites if that is likely. I check for all appropriate agents (bacteria, mycobacteria, fungi, viruses, and parasites). I notify my microbiology laboratory that the specimens are from a patient with chronic meningitis so that they carry out prolonged incubations and special procedures (anaerobic culture for *Actinomyces* and *Arachnia*, increased CO_2 for *Brucella*, Sabouraud's agar for fungi). Among fungi, only *Candida* and *Cryptococcus* have a high yield of positive CSF cultures.

I request antibodies on paired CSF and serum samples in order to maximize information about intrathecal antibody production. There are reliable serologies to test for bacteria (*B.burgdorferi, Brucella, Leptospira*, syphilis, possibly *Nocardia*), fungi (*Coccidioides, Histoplasma, Sporothrix*, possibly *Aspergillus, Blastomyces, Candida, Cryptococcus*, and *Paracoccidioides*), parasites (*Cysticercus, Toxoplasma*), and viruses (HIV-1, HTLV-1).

There are certain infectious agents for which antigen assays are available. I check cryptococcal polysaccharide antigen in CSF and serum. CSF antigen is positive in over 90 percent of meningitis cases. If *Histoplasma* infection is possible, I try to obtain histoplasma polysaccharide antigen studies on CSF, serum,

Table 5 Suggestive Cerebrospinal Fluid Patterns in Chronic Meningitis

Cell count
  Less than 50/mm³
    Noninfectious
  Neutrophil predominance
    Bacteria (*Actinomyces, Arachnia, Brucella, Nocardia*, early TB)
    Fungi (*Aspergillus, Blastomyces, Candida, Cladosporium, Coccidioides, Histoplasma, Pseudoallescheria, Mucormycetes*)
    Parasites (acanthamoeba)
    Noninfectious (chemical, systemic lupus, vasculitis)
  Eosinophil predominance
    Parasites (angiostrongylus, cysticercus)
    Coccidioides
    Noninfectious (lymphoma, polyarteritis, chemical)
  Plasma cells
    Lyme disease

Protein
  High level
    TB

Table 6 Differential Diagnosis of the Chronic Meningitis Syndrome

Encephalitis
Acute meningitis
  Aseptic
  Recurrent
  Partially treated
Reactive CSF due to a variety of processes
Giant cell arteritis
Metabolic/toxic encephalopathy
Multiple sclerosis
Postinfectious encephalitis
Systemic lupus erythematosus
Thrombotic thrombocytopenic purpura

Table 7 Causes of the Recurrent Meningitis Syndrome

Anatomic defects
  Congenital
  Postoperative
  Traumatic
Behçet's disease
Chemical meningitis
Collagen vascular diseases
Drug induced
Familial Mediterranean fever
Immune defects
  Antibody deficiency
  Complement deficiency
  Splenectomy
Migraine with pleocytosis
Mollaret's
Parameningeal infection with seeding
Recurrent bacterial/viral infections
Vogt-Koyanagi-Harada disease

Table 8 Causes of Chronic Meningitis in the Patient Infected with HIV-1

HIV-1
Opportunistic
  Cryptococcus (affects 10%)
  Other fungi (*Coccidioides, Histoplasma*)
  Mycobacteria
    TB (in Haitians, intravenous drug users)
    Atypical
  Syphilis
  Listeria
  Prototheca wickerhamii (alga)
Neoplastic
  Metastatic systemic lymphoma
  Primary CNS lymphoma

and urine. *Aspergillus, Candida,* and *Coccidioides* are other fungi for which antigen assays are being evaluated.

I plant an anergy panel and intermediate strength purified protein derivative (PPD) on all chronic meningitis patients. If the PPD is negative, I repeat it 2 to 4 weeks later. I then perform a second strength PPD, if the patient is not anergic. I do not plant any fungal skin tests, since they interfere with serologies.

With regard to imaging studies, I pay particular attention to the chest film to look for a lung mass (tumor, granuloma, abscess) or hilar adenopathy. For neuroimaging, I prefer contrast magnetic resonance imaging (MRI) to contrast computed tomography. I look for meningeal enhancement, basilar exudate, hydrocephalus, and associated focal lesions such as abscesses or strokes. If strokes are evident or vasculitis is a possibility, I proceed to angiography. If I suspect any spinal cord disease, I image the spine using MRI.

I biopsy any suspicious skin, lung, or paranasal sinus lesion for tissue, culture, and stain. If there is evidence of bone marrow or liver involvement, which occurs in particular with TB and *Histoplasma,* I proceed to biopsy this site if I have no diagnosis. Leptomeningeal/brain biopsy has a low yield (21 percent) but can be diagnostic,

especially for neoplastic meningitis and primary CNS vasculitis. I proceed to leptomeningeal/brain biopsy in the undiagnosed patient who continues to deteriorate, who does not respond to empiric therapeutic trials, or who is to undergo a neurosurgical procedure such as shunt insertion or ventricular tap.

DIFFERENTIAL DIAGNOSIS

A differential diagnosis for chronic meningitis is listed in Table 6. The two conditions most commonly misdiagnosed as chronic meningitis are the acute neurologic infections (encephalitis or meningitis) and a variety of processes that affect the brain to produce reactive CSF. Recurrent meningitis involves repeated attacks of acute meningitis, but in between attacks the patient is well and the CSF is normal. Recurrent meningitis should not be confused with chronic meningitis, because it has distinct causes (Table 7). Some cases of encephalitis, and acute and partially treated meningitis, still show CSF abnormalities 1 month after onset. However, the clinical picture and the CSF profile are

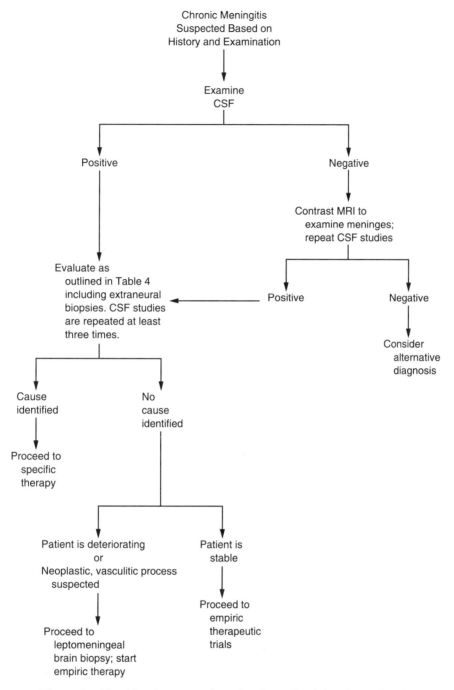

Figure 1 Algorithm for approach to the diagnosis of chronic meningitis.

improving over that time period. This is the key to distinguishing them from chronic meningitis. Processes as diverse as brain tumor, endocarditis, parameningeal infection, subarachnoid hemorrhage, and subdural hematoma may all produce a CSF pleocytosis in addition to other CSF changes. However, a careful assessment using history, examination, and laboratory evaluation quickly clarifies the diagnosis. These conditions are only missed in the patient with presumed chronic meningitis who is *not* properly worked up.

There are certain pitfalls that lead to misdiagnosis. One is the absence of CSF pleocytosis. In rare cases, a patient with a chronic meningitis may have a normal CSF cell count. Serial CSF examinations subsequently reveal a pleocytosis, or neuroimaging documents meningeal enhancement consistent with an inflammatory process. Meningitis is defined by inflammation of the meninges, and although CSF pleocytosis is almost invariable, in rare cases the cell count may be normal. TB is currently on the rise in the United States. TB meningitis is often thought of as a severe subacute infection that, if untreated, steadily worsens to a moribund state within weeks. This is not always true, and untreated TB meningitis sometimes takes a chronic course lasting months. The usual clinical picture is that of a dementia, so that I never rule out TB meningitis because of an extended clinical course. In the case of neoplastic meningitis, a negative cytology does not rule out the diagnosis. It may take five or six lumbar punctures to obtain a positive cytology, and cytology remains negative in about 10 percent of cases. Finally, I never hesitate to proceed to leptomeningeal/brain biopsy in worrisome patients. The risk is relatively low for this procedure, and it may provide a definitive diagnosis to guide therapy.

HIV-1 infection is discussed in detail in the chapter *Central Nervous System HIV and Related Opportunistic Infections*. Chronic meningitis in the patient with HIV-1 infection has a distinct clinical profile (Table 8).

An algorithm for my diagnostic approach to chronic meningitis is outlined in Figure 1.

SUGGESTED READING

Anderson NE, Willoughby EW. Chronic meningitis without predisposing illness: A review of 83 cases. Q J Med 1987; 63:283–295.
Chang KH, Han MH, Roh JK, et al. Gd-DTPA–enhanced MR imaging of the brain in patients with meningitis: Comparison with CT. AJNR Am J Neuroradiol 1990; 11:69–76.
Ellner JJ, Bennett JE. Chronic meningitis. Medicine 1976; 55:341–369.
Hopkins AP, Harvey PKP. Chronic benign lymphocytic meningitis. J Neurol Sci 1973; 18:443–453.
Katzman M, Ellner JJ. Chronic meningitis. In: Mandell GL, Douglas RG Jr, Bennett JE, eds. Principles and practice of infectious disease. 3rd ed. New York: Churchill Livingstone, 1990:755.
Peacock JE Jr, McGinnis MR, Cohen MS. Persistent neutrophilic meningitis. Medicine 1984; 63:379–395.
Tucker T, Ellner JJ. Chronic meningitis. In: Scheld WM, Whitley RJ, Durack DT, eds. Infections of the nervous system. New York: Raven, 1991:703.
Wilhelm CS, Marra CM. Chronic meningitis. Semin Neurol 1992; 12:234–247.

SUBDURAL EMPYEMA

MATT J. LIKAVEC, M.D.

Subdural empyema is rare but does account for about 15 percent of localized intracranial bacterial infections. Subdural empyema is a fulminant purulent infection that spreads over and between the cerebral hemispheres and, rarely, beneath the tentorium. The dura and the arachnoid encompass a potential space crossed by numerous small veins. Anatomic barriers to this space exist at the falx, the tentorium, the base of the brain, and the foramen magnum. These barriers divide the subdural space into compartments that confine the infection and consequently cause the infection to behave as an expanding mass lesion.

The cause of subdural empyema is usually the spread of infection through emissary veins or by contiguous infections in the skull. In children under 5 years of age, subdural empyema typically follows bacterial meningitis.

The key to the diagnosis is a knowledge of the patients at risk. Infection in the paranasal sinuses is the most common source of infection in the adult. Middle ear and mastoid infections follow next in frequency. Infections of the scalp and skull may also lead to subdural empyema. Trauma and surgical procedures, including insertion of ventricular shunts and intracranial pressure monitors, have been identified as a source of subdural empyema. Infection of a pre-existing chronic subdural hematoma has been reported as a cause. Last, in children, subdural empyema can evolve after bacterial meningitis.

Symptoms may develop with a short fulminating course, or they may evolve over a period of weeks. Prior use of antibiotics makes the symptoms present in a more indolent and insidious manner. Definitive diagnosis is more difficult in these patients.

The symptoms include headache (first focal, later generalized), fever, malaise, nausea, vomiting, irritability, stiff neck, and lethargy. Mental status may show insidious deterioration, but seizures, focal neurologic deficits, and coma can occur rapidly.

DIAGNOSIS

The signs on physical exam include fever, photophobia, meningismus, localized skull tenderness, delirium, localized neurologic deficits, decreased mental status, and coma. Meningeal signs associated with a focal neurologic deficit should raise the suspicion of subdural empyema.

The systemic and cerebrospinal fluid (CSF) laboratory evaluation is often abnormal but rarely diagnostic. The peripheral white blood count can be elevated but is not always. Fever may or may not be present. Lumbar puncture is typically contraindicated for fear of causing herniation. Nonetheless, a lumbar puncture has often been performed in the course of the workup. The CSF pressure may be normal or high. The CSF glucose is most often normal. The CSF protein can vary from normal to slightly elevated. The CSF white blood cell count is most often elevated, and can exhibit either polymorphonuclear or monocyte predominance. In summary, the results of the lumbar puncture are often abnormal, never diagnostic, and possibly dangerous.

The diagnosis of subdural empyema is made by a computed tomography (CT) scan with contrast, or a magnetic resonance imaging (MRI) of the head. Uncontrasted CT scans may miss the diagnosis because of the small size of the collection or its anatomic location, particularly in the parafalcine, subfrontal, or posterior fossa areas. Coronal CT may suggest the diagnosis because of underlying bone destruction, opacification of the sinuses, midline shift, or edema out of proportion to the subdural collection. However, a contrasted CT scan should detect the enhancing membranes associated with subdural empyema. The MRI provides better anatomic definition and identifies collections at the base of the brain, along the falx, and in the posterior fossa, the blind spots of CT.

In rare cases the diagnosis of subdural empyema is made only at surgery. It is of note that subdural empyema has been reported in rare instances to occur along the spinal axis.

The major pitfalls in the diagnosis include patients with atypical presentations, intercurrent use of antibiotics, failure to obtain the appropriate radiologic study, improper interpretation of the radiologic study, and the danger and lack of diagnostic accuracy of the lumbar puncture.

Therapy for a subdural empyema should not be delayed to obtain an MRI "the next morning." If the diagnosis is entertained, prompt neurosurgical consultation is mandated. Antibiotic coverage should be instituted while awaiting definitive surgery.

The prognosis for patients with subdural empyema is poor, with a 15 percent mortality rate. Only with knowledge of the patients at risk, expeditious acquisition of appropriate radiologic studies, and prompt therapeutic intervention can the prognosis for subdural empyema be improved.

SUGGESTED READING

Courville CB. Subdural empyema secondary to purulent frontal sinusitis. Arch Otolaryngol 1944; 39:211–230.
Dunker RO, Khaako RA. Failure of computer tomographic scanning to demonstrate subdural empyemas. JAMA 1981; 246:235–238.
Fraser RAR, Ratzen K, Wolpert SM, Weinstein L. Spinal subdural empyema. Arch Neurol 1973; 28:235–238.
Hockley AD, Williams B. Surgical management of subdural empyema. Child's Brain 1983; 10:294–300.
Kaufman DM, Miller MH, Steigbigel NH. Subdural empyema: Analysis of 17 recent cases and review of the literature. Medicine 1975; 54:485–498.
Mosley IF, Kendall BG. Radiology of intracranial empyema. Neuroradiology 1984; 26:333–345.
Renaudin JW, Frazee J. Subdural empyema: Importance of early diagnosis. Neurosurgery 1980; 7:477–479.

SPINAL EPIDURAL ABSCESS

ALLEN J. TEMAN, M.D.

Early detection of spinal epidural abscess (SEA) is imperative because delays in treatment may result in irreversible neurologic damage or death. SEA may present as an acute or chronic syndrome. The acute syndrome is defined as the presence of symptoms for less than 2 weeks and typically is associated with fever and leukocytosis. Patients with a chronic SEA may not seek medical attention for months. Usually their only complaint is of back pain associated with myelopathy or radiculopathy. Patients with a chronic abscess are often afebrile and have a normal serum white blood cell count. Compared to the acute syndrome, the chronic syndrome is nearly as prevalent, may be equally devastating, and is more frequently misdiagnosed.

The incidence of SEA is approximately one out of every 20,000 hospital admissions. The rarity of an SEA contributes to the likelihood of its being overlooked. Predisposing factors are intravenous drug abuse, immu-

nosuppression, diabetes, alcohol abuse, and back trauma. Back trauma includes prior spinal surgery, lumbar puncture, and blunt trauma. Blunt trauma may induce an epidural hematoma that will serve as a nidus for infection from transient bacteremia.

SEA most commonly occurs in the thoracic or lumbar spine. Pathophysiologically the width of the epidural space relates to the probability that an abscess will occur within a certain region of the spine. The epidural space of the thoracic spine measures from 0.5 to 0.75 cm, while that of the cervical spine is only approximately 0.1 cm. The epidural regions from T4 to T8 and L2 to L5 are the largest. Also important anatomically is the extensive epidural venous plexus within the thoracic and lumbar spine. The venous plexus provides a pathway for infective organisms to reach the epidural space.

Symptomatically, all patients with an SEA will present with back pain. Neurologic dysfunction, if any, corresponds to the location of the abscess and the amount of compression upon the adjacent nerve roots and spinal cord. Frequently, the chronic syndrome may present only with persistent unexplained back pain. Patients with the acute syndrome present more dramatically with fever and leukocytosis. Even without obvious cord compression at the time of initial examination, chronic abscesses can lead to sudden demise by venous infarction of the spinal cord.

The length of an SEA may span several vertebrae. Typically an SEA will have a single epicenter at which spinal cord and nerve root damage will occur. Rarely, the infection may span the entire length of the spine. Most infections are located dorsally since ventrally the dura is tightly adherent to the posterior longitudinal ligament. Hematogenous spread of organisms typically leads to a dorsally located abscess. Vertebral osteomyelitis may spread to the ventral epidural space and lead to a spinal epidural abscess. Clinically, a ventral abscess may present with back pain for a longer period of time before the onset of neurologic dysfunction.

Spread of infection from an SEA to the subarachnoid space is rare. The dura provides an excellent barrier against the passage of organisms into the cerebrospinal fluid (CSF). Acute bacterial meningitis is thus a rare occurrence. In cases without meningitis, CSF usually reveals an elevated protein concentration and a mononuclear pleocytosis. CSF glucose is only low in cases of active bacterial or tuberculous meningitis. The main disadvantage of collection of CSF for analysis is the possibility of inadvertent puncture of an SEA, leading to seeding of the CSF with organisms. I thus recommend against the routine evaluation of CSF in patients with a possible SEA.

DIAGNOSIS

The most accurate way to make the diagnosis of SEA is with magnetic resonance imaging (MRI) (Fig. 1). The comparison of T1, T2, and contrast-enhanced T1 weighted images performed in the sagittal and axial planes will lead to the correct diagnosis in most cases. MRI allows direct visualization of the upper and lower extent of the abscess as well as its involvement of adjacent structures. MRI can be used to determine if osteomyelitis is present and may be easily repeated to follow the response to therapy (Fig. 2).

The differential diagnosis of any process extending into the epidural space includes infection and tumor. Typically, tumor does not invade the disk space, though infection does not respect such anatomic boundaries. Any process that invades the disk space in addition to adjacent bone must be considered an SEA until proven otherwise. The usual MRI scan of the spine may not include T2 sagittal or T1 contrast-enhanced images. When an SEA is considered in the differential diagnosis, these extra sequences must be performed. Infection appears as a low signal abnormality on T1 weighted images and high signal on T2. Normal epidural fat is high signal on T2 but typically decreases in signal intensity on more progressively weighted T2 images. Infected fat or pure abscess will remain high signal despite changes in T2 weighting. Gadolinium is a paramagnetic substance that will readily enhance areas of infection on T1 weighted images. Gadolinium is a nontoxic, intrave-

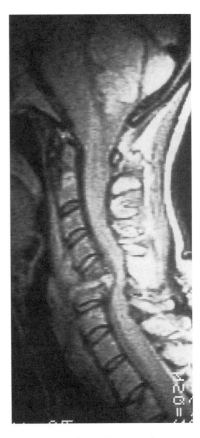

Figure 1 Sagittal T2 weighted magnetic resonance imaging reveals spinal epidural abscess at the C5–C6 level producing marked spinal cord compression (T2, 2,500 milliseconds; TE, 38 milliseconds).

nously injected material that is currently widely available and should be used in all suspected cases of SEA.

Myelography is only indicated when MRI is not available or in selected cases of acute bacterial meningitis. Patients with bacterial meningitis may require myelography in conjunction with computed tomography, since in this setting MRI does not distinguish the subarachnoid space from the infected epidural tissue. The drawbacks of myelography include the inadvertent seeding of the CSF with bacteria during lumbar puncture, inability to define the upper and lower borders of an SEA in patients with complete block of CSF flow, and the risk of clinical deterioration after removal of CSF in patients with a complete CSF block. Other radiographic studies such as indium or gallium scans need not be performed in patients suspected to harbor an SEA, since they cause further delay until treatment.

Treatment of SEA is usually surgical. Surgery should be performed in all patients except those unable to survive an operation or those who are plegic for more than 72 hours. Patients completely paralyzed for more than 3 days should have a needle biopsy to provide culture material, and MRI may be used to follow the response to treatment. In most patients, surgery can be used to obtain culture material, decompress the spinal cord and nerve roots, and remove infected material from

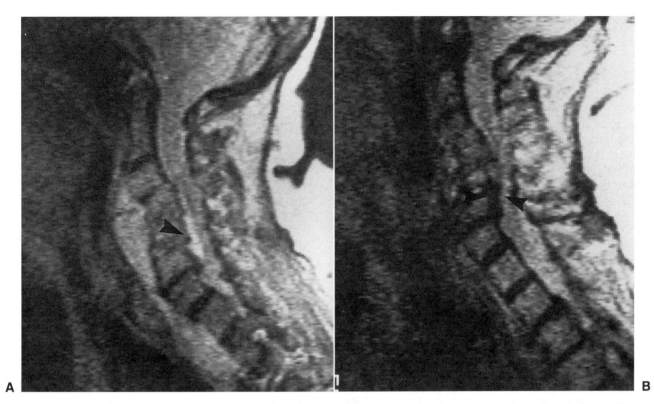

A   B

Figure 2 *A,* Sagittal T2 weighted magnetic resonance imaging reveals ventral epidural abscess with cord compression (T2, 2,500 milliseconds; TE, 75 milliseconds). *B,* After treatment, T2 weighted image shows resolution of high signal emanating from ventral epidural space (TR, 2,500 milliseconds; TE, 76 milliseconds).

around vascular channels. Material should be sent for Gram stain, cultures for bacteria and fungi, and acid fast staining to evaluate for *Mycobacterium tuberculosis.*

In all studies to date, *Staphylococcus aureus* has been the most commonly encountered organism, though a significant number of infections may be caused by gram negative rods. In my studies of patients with spinal epidural abscesses, I have encountered a few patients in whom a chronic abscess is present months after a urinary tract infection. Blood cultures should be drawn in all patients before the initiation of antibiotics. Antibiotic coverage should be adjusted once results from epidural cultures are obtained. It is not exceedingly unusual for an abscess to consist of multiple organisms. Patients suspected to have Pott's disease should be started on antituberculous therapy.

COMMENTS

Physicians should maintain a high index of suspicion for SEA in any patient with back pain and a recent febrile illness. Those patients who are immunosuppressed or have predisposing factors for SEA pose additional cause for concern. Patients suspected to harbor an SEA require urgent radiologic confirmation

with gadolinium MRI. All patients with MRI findings of any epidural mass involving bone and extending into the disk space should be restudied using gadolinium-enhanced T1 images and sagittal T2 weighted images. After radiologic confirmation, surgery should be performed immediately and broad spectrum antibiotic coverage initiated.

SUGGESTED READING

Baker AS, Ojemann RG, Swartz MN, Richardson EP. Spinal epidural abscess. N Engl J Med 1975; 293:463–468.

Hakin RN, Burt AA, Cook JB. Acute spinal epidural abscess. Paraplegia 1979-1980; 17:330–336.

Kaufman DM, Kaplan JG, Litman H. Infectious agents in spinal epidural abscess. Neurology 1980; 30:844–850.

Koppel BS, Tuchman AJ, Mangiardi JR, et al. Epidural spinal infection in intravenous drug abusers. Arch Neurol 1988; 45:1331–1337.

Larsson EM, Holtas S, Crunqvist S. Emergency magnetic resonance examination of patients with spinal cord symptoms. Acta Radiol 1988; 29:69–75.

Phillips GE, Jefferson A. Acute spinal epidural abscess: Observations from fourteen cases. Postgrad Med J 1979; 55:712–715.

Post M, Donovan J, Quencer RM, et al. Spinal infection: Evaluation with MR imaging and intraoperative ultrasound. Radiology 1988; 169:765–771.

Teman AJ. Spinal epidural abscess: Early detection with gadolinium magnetic resonance imaging. Arch Neurol 1992; 49:743–746.

LYME DISEASE

PATRICIA K. COYLE, M.D.

Lyme disease now accounts for 91 percent of vector-borne infections in the United States. Numerically it is the leading new infectious problem after acquired immunodeficiency virus, with over 40,000 cases reported to the Centers for Disease Control and Prevention (CDCP) in the last decade. Lyme disease is caused by a spirochete, *Borrelia burgdorferi,* which infects Ixodes (hard body) ticks. Up to 50 percent of *B. burgdorferi* infections are asymptomatic. Symptomatic infection leads to a range of acute and chronic clinical syndromes that target specific body organs to produce skin, joint, heart, eye, and nervous system problems. Clinical disease may occur in different stages of the infection, punctuated by silent periods. Disease may occur as early local infection, during early dissemination, or months to years later as chronic persistent infection. Spirochetes are inoculated into the skin of a person while an attached infected tick is feeding. Organisms then disseminate to multiple organs by cutaneous, lymphatic, and hematogenous pathways. Infection with *B. burgdorferi* is chronic, and spirochetes can be isolated from various body tissues and fluids months to years after the onset of symptoms.

Lyme disease is geographically restricted. It is endemic in regions inhabited by Ixodes ticks in North America, Europe, and Asia. In North America the disease is concentrated in the coastal northeast, north-central states, northern California, and southeastern Ontario Province. Ten states account for 88 percent of Lyme cases: in particular, New York (40 percent), followed by Connecticut, New Jersey, Pennsylvania, Rhode Island, Massachusetts, Maryland, Wisconsin, Minnesota, and California. Within these states the distribution of Lyme disease is quite focal, with the highest endemic areas showing incidence rates as high as 150 per 100,000 population. Lyme disease is increasing as the tick vector spreads and the endemic tick infection rate rises. There has been a 19-fold increase in annual cases since 1982. In 1992 over 9,600 cases were reported from 45 states. This is a 19 percent increase from 1990, and it is likely this trend will continue. Lyme disease is an important treatable infection, which needs to be included in the differential diagnosis of many central nervous system (CNS) and peripheral nervous system (PNS) syndromes.

HISTORY

Table 1 lists the key historical features I look for in Lyme disease. The most important is the occurrence of the skin lesion erythema migrans (EM), a pathogno-

Table 1   Key Historical Features in the Diagnosis of Neurologic Lyme Disease

Erythema migrans

Exposure to endemic region

Antecedent tick bite
   Type of tick
   Likelihood of infection
   Duration of tick attachment
   Engorgement

Antecedent flulike illness

Suggestive extraneural features
   Joint involvement
   Jaw pain
   Myalgias
   Prominent fatigue
   Cardiac features
   Ocular features

Typical neurologic syndromes

monic marker for infection. Unfortunately, only 60 to 80 percent of Lyme patients develop or notice EM. This expanding red lesion occurs at the site of the tick bite an average of 8 to 9 (range 2 to 28) days after infection. Its characteristic feature is that it enlarges over several days up to 4 to 42 cm in diameter. EM begins as a macule, which becomes a papule and then an annular erythematous plaque. Variations include a bull's-eye pattern, and a vesicular, crusted, or edematous center. The skin lesion is generally asymptomatic, but can be warm to the touch, pruritic, or even painful. EM occurs most commonly on the trunk or legs, and in children occurs especially on the head and neck. In 6 to 48 percent of cases multiple EM lesions develop, a sign that spirochetes have disseminated from their local infection site. The major differential diagnoses for EM include fixed drug eruption, ringworm, cellulitis, contact dermatitis, cutaneous arthropod reactions, and erythema multiforme.

A second key historical point is the infection's geographic restriction. I expect patients to have a history of exposure to an endemic region based on where they live or where they have traveled. It is very difficult to make a case for Lyme disease in someone from Alaska or New Mexico, states that do not contain the tick vector and have never had an indigenous case. My index of suspicion is always higher for outdoor workers, or for people who spend a lot of leisure time outdoors. However, infected ticks are not limited to shrubbed and wooded areas. They can be plentiful on suburban lawns and have been found in parks in Baltimore and Philadelphia.

A third useful historical clue is antecedent tick bite, but less than 50 percent of neurologic Lyme patients report this. I try to determine the type of tick, since Ixodes ticks are virtually the only vector for Lyme disease and bites from other ticks are not a risk factor. Ixodes ticks are very small, the size of poppy seeds, and are much more likely to be overlooked than the larger and very common dog tick *(Dermacentor variabilis)*. Possible transmission cases have been linked to another tick, *A. americanum,* as well as horse flies, but these are exceptional cases. The smaller nymphal Ixodes ticks are much more likely than adult ticks to be infected and to bite humans. They feed in late spring and early summer. The likelihood of an Ixodes tick being infected with *B. burgdorferi* depends on the geographic area. In the northeast and midwest, *I. dammini* (deer tick) is the principal vector, and nymphal ticks have infection rates of 30 to 60 percent in the northeast and 10 to 16 percent in the midwest. In the west, *I. pacificus* (western black legged tick) is the vector of Lyme disease,but this tick has much lower infection rates (1 to 6 percent) than *I. dammini. I. scapularis* is another Ixodes tick strain, which is endemic in the south. This tick has been shown experimentally to transmit *B. burgdorferi,* but it has a low infection rate and rarely feeds on humans.

Ticks probably have to be attached and feeding for at least 24 to 48 hours to transmit *B. burgdorferi.* Engorgement is a sign that the tick has been feeding for an extended period, and increases the likelihood of transmission.

In the history, I always ask whether a systemic illness preceded neurologic complaints. Acute infection with *B. burgdorferi* may be associated with a flulike or viral syndrome, with or without EM, characterized by fever, chills, headache, stiff neck, malaise, and muscle and joint pains. Generally symptoms are mild, but occasionally patients describe a quite severe constitutional syndrome.

Since Lyme disease is a systemic infection, I look for extraneural features in the history. Over 40 percent of patients note arthralgias and myalgias, and in fact a syndrome virtually indistinguishable from fibromyalgia may occur. Joint pain is frequently migratory, involves one or two regions at a time, and then resolves over hours to days. In late infection the patient may give a history consistent with inflammatory arthritis, with intermittent asymmetric synovitis of one or more large joints. The most common joint involved in Lyme disease is the knee, followed by the shoulder, ankle, elbow, wrist, hip, finger, toe, and sternoclavicular joint. Swelling is typically painless. The temporomandibular joint is involved in up to 25 percent of patients, so that a history of jaw pain, a somewhat unusual symptom, suggests Lyme disease.

Although it is clearly nonspecific, prominent fatigue suggests Lyme disease. Fatigue and malaise are frequent in all stages of this infection, and in various studies 39 to 85 percent of untreated symptomatic patients complained of fatigue. Fatigue is generally persistent and can be so severe as to mimic a chronic fatigue syndrome. However, it is accompanied by other complaints suggestive of Lyme disease.

Since the heart and eye can be involved in Lyme disease, I specifically ask about arrhythmias, eye irritability, and photophobia in the history.

Finally, there are typical neurologic syndromes associated with Lyme disease (Table 2). Neurologic

Table 2 Characteristic Neurologic Syndromes Seen in Different Stages of Lyme Disease

Early local infection
  Asymptomatic central nervous system seeding
  Headache with or without stiff neck

Early dissemination
  "Aseptic" meningitis/meningoencephalititis
  Cranial nerve palsy (especially Bell's palsy)
  Radiculoneuritis

Late persistent infection
  Encephalopathy
  Polyneuropathy
  Meningoencephalomyelitis

features particularly suggestive are viral meningitis with facial nerve and radicular involvement, bilateral Bell's palsy, a Guillain-Barré–like syndrome with cerebrospinal fluid (CSF) pleocytosis, and mild polyneuropathy with limb paresthesias. It is harder to make a case for Lyme disease when the patient has an atypical syndrome. However, I always keep an open mind since we have not defined the full clinical spectrum of North American Lyme disease. I have seen a variety of unusual neurologic features that I believe are due to this infection. One striking pediatric disorder is a pseudotumor-cerebri–like syndrome, with headache and papilledema. In these children and adolescents, the CSF generally shows mild abnormalities.

EXAMINATION

Cutaneous markers for Lyme disease are EM and two lesions seen particularly in Europe: borrelial lymphocytoma during early infection, and acrodermatitis chronica atrophicans (ACA) during late infection. Lymphocytoma is a bluish-red tumorlike lesion with a predilection for the earlobe in children and the areolar region in adults. ACA is most common in women. It occurs on the lower extremity as a bluish-red skin lesion that evolves into a fibrotic lesion with skin atrophy.

Joint examination in the Lyme patient is frequently normal, despite subjective complaints. However, patients may have a frank synovitis, which is episodic or chronic. Typically there is a relatively painless knee effusion with a Baker's cyst. Occasionally a joint is red and hot and mimics septic arthritis. Less than 10 percent of Lyme patients show symmetric joint involvement reminiscent of rheumatoid arthritis.

Ophthalmologic examination may show conjunctivitis (11 percent) or periorbital edema (3 percent) in early infection, and keratitis or uveitis in late infection. Cardiac examination may suggest conduction abnormalities or a myopericarditis.

There are no unique features on the neurologic examination, but peripheral facial weakness (particularly if it is bilateral) or an unexpected finding of a carpal tunnel syndrome or distal mild sensory loss would support Lyme disease.

LABORATORY EVALUATION

The CDCP has created a case definition for Lyme disease for surveillance purposes (Table 3). It relies very heavily on laboratory criteria. In reality, there are many true cases that do not fulfill such strict criteria. I make the diagnosis of neurologic Lyme disease based on my clinical suspicion, and I use laboratory tests to provide supportive and baseline data (Table 4). The most important laboratory screening test is serum anti–*B. burgdorferi* antibodies. Positive serology documents exposure to the Lyme agent but says nothing about whether infection is active. Most antibody assays now use enzyme-linked immunosorbent assay (ELISA) technology rather than immunofluorescence. Unfortunately, there is still a quality control problem involving both inter- and intralaboratory consistency. It is important to use a reliable laboratory. I use the Clinical Immunology Laboratory at University Hospital, Stony Brook, which has a very good assay and also runs outside samples in bulk quantities. If there is any question about reliability, I recommend repeat serology in a different laboratory. The role of Western blot in Lyme disease is controversial since results are somewhat variable and not standardized. It is not a gold standard to document reactivity. I use Western blot to pursue a suspected false-positive ELISA. I do not pursue Western blot when reliable ELISA is negative. I also do not use lymphocyte proliferation to *B. burgdorferi* as a diagnostic test. I consider this cell-mediated immunity assay to be a research tool.

Up to 95 percent of neurologic Lyme patients are seropositive, but certain factors may contribute to false-negative and false-positive serologies (Table 5). Since it takes several weeks to mount sufficient amounts of antibodies to be detected, patients with very recent infections are likely to be seronegative. Early treatment may block the mature antibody response. When I have a patient with presumed late infection who is seronegative, I probe very carefully in the history looking for antibiotic use around the time they were infected. Legitimate false-positive serologies can occur due to cross-reactivity since several major *B. burgdorferi* antigens are shared by other organisms. For example, nonpathogenic oral treponemes cross-react with *B. burgdorferi*. When I suspect a false-positive serology, I specifically ask about gum disease and recent dental work. I will check for syphilis, elevated immunoglobulin levels, and autoantibodies.

Other than Lyme serology and studies performed to exclude other conditions, blood tests are generally not helpful in diagnosis. In early symptomatic infections, most patients show elevated levels of circulating immune complexes, and over 50 percent have an elevated erythrocyte sedimentation rate. A minority show mildly increased liver function tests and serum IgM levels. I

Table 3 Centers for Disease Control and Prevention Case Definition for Neurologic Lyme Disease

Physician-diagnosed EM (at least 5 cm)

or

Late manifestation
  Meningitis
  Cranial neuritis
  Radiculoneuropathy
  Encephalomyelitis with intrathecal antibody production

and

Laboratory confirmation
  Culture
  Serum or CSF antibodies
  Rising titers on acute and convalescent sera

EM = erythema migrans; CSF = cerebrospinal fluid.

Table 4 Key Laboratory Tests in the Diagnosis of Neurologic Lyme Disease

Positive serology (anti–*B. burgdorferi* antibodies)
  ELISA
  Western blot

Other blood tests
  Immune complexes
  Erythrocyte sedimentation rate
  Liver function tests
  IgM

Cerebrospinal fluid studies
  Anti–*B. burgdorferi* antibodies
  Intrathecal production of specific antibodies
  Cell count
  Protein and glucose
  VDRL
  Research studies (antigen, culture, immune complexes, nucleic acid)

Ancillary studies
  Neuroimaging
  Neurophysiologic tests
  Neuropsychological tests

Other studies
  Electrocardiogram
  Synovial fluid
  Biopsy
  Culture

always test for syphilis because it can cause a false-positive Lyme serology. I use a nontreponemal test since Lyme disease itself can produce a false-positive FTA-ABS.

I always examine CSF in suspected neurologic infections, even when the syndrome appears limited to the PNS, since the results affect how I treat the patient. CSF abnormalities are most marked in the meningitis syndrome, less striking in the other CNS syndromes, and generally normal in PNS syndromes unless there is radicular involvement. Overall, North American Lyme disease patients are less likely to have inflammatory CSF changes than European patients. Therefore I find abnormal CSF helpful when present to document neurologic infection, but I do not use normal CSF to

Table 5 Causes of a False-Positive and False-Negative
Lyme Serology

False-positive
 Cross-reactive spirochetal infection (e.g., mouth treponemes,
  syphilis, leptospirosis, relapsing fever)
 Severe bacterial infections
 Hypergammaglobulinemia
 Epstein-Barr virus
 Autoimmune disorders with high autoantibody titers
 Human immunodeficiency virus infection
 Unreliable assay
False-Negative
 Too early in the infection
 Early antibiotics with blunted humoral response
 Unreliable assay

exclude neurologic Lyme disease. Of available tests, intrathecal production of specific antibodies (CSF Lyme antibody index) is the best documentation for infection. This is offered commercially by several laboratories, including the Clinical Immunology Laboratory at Stony Brook. Other CSF abnormalities that can be seen include a low-grade mononuclear pleocytosis, plasma cells or atypical lymphocytes, and mildly elevated CSF protein. Glucose is normal in almost all Lyme cases, and CSF oligoclonal bands or increased IgG index are unusual. CSF myelin basic protein is never positive. I always check a CSF Venereal Disease Research Laboratory, since Lyme disease does not cause a false-positive nontreponemal test.

Several research tests are being applied to CSF of Lyme patients. These include detection of *B. burgdorferi* antigens and nucleic acids (polymerase chain reaction), Borrelia-specific immune complexes, and enhanced culture techniques. Although currently these tests are only available at specialized research centers, it is reasonable to save frozen CSF on very interesting patients for possible future testing.

Ancillary tests may be diagnostically helpful. Neuroimaging (magnetic resonance imaging [MRI] is superior to computed tomography) is abnormal in about 25 percent of neurologic Lyme patients. Abnormalities are nonspecific. When there are subcortical white matter lesions, they tend to be smaller than those seen in multiple sclerosis (MS). Nerve conduction tests may indicate a multifocal axonal neuropathy, which is very suggestive for Lyme disease. In the rare cases of muscle involvement due to Lyme disease, electromyogram studies may show a myopathic pattern. Electroencephalogram may be abnormal in encephalitis cases, but the slowing is nonspecific. Overall, seizures are rare in Lyme disease. Evoked potential tests are normal in Lyme disease. Formal cognitive function tests are helpful to document suspected encephalopathy. They also provide a quantitative baseline assessment that can be repeated after treatment.

Other helpful laboratory tests include electrocardiogram to look for heart block (third-, second-, or first-degree atrioventricular block; sinoatrial block), and synovial fluid examination (intrathecal antibody pro-

duction may be seen). Biopsy yield in Lyme disease is low, with the exception of the expanding edge of the EM lesion. Culture yield is also very low, and culture attempts are only made at specialized research centers.

DIFFERENTIAL DIAGNOSIS

There is nothing unique about the neurologic syndromes caused by *B. burgdorferi*. I consider the usual wide differential diagnosis list, in addition to Lyme disease, when faced with a patient with aseptic meningitis, Bell's palsy, isolated cranial nerve palsy, encephalopathy, neuropathy, radiculoneuropathy, or encephalomyelitis. Since Lyme disease occasionally produces atypical syndromes such as vasculitis, psychiatric disorders, dementia syndromes, and myopathies, I also consider Lyme disease in the differential diagnosis of such patients. Some aspects of Lyme disease may mimic a chronic fatigue or fibromyalgia syndrome. However, I expect such patients to have other features that suggest Lyme disease, in addition to their nonspecific complaints.

One differential diagnosis that is mentioned frequently with Lyme disease is MS. I rarely find it difficult to distinguish these two disorders. The history, examination, and laboratory data are distinct. In Lyme disease I expect extraneural features and frequent PNS involvement. CSF of Lyme patients infrequently shows oligoclonal bands or increased IgG index, which are found in 90 to 95 percent and 70 to 90 percent of MS patients, respectively. CSF from Lyme patients is much more likely to show mild pleocytosis and protein elevation. Elevated myelin basic protein is not found in Lyme disease but may be seen in MS relapses. MRI abnormalities are uncommon in Lyme disease but are seen in 90 percent of MS patients. When present, white matter lesions in Lyme disease tend to be smaller and more like a "vasculitic" pattern than a demyelinating pattern. Evoked potentials are normal in Lyme disease but are abnormal in about 50 percent of MS patients. Of course, in some cases I make a dual diagnosis: an MS patient can certainly be infected with *B. burgdorferi*.

Certain pitfalls lead to overdiagnosis of Lyme disease (Table 6). Clearly, when up to 50 percent of infections are asymptomatic, the finding of a positive serology in a patient with a common complaint (headache, dizziness, pain) does not mean the complaint is due to Lyme disease. In such cases I look for substantiating data for the diagnosis using history, examination, and laboratory evaluations. It is also common for complaints such as fatigue, headache, muscle and joint pain to linger for a period of time after treatment. Such postinfectious syndromes are particularly likely when treatment is given later in the infection and when infection has produced marked constitutional symptoms. This postinfectious syndrome is not necessarily evidence for ineffective therapy requiring further antibiotics if the trend over time is improvement of the complaints. I counsel my patients that it may take from months to nearly a year or

Table 6 Major Pitfalls in the Diagnosis of
Neurologic Lyme Disease

The patient must have active Lyme disease because:
• They have a positive Lyme serology.
• Although they were treated for Lyme disease, they still have complaints.
• They are seronegative, but Lyme disease may explain their complaints (headache, fatigue, myalgias, arthralgias, cognitive problems).

The patient cannot have active Lyme disease because:
• They are seronegative.
• They were treated for Lyme disease.
• It is not summertime.
• They were not bitten by a tick.
• Their CSF is normal.

two for them to fully recover. If I become concerned about the severity or pattern of a postinfectious syndrome, I re-evaluate the patient, including CSF examination. My index of concern is highest for postinfectious encephalopathy. Some of these patients do have a persistent infection. Finally, Lyme disease is never blindly applied as a diagnosis when patients complain of nonspecific symptoms and there is no other clearcut cause. It is tempting to assign a treatable condition to desperate patients, but it is a disservice to do this without supportive data.

Certain pitfalls also lead to underdiagnosis (see Table 6). Not all Lyme patients are seropositive, and legitimate seronegative patients exist. I evaluate such patients as seriously as those who have a positive ELISA. Some postinfectious syndromes represent persistent infection. Reinfections can also occur. Therefore I periodically reassess my thinking in treated patients who have continued complaints. I never use the time of year to exclude the possibility of Lyme disease. Although there is a seasonal pattern, particularly in the northeast, cases can be seen all year round. Patients can present clinically at different periods after the infection. It is also true that winters have been milder, so that tick bites may occur beyond just the summer months. Most neurologic Lyme patients will not give a history of tick bite, so this is never used to exclude Lyme disease. Finally, abnormal CSF is diagnostically useful when present, but normal CSF does not rule out neurologic Lyme disease. Although in the future, CSF research tests are likely to enhance our ability to establish a diagnosis, none of these tests are 100 percent accurate for infection.

SUGGESTED READING

Coyle PK. Neurologic Lyme disease. Semin Neurol 1992; 12:200–208.
Coyle PK, ed. Lyme disease. St. Louis: Mosby–Year Book, 1993.
Logigian EL, Kaplan RF, Steere AC. Chronic neurologic manifestations of Lyme disease. N Engl J Med 1990; 323:1438–1444.
Rahn DW, Malawista SE. Lyme disease: Recommendations for diagnosis and treatment. Ann Intern Med 1991; 114:472–481.
Reik LR Jr. Lyme disease and the nervous system. New York: Thieme, 1991.
Steere AC. Lyme disease. N Engl J Med 1989; 321:586–596.

NEUROSYPHILIS

LARRY E. DAVIS, M.D.

Neurosyphilis is due to infection of the central nervous system (CNS) by *Treponema pallidum*. *T. pallidum* is a spirochete with Homo sapiens as its only known natural reservoir. The spirochete replicates slowly, with a division occurring every 30 to 35 hours. The slow division time accounts in part for the chronic nature of this disease. To date, continued in vitro growth in tissue culture of *T. pallidum* has not been successful. However, the organism will replicate in the testes of rabbits, and animal inoculations have successfully isolated *T. pallidum* from human cerebrospinal fluid (CSF).

Syphilis is acquired primarily through sexual contact. The primary site of infection is usually the vagina, penis, or rectum. Transmission can also occur to a fetus following spirochete passage through the placenta. After *T. pallidum* penetrates the skin or mucous membranes, the spirochetes replicate locally and enter the lymphatics and bloodstream to disseminate throughout the body. A genital chancre develops about 3 weeks after the initial infection. Secondary syphilitic lesions usually occur several weeks later. At this stage, spirochetes invade the CNS in up to 40 percent of individuals. The CNS infection is reflected by abnormalities in the CSF. The patient may be asymptomatic (asymptomatic neurosyphilis) or symptomatic (acute syphilitic meningitis). Even in the absence of treatment, this stage usually subsides and a latent period ensues. Months to years later, some patients experience tertiary CNS manifestations of the infection. Although the clinical manifestations of neurosyphilis are varied, most can be viewed as consequences of a low-grade persistent meningitis.

Tertiary neurosyphilis has generally been divided into three broad types: meningovascular syphilis, parenchymatous neurosyphilis (paretic neurosyphilis or general paresis), and tabes dorsalis. In meningovascular syphilis, the chronic meningitis results in arteritis and occlusions of small meningeal blood vessels, producing brain stem or cerebral cortex infarctions. In parenchymatous neurosyphilis, spirochetes invade the brain causing a low-grade encephalitis resulting in neuropsychiatric abnormalities, pupillary abnormalities, and progressive dementia. In tabes dorsalis, abnormalities of the spinal cord predominate, with sensory ataxia, painful paresthesias, and loss of deep pain sensation in the legs. Optic atrophy and Argyll Robertson pupils may also occur. The signs and symptoms of these types of neurosyphilis are well described in most neurology textbooks and are beyond the scope of this chapter. Although this chapter will not discuss the diagnosis of congenital neurosyphilis in detail, the signs, symptoms, and serology are fairly similar to those of acquired neurosyphilis except that they occur at a younger age.

CEREBROSPINAL FLUID IN NEUROSYPHILIS

Invasion of the meninges by *T. pallidum* produces characteristic CSF abnormalities typical of a chronic meningitis (Table 1). These CSF changes are present in all stages of neurosyphilis. The CSF demonstrates a mild lymphocytic pleocytosis, moderately elevated protein, and normal glucose level. In response to the chronic meningitis, B lymphocytes migrate into the meninges producing an increased synthesis of CSF immunoglobulins. Electrophoresis of CSF usually shows an increase in the percentage of gamma globulin and several oligoclonal bands in the gamma globulin region. In acute syphilitic meningitis, spirochetes may occasionally be seen by dark field or direct fluorescent antibody microscopy of CSF sediment. One should not see the CSF changes of acute pyogenic meningitis, such as glucose levels below 35 mg per deciliter, protein levels above 250 mg per deciliter, or bacteria on Gram's stain of CSF sediment. *T. pallidum* spirochetes are too narrow to be seen by light microscopy unless special silver stains are used.

Examination of the CSF should be performed on all patients with reactive serum syphilis serology who have neurologic signs compatible with neurosyphilis, or in patients with previously treated neurosyphilis in whom there is a possibility of a relapse.

CSF SEROLOGIC TESTS FOR SYPHILIS

A definitive diagnosis of neurosyphilis can be made by isolation of *T. pallidum* from brain, meninges, or CSF. In practice this is seldom done, because animal inoculation is required and small numbers of spirochetes are present in the tertiary stage of neurosyphilis. Thus, serologic tests have become the standard for diagnosing neurosyphilis.

To diagnose syphilis, one wants the most sensitive and specific test available to detect any *T. pallidum* antibody in blood produced by the patient in response to the infection. To diagnose neurosyphilis, one wants a CSF test that can distinguish between *T. pallidum* antibody that passively enters the CSF through the choroid plexus and *T. pallidum* antibody that is locally produced in the brain and meninges by B cells that have migrated into the CNS in response to a local spirochetal infection. Therefore, an extremely sensitive serologic test may not be helpful in diagnosing neurosyphilis.

Table 1 Cerebrospinal Fluid in Neurosyphilis

CSF Measure	Value
Percent with elevated opening pressure	<10%
Total white blood cells	5–500/mm^3
Percent lymphocytic cells	50%–99%
Total red blood cells	0–5/mm^3
Glucose level	35–75 mg/dl
Total protein level	30–250 mg/dl
Percent with elevated gamma globulin level (>11% of total protein)	50%–80%
Percent with oligoclonal bands	>50%
Percent with reactive CSF VDRL test	50%–85%
Percent with reactive CSF FTA-ABS test	75%–95%

CSF = cerebrospinal fluid, VDRL = Venereal Disease Research Laboratory, FTA-ABS = fluorescent treponemal antibody absorption.

The CSF-Venereal Disease Research Laboratory (CSF-VDRL) test is a widely used nontreponemal test. In this test, CSF is evaluated for its ability to flocculate a suspension of cardiolipin-cholesterol-lecithin antigen. Although false-positive VDRL tests occur in serum, they are rare in CSF. Therefore, the presence of a reactive CSF-VDRL test is virtually diagnostic of neurosyphilis. An advantage of the CSF-VDRL test is that the amount of antibody present in the CSF can be titered. Since the CSF-VDRL titer falls after appropriate antibiotic treatment, the response to treatment can be followed with this test. Unfortunately, the CSF-VDRL test is not sufficiently sensitive to diagnose all cases of neurosyphilis. Several studies have reported the test sensitivity to be from 50 to 85 percent. Thus, exclusive use of the CSF-VDRL test to diagnose active neurosyphilis will miss up to one-half of the patients.

Another nontreponemal test, the rapid plasma reagin (RPR) test, is widely used as a screening test on serum. However, this test has frequent false-positive reactions in CSF and should not be used.

Several specific treponemal serological tests can be used on CSF. The most commonly used are the fluorescent treponemal antibody absorption (CSF-FTA-ABS) test and the microhemagglutinin assay for antibodies to *T. pallidum* (CSF-MHA-TP). In the CSF-FTA-ABS test, CSF is mixed with sorbent (sonicate of Reiter treponemes and other appropriate material) to remove low-grade nonspecific antibody and then incubated on slides containing *T. pallidum* antigen. Fluorescein-labeled antihuman globulin is applied to the slides, which are examined under a fluorescent microscope. In the CSF-MHA-TP test, CSF is tested for its ability to agglutinate sensitized sheep erythrocytes that are coated with lysed *T. pallidum*. In a recent comparison, the CSF-FTA-ABS test was found to be superior in sensitivity and specificity.

The CSF-FTA-ABS test has several major disadvantages. It is a qualitative test and does not yield a titer. Thus the test cannot be used to follow response to treatment. Furthermore, like the blood FTA-ABS test, the CSF-FTA-ABS test usually remains reactive for many years, even after appropriate treatment. Finally, the test is so sensitive that small amounts of serum or blood leakage into CSF via a traumatic lumbar puncture or break in the blood-brain barrier may produce a false-positive test. These limitations mean that a reactive CSF-FTA-ABS test can indicate several things: active neurosyphilis, asymptomatic neurosyphilis, treated neurosyphilis, or a false-positive reaction. Additional clinical and laboratory information is needed to determine which is correct. On the other hand, a nonreactive CSF-FTA-ABS or serum FTA-ABS test rules out neurosyphilis, except in the patient with acquired immunodeficiency syndrome (AIDS).

DIAGNOSIS OF ACTIVE NEUROSYPHILIS

The diagnosis of active neurosyphilis requires fulfillment of three criteria—compatible clinical history, characteristic CSF abnormalities, reactive syphilis serologic tests—and no other explanation for the neurologic signs and CSF abnormalities.

1. *Compatible clinical history:* While neurosyphilitic signs and symptoms may be varied, they are usually of recent onset (less than 1 year) and progressive. In addition, one or more of the following are usually present:
   - Decrease in cognitive function
   - Unexplained personality change
   - Stroke
   - Irregular or Argyll Robertson pupils
   - Chorioretinitis or optic nerve dysfunction
   - Dizziness or hearing loss attributable to inner ear dysfunction
   - Loss of position sense in feet with preserved pain and temperature sense

2. *Characteristic CSF abnormalities:* Typical CSF changes are outlined in Table 1. In general, the CSF should contain:
   - Pleocytosis with 5 to 250 lymphocytes per cubic millimeter
   - Protein level below 250 mg per deciliter
   - Glucose level above 35 mg per deciliter

It is well recognized that active neurosyphilis can occasionally occur when the CSF lacks a pleocytosis or the protein level is normal.

3. *Reactive syphilis serologic tests:*
   - Reactive serum FTA-ABS test
   - Reactive serum RPR test
   - Reactive CSF-VDRL test

4. As previously discussed, some patients with active neurosyphilis have a nonreactive CSF-VDRL test. In this situation, the patient should have a reactive CSF-FTA-ABS test, elevated CSF immunoglobulin G levels, or oligoclonal

bands in the gamma globulin region of electrophoresed CSF.

DIAGNOSIS OF ASYMPTOMATIC NEUROSYPHILIS

Asymptomatic neurosyphilis implies a *T. pallidum* infection of the meninges without compatible neurologic signs and symptoms. Therefore one would expect to find reactive syphilis serologic tests and CSF abnormalities. The CSF abnormalities are usually mild, and a CSF pleocytosis may not be present.

DIAGNOSIS OF TREATED NEUROSYPHILIS

Neurosyphilitic patients who are adequately treated with antibiotics may have permanent neurologic damage with persistence of neurologic signs and CSF abnormalities. In general, adequately treated patients should meet the following criteria:

1. *History of adequate treatment with appropriate antibiotics*
2. *Lack of new or progressive neurologic signs:* While this criterion holds true for acute syphilitic meningitis, meningovascular syphilis and parenchymatous neurosyphilis, occasional patients with tabes dorsalis may develop progressive neurologic signs in the face of adequate treatment.
3. *Improvement in CSF abnormalities over time:* By 3 to 6 months after adequate antibiotic treatment, the CSF cell count should be normal and the protein level at or near normal. The CSF-VDRL titer should have fallen from its initial level. By 2 years, the CSF should be normal and the CSF-VDRL test nonreactive or reactive at a very low titer. The CSF-FTA-ABS test usually remains reactive for indefinite periods of time and cannot be used to evaluate the treatment status.

Patients who have been previously treated for syphilis but fail to meet the above criteria should be considered to have been inadequately treated and should be retreated with antibiotics. One should be particularly careful about patients who did not receive penicillin, because the relapse rate for second line antibiotics is considerably higher.

NEUROSYPHILIS IN A PATIENT INFECTED WITH HUMAN IMMUNODEFICIENCY VIRUS

There are several reasons why neurosyphilis is more difficult to diagnose in HIV-infected patients. First, HIV-infected individuals have an impaired cellular immune system, particularly in the later stages of the infection. As a consequence, *T. pallidum* infections often progress at a faster rate and produce more unusual clinical features than normally expected. This is particularly notable in secondary syphilis where CNS manifestations are frequent. Second, serum and CSF syphilis serologic tests may be nonreactive in these patients even though *T. pallidum* has been recovered from CSF. Nonreactive syphilis serologic tests have usually occurred in patients with secondary syphilis rather than tertiary syphilis. However, the majority of HIV-infected patients with active neurosyphilis have reactive serum and CSF treponemal and nontreponemal tests. Third, the HIV infection may cause a chronic meningitis that mimics the CSF changes seen in neurosyphilis. In particular, CSF pleocytosis, elevated protein level, and elevated immunoglobulin G level may be present in HIV-infected patients. Fourth, AIDS may cause a progressive dementia and myelopathy that mimics the signs of neurosyphilis. However, Argyll Robertson pupils have not been seen in AIDS.

The CSF should be examined in all HIV-infected patients with clinically suspected neurosyphilis. If the patient meets the criteria for active neurosyphilis, even though the CSF abnormalities could be due to HIV, a presumptive diagnosis of active neurosyphilis should be made and the individual should be treated with long-term high-dose penicillin.

SUGGESTED READING

Davis LE. Neurosyphilis in the patient with human immunodeficiency virus. Ann Neurol 1990; 21:211–212.

Davis LE, Schmitt JW. Clinical significance of cerebrospinal fluid tests for neurosyphilis. Ann Neurol 1989; 25:50–55.

Hart G. Syphilis tests in diagnostic and therapeutic decision making. Ann Intern Med 1986; 104:368–376.

Larsen SA, Hamble EA, Wobig GH, Kennedy EJ. Cerebrospinal fluid serologic test for syphilis: Treponemal and nontreponemal tests. In: Morisset R, Kurstak E, eds. Advances in sexually transmitted diseases. Utrecht: VNU Science Press, 1987:157.

Lukehart SA, Hook EW, Baker-Zander SA, et al. Invasion of the central nervous system by *Treponema pallidum*: Implications for diagnosis and treatment. Ann Intern Med 1988; 109:855–862.

Merritt JJ, Adams RD, Solomon HC. Neurosyphilis. New York: Oxford University Press, 1946.

Nordenbo AM, Sorensen PS. The incidence and clinical presentation of neurosyphilis in greater Copenhagen 1974 through 1978. Acta Neurol Scand 1981; 63:237–246.

Simon RP. Neurosyphilis. Arch Neurol 1985; 42:606–613.

TUBERCULOSIS OF THE NERVOUS SYSTEM

NAGAGOPAL VENNA, M.D.
THOMAS D. SABIN, M.D.

The resurgence of tuberculosis in the United States during the past decade is largely due to acquired immunodeficiency syndrome (AIDS), but the expanding reservoir of tuberculosis has heightened the risk of infection in the general community as well. About 15 percent of patients with tuberculosis have extrapulmonary disease, and about 6 percent of these have neurologic involvement. These proportions are substantially larger in patients with AIDS.

Table 1 A Classification of Neurotuberculosis

Intracranial Tuberculosis
  Cranial meningitis with cranial neuropathies and
    encephalopathies
  Intracerebral tuberculoma
  Tuberculous allergic encephalopathy

Intraspinal Tuberculosis
  Vertebral tuberculosis with compressive myelopathy and
    radiculopathy (Pott's disease)
  Spinal meningitis with myeloradiculopathy

Tuberculosis affects the nervous system in several patterns (Table 1), the most common being tuberculous meningitis, but the neurologist must be vigilant for unusual forms such as spinal meningitis, cerebral tuberculomas, and overlapping syndromes.

CLINICAL EPIDEMIOLOGY OF NEUROTUBERCULOSIS

A high index of suspicion is essential for the diagnosis of neurotuberculosis because the neurologic manifestations are protean and alarmingly nonspecific. High-risk groups include patients with human immunodeficiency virus (HIV) infection, especially IV drug abusers; immigrants from areas such as Asia, the Caribbean, and the Pacific islands where tuberculosis is highly endemic; persons exposed to patients with tuberculosis at home or at work, including physicians and nurses; persons with alcoholism and malnutrition; people in prisons, shelters for the homeless, nursing homes, and psychiatric institutions; the elderly; and Native Americans. Patients who are immunosuppressed by chronic corticosteroid therapy or by treatment for organ transplantation are also at increased risk. Neurologic tuberculosis may still emerge in the patient already receiving drugs for treatment of extraneural tuberculosis because of an inadequate regimen of drugs, poor compliance by the patient with the treatment, resistance of the mycobacteria to conventional drugs, or because not enough time has elapsed for the drugs to be effective.

TUBERCULOUS CRANIAL MENINGITIS

Tuberculous meningitis (TBM) is the most common form of neurologic tuberculosis, with about 4,000 new cases per year in the United States alone. Extensive gelatinous exudate fills the cisterns at the base of the brain and the sylvian fissures, leading to entrapment of the cranial nerves and occlusive vasculitis of the circle of Willis and the middle cerebral arteries, with consequent multifocal cerebral infarctions, especially in the basal ganglia. Obliteration of the basal cisterns and blockage of the foramina of the fourth ventricle by the exudate, tuberculous ventriculitis, and occasionally an aqueductal tuberculoma conspire to cause obstructive hydrocephalus. The optic nerves, chiasm, and hypothalamus are frequently severely affected.

Clinical Features

An often nonspecific prodrome of up to 2 weeks consists of subacute intermittent headache, malaise, and lassitude mingled with periods of confusion and agitation. A low-grade fever may accompany this but frequently without symptoms of meningeal irritation. The patient may complain of an unduly prolonged flulike illness, and friends and family may remark on a change of personality with withdrawal and irritability.

Inexorably, the meningitic phase ensues, with increasing headache, neck pain, and stiffness and deepening lethargy. Symptoms of cranial neuropathy such as blurring of vision or double vision are often obscured by stupor. Patients tend to deteriorate over days or weeks into coma with decerebrate or decorticate postures. The course is punctuated by focal or generalized seizures and an accumulation of focal neurologic signs such as hemiplegia due to brain infarction. Cranial nerve abnormalities include blindness and occular and facial palsies. Hypothermia and diabetes insipidus due to hypothalamic injury further complicate the clinical picture. The course of the illness is steadily downhill over about 4 to 6 weeks, death being the rule if the patient is not treated.

Other patterns of TBM are infrequent. An acute meningitic form that evolves over hours or a few days closely resembles acute purulent bacterial meningitis. At the other extreme, some patients present with a brain-tumor–like picture of increasing headaches, changes in mental function, and gait disturbance due to a quietly developing hydrocephalus with hardly a hint of the underlying meningitis. A stroke syndrome such as an acute hemiplegia can be the presenting symptom.

Patients usually appear ill, with a low-grade fever and neck stiffness, but these features may be absent. The body temperature may actually be subnormal due to hypothalamic injury. Large pupils that react poorly to light are a curious diagnostic feature and have been attributed to involvement of the pupilloconstrictor fibers on the surface of the third cranial nerves by the meningitis. Internuclear ophthalmoplegia has been attributed to the ischemia in the territory of the penetrating arteries of the brain stem secondary to the meningitic vasculitis. Scrupulous general physical examination may reveal evidence of tuberculosis elsewhere and should include a search for choroidal tubercles by ophthalmoscopy. Ileocecal masses of tuberculous enteritis, especially in patients of Asian origin, and matted, enlarged lymph nodes with cold abscess or fistula are other highly diagnostic clues.

Diagnosis

Only a high degree of clinical suspicion will permit diagnosis early enough to avert otherwise inevitable major neurologic morbidity or mortality. This requires that an examination of the cerebrospinal fluid (CSF) be performed with fairly nonspecific symptoms when the clinical context is suggestive. The diagnosis should also be considered when the clinical and CSF profile indicate partially treated pyogenic meningitis or an acute viral meningitis. Table 2 lists clinical syndromes where TBM should be in the differential diagnosis.

Laboratory Aids in Diagnosis

Brain Scan. Although CSF examination is the critical test, it is probably unrealistic to expect this to be done prior to computed tomography (CT) or magnetic resonance imaging (MRI) of the brain in most hospitals in the United States at present, especially in a subacute illness. In our experience the neurologist is typically consulted after brain imaging. This practice is acceptable as long as the brain is scanned urgently and the lumbar puncture (LP) is not postponed unduly while awaiting the scan. The scan should not replace the CSF examination, because it only shows the effects of the meningitis on the brain or sometimes reveals alternative diagnoses. The scan does not permit the specific diagnosis of TBM itself. The contrast-enhanced CT scan may be normal, indicating a good prognosis because secondary damage to the brain has not yet occurred. In about 10 percent of cases, tuberculomas may appear as focal enhancing lesions with or without calcification and provide good supportive evidence of a tuberculous process. In many cases there is nonspecific enhancement of the basal cisterns, indicating inflammation of the meninges. Later, hydrocephalus may appear. Dilation of the temporal horns in particular suggests a rapidly evolving obstructive hydrocephalus. Infarctions may be seen as hypodense areas in the basal ganglia or on the surface of the brain in the perisylvian regions. MRI scans show the same abnormalities but with greater precision and

Table 2 Syndromes in Which TBM Should Be Considered

Subacute meningitis
Subacute encephalopathy: with confusion, agitation, psychosis, personality changes
Subacute coma
Acute meningitis; partially treated pyogenic meningitis
Stroke syndrome preceded by constitutional prodrome
Subacute multiple cranial neuropathies

sensitivity (Fig. 1). The basal meningeal enhancement and ventricular ependymal enhancement with gadolinium are demonstrated exquisitely. Some tuberculomas and hypothalamic involvement are well seen even when they are not apparent on CT scans. The MRI scan is more sensitive than the CT scan in delineating ischemic lesions. On the other hand, the telltale clue of calcification in the tuberculomas may be missed on the MRI while being readily visible on the CT scans.

Cerebrospinal Fluid Examination. This crucial test should be done promptly and repeated on several occasions in the first few days if initial examination is inconclusive. The typical profile is highly suggestive of the diagnosis but is nonspecific. The CSF may be xanthochromic due to marked increase in the protein, and it tends to form a cobweb on standing. The predominantly lymphocytic pleocytosis is between 100 and 500 cells per cubic millimeter. Protein is often increased to 100 to 500 mg per deciliter and glucose reduced to less than 45 mg per deciliter, or to less than 40 percent simultaneous blood glucose in patients with hyperglycemia. Atypical initial CSF profiles include predominantly polymorphonuclear cell increase in about 15 percent of patients, with only mildly increased protein and normal glucose. Gradual transition of the cells to lymphocytes from polymorphonuclear cells and gradual decline in the glucose on serial taps are characteristic. The protein may reach levels of 1 to 2 g per deciliter. On the other hand, the initial CSF may, rarely, be acellular, while subsequent spinal taps reveal typical abnormalities.

Because culture of the CSF requires up to 6 or 8 weeks, diagnosis depends on immediate detection of the bacilli. Although the acid-fast bacilli (AFB) stain may be negative in more than 50 percent of cases, the yield can be maximized by the following techniques. Large volumes (10 to 30 ml) of the CSF should be obtained. Smears should be obtained from both the sediment and the pellicle after the CSF is centrifuged for about 20 minutes. The multiple drop method, in which several sequential drops of the spinal fluid are allowed to dry, is another technique to enhance the yield. Repeating the LP over the next 3 to 4 days despite starting antituberculous therapy is an important way to find positive stains. Prolonged scrutiny of the smears for at least 30 minutes is useful because of the paucity of the AFB in the CSF.

Cerebrospinal Fluid Cultures for Mycobacteria. Culture is the gold standard for TBM, but it may be negative in about 20 percent of patients and requires 6 to 8 weeks. This makes the diagnosis retrospective, but correct diagnosis remains important in the management of the patient facing 1 to 2 years of multiple drug therapy. As with the AFB stains, the culture yield is increased by using large volumes of CSF and repeating the LP on several occasions in the first few days. Determination of drug sensitivities is also important, because ever more cases are caused by resistant strains. Drug sensitivity assays are available in only a few centers in the United States at the present time, an example of which is the National Jewish Center for Immunology and Respiratory Medicine in Denver, Colorado.

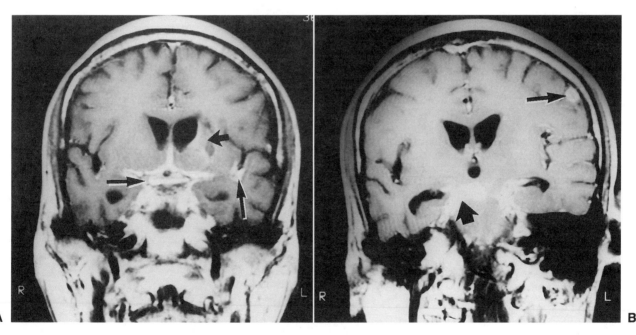

Figure 1 Tuberculous meningitis. This young man from Vietnam developed tuberculous meningitis while being treated for pulmonary tuberculosis caused by multidrug-resistant organisms. He was HIV negative. *A,* Coronal brain magnetic resonance imaging with gadolinium. Long arrows show intense enhancement of the meninges in the suprasellar cisterns and sylvian fissure. Short arrow shows low signal in the basal ganglia and ipsilateral dilation of the frontal horn due to lenticulostriate territory infarction and focal volume loss. *B,* Long arrow shows focal, rounded high signal in left cerebral cortex consistent with tuberculoma. Short arrow indicates extensive basal meningeal enhancement.

Rapid Diagnostic Tests in Cerebrospinal Fluid. Even in this age of biotechnology, bacteriologic diagnosis of TBM remains slow and uncertain, but newer methods are being developed. These include estimation of levels of adenosine deaminase, detection of the products of mycobacterial tuberculostearic acid by spectroscopy, detection of mycobacterial antigens by immunologic methods, and amplification of bacterial DNA by polymerase chain reaction (PCR). Another promising technique is the use of bacteriophages (luciferases) that specifically infect *Mycobacterium tuberculosis* and are easily detected by their fluorescence.

Meningeal/Brain Biopsy. Rarely, TBM has been inadvertently diagnosed by biopsy of the meninges or the brain in cases thought to be due to obscure meningoencephalitis. However, the biopsy may be inconclusive since the basal surface is most severely affected by TBM, rather than the convexity surface, which is usually biopsied.

Laboratory Evidence of Extraneural Tuberculosis. Because the clinical, CSF, and brain imaging picture of TBM is nonspecific, extraneural tuberculosis provides important supportive evidence for the diagnosis. Scrutiny of chest films for infiltrates, cavitation, fibrosis, pleural effusion, hilar and mediastinal adenopathy, and miliary tubercles is useful. These tests may be negative in about 50 percent of patients. Sputum should be examined thoroughly for AFB even if a chest film is negative. The skin purified protein derivative (PPD) test is useful but may be negative in about 50 percent of patients, sometimes temporarily, because of the meningitis. Conversion of the skin test from negative to positive as documented in military personnel or in prisoners is useful supportive evidence, as in one of our recent patients with spinal tuberculosis. The tuberculous nature of the infection can be established sometimes by biopsy of an abnormal lymph node, bone marrow, a cold abscess, or an ileocecal mass.

Table 3 Causes of Difficulty in the Clinical Diagnosis of Tuberculous Meningitis

Lack of high index of clinical suspicion
Presentation as acute meningitis
Presentation with prominent changes in mental functions and little to indicate meningeal irritation so that CSF analysis is not done or delayed
Frequent absence of neck stiffness and/or fever. Complexity of clinical picture once meningitis is complicated by cranial nerve palsies, hypothalamic derangement, brain infarctions, hydrocephalus, and seizures
Stroke presentation with a mild constitutional prodrome
Neurologic picture obscured by intercurrent illness such as alcohol withdrawal or head trauma
Neurologic syndrome evolving while patient is on antituberculous chemotherapy
Frequent absence of clinical and laboratory evidence of extraneural tuberculosis
Therapeutic response to antituberculous drugs not always predictable as a diagnostic test

Differential Diagnosis

The diagnosis of TBM is often straightforward, but can severely test the acumen of even seasoned clinicians. Tables 3 and 4 list the reasons for the complexity of the diagnosis. Table 5 lists some of the conditions that should be considered in the differential diagnosis.

Ruling out other infections causing subacute meningitis is the most pressing problem and usually can be performed by a combination of clinical and laboratory methods. Fungal meningitis, most often due to cryptococci and in certain geographic areas histoplasmosis and blastomycosis, may mimic TBM closely. Identification of the fungi on stains, estimation of fungal antigens or antibodies, and culturing the organisms from the CSF provide fairly rapid diagnosis. The acute aseptic meningitis of secondary stage and the stroke and dementia syndromes of tertiary syphilis can resemble TBM both clinically and in the CSF profile, but the serum and CSF-VDRL and specific treponemal antibody tests

Table 4 Causes of Difficulty in the Laboratory Diagnosis of Tuberculous Meningitis

Rare cases of initially normal CSF
CSF may initially show a predominantly polymorphonuclear pleocytosis (15% of cases)
CSF glucose may be normal initially so that the initial diagnosis is "aseptic meningitis"
AFB are found in CSF smears in less than 50% of cases as usually examined
Culture of AFB in CSF may take 4 to 6 weeks
Typical profile of CSF abnormalities is nonspecific
CT, MRI appearance are often nonspecific, indicating only basal meningitis

Table 5 Differential Diagnosis of Tuberculous Meningitis

Subacute meningeal infections
  Fungal meningitis
    Cryptococcosis
    Coccidioidomycosis
    Histoplasmosis
    Blastomycosis
  Syphilis
    Aseptic meningitis of secondary stage
    Meningovascular syphilis of tertiary stage
  Partially treated bacterial pyogenic meningitis
    Neurobrucellosis
    Lyme meningoencephalitis

Parameningeal infections
  Pyogenic infections
    Epidural abscess
    Brain abscess
    Subdural empyema

Viral infections
  Herpes simplex encephalitis

Noninfectious causes
  Sarcoidosis
  Neoplastic meningitis

establish the diagnosis. In the appropriate epidemiologic context, Lyme disease and brucellosis need to be ruled out by serologic tests. Partially treated pyogenic meningitis is difficult to distinguish from TBM because antibiotics often eradicate the organisms from the CSF smears and cultures and modify its profile to resemble TBM. However the cell type is predominently polymorphonuclear, cell counts are usually in the thousands per cubic millimeter, and the protein is elevated only modestly. Counterimmunoelectrophoresis may rapidly detect the bacterial antigens commonly causing meningitis, but negative tests do not rule out the infection. In practice it is not uncommon for the patient to be treated empirically with antibiotics for the usual causes of bacterial meningitis until the picture becomes clearer. Herpes encephalitis also resembles TBM, but the images by CT or MRI performed sequentially reveal the characteristic evolving focal abnormalities in the frontal and temporal lobes with mass effect. Definite diagnosis may require a brain biopsy. The CSF in cases of parameningeal infection such as a brain abscess, intracranial subdural empyema, or a spinal epidural abscess can resemble the picture of TBM, but the CSF glucose is normal. The clinical picture and appropriate imaging usually identify the parameningeal infection rapidly.

Noninfectious causes such as sarcoidosis and neoplasms can produce clinical and CSF pictures similar to those of TBM. The neoplastic meningitis caused by lymphomas and carcinomas is established by repeated cytologic examination of large volumes of CSF. The diagnosis of sarcoid meningitis is established by biopsy of tissues such as lymph nodes, liver, or skeletal muscle.

Therapeutic Diagnostic Tests

Even when the CSF does not reveal AFB on stain, antituberculous therapy with at least three drugs such as isoniazid (INH), rifampin, and pyrazinamide, which have good penetration into the CSF, should be started when the clinical and laboratory abnormalities are strongly suggestive and no alternative diagnosis can be established rapidly. The CSF should continue to be studied for at least 3 to 4 days after starting antituberculous therapy so that the organism can be cultured or found in smears. When the information does not sharply support one diagnosis, empirical therapy for tuberculosis, syphilis, herpes simplex, and acute bacterial meningitis may be used in various combinations depending upon the clinical context. As more information becomes available, some of these treatments can be discarded.

Therapeutic response to antituberculous drugs is gratifying, provided diagnosis is made early. Improvement in alertness and clearing of confusion are paralleled by falling cell counts and rising glucose in the CSF in a few weeks, but protein levels often take longer to improve. However, the therapeutic response can be confusing when the treatment is initiated after the meningitis is well established, because the drugs may not promptly stop the pathologic cascade set in motion by

the adhesive meningitis. Despite appropriate drug therapy, the patient may continue to deteriorate, with the development of strokes, cranial neuropathies, and obstructive hydrocephalus. Rarely, a tuberculoma, previously unrecognizable, may appear in the brain and enlarge, causing further neurologic impairment despite antituberculous therapy. Exceptionally, an acute neurologic worsening with stupor can occur with the initiation of therapy, associated with diffuse brain edema as an allergic reaction to the tubercular protein. Both these paradoxical responses can be controlled with judicious use of dexamethasone.

Tuberculous Meningitis in AIDS

Extrapulmonary tuberculosis occurs in about 25 to 40 percent of AIDS patients, about 10 percent of them having tuberculous meningitis. TBM is an AIDS-defining diagnosis that tends to occur in the earlier phases of immunodeficiency, with CD4 T cell counts of about 400 per cubic millimeter. The spectrum of clinical, CSF, and brain imaging manifestations of TBM in AIDS patients is very similar to that in patients without HIV infection. However, the supportive evidence of extra-neurotuberculosis is quite different in AIDS patients. The PPD skin test tends to be less frequently positive, even when induration of over 5 mm is considered to be abnormal. The chest films show unusual patterns, such as infiltrates in many lobes of the lungs, lack of cavitation, and frequent hilar and mediastinal adenopathy. The chest film may be normal yet the sputum may show abundant AFB. Most AIDS patients with TBM respond to antituberculous drugs, like patients without AIDS, although when the CD4 T cell counts fall below 200 per cubic millimeter the prognosis is poor. Most tuberculous infections resistant to conventional drugs occur in AIDS patients, so that whenever possible their CSF and sputum should be assayed for drug sensitivities.

TUBERCULOMAS OF THE BRAIN

Caseating granulomas made up of epithelioid cells and macrophages containing mycobacteria occur in the brain as single or multiple focal lesions and may become calcified. Rarely, extensive caseating necrosis forms a tuberculous (cold) abscess, especially in patients with AIDS. Both of these lesions usually occur without meningitis.

Clinical Features

Calcified granulomas in the brain may be seen as incidental findings in brain scans obtained for unrelated reasons, especially in endemic areas. Tuberculomas are an important consideration in the evaluation of new onset seizures, whether the seizures are focal, generalized, or, rarely, in the form of status epilepticus. Interictal neurologic examination is often completely normal but may show focal signs depending on the location and size of the lesions. More commonly tuberculoma has a brain-tumor–like presentation, with gradually worsening headaches over weeks or months, accompanied by seizures, emerging focal neurologic impairments, and eventually progressive obtundation due to increasing mass effect. Examination may reveal papilledema, sixth nerve palsies (secondary to raised intracranial pressure), hemiparesis, visual field defects, and facial myokymia or hemiparkinsonism depending on the location of the lesion. In some, there are only signs of raised intracranial pressure resembling pseudotumor cerebri. On general physical examination the patients usually look remarkably well, without evidence of extraneural tuberculosis.

Laboratory Tests

CT or MRI scan of the brain with contrast material is essential for the diagnosis, although the appearances are not pathognomonic. Tuberculomas appear as single or multiple lesions of varying sizes, affecting virtually any part of the brain, and often have a rim of calcification. Enhancement of the periphery of the lesion by contrast material is characteristic, but diffuse enhancement of the lesion or lack of the enhancement do not rule out the diagnosis. Surrounding edema may be minimal or massive enough to cause brain herniation. Occasionally the lesions can be large, with a markedly hypodense

loculated center indicating abscess formation. MRI scan appearances are very similar but may show additional lesions not visible on CT scans. However, the telltale calcification may be missed. This is readily visible on CT scans. Unless there is danger of herniation, CSF examination by LP can be performed and usually is normal. It serves to detect alternative diagnoses.

Diagnosis

Identification of the focal brain lesions as tuberculoma is based primarily on clinical and epidemiologic circumstances, the brain images being consistent or suggestive only and the CSF providing no positive evidence. The occurence of these lesions in a patient at risk for tuberculosis, as outlined in the section on TBM, is the single most important clue. In a patient we saw with hemisensory dysesthesias due to a thalamic calcific mass, the history of working in a sanitorium years previously provided the correct clue to its tuberculous nature. Evidence of extraneural tuberculosis should be sought as outlined in the section on TBM. The PPD skin test is usually positive, but negative tests do not rule out the diagnosis.

Next to clinical suspicion, the most important diagnostic test is the response to antituberculous therapy. This can be used in most patients in lieu of brain biopsy. When a combination of drugs such as INH, rifampin, and pyrazinamide, which have good penetra-

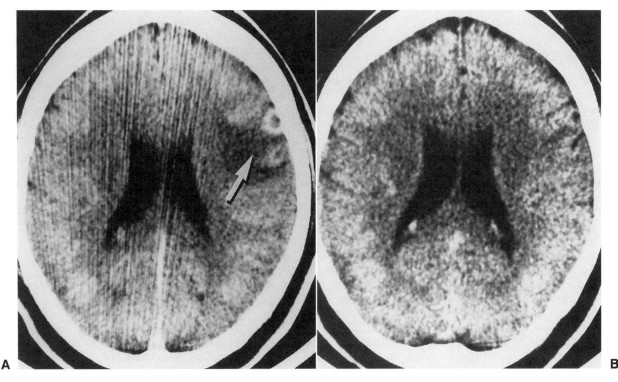

A   B

Figure 2 *A,* Brain tuberculoma. A young Haitian man presented with a grand mal seizure. Neurologic examination, chest films, and HIV test were negative. Purified protein derivative skin test was strongly positive. *B,* Brain computed tomography scan with contrast. Scan on left shows two cortical lesions with ring enhancement and surrounding edema. Scan on right, 4 weeks after triple antituberculous drugs, shows resolution of the lesions.

tion into the brain, is given, the clinical and radiologic response is generally excellent and occurs over a few weeks. In one of our recent patients with a parasagittal tuberculoma, the chief symptoms—foot paresthesias and clumsiness—improved strikingly within days of therapy. The brain scans are useful in documenting the complete regression of the lesion after several months of therapy, though areas of calcification may remain (Fig. 2). Corticosteroids should be avoided unless there is life-threatening brain edema, so that the specificity of response to chemotherapy is not obscured. Rarely, there is a paradoxical expansion of the tuberculoma while being treated with antituberculous drugs. This is presumed to be due to release of tuberculoproteins as the mycobacteria are killed by the drugs. Judicious use of dexamethasone may help tide the patient over this period of apparent clinical decline. When circumstantial evidence for tuberculosis is strong, brain biopsy can be withheld, especially when the main differential diagnosis is a malignant neoplasm, where a few weeks delay rarely makes much difference.

INTRASPINAL TUBERCULOSIS

Tuberculosis of the spine affects the same population that is at risk for other forms of neurotuberculosis, but it is decidedly less common than intracranial disease. The primary process consists of caseating necrosis and granulation tissue causing destruction of the intravertebral disks and the vertebral bodies and extending into the epidural space, with secondary compression of the spinal cord and the nerve roots. This is most common in the thoracic spine, but the lumbar and the cervical spine may also be affected.

Clinical Picture

Localized, persistent pain over the spine worsened by weight bearing and activity, progressively increasing over weeks to months, is the cardinal symptom, usually accompanied by fevers, night sweats, malaise, anorexia, and weight loss. Later, symptoms of spinal cord or lumbosacral root compression emerge, with weakness of the lower extremities, spasms of the legs, tingling, numbness, and pains in the legs and perineal area, eventually leading to difficulty with bladder and bowel function. Neurologic examination reveals signs of myelopathy in the form of spastic paraparesis, often with a transverse sensory level. In cases where the epidural process affects the cauda equina, a lower motor neuron type of areflexic paraparesis with saddle hypesthesia and loss of anal sphincter tone may be found. Not uncommonly, the examination shows combinations of spinal cord and cauda equina dysfunction (myeloradiculopathy).

A spinal gibbus, localized area of extreme spinal tenderness and painful limitation of spinal mobility are characteristic findings. The thigh may be held flexed because of spasm of the psoas muscle by the overlying tuberculous abscess. Paraspinal soft tissue swelling may be palpable, and the abscesses may track down the psoas and present as an inguinal mass. The patient usually appears chronically ill.

Laboratory Tests

Plain films of the spine characteristically show destruction of the intervertebral disks and lucencies in the adjacent, partially collapsed vertebral bodies. Paraspinal soft tissue masses and masses along the psoas muscles are highly suggestive of tuberculosis. CT and MRI scans of the spine delineate these findings even better, especially the unilateral or bilateral psoas abscesses. The MRI scan with gadolinium exquisitely delineates the effects of the spinal and epidural mass on the cord and nerve root (Fig. 3A and 3B). MRI is also useful in excluding the rare intramedullary tuberculoma. The combination of the clinical picture and the spinal images, especially with bilateral psoas abscesses (Fig. 3C), in this context, is almost pathognomonic of tuberculosis. Further evidence for extraneural tuberculosis should be sought by chest film and skin PPD testing.

Diagnosis

A strong presumptive diagnosis of compressive myeloradiculopathy due to tubercular spondylitis can be made by clinical and laboratory findings in the appropriate epidemiologic context. LP is generally not advisable or useful. Rarely, the psoas abscess may be drained under radiologic monitoring to confirm the diagnosis by finding mycobacteria and to determine sensitivities of the organisms.

Empirical antituberculous therapy should be started promptly with the presumptive diagnosis. Back pain and constitutional symptoms improve rapidly with a sense of well-being. Neurologic impairments usually do not worsen and improve gradually over several weeks, but the bone healing takes many months. The seemingly impossible psoas abscesses resolve completely over a few months. Exceptionally, sudden paraplegia may occur despite prompt therapy, probably due to tuberculous arteritis causing cord infarction.

TUBERCULOUS MENINGOMYELITIS

This is the least common form of neurotuberculosis, seen mostly in highly endemic areas, but it has been described in AIDS patients in the United States. The basic process is not in the spine but is an infection of the spinal leptomeninges, forming thick, tubular exudates and tubercles that engulf the emerging nerve roots and encase the spinal cord.

Clinical Picture

The illness evolves subacutely over several weeks, with back pain, paresthesias, and weakness of the lower

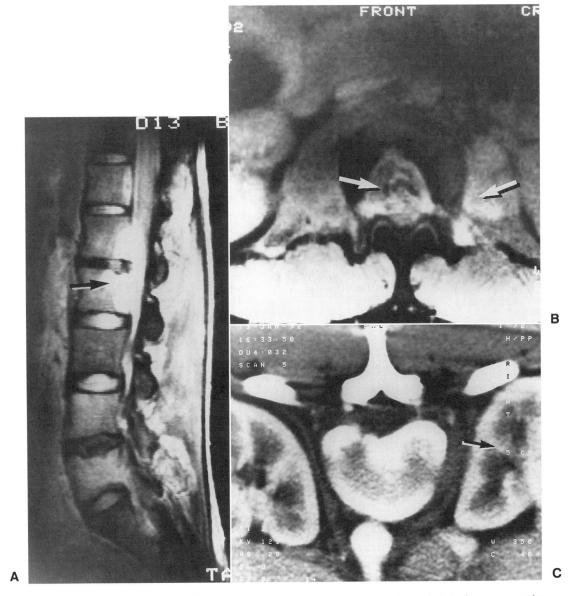

Figure 3 Spinal tuberculosis. This young man presented with back pain and right lower extremity polyradiculopathy. Purified protein derivative skin reaction, negative when tested 1 year previously in the National Guard, converted to positive, but chest film was normal. *A,* Sagittal magnetic resonance imaging of the lumbar spine with gadolinium shows high signal in L1–L2 vertebral bodies across the disk space. The mass extends epidurally, impinging on the cauda equina. *B,* Transverse image at L2 vertebra with gadolinium. Central arrow shows high signal in the body encroaching epidurally into spinal canal. Lateral arrow shows high signal in the psoas, indicating inflammation. *C,* Computed tomography scan of upper lumbar spine. Arrow indicates multiloculated cold abscess formation in the psoas.

extremities, often accompanied by loss of bladder and bowel control. Fever, malaise, and anorexia may be absent. The examination reveals a combination of nerve root and spinal cord dysfunction without deformity or tenderness over the spine. Rarely, the presentation is one of a slowly progressive myelopathy indistinguishable from a spinal cord tumor.

Laboratory Tests

Radiographs and MRI scans of the spine may be normal. CSF is markedly abnormal, with extremely high proteins, sometimes reaching 2 to 3 g per deciliter, but only 15 to 50 lymphocytes per cubic millimeter, glucose being frequently normal. AFB stains of the spinal fluid are rarely positive, and dry taps are not uncommon on

LP. Myelography and MRI with gadolinium may reveal nonspecific patchy enlargement of the nerve roots and some swelling of the spinal cord.

Diagnosis

In nonendemic areas, the diagnosis is difficult. In AIDS patients, a similar syndrome is commonly produced by cytomegalovirus, schistosomiasis, and less commonly by cryptococcosis, syphilis, and lymphoma. These can be diagnosed by appropriate microbiologic and serologic tests and by cytology for malignant cells. When these more common causes of the myeloradiculopathy syndrome cannot be confirmed in AIDS patients, empirical therapy with antituberculous drugs is reasonable. Occasionally a laminectomy and meningeal biopsy may be needed to establish the diagnosis.

TUBERCULOUS ENCEPHALOPATHY

This rare entity has been described mainly in children from areas where tuberculosis is prevalent, in association with various forms of neurologic and extraneural tuberculosis. Diffuse brain white matter edema and perivascular hemorrhages develop acutely, sometimes in association with diffuse scattered tubercles in the meninges, felt to be an allergic reaction to the release of tuberculoprotein. Clinically the patient presents with an acute encephalopathy with depressed level of consciousness and seizures. The CSF may be normal or show mild increase in lymphocytes. High-dose steroid therapy may be useful in this difficult-to-diagnose syndrome, suspected by the clinical picture occuring in the context of active tuberculosis in the brain or elsewhere.

SUGGESTED READING

Bergenguer J, Moreno S, Laguna F, et al. Tuberculous meningitis in patients infected with human immunodeficiency virus. N Engl J Med 1992; 326:668–672.
Chambers ST, Record C, Hendricke WA, et al. Paradoxical expansion of intracranial tuberculomas during chemotherapy. Lancet 1984; 181–184.
Kocen RS, Parsons M. Neurological complication of tuberculosis: Some unusual manifestations. Q J Med 1970; 39:17–30.
Leonard JM, DesPrez RM. Tuberculous meningitis. Infect Dis Clin North Am 1990; 4:769–787.
Ogaura SK, Smith MA, Brennessell DJ, Lowy FD. Tuberculous meningitis in an urban medical center. Medicine 1987; 66:317–326.
Snider DE, Roper WC. The new tuberculosis. N Engl J Med 1992; 326:703–705.
Udani PM, Dastur DK. Tuberculous encephalopathy with or without meningitis. J Neurol Sci 1970; 10:541–561.
Vengsarkar US, Pisipaty RP, Parek B, et al. Intracranial tuberculoma and the CT scan. J Neurosurg 1986; 64:568–574.
Villoria MF, dela Torre J, Rortea F, et al. Intracranial tuberculosis in AIDS: CT and MRI findings. Neuroradiology 1992; 34(1):11–14.
Woolesey RM, Chambers TJ, Chung HD, McGarry JD. Mycobacterial meningomyelitis associated with human immunodeficiency virus infection. Arch Neurol 1988; 45:691–693.

CYSTICERCOSIS

OSCAR H. DEL BRUTTO, M.D.

Cysticercosis is the most common parasitic disease of the central nervous system, affecting thousands of people in developing countries of Asia, Africa, and Latin America. In addition, massive immigration of people from endemic to nonendemic areas has recently produced a significant increase in the prevalence of cysticercosis in the United States and other industrialized countries. The disease occurs when humans become the intermediate host in the life cycle of the tapeworm *Taenia solium* by ingesting its eggs from contaminated water or food. Cysticerci may invade almost every tissue of the host, but clinically relevant disease is usually related to involvement of the nervous system.

Neurocysticercosis (NCC) is highly pleomorphic due to individual differences in the number and topography of the lesions and to variations in the degree of the host immune response against the parasites. Indeed, NCC has been considered in endemic areas as the "great imitator" because it may mimic almost any neurologic disorder. A single diagnostic approach is not useful for every patient with suspected NCC, but in general terms, three orderly steps—clinical, radiologic, and immunologic—permit an accurate diagnosis in most cases.

CLINICAL DIAGNOSIS

Epidemiologic data including the place of birth, country of residence, and travel history provide important information when evaluating patients with suspected NCC. Nevertheless, it must be remembered that this disease has been reported in persons born in the United States and European countries who have never traveled to endemic regions. Likewise, personal or family history of intestinal taeniasis should also be investigated, but its absence does not exclude the diagnosis, since only a small percentage of patients with NCC have such a history.

The clinical picture of NCC is varied and nonspecific. Epilepsy, focal neurologic deficits, intellectual deterioration, and increased intracranial pressure, the most common clinical manifestations of NCC, are also observed in many other infectious or neoplastic diseases of the central nervous system. In addition, many patients

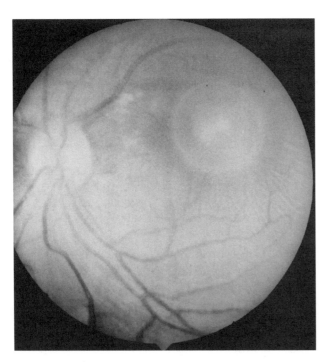

Figure 1 Ophthalmoscopic appearance of subretinal cysticercus.

with NCC complain of only vague symptoms, such as headache and dizziness, and show normal results on neurologic examination. These facts emphasize the need for performing complementary studies in every patient with suspected NCC to confirm the diagnosis.

While NCC may occur from birth to senility, its peak incidence is in the third and fourth decades. Therefore, the recent onset of seizures or progressive neurologic signs in otherwise healthy middle-aged individuals from endemic areas is highly suggestive of NCC. This parasitic disease should also be considered in the differential diagnosis of cerebral infarcts in young adults with no obvious risk factors for cerebrovascular disease, and in patients with an unexplained syndrome of intracranial hypertension of subacute onset with or without localizing signs. Dementia is also a rather frequent form of presentation of NCC. Unfortunately, most of these patients are chronic inhabitants of mental hospitals before the correct diagnosis is suspected.

Cysticerci outside the central nervous system are seldom associated with clinical manifestations, but can be a great aid to the diagnosis of NCC in patients who also have neurologic complaints. Ophthalmoscopic examination provides the unique opportunity to visualize in vivo the movements of ocular cysticerci. They are most often located in the subretinal space over the macular region and have a white or yellowish color with a central dark zone representing the scolex (Fig. 1). Soft tissue cysticerci appear as subcutaneous or muscular nodules that are firm and nontender at palpation. These lesions are rare except in patients from the Indian subcontinent.

RADIOLOGIC DIAGNOSIS

Modern neuroimaging techniques have greatly improved our diagnostic accuracy for NCC by providing objective evidence about the topography of the lesions and the degree of the host inflammatory response against the parasites. Both computed tomography (CT) and magnetic resonance imaging (MRI) have largely replaced previous radiologic procedures, such as plain x-ray films of the skull or pneumoencephalograms, which were once considered to be of diagnostic value. They now have only historical significance.

Computed Tomography

CT findings in parenchymal NCC depend on the stage of development of the cysticerci. Vesicular cysts (viable cysticerci) appear as small and rounded areas of low density without perilesional edema and with little or no enhancement after contrast medium administration. Colloidal cysts (dying cysticerci) are visualized as single or multiple ill-defined hypodense or isodense lesions surrounded by edema, showing ringlike or nodular enhancement after contrast medium administration. Finally, calcified lesions (dead cysticerci) appear as hyperdense nodules without perilesional edema or abnormal enhancement after contrast medium administration (Fig. 2). While these CT patterns are highly characteristic of parenchymal NCC, the differential diagnosis with other infectious or neoplastic diseases may prove difficult in selected cases. The main problem arises with single or multiple ringlike enhancing lesions, since pyogenic brain abscesses, fungal abscesses, tuberculomas, toxoplasma abscesses, torulomas, and primary or metastatic brain tumors may produce similar findings on CT. In such cases, the presence of fever, weight loss, and signs of meningeal irritation (very rare in NCC), together with data provided by x-ray films of the chest, cerebrospinal fluid (CSF) analysis, and other complementary studies, usually permit an accurate diagnosis.

Occasionally the CT of patients with parenchymal NCC shows only diffuse brain swelling and no areas of abnormal enhancement or cystic lesions. Moreover, in some other cases, the CT may be normal or may show only small lateral ventricles. These patients usually have a clinical syndrome of increased intracranial pressure without localizing signs. Therefore they may mimic a syndrome of pseudotumor cerebri. In those cases, CSF analysis provides clues to the correct diagnosis.

CT findings in subarachnoid NCC include hydrocephalus, abnormal enhancement of the leptomeninges at the base of the skull, subarachnoid cysts, and cerebral infarcts. Most of these findings, with exception of cystic lesions, are also observed in tuberculous or fungal meningitis. Cornerstones for differential diagnosis between tuberculous, fungal, and cysticercotic meningitis are the neurologic examination and the results of CSF analysis. As previously noted, patients with NCC rarely, if ever, have fever or signs of meningeal irritation.

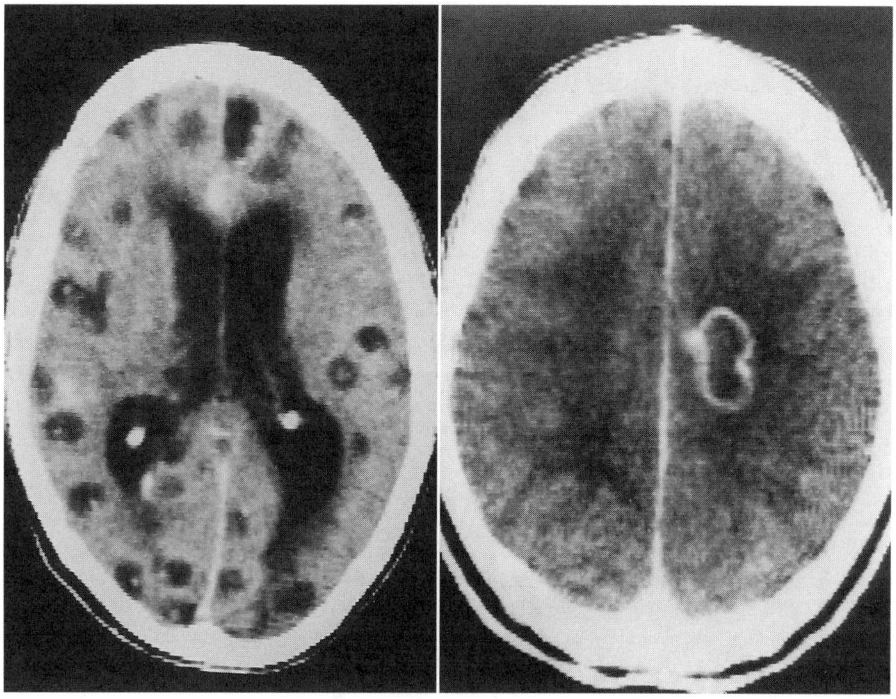

Figure 2 Contrast-enhanced computed tomographic scans of brain parenchymal cysticerci. *A,* Multiple vesicular cysts. *B,* Single colloidal cyst.

Likewise, CSF glucose levels are almost always normal in patients with cysticercotic meningitis. In contrast, fungal and tuberculous meningitis usually produce fever, neck stiffness, and decreased CSF glucose levels. The tuberculin skin test may also be useful for the diagnosis of tuberculous meningitis in areas of the world where tuberculosis is not endemic. Unfortunately, in developing countries both tuberculosis and cysticercosis are endemic, and this test could not be used as a reliable indicator of active tuberculous disease.

Subarachnoid cysts may be small and scattered if they are located within cortical sulci or may reach a large size if they are within cisterns of CSF. The most common locations of giant cysts are the sylvian fissure, the ambiens cistern, and the cerebellopontine angle cisterns. Occasionally these lesions may be confused with leptomeningeal cysts. In such cases, the absence of bone erosion and the multilobulated appearance of the cyst favor the diagnosis of NCC (Fig. 3). Hydatid disease may also resemble a giant subarachnoid cysticerci, but hydatidoses is most prevalent in Argentina and Moslem countries where cysticercosis is very rare.

Ventricular cysticerci are usually isodense with CSF. Therefore their recognition with CT may prove difficult and the diagnosis of ventricular NCC may only be inferred in patients showing asymmetric hydrocephalus. In other cases, the wall of the cyst is visualized within the ventricular system and the diagnosis is easier. This finding is observed in patients who, besides ventricular cysts, have granular ependymitis. The administration of iodinated contrast medium through a ventricular or spinal puncture usually allows precise visualization of ventricular cysticerci.

Cysticerci located within the sellar region are visualized on coronal CT scans as hypodense lesions that displace and flatten the pituitary gland on the sellar floor. These lesions may be completely hypodense or may show ringlike enhancement after contrast medium administration. In every case, CT findings are nonspecific and may simulate either a cystic pituitary tumor or an arachnoid cyst. CSF findings are also nonconclusive in patients with sellar NCC. The diagnosis is usually made at surgery.

Magnetic Resonance Imaging

MRI is very useful for the evaluation of patients with suspected NCC who have inconclusive CT findings. These findings include ventricular cysts, small subarachnoid cysts over the convexity of cerebral hemispheres, ring-enhancing lesions, and spinal cysticerci.

Parenchymal viable cysts appear on MRI as rounded lesions with signal properties similar to those of CSF on both T1- and T2-weighted images. The scolex is visualized on T1-weighted images as a high-intensity nodule within the cyst producing a pathognomonic "hole-with-dot" image (Fig. 4). The wall of the cyst cannot be visualized but may be inferred because of the sharp demarcation of the cyst from the surrounding brain parenchyma. The appearance of colloidal cysts is quite different because proteins from the degenerated scolex combine with the vesicular fluid and the whole cysticerci becomes isointense with the brain parenchyma in the T1-weighted images. Therefore the cyst is better or perhaps only discernible on T2-weighted images. In addition, the wall of the cyst becomes thick and

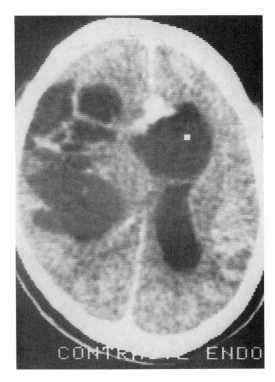

Figure 3 Computed tomography showing a large subarachnoid cysticerci in the sylvian fissure. Note the multilobulated appearance of the cyst and the absence of bone erosion.

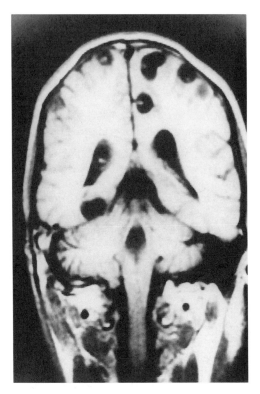

Figure 4 T1-weighted magnetic resonance imaging showing vesicular cysticerci with their characteristic "hole-with-dot" appearance.

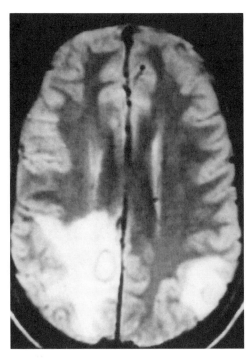

Figure 5 T2-weighted magnetic resonance imaging of a colloidal cyst with a thick hypointense capsule and marked perilesional edema.

hypointense, and there is perilesional edema (Fig. 5). Calcified cysticerci are visualized as areas of signal void on both T1- and T2-weighted images. This form of parenchymal NCC represents the most important shortcoming of MRI for the diagnosis of NCC since small calcifications may escape detection if only MRI is performed.

MRI provides an excellent opportunity to visualize small subarachnoid cysticerci over the convexity of cerebral hemispheres. Before the introduction of MRI these lesions on CT scans were considered to be within the brain parenchyma. This misinterpretation had therapeutic implications since anticysticercal drugs are more effective in parenchymal than in subarachnoid cysticerci. Some of the failures of praziquantel reported in the first studies on this subject could have been related to incorrect CT interpretation of the location of the cysts.

One of the greatest advances produced by MRI in the diagnosis of NCC is the noninvasive recognition of ventricular cysticerci. Using MRI, most ventricular cysts are detected because the scolex is better visualized than with CT. In addition, cyst mobility within ventricular cavities related to movements of the patient's head can be better observed with MRI than with CT. This sign of "ventricular migration" has been considered pathognomonic of cysticercosis.

As previously noted, CT does not permit an accurate differential diagnosis of single or multiple ring-enhancing lesions. Using MRI, however, some signal changes within lesions may provide clues to the correct diagnosis. While the fluid of most cysticerci has homogeneous signal properties, tuberculomas, pyogenic abscesses, tumors, and other conditions with ring-enhancing lesions on CT will show heterogeneous signal changes on MRI.

Another advance permitted by MRI in the diagnosis of NCC is the recognition of spinal cysts. Cysticerci within the spinal cord parenchyma or in the spinal subarachnoid space are better visualized with MRI than with CT. Nevertheless, some spinal leptomeningeal cysts may escape MRI detection if they are small or unaccompanied by inflammatory changes. In these cases myelography is still of diagnostic value because it shows multiple filling defects in the column of contrast medium.

IMMUNOLOGIC DIAGNOSIS

Experimental studies have documented the existence of different cysticercal antigens. Some of these antigens stimulate the production of specific antibodies, which represent the basis for the immunologic diagnosis of NCC. Nevertheless, the percentage of patients with NCC who have detectable titers of antibodies against cysticerci depends on the immunologic technique employed and on whether the test is performed in serum or CSF. In addition, the location of the parasites within the central nervous system and the viability of cysticerci are major determinants for the positivity of such tests. In my opinion, immunologic studies are a valuable complement to neuroimaging in the evaluation of patients with suspected NCC and inconclusive CT or MRI findings, but they should never be used alone to exclude or confirm the diagnosis of NCC.

A number of tests have been developed for the detection of anticysticercal antibodies in serum. Among these are immunoelectrophoresis, indirect hemagglutination, complement fixation, and enzyme-linked immunosorbent assay (ELISA). Unfortunately, most of these tests give controversial results due to the high number of false-positive and false-negative cases. False-positive results may be related to previous contact with the adult *Taenia solium* or to cross-reactivity with other microorganisms. False-negative results are due to the local production of specific antibodies within the central nervous system without a parallel increase of antibodies in peripheral blood.

Recently an improved specificity of antibody detection in serum has been possible through the discovery that anticysticercal antibodies can be demonstrated by immunoblot. Nevertheless, to asses the reliability of serologic diagnosis of NCC by immunoblot, the technique must first be tested in a large and unbiased group of neurologic patients in an endemic area of cysticercosis in whom the diagnosis of NCC has definitively been proved or ruled out. Such a study has not been performed.

Immunologic techniques for the detection of anticysticercal antibodies in CSF are more reliable than those performed in serum. It must be remembered, however, that the positivity of such tests is directly related to the contact of cysticerci with the subarachnoid space and to whether the cytochemical analysis of CSF shows inflammatory changes (pleocytosis, increased protein, or both). For example, the complement fixation test has 83 percent sensitivity in patients with inflammatory CSF and 22 percent sensitivity when no evidence of inflammation is found in the CSF. A method that measures IgM antibodies against cysticerci by ELISA has the advantage of recognizing cases in which the CSF is not inflammatory. The test has 87 percent sensitivity and 95 percent specificity in patients with active NCC. Simultaneous detection of IgG and IgM antibodies further increases the sensitivity of the ELISA. Both the ELISA and the complement fixation test are usually negative in patients with inactive NCC or in patients with parenchymal viable cysts that are not in contact with the subarachnoid space.

SUGGESTED READING

Cameron ML, Durack DT. Helminthic infections of the central nervous system. In: Scheld WM, Whitley RJ, Durack DT, eds. Infections of the central nervous system. New York: Raven Press, 1991:825–858.

Del Brutto OH. Cysticercosis and cerebrovascular disease: A review. J Neurol Neurosurg Psychiatry 1992; 55:252–254.

Del Brutto OH, Santibañez R, Noboa CA, et al. Epilepsy due to neurocysticercosis: Analysis of 203 patients. Neurology 1992; 42: 389–392.

Del Brutto OH, Sotelo J. Neurocysticercosis: An update. Rev Infect Dis 1988; 10:1075–1087.

Martinez HR, Rangel-Guerra R, Elizondo G, et al. MR imaging in neurocysticercosis: A study of 56 cases. AJNR Am J Neuroradiol 1989; 10:1011–1019.

Ramos-Kuri M, Montoya RM, Padilla A, et al. Immunodiagnosis of neurocysticercosis. Arch Neurol 1992; 49:633–636.

Richards F Jr, Schantz PM. Laboratory diagnosis of cysticercosis. Clin Lab Med 1991; 11:1011–1028.

CREUTZFELDT-JAKOB DISEASE

WILLIAM W. PENDLEBURY, M.D.

Creutzfeldt-Jakob disease (CJD) is a rapidly progressive, transmissible disease of the central nervous system (CNS) caused by an unusual agent that has been designated as the *prion* (*pro*teinaceous *in*fectious particle). CJD presents in middle life. However, patients as young as 27 years and as old as 78 years have been reported. The onset of the disorder is often subtle, with vague symptoms of insomnia, confusion, peculiar sensations, and visual complaints. Within weeks to months, a profound, progressive dementia develops, often accompanied by evidence of cerebellar, basal ganglia, focal motor, or lower motor neuron involvement. Myoclonus provoked by startle is a prominent feature of the disease. Death generally occurs within 1 year. About 10 percent of cases of CJD occur in a pattern consistent with autosomal dominant inheritance. There are no laboratory or radiologic findings specific for CJD, and in fact the evaluation of a patient suspected of having the disease usually produces normal findings. Therefore the diagnosis is one of exclusion made on the basis of a careful history and physical examination. Confirmation of the diagnosis is achieved by postmortem examination of the brain.

HISTORICAL PERSPECTIVE

CJD was first described by Creutzfeldt (one case) and Jakob (five cases) in the early 1920s. Although only two of their original six cases are classified as examples of CJD using current diagnostic criteria, the disease continues to bear the eponym that recognizes Creutzfeldt and Jakob's original contribution. For much of the twentieth century, CJD remained a medical curiosity and was felt to represent a rare degenerative disease of the CNS. However, in 1968 Gibbs, Gajdusek, and co-workers reported the successful transmission of CJD to the chimpanzee by intracerebral inoculation of brain tissue obtained from patients with the disorder. This landmark observation established CJD as one of the eight transmissible encephalopathies of animals and humans. Subsequent studies have demonstrated the ability to transmit the disease using cerebrospinal fluid (CSF), kidney, liver, lung, and lymph nodes from affected individuals. Transmission has not been accomplished following inoculation of ovary, testes, semen, hair, skin, saliva, feces, urine, sweat, tears, milk, or placenta from affected cases. Transmission to susceptible primates has been reported through inoculation via the intravenous, intramuscular, subcutaneous, intradermal, corneal, and oral routes, although only with extremely high doses of affected tissue via the oral route.

An understanding of the characterization of CJD as an unconventional transmissible agent disease requires a brief consideration of two related conditions, the human condition kuru and the animal condition scrapie. Kuru, first described by Gajdusek and Zigas in 1957 following their examination of 114 cases of the disorder, causes a progressive cerebellar ataxia in the people of the Fore linguistic group living in the Eastern Highlands of Papua New Guinea. Very few new cases of kuru have been reported in recent years due to the elimination of its vector, cannibalism. Scrapie, a cerebellar disease of sheep and goats, was known to be a transmissible disorder based on studies that took place in the 1930s and 1940s. In 1959 Thomas Hadlow, a veterinarian who was aware of the transmissible nature of scrapie, recognized the clinical and pathologic similarities between it and kuru. This recognition, combined with the observation by pathologist Igor Klatzo that the neuropathology of scrapie, kuru, and CJD are all strikingly similar, led to the transmission experiments that proved the true nature of CJD in 1968.

Other disorders now considered to be unconventional transmissible agent diseases include bovine spongiform encephalopathy ("mad cow disease"), chronic wasting disease in mule deer and elk, transmissible mink encephalopathy, the recently described fatal familial insomnia, and the Gerstmann-Sträussler syndrome (Table 1). The latter two entities, like kuru and CJD, use the human as their naturally occurring host. The eight diseases share common features that are listed in Table 2. Although other organ systems, particularly the reticuloendothelial system, may harbor the agent, the signs and symptoms of disease are restricted to the

Table 1 Unconventional Transmissible Agent (Prion) Diseases in Animals and Humans

Disease	Host
Bovine spongiform encephalopathy	Cattle
Chronic wasting disease	Mule deer and elk
Scrapie	Sheep and goats
Transmissible mink encephalopathy	Mink
Creutzfeldt-Jakob disease	Humans
Fatal familial insomnia	Humans
Gerstmann-Sträussler syndrome	Humans
Kuru	Humans

Table 2 Characteristics of Unconventional Transmissible Agent (Prion) Diseases

1. The signs and symptoms of the disease are restricted to the central nervous system.
2. There is a long incubation period (months to years) prior to the onset of symptoms.
3. Following its onset, the disorder is progressive leading to death.
4. The pathology is characterized by spongiform change, neuronal loss, astrocytosis, and gliosis in selected brain regions.
5. The transmissible agent (prion) has unusual properties that distinguish it from viruses, viroids, and other infectious agents.

CNS. Exposure to the transmissible agent may take place months to years before the development of symptoms, but once symptoms are present there is a rapid progression to death, usually in 6 months to 1 year. The neuropathology is strikingly uniform in both humans and animals, although a distinctive topography of the lesion is found in the brain in each disorder. All eight entities are thought to be due to an unconventional transmissible agent, the prion, that has been best characterized in experimental models of scrapie and will be further described below.

EPIDEMIOLOGY

CJD is a form of rapidly progressive dementia that represents the only unconventional transmissible agent disease of humans that is seen worldwide. The disease occurs with an annual incidence of approximately 0.5 to 1.0 case per million people per year. Subtypes of CJD that have been described include an amyotrophic form, a so-called Heidenhain variant characterized by prominent, early visual symptoms, and a variant with extensive white matter involvement. Until the exact nature of the causative agent is known, there is no rationale for considering these subtypes to represent separate diseases.

CJD usually presents in middle life in the sixth decade. However, cases occurring in the third and eighth decades have been reported. In one large series, the average age of onset was 60 years and the mean duration of illness 7.6 months. Men and women are affected equally, although large series from several countries suggest a slight female predominance. Approximately 10 percent of all cases of CJD are familial, with a pattern consistent with autosomal dominance inheritance, and another 5 to 10 percent have a clinical course that continues for 2 years or more. These latter cases tend to be familial and to have a younger age of onset, although the pathology does not differ from more typical CJD. Race does not appear to predispose to the development of CJD.

CLINICAL FEATURES

The following clinical case from my own file illustrates the salient features of CJD. The patient was a 63-year-old man who first noticed difficulty completing the Sunday *New York Times* crossword puzzle. He usually finished the puzzle in a few hours, and now the task took him at least 3 days to accomplish. Within 2 to 4 weeks, he was no longer able to balance his checkbook. He also developed increasing difficulty using his right hand, followed by unsteady walking. On admission to the hospital for neurologic evaluation, the patient was disoriented in three spheres and showed prominent memory loss. Snout, grasp, and suck reflexes were elicited and occasional myoclonic jerks were noted. CSF was clear and colorless, under normal pressure, and

without cells or other abnormalities. Cerebral angiogram, radionucleotide brain scan, and computed tomographic (CT) scan were all normal. The electroencephalogram (EEG) had delta and theta background activity with rhythmic bursts of spike wave complexes. Over the next 3 months the patient deteriorated markedly until he was no longer able to feed himself or ambulate. He became incontinent of urine and feces and displayed repeated jerking movements of his arms and legs. The patient died of pneumonia 5 months after the initial manifestations of his illness. An autopsy restricted to examination of the brain confirmed the diagnosis of CJD.

CJD is characterized clinically by prominent, profound dementia, myoclonus, and a characteristic EEG abnormality. The onset of CJD is often subtle, with vague presenting symptoms of insomnia, confusion, peculiar sensations, and visual complaints. Patients frequently believe they are overtired due to stress, physical exertion, or a viral illness, or think they are mildly depressed. Following this, there is a progressive dementia that is unusual and distinctive because of its extraordinary rapidity. Patients often evolve from a relatively normal state to being comatose in as little as 4 months. As with other forms of dementia, previously acquired cognitive abilities and memory are lost, and as the disease progresses there is also a loss of language function. Patients are usually mute in the terminal stages of CJD. Early pathologic involvement of the occipital cortex may lead to blindness (Heidenhain variant), and loss of anterior horn cells may cause significant weakness (amyotrophic variant). In both of these, however, dementia becomes the predominant clinical feature.

The physical sign of greatest constancy in CJD is that of myoclonus since it is present in more than 80 percent of patients. The myoclonic jerking is not specific for CJD and has been described in other neurologic conditions including Alzheimer's disease (AD). However, this feature in combination with a rapidly progressive dementia should cause one to strongly suspect the diagnosis of CJD. The myoclonus is more prominent as the disease progresses but becomes less prominent and disappears terminally. It has been described frequently as a response to startle that may affect the entire body, or the jerking may be restricted to a single limb. Other physical findings that are seen less commonly include pyramidal and extrapyramidal signs, cerebellar signs, a lower motor neuron syndrome, and seizures.

Laboratory and radiologic studies, with the exception of the EEG, are normal or nonspecific in CJD. Complete blood count and metabolic studies are unremarkable. Examination of CSF infrequently discloses a mild elevation of protein. In patients in whom cerebral angiography has been performed, no abnormalities have been reported. CT scanning may show cortical atrophy or enlargement of the ventricles, but this is a nonspecific finding that in most cases is minimal in degree. Magnetic resonance imaging (MRI) and positron emission tomography are of no proven usefulness in the diagnosis of CJD. The EEG is usually abnormal, revealing either

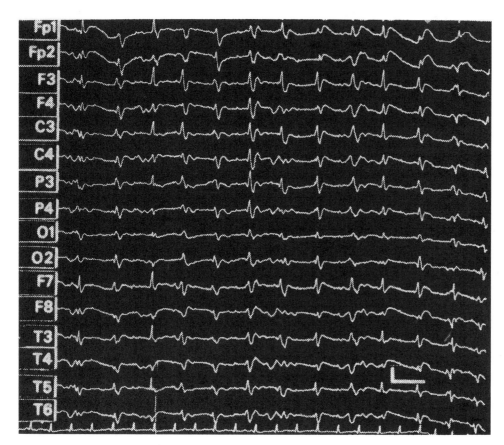

Figure 1 Electroencephalogram from a patient with Creutzfeldt-Jakob disease showing pseudoperiodic sharp-wave complexes appearing synchronously at regular intervals from all head regions. The calibration is 1 second and 50 microvolts. (From Case records of the Massachusetts General Hospital: Case 43-1977. N Engl J Med 1977; 297:930; with permission.)

generalized slowing or more characteristically pseudoperiodic sharp-wave activity (Fig. 1).

NEUROPATHOLOGY

The neuropathology of CJD is extraordinary and highly typical of the disease. Grossly, the brain appears normal or shows generalized cortical atrophy with ventricular enlargement. The degree of atrophy is closely linked to the length of the clinical course. There is nothing characteristic about the gross appearance that distinguishes CJD from other causes of brain atrophy, including AD and normal aging. The cerebellum may or may not be involved in the atrophic process. Microscopically, the prominent features include astrogliosis, varying degrees of neuronal loss, and spongiform change. All regions of the cortical ribbon are involved, but the degree of involvement varies from case to case. In fact the absence of spongiform change is not incompatible with the diagnosis of CJD, since brain tissue from such atypical cases has been used to transmit the disease to experimental animals.

In typical cases of CJD, the lesions involve the neocortex, striatum, thalamus, grey matter of the brain stem, and cerebellum. Interestingly, the hippocampus is usually relatively spared. The spongiform change is cell associated (Fig. 2A), distinguishing it from the microcystic change or the spongy state caused by hypoxic/ischemic damage and edema, or from perineuronal vacuolation caused by tissue processing. Much of the appearance of spongiform change is caused by neuronal intracytoplasmic vacuoles that often leave neurons with only a nucleus and fine wisps of cytoplasm (Fig. 2B). The astrogliosis is usually striking and is particularly prominent in areas of the brain where neuronal loss is severe. Electron microscopy reveals intracytoplasmic membrane–bounded vacuoles that contain swollen cell processes.

PATHOGENESIS

The pathogenesis of CJD is not completely understood. The agent that causes the disease, an entity that is transmissible, elicits neither a cellular nor a humoral immunologic response in patients with the disorder. In fact an inflammatory response is entirely absent in the brain, and patients remain afebrile throughout the course of their illness. After exposure to the agent, an incubation period lasting months to years may ensue before the onset of clinical illness. The agent is unusual in that it is resistant to inactivation by formalin, heat, and ionizing and ultraviolet irradiation. It is also resistant to procedures that modify nucleic acids, and therefore has properties that are different from those of viuses and viroids. Following a series of experiments spanning a number of years, Prusiner and his colleagues in 1982

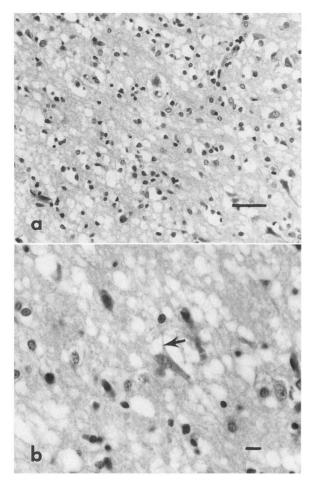

Figure 2 *a*, Section of cerebral cortex from a patient with Creutzfeldt-Jakob disease showing marked spongiform change, neuronal loss, and astrogliosis. *b*, Higher power shows that the spongiform change is cell associated. The neuron in the center clearly shows the intracytoplasmic nature of the spongiform change with a fine strand of cytoplasm *(arrow)* remaining. Hematoxylin and eosin stain. Calibration bar in *a* is 50 micrometers and in *b*, 10 micrometers. (From Bradley WG, Daroff RB, Fenichel GM, Marsden CD, eds. Neurology in clinical practice. Boston: Butterworth-Heinemann, 1991:1115; with permission.)

function is unknown. The isoform that is transmissible is designated PrP^{Sc}. The two isoforms are functionally different in that PrP^C is protease-sensitive, whereas PrP^{Sc} is protease-resistant. No other component of the prion, such as a nucleic acid, has been found to date. Although the pathogenesis of CJD is not yet completely understood, evidence is accumulating to suggest that PrP^{Sc} is a post-translational conformational modification of the normal host protein PrP^C. This modified form is capable of interacting with susceptible hosts, such as those harboring point or missence mutations of the prion protein gene, to cause disease. Current evidence would suggest, therefore, that CJD is both transmissible and genetic, if not infectious.

CJD is not contagious but is highly transmissible, and a number of instances of iatrogenic contamination have been described. These included a patient who received a corneal implant from a donor with CJD, two patients who were exposed to EEG depth electrodes that were contaminated although sterilized by conventional methods, several patients who received growth hormone from contaminated autopsy pituitary glands, and a patient who received a contaminated cadaveric dura mater graft. Because of the known transmissible nature of CJD, strict criteria for precautions in the handling of tissues and other contaminated materials from patients with CJD have been developed. Methods thought to be fully effective for inactivation of the unconventional transmissible agent include steam autoclaving for 1 hour at 132°C and immersion in 1N sodium hydroxide for 1 hour at room temperature.

SUGGESTED READING

Bastian FO, ed. Creutzfeldt-Jakob disease and other transmissible spongiform encephalopathies. St Louis: Mosby–Year Book, 1991.

Brown P, et al. Potential epidemic of Creutzfeldt-Jakob disease from human growth hormone therapy. N Engl J Med 1985; 313:728–731.

Brown P, et al. The epidemiology of Creutzfeldt-Jakob disease: Conclusion of a 15-year investigation in France and review of the world literature. Neurology 1987; 37:895–904.

Gajdusek DC, Zigas V. Degenerative disease of the central nervous system in New Guinea: The endemic occurrence of "Kuru" in the native population. N Engl J Med 1957; 257:974–978.

Medori R, et al. Fatal familial insomnia, a prion disease with a mutation at codon 178 of the prion protein gene. N Engl J Med 1992; 326:444–449.

Prusiner SB. Molecular biology of prion diseases. Science 1991; 252:1515–1522.

Prusiner SB, McKinley MP, ed. Prions: Novel infectious pathogens causing scrapie and Creutzfeldt-Jakob disease. New York: Academic Press, 1987.

Rosenberg RN, et al. Precautions in handling tissues, fluids, and other contaminated materials from patients with documented or suspected Creutzfeldt-Jakob disease. Ann Neurol 1986; 19:75–77.

designated the prion as the likely transmissible agent causing CJD and scrapie. Over the past decade, a partial understanding of the molecular nature of the prion and its relationship to the pathogenesis of CJD have been forthcoming.

The prion appears to be composed primarily of a protein, referred to as prion protein (PrP), coded for by a gene that resides on chromosome 20. The normal isoform of the protein is designated PrP^C, but its

NEOPLASTIC DISEASES

LOW-GRADE ASTROCYTOMA

MARK T. BROWN, M.D.
S. CLIFFORD SCHOLD Jr., M.D.

Astrocytic neoplasms are the most common primary brain tumors in adults. They can be classified pathologically according to their degree of histologic differentiation (poorly differentiated malignant lesions such as anaplastic astrocytoma and glioblastoma multiforme versus well-differentiated astrocytomas), as well as their cellular morphology (fibrillary versus pilocytic). In this chapter we focus on the diagnosis of low-grade fibrillary astrocytoma.

PATHOLOGY

Defining astrocytoma pathology is essential in guiding rational clinical evaluation and management strategies. Over the years, investigators have devised various schemes of classifying astrocytic brain tumors. Bailey and Cushing's system, developed in 1926, relied on cytologic characteristics and reflected variations in the developmental morphology of normal glial cells. On this morphologic basis, astrocytomas were characterized as fibrillary or protoplasmic. Pilocytic and gemistocytic forms were later described. This classification system was based on cytologic characteristics, not biologic behavior, and was not optimal in clinical applicability.

In 1949 Kernohan proposed a classification system that became more widely accepted. Kernohan observed that fibrillary astrocytomas show various degrees of cytologic malignancy, with progressive dedifferentiation of the mature astrocyte in the course of neoplastic transformation. His classification included a numeric grading system based on increasing grades of malignancy from grade I to grade IV. Grades I and II fibrillary tumors were the better differentiated astrocytomas, while grades III and IV were the more anaplastic astrocytic tumors.

In 1950 Ringertz introduced a three-tiered system that has become widely used for classification. Under this system, fibrillary astrocytic neoplasms are assigned to one of three categories: well-differentiated astrocytoma, anaplastic astrocytoma, and glioblastoma multiforme. Nonfibrillary lesions, such as pilocytic astrocytomas, make up less than 10 percent of astrocytic neoplasms and are considered pathologic and clinical entities separate from fibrillary astrocytic tumors. In this discussion, the term *astrocytoma* will refer to the well-differentiated, fibrillary astrocytic neoplasm.

Grossly, astrocytomas are indistinct, poorly demarcated, diffusely infiltrating lesions. These lesions have a pink-gray appearance and are generally solid with a gelatinous texture, though some have associated cystic or calcified regions. They may occur anywhere in the brain with an incidence that varies in rough proportion to the white matter content of the region. Microscopically, astrocytomas diffusely infiltrate gray and white matter, though the cellularity may be only slightly greater than that of normal brain. The astrocytes have nuclei that are more varied in shape and size than normal and often have delicate eosinophilic cytoplasmic processes, which form a fibrillary background. Vascular proliferation and necrosis are noted in the high-grade astrocytomas but are usually lacking in well-differentiated astrocytomas.

CLINICAL PRESENTATION

Although astrocytomas can present at any age, most become symptomatic in the third or fourth decade. Astrocytomas are usually slow-growing tumors whose symptoms may be insidious in onset and evolution. Several series document substantial proportions of patients in whom symptoms were present for months or years before diagnosis. However, these tumors have a propensity to acquire a more anaplastic histologic appearance and more rapid growth rate over time. Regardless of the exact symptoms, a subacute progressive clinical course, highly characteristic of astrocytomas, should prompt a thorough clinical evaluation.

Seizures, the most common presenting symptoms of astrocytomas, occur in 55 to 65 percent of patients in most studies. Generalized seizures are more common than focal seizures, but focal seizures may point to an underlying structural cause such as an astrocytoma. Headaches, the second most common symptoms of astrocytomas, occur in 35 to 45 percent of patients at presentation. The headaches are usually intermittent and may localize to the side of the tumor. Their frequency and severity often increase as the tumor progresses. When the tumor causes increased intracranial pressure, nausea and vomiting may accompany the headache. The presence of focal symptoms such as hemiparesis, unilateral sensory disturbances, visual field abnormalities, or aphasia depends on the location of the lesion. Such focal abnormalities are presenting symptoms in roughly 5 to 15 percent of patients. Finally, progressive behavioral and personality changes, such as memory difficulty, impaired attention, and increasing apathy, may be symptomatic of astrocytomas, though less frequently than seizures or headaches.

Neurologic signs in patients with astrocytoma at presentation include papilledema, hemiparesis, cognitive changes, and cranial nerve abnormalities. A large retrospective study of 615 gliomas of all types conducted by McKeran and Thomas from 1955 to 1975 assessed the physical findings in astrocytomas at diagnosis. Cranial nerve signs (65 percent), papilledema (50 percent), hemiparesis (45 percent), and mental changes (39 percent) were most common. Less common signs (present in 20 to 35 percent) included dysphasia, hemianopsia, and hemianesthesia. Although this study generally supports observations of other investigators, it was conducted before the era of computed tomography (CT) scanning. The subsequent advent of sensitive neuroimaging techniques permits earlier detection of these tumors. Today we less often see signs of advanced tumor progression, such as papilledema, and often find a normal exam in a young person who has presented with a seizure. There has not been a comparable systematic study reviewing presenting symptoms in patients with astrocytomas in the modern imaging era.

DIAGNOSTIC STUDIES

In the pioneering days of neurosurgery, localization of a tumor depended on the emergence of focal signs and symptoms. Leading technological diagnostic tools included radiographs of the skull and pneumoventriculography, although they were helpful in only a limited number of cases. Electroencephalography and angiography contributed to tumor localization but were, and have remained, valuable primarily as supportive information in tumor diagnosis.

With the advent of CT scanning in the mid 1970s, the neurologist and neurosurgeon gained a powerful new tool, which quickly became the cornerstone in the diagnosis and management of patients with brain tumors. The CT scan has proven to be an outstanding diagnostic tool in detecting and precisely localizing intracranial tumors. It generally shows a mass of abnormally decreased tissue attentuation (low density), often with indistinct margins. Distinguishing astrocytoma from tumor edema may be difficult or impossible, though low-grade lesions usually lack the prominent

edema associated with malignant astrocytomas or metastases. Occasionally, one or more areas of calcification within the lesion are seen as inhomogeneous regions of hyperdensity. These tumors may contain one or more cysts. Astrocytomas usually show minimal or no enhancement following intravenous contrast administration. Occasionally the tumor may present as a well-defined, sharply outlined focus of low density. In such instances, distinguishing the lesion from a simple cyst or an infarct may be difficult. Despite the sensitivity of the CT scan, some astrocytomas are isodense with surrounding brain tissue and escape detection by CT.

Magnetic resonance imaging (MRI), developed for widespread clinical use in the 1980s, is a more sensitive neuroimaging technique than CT scanning. In our opinion, MRI is the imaging modality of choice in the diagnosis and management of astrocytomas (Fig. 1). Patients strongly suspected of having an underlying neoplasm should be imaged with MRI, even if CT fails to demonstrate a lesion. MRI is more sensitive in detecting tumors that appear isodense on CT and may show the tumor to be larger than appreciated on CT. Astrocytomas generally appear as low signal intensity (dark) lesions on T1 weighted MRI images and as high signal intensity (bright) lesions on T2 weighted images. While intravenous contrast agents such as gadolinium demonstrate little if any enhancement on T1 weighted images of astrocytomas, enhancement is more often seen with MRI than CT. As with CT, distinguishing tumor from edema using MRI may be difficult, but techniques such as diffusion gradient MRI may help overcome this limitation in the future.

Positron emission tomography (PET) scanning, a new imaging modality, examines the metabolic activity of the normal brain and brain tumor using fluorinated-deoxyglucose (FDG) uptake to measure metabolic activity. In our experience, nearly all well-differentiated astrocytomas have less metabolic activity than gray matter. When FDG uptake is greater than gray matter, a more aggressive clinical course often ensues. PET may help identify the most anaplastic area to biopsy.

TISSUE DIAGNOSIS

Despite the dramatic advances of neuroimaging techniques, the images do not provide histologic diagnoses. Histologic evaluation of tumor tissue remains the only definitive method of diagnosis. Diagnostic surgical procedures include biopsy (stereotactic or open biopsy) or resection (subtotal or gross total). Open, free-hand biopsy is rarely utilized today. In the past, open biopsy, which carried a high morbidity and mortality rate, was generally reserved for patients too ill to tolerate a more extensive resection. Stereotactic biopsy is substantially safer than previous biopsy procedures, and in skilled hands should have a morbidity rate of about 1 percent. This procedure provides a small tissue sample of between one and six 1 mm^3 specimens from a target predetermined on the patient's CT or MRI. Usually this

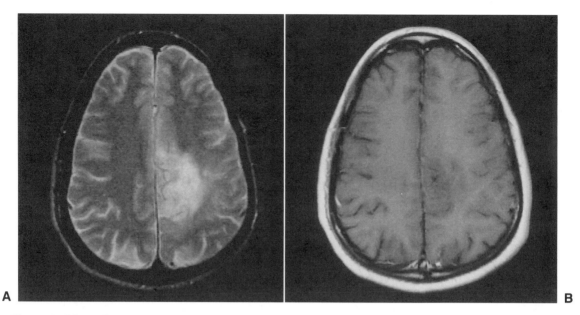

A   B

Figure 1 Magnetic resonance scan of a patient with a well-differentiated astrocytoma. *A,* The T2 weighted image shows a high signal abnormality. *B,* The T1 weighted image shows a more subtle reduced signal abnormality in the same area.

is adequate for diagnosis, particularly if the neuropathologist is providing on-site consultation in the operating room. However, the correlation between diagnosis from biopsy and from resected larger specimens is imperfect. Occasionally, adequate tissue for a definitive diagnosis is not obtained. In a few cases, serious diagnostic errors from biopsy can result in clinical mismanagement. Nevertheless, studies in the mid-1980s demonstrated that pathologists made an accurate histologic diagnosis in 82 to 95 percent of cases when frozen section specimens from needle biopsies were compared with the permanent section. Comparison of biopsy results and resected surgical specimens has shown that stereotactic biopsy samples generally provide histologic diagnoses appropriate for clinical management.

Surgical resection, the other means of obtaining a tissue diagnosis, provides more tissue for making a histologic diagnosis and contributes to the treatment of the tumor by removing a portion of it. A major goal of neurosurgery, when possible, has been gross total resection of well-differentiated astrocytomas. Subtotal resection is the more common operation, chiefly because tumor size or location precludes total excision without serious risk of debilitating neurologic sequelae. Most investigators believe that more extensive resection of astrocytomas contributes to a better outcome.

Weir and Grace, in a 1976 study of 107 patients with well-differentiated astrocytomas, analyzed clinical data collected between 1960 and 1970 for the relative significance of different factors affecting survival. They found that the extent of surgical removal of well-differentiated astrocytomas was important for survival. The survival rate was greater for subtotal resection than total resection for the first 9 months postoperatively, but

thereafter it was greater for total resection. Both subtotal and total resection were associated with longer survival than needle biopsy. Average postoperative survival for all patients with grade I astrocytomas was 52 ± 39 months, while for patients with grade II tumors survival was 30 ± 34 months.

In a 1984 retrospective analysis of 461 cases of grade I or II supratentorial astrocytomas, Laws and colleagues found that a number of factors influenced the overall 5 year postoperative survival rate of 36.5 percent, including gross total excision, lack of major postoperative deficit, and the performance of surgery after the year 1950. Patients whose tumors were totally resected had a higher survival rate (61 percent 5 year survival) than patients whose tumors were subtotally resected or biopsied (44 percent and 32 percent 5 year survivals, respectively). Regression analysis of various patient characteristics and treatment variables reduced the importance of surgery type. Total excision appeared consistently better than subtotal removal, but the difference was statistically significant only in younger patients. Laws concluded that "the data generally support a philosophy of radical surgical removal whenever possible."

In each case, the physician must analyze the potential for surgical treatment. We suggest aggressive use of diagnostic tests to establish as accurately as possible whether a lesion is anatomically resectable and to estimate, in conjunction with clinical experience, the risk of significant neurologic impairment as a result of surgery. Based on the results of the most sensitive imaging techniques (MRI and CT) and appropriate testing of cerebral dominance by Wada tests, we may reasonably regard as unresectable those tumors in direct proximity to the patient's language or motor cortex centers, tumors with extensive hemispheric involvement of multiple lobes, tumors that cross the midline via the corpus callosum, and tumors with deep extension to the internal capsule, basal ganglia, thalamus, or brain stem.

Aside from the question of resectability, the problem of when to resect may be significant. Little has been written about the appropriate timing for resection. Obviously, the physician should waste no time when a lesion is likely to be totally resectable with relatively small neurologic risk to the patient. In patients whose lesions are questionably resectable or resectable with a significantly greater risk of postoperative neurologic impairment, adopting a "wait and watch" attitude with careful and frequent follow-up imaging studies may be in the patient's best interest, provided symptoms can be controlled adequately. This approach recognizes that despite the various statistical methods of estimating prognosis, a given patient may not follow the predicted clinical pattern, especially since these tumors are notoriously variable in their clinical courses. This approach would postpone a questionably beneficial operation that carries a substantial risk of impairment until the progression of the patient's symptoms or tumor size on imaging studies force intervention.

In both questionably resectable and obviously unresectable tumors, CT guided stereotactic biopsy is warranted in nearly all cases to definitively establish an accurate histopathologic diagnosis. Purely intrinsic brain stem tumors continue to be an exception to this practice. Presumptive diagnosis of a brain tumor based on results from neuroimaging studies is no longer acceptable in most cases. Both treatment and prognosis should be based on the precise diagnosis because the morbidity of obtaining diagnostic tissue is low. An accurate diagnosis, with either surgical resection or stereotactic biopsy, should be made in the great majority of patients with astrocytomas before treatment begins.

SUGGESTED READING

Baily P, Cushing H. A classification of the tumors of the glioma group on a histogenic basis with a correlated study of prognosis. Philadelphia: JB Lippincott, 1926.

Bradley WG Jr, Waluch V, Yadley RA, Wycoff RR. Comparison of CT and MR in 400 patients with suspected disease of the brain and cervical spinal cord. Radiology 1984; 152:695–702.

Brown MT, Hoffman JM, Schifter T, et al. Positron emission tomography (PET) findings in well-differentiated astrocytomas. Neurology 1992; 42(suppl 3):191.

Burger PC, Scheithauer BW, Vogel FS. Brain: tumors. In: Surgical pathology of the nervous system and its coverings. 3rd ed. New York: Churchill Livingstone, 1991:193.

Chandrasoma PT, Smith MM, Apuzzo MLJ. Stereotactic biopsy in the diagnosis of brain masses: Comparison of results of biopsy and resected surgical specimen. Neurosurgery 1989; 24:160–165.

Laws ER Jr, Taylor WF, Clifton MB, Okazaki H. Neurosurgical management of low-grade astrocytomas of the cerebral hemispheres. J Neurosurg 1984; 61:665–673.

McKeran RO, Thomas DGT. The clinical study of gliomas. In: Thomas DGT, Graham DI, eds. Brain tumours: Scientific basis, clinical investigation, and current therapy. Boston: Butterworths, 1980:194.

Ringertz N. Grading of gliomas. APMIS 1950; 27:51–64.

Rosenblum ML. General surgical principles, alternatives, and limitations. Neurosurg Clin North Am 1990; 1:19–36.

Weir B, Grace M. The relative significance of factors affecting postoperative survival in astrocytomas, grades one and two. Can J Neurol Sci 1976; 3:47–50.

PARANEOPLASTIC SYNDROMES

ROBERT B. DARNELL, M.D., Ph.D.*

AN APPROACH TO DIAGNOSIS

The paraneoplastic neurologic disorders (PND) are a diverse set of syndromes for which clinical experience and appropriate laboratory tests will lead to definitive diagnosis in the majority of cases. In this chapter I will review features of these disorders that alert the clinician to the possibility of PND. I will focus on clinical syndromes defined well enough to warrant their inclusion in a differential diagnosis and permit laboratory confirmation of their diagnosis.

PNDs are antibody-mediated disorders in which specific antigens are targeted. This observation has led to

*Supported in part by Clinical Investigator Development Award, #1 KO8 NS01461-01, and ACS grant #VM-30.

the development of specific laboratory testing that confirms the clinical diagnosis. These tests include paraneoplastic cerebellar degeneration (PCD)—the Yo syndrome; paraneoplastic encephalomyelitis/sensory neuropathy (PEM/SN)—the Hu syndrome; paraneoplastic opsoclonus/ataxia—the Ri syndrome; and paraneoplastic retinal degeneration. A number of other paraneoplastic syndromes have been described, but their causes are unclear, precluding a definitive diagnosis. Whether they are infectious, nutritional, or immune-mediated remains to be determined.

How frequently can the clinician expect to encounter patients with PND? For the general oncologist, the answer is rarely. PNDs are thought to occur in perhaps only 0.1 percent of cancer patients. However, these syndromes are more frequently considered and diagnosed by the neurologist, for several reasons. First, most patients with PND present with neurologic disease, not cancer. Second, the neurologic symptoms of many of the PNDs are relatively common to the neurologist: for example, sensory neuropathy, idiopathic cerebellar dysfunction, obscure visual complaints. Finally, because the paraneoplastic syndromes are so distinctive, as discussed below, they compete in the differential diagnosis with only a limited number of disorders, many of which can be tested for and ruled out, leaving a high clinical suspicion of PND. For example, a young woman presenting with subacute cerebellar dysfunction, normal magnetic resonance imaging (MRI), and no obvious cause has roughly a 50 percent chance that an underlying malignancy accounts for her symptoms. Similarly, unexplained sensory neuropathies have a 20 percent chance of being associated with malignancy. Thus the PNDs are important for neurologists to understand and include effectively in their array of differential diagnoses.

Certain features are common to all of the PNDs and serve to alert the clinician to consider them in a differential diagnosis (Table 1). Despite the link of PND with malignancy, an established tumor diagnosis is not typical in patients presenting with neurologic symptoms associated with PND. The great majority of PND patients present to clinicians with neurologic symptoms prior to the discovery of a malignancy: 49 of 59 (83 percent) Hu syndrome patients in whom tumors were diagnosed developed neurologic disease prior to the diagnosis of tumors. Similarly, 34 of 52 (65 percent) Yo syndrome patients presented with neurologic disease. Thus the neurologic picture, not the oncologic disease, defines the early approach to diagnosis.

PNDs are associated with specific tumor types. Small cell lung cancer (SCLC) or gynecologic tumors are the most frequent malignancies associated with PND, and their identification or suspicion in a patient with undiagnosed neurologic disease would be an important clue to suspecting a diagnosis of PND. Much less clear is the relationship of non-SCLC, germ cell tumor, or Hodgkin's disease to PND. Other tumors, such as leukemias, primary brain tumors and sarcomatous tumors, are rarely, if ever, associated with PNDs.

The temporal profile of the PNDs is characterized by the rapid onset of symptoms. Patients may develop a severe neurologic syndrome over the course of hours, although more frequently over the course of days to weeks. This is a critical point in suspecting PNDs, since most other neurodegenerative disorders develop much more gradually.

Routine laboratory studies are typically unremarkable in PND. Perhaps most importantly, nearly all patients have normal cranial MRI at the time of presentation. Some exceptions exist. Patients with limbic encephalopathy may have high T2 signals in the temporal lobes, and patients with long-standing PND may show evidence of cortical or cerebellar atrophy. Generally, however, cranial MRI is useful for excluding a diagnosis of PND since radiologic abnormalities that correlate with clinical findings should prompt another diagnosis.

The most significant finding common to PND patients is the presence of autoantibodies. These reflect the presumed pathogenesis of the disorder. The antibodies recognize antigens in tumor cell that are normally expressed in clinically affected areas of the nervous

Table 1 Common Features of the Paraneoplastic Neurologic Diseases

Neurologic presentation in the majority of patients
Common tumor types: small cell lung cancer or gynecologic cancer
Rapid clinical presentation and course
Antineuronal antibodies in serum and cerebrospinal fluid

system. The characterization of these antigens has allowed the development of specific diagnostic criteria for some of the PNDs, as discussed below.

It should be noted, however, that some antibody assays provide much greater specificity than others. Antibody assays that rely solely on immunohistochemical detection of antigen are unable to discriminate between two antigens that are expressed in the same distribution within a neuron but are entirely different proteins. There are numerous examples of similar appearing, but distinct, paraneoplastic antigens. Thus the neurologist must rely on assays that include either Western blot or analysis of cloned PND antigens to make a specific diagnosis. For example, Hu and Ri PND antibodies both stain neuronal nuclei but recognize completely different proteins, which are distinguishable by Western blot. Similarly, Yo antibodies are but one of a number of anti-Purkinje cell antibodies defined immunohistochemically that can only be distinguished by Western blot analysis. These distinctions are not trivial. Diagnosis of an Hu antibody directs a search for SCLC, while an Ri antibody suggests occult breast cancer. Only the Yo antibody, of all Purkinje antibodies described, mandates an aggressive search for an occult gynecologic tumor.

It should be noted that when one of the PND antibodies cannot be found, a PND is not absolutely excluded. The repertoire of PNDs continues to expand. In some cases, sera negative for typical PND antibodies on routine testing have still been found to recognize neuronal antigens by immunohistochemistry or more specific Western blot techniques. Thus when a PND remains likely despite a negative screen for typical PND antibodies, further evaluation of serum in a research laboratory is an important asset for the clinician and a necessary route to expanding our knowledge of the spectrum of these disorders.

SPECIFIC PARANEOPLASTIC NEUROLOGIC DISORDER SYNDROMES

Paraneoplastic Cerebellar Degeneration: The Yo Syndrome

Like all the PNDs, PCD is a spectrum of disorders. By far the majority of these patients have underlying gynecologic malignancy and the Yo antibody. Because of the strong association with breast or ovarian carcinoma, all of these patients are women (55 of 55 in one study). The neurologic disease is believed to relate to Purkinje neuronal loss in the cerebellum, which remains subclinical until a critical threshold is crossed, leading to the abrupt onset of severe cerebellar symptoms. These symptoms typically plateau and are irreversible soon after onset, presumably because of the loss of Purkinje neurons. The clinical symptoms are severe pancerebellar dysfunction. Many patients cannot feed themselves, nearly all cannot walk, and many have unintelligible speech due to dysarthria. A number of minor symptoms may be associated with PCD but do not localize to the cerebellum, including diplopia (with or without demonstrable ocular palsies) and sensory symptoms. On examination, all patients have nystagmus, most with a vertical component. Typically, patients have severe scanning dysarthria and both midline and appendicular ataxia. Routine laboratory studies are unrevealing, including a normal cerebrospinal fluid (CSF) and cranial MRI, although some patients may have a mild, nonspecific CSF pleocytosis at presentation and evidence of cerebellar atrophy late in the course of the illness.

The clinical picture is characteristic enough to lead the clinician to suspect the possibility of PCD in most instances. Parenchymal lesions such as tumor, hemorrhage, or infarct are ruled out by clinical presentation and MRI scan. Hereditary cerebellar degeneration, slow virus (particularly the Gerstmann-Straussler variant of Creutzfeld-Jacob disease), metabolic disease, and alcoholic cerebellar degeneration differ from PCD in their mode of onset, usually with a more gradual temporal profile. Leptomeningeal disease, particularly that associated with primary central nervous system lymphoma, can be difficult to distinguish from PCD. For each of these disorders, a careful history, close clinical follow-up, watching especially for the time course of progression and the development of extracerebellar neurologic signs, and serial CSF studies including cytology and tumor markers are able in most cases to distinguish PCD from other causes of cerebellar dysfunction.

The diagnostic test of choice to establish a suspected diagnosis of PCD is a serum assay for the presence of Yo antibodies. Approximately 50 percent of PCD patients are positive. The specificity of this test is important since a positive Yo antibody should prompt a detailed search for a gynecologic malignancy. Conversely, a number of PCD patients who are Yo negative may harbor other antineuronal antibodies by immunohistochemistry or Western blot, some of which may lead to specific diagnoses. In particular, patients with Hu antibodies or Ri antibodies can present with purely cerebellar dysfunction, and these diagnoses must be considered in Yo-negative patients. Less well-defined antibodies in Yo-negative PCD patients include antibodies against voltage-gated calcium channels or neuronal adaptin proteins. Currently, distinctions between typical Yo and these atypical PCD antisera can be made only by referring Yo-negative sera to the research laboratory.

Paraneoplastic Encephalomyelitis/Sensory Neuropathy: The Hu Syndrome

The diversity of patients with anti-Hu-associated PEM/SN is so broad as to appear initially to be a source of confusion. Perhaps the reason for this diversity is that the Hu antibody binds to all neurons of the nervous system. However, certain common features stand out and allow the diagnosis to be suspected. While over 80 percent of patients present with neurologic and not lung disease, a history or suspicion of lung cancer (for example, a strong smoking history or abnormal chest x ray) are common in Hu patients; over three-fourths are ultimately found to harbor SCLC. Sixty percent of patients present with sensory symptoms. Thus an unexplained sensory neuropathy should raise the suspicion of PEM/SN. Typically, this is a painful neuropathy, involving both large and small fibers. Many patients progress to severe dysfunction, with loss of all sensory modalities. This is an important point distinguishing Hu patients from patients with cancer and chemotherapy-induced (e.g., cisplatin) large fiber neuropathies.

Forty percent of Hu patients present with diverse neurologic signs, including limbic symptoms, cerebellar dysfunction, motor weakness, brain stem dysfunction, or autonomic dysfunction (orthostasis). In these patients the diagnosis can be more difficult, but the outstanding clinical features common to such Hu patients are a normal cranial MRI and an inexorable progression of signs and symptoms. The CSF may show a mild, nonspecific pleocytosis and elevated protein. Sensory nerve conduction may be abnormal, even in asymptomatic patients. The electroencephalogram may reveal temporal slow wave or spike foci in cases in which limbic dysfunction is evident. The diagnosis for all Hu patients is established by assaying serum or CSF for the presence of Hu antibodies, using the cloned Hu antigen as a purified reagent in a Western blot.

The progression of symptoms following diagnosis is often rapid. The average time from neurologic diagnosis to death is 7 months. Frequently, multiple areas of the nervous system are involved, despite unifocal neurologic presentations. Most of those with unifocal symptoms throughout their illness have sensory neuropathies. While the identification of an Hu antibody should lead to an aggressive search for and treatment of SCLC, these patients await the development of a successful treatment approach for the neurologic illness.

Paraneoplastic Opsoclonus/Ataxia: The Ri Syndrome

Paraneoplastic opsoclonus/myoclonus is a misnomer for this syndrome when it occurs in adults. In childhood, opsoclonus associated with limb and truncal myoclonus and occasionally seizures is a syndrome with a high (perhaps up to 50 percent) association with neuroblastoma but with an obscure pathophysiology. In adults, eight patients have been reported in whom a defined antitumor and antineuronal antibody (anti-Ri) has been defined. The two outstanding features of these patients are opsoclonus (six of eight) and truncal ataxia (seven of eight). Only a small minority had myoclonus or appendicular ataxia.

Opsoclonus can be recognized clinically by the presence of spontaneous, large-amplitude saccades oc-

Table 2 Features of the Paraneoplastic Neurologic Disorders

Syndrome	History	Clinical Onset	Early Symptoms	Early Signs	Clinical Course	Clinical Tests	Antibody Tests
Yo	Female	Rapid (days–weeks)	Pancerebellar, diplopia	Pancerebellar	Plateau with severe deficit	Normal cranial MRI	+ Yo fusion protein
Hu	Smoker	Subacute (weeks–months)	Sensory (60%), other (40%)	Large and small fiber neuropathy, other	Inexorably progressive, multifocal	Normal cranial MRI, may have abnormal NCV	+ Hu fusion protein
Ri	Likely female	Rapid (days–weeks)	Gait difficulty, visual disturbance	Midline cerebellar dysfunction, opsoclonus, myoclonus	50% remission	Normal cranial MRI	+ Ri fusion protein
CAR	Smoker	Subacute (weeks–months)	Bizarre visual obscurations, night blindness	Visual loss, central sparing	Inexorably progressive to blindness	Abnormal ERG	+ photoreceptor antibody

CAR = cancer-associated retinopathy; NCV = nerve conduction velocities; ERG = electroretinography.

curring in all directions of gaze, exacerbated by voluntary saccadic movements or attempts at visual pursuit. The dyad of opsoclonus and truncal ataxia occurs with an abrupt onset and is associated with occult breast cancer in most patients. We have followed one Ri patient with opsoclonus, truncal ataxia, and myoclonus who had SCLC. Cranial MRI is normal, and the CSF may show a mild pleocytosis and protein elevation. To establish the diagnosis, one must assay serum or CSF for the Ri antibody. When the cloned Ri antigen is used, Ri antibodies can be detected at serum dilutions of well over 1:10,000.

An important clinical feature of the Ri syndrome that further distinguishes it from either Yo or Hu is that symptoms may substantially improve in Ri patients. Half of the reported Ri-positive patients showed substantial or near complete improvement of their neurologic syndrome with time. One of our patients, wheelchair bound and suffering from disabling opsoclonus, recovered to nearly normal function after the identification and treatment of an occult malignancy. These observations stress the importance of recognizing this disorder, because it is typically associated with treatable limited stage tumors. These patients may have a particularly favorable neurologic and oncologic prognosis.

Cancer-Associated Retinopathy

Blindness as a paraneoplastic disease is associated with SCLC and antibodies to retinal photoreceptors, particularly rod neurons. The early clinical picture is suggestive of a specific rod cell disorder. Patients typically present with night blindness and bizarre visual obscurations prior to detection of their tumors. Examination early in the course of the disorder may reveal ring scotomata with preservation of visual acuity. Symptoms may present in one eye, but inevitably both eyes become involved. Electroretinography is the most useful physiologic test, allowing confirmation of a retinal defect. Weeks or months after the onset of symptoms patients progress inexorably to blindness. An antibody that reacts with a photoreceptor rod protein termed recoverin, has been described in these patients.

DISCUSSION

The diagnostic approach to the PNDs (Table 2) is based upon (1) the history, most notably abrupt onset of neurologic disease in previously well patients, (2) the physical examination, with characteristic findings for each syndrome, (3) the clinical course, typically inexorable progression to severe disability, and (4) laboratory tests, most specifically the assay for antibodies against defined neuronal antigens. In most cases, attention to the first three features will lead physicians to suspect PND, which can be definitively diagnosed by antibody testing. Patients with positive antibody assays need careful evaluation for malignancy, depending on which antibody is detected.

Most patients who are antibody-negative will have an alternative explanation for their disease. When physicians remain highly suspicious of a PND despite negative commercial tests for antibodies, serum or CSF should be forwarded to a research laboratory. The complete spectrum of the PNDs remains to be defined.

SUGGESTED READING

Anderson NE, Cunningham JM, Posner JB. Autoimmune pathogenesis of paraneoplastic neurological syndromes. In: Roses A, ed. Critical review in clinical neurobiology. Boca Raton, Fl.: CRC Press, 1987:245.

Dalmau J, Graus F, Rosenblum MK, Posner JB. Anti-Hu-associated paraneoplastic encephalomyelitis/sensory neuronopathy: A clinical study of 71 patients. Medicine 1992; 71:59–72.

Darnell RB, Posner JR. Cloning and characterization of the neuronal antigen recognized in paraneoplastic opsoclonus-myoclonus. Neurology 1991; 41(suppl):363.

Darnell RB, Furneaux HM, Posner JR. Antiserum from a patient with cerebellar degeneration identifies a novel protein in Purkinje cells, cortical neurons, and neuroectodermal tumors. J Neurosci 1991; 11:1224–1230.

Fathallah-Shaykh H, Wolf S, Wong E, et al. Cloning of a leucine-zipper protein recognized by the sera of patients with antibody-associated paraneoplastic cerebellar degeneration. Proc Natl Acad Sci U S A 1991; 88:3451–3454.

Luque FA, Furneaux HM, Ferziger R, et al. Anti-Ri: An antibody associated with paraneoplastic opsoclonus and breast cancer. Ann Neurol 1991; 29:241–251.

Peterson K, Rosenblum MK, Kotanides H, Posner JB. Paraneoplastic cerebellar degeneration: I. A clinical analysis of 55 anti-Yo antibody-positive patients. Neurology 1992; 42:1931–1937.

Polans AS, Buczylko J, Crabb J, Palczewski K. A photoreceptor calcium binding protein is recognized by autoantibodies obtained from patients with cancer-associated retinopathy. J Cell Biol 1991; 112:981–989.

Posner JB, Furneaux HM. Paraneoplastic syndromes. In: Waksman BH, ed. Immunologic mechanisms in neurologic and psychiatric disease. New York: Raven Press, 1990.

Szabo A, Dalmau J, Manley G, et al. HuD, a paraneoplastic encephalomyelitis antigen contains RNA binding domains and is homologous to Elav and sex lethal. Cell 1991; 67:325–333.

PRIMARY CENTRAL NERVOUS SYSTEM LYMPHOMA

LISA M. DeANGELIS, M.D.

Non-Hodgkin's lymphoma (NHL) is called primary central nervous system lymphoma (PCNSL) when it arises within and is confined to the nervous system. Histologically identical to intermediate and high-grade systemic NHL, PCNSL is not associated with systemic disease and is different from metastatic lymphoma to the central nervous system. PCNSL is a brain tumor and presents as an intracranial mass, whereas metastatic lymphoma involves the leptomeninges primarily and rarely forms parenchymal brain lesions. Like comparable systemic NHLs, PCNSL is virtually always a B-cell neoplasm. True T-cell PCNSLs are rare and do not differ biologically from the usual B-cell tumors.

PCNSL accounts for only 1 percent of all intracranial neoplasms but is more common among patients with congenital or acquired immunodeficiency syndromes, particularly those with AIDS. However, most patients with PCNSL are not identifiably immunocompromised. PCNSL is receiving increasing attention because its incidence in the otherwise normal population has risen at least three-fold in the past 15 years. The explanation for this epidemiologic change is unknown. Nevertheless, physicians will see patients with PCNSL more frequently than ever before, and need to appreciate its diagnostic pitfalls.

Although PCNSL is uncommon, its specific features are important because new treatment approaches have improved patient survival, and the treatment is different from that for other brain tumors. Thus accurate diagnosis is essential and must be established before cytotoxic therapy can begin. If PCNSL seems a likely diagnosis based on the patient's initial clinical symptoms and the radiographic appearance of the lesions, the physician's approach to establishing the diagnosis differs from that for other brain tumors. Unlike either primary or metastatic tumors, the diagnosis of PCNSL can be obscured by usual measures undertaken during the initial evaluation of an intracranial mass lesion, such as the early institution of corticosteroids. In addition, because PCNSL frequently presents with multiple lesions and is often confused with brain metastases, the physician may prescribe cranial radiotherapy (RT) without a histologic diagnosis, losing the opportunity to treat PCNSL with more effective regimens employing chemotherapy initially. Furthermore, PCNSL can mimic other conditions that are not neoplasms, such as multiple sclerosis and sarcoidosis, which demand completely different therapy.

CLINICAL DIAGNOSIS

The clinical presentation of PCNSL in immunocompetent and immunocompromised patients is similar, and the following descriptions apply to both populations. Most patients with a PCNSL present with symptoms of an intracranial mass lesion, such as increased intracranial pressure, alterations in intellect, and lateralizing signs. PCNSL usually involves the brain as single (60 percent) or multiple tumor(s) (40 percent). Patients with parenchymal PCNSL have at least a two-thirds chance of having coexistent leptomeningeal infiltration. However, this meningeal involvement is usually clinically silent, evident only on cerebrospinal fluid (CSF) cytologic examination. The eye, being an extension of the nervous system, can also be involved by PCNSL. A few patients present with isolated ocular, leptomeningeal, or spinal cord lymphoma. Each of these areas is discussed individually.

Brain

PCNSL is a multifocal disease in approximately half of patients, and at least one lesion will involve the deep periventricular structures. The frontal lobe is the most commonly affected region of the brain, followed by the basal ganglia. These areas of involvement are reflected in the usual constellation of symptoms and signs seen in patients with PCNSL. Behavioral and mental status changes are common, seen in at least two-thirds of patients, and may be the only clinical manifestation of this disease in a significant minority. These symptoms are less common in other types of brain tumors such as gliomas and meningiomas. Lateralizing signs such as hemiparesis, aphasia, and visual field defects are presenting complaints in about half of patients. Seizures are the presenting symptom in only 10 percent of patients, compared to 25 percent of those with gliomas or metastatic brain tumors. The lower incidence of seizures can be explained by the deep location of most PCNSL lesions. Depending on the area of involvement, cerebellar or brain stem signs are occasionally apparent.

Eye

Patients with ocular lymphoma usually have mild, nonspecific visual complaints, such as visual blurring, floaters, or visual loss, or may be asymptomatic. Symptoms may be unilateral or bilateral, although they are typically asymmetric when both eyes are affected. Ocular lymphoma usually involves the vitreous, choroid, or retina and may present as a chronic uveitis that is unresponsive to therapy. A poor therapeutic response to uveitis treatment may be the first clue that the ocular process is due to lymphoma. A slit-lamp examination and indirect ophthalmoscopy are essential for the diagnosis of ocular lymphoma. Cells in the vitreous are detected on the slit-lamp examination, and choroidal masses and retinal detachments due to tumor underneath the retina are often appreciated only on indirect examination. The diagnosis is established by vitrectomy or a vitreous aspirate. Every patient with confirmed PCNSL should have a complete ophthalmologic evaluation at diagnosis and at the time of tumor recurrence even if the patient does not have visual symptoms.

PCNSL may involve the eye either in conjunction with cerebral disease or as the sole site of tumor. The majority (50 to 80 percent) of patients who have ocular lymphoma as their first manifestation of disease go on to develop cerebral lymphoma at some point in the course of their illness. There may be a latency of several years before CNS lymphoma becomes apparent, but this high incidence means that a neurologic evaluation, cranial magnetic resonance imaging (MRI), and lumbar puncture should be performed in any patient with confirmed ocular lymphoma. Occasionally ocular lymphoma can be very indolent, with slowly progressive disease for several years before cerebral lymphoma or rapidly progressive ocular disease develops. Conversely, patients with PCNSL have a 15 to 20 percent incidence of coexistent ocular disease. These patients may have ocular symptoms or may have clinically silent ocular involvement that is appreciated only on slit-lamp examination.

Leptomeninges and Spinal Cord

PCNSL rarely presents as primary leptomeningeal lymphoma (i.e., tumor confined to the meninges) or primary spinal cord lymphoma. Leptomeningeal lymphoma presents with a chronic meningitis and often with symptoms of increased intracranial pressure, with headache, nausea and vomiting, cranial nerve palsies, and multiple radiculopathies usually involving the lumbar and cervical roots. Spinal cord involvement by PCNSL is even less common than primary leptomeningeal lymphoma, and may occur in association with cerebral lymphoma. It usually presents as a painless, rapidly progressive myelopathy. The lesion usually affects the thoracic cord, and therefore symptoms and signs are restricted to the legs.

LABORATORY STUDIES

PCNSL cannot be diagnosed with certainty by clinical signs or symptoms alone. While the general concepts outlined above are helpful, they are not specific, particularly for the individual patient. These clinical features indicate the presence of an intracranial mass lesion that requires further definition. When patients present with any of the above symptoms or signs, the first test that should be obtained is cranial MRI with gadolinium. If MRI is not available, a computed tomography (CT) scan with contrast should be obtained, but the greater sensitivity of the MRI makes it preferable even though it is more costly. An initial MRI often saves money since it avoids duplication when an MRI is required after a mass is seen on CT scan.

Radiologic Features

The radiologic features of PCNSL are similar on CT or MRI. On precontrast CT or MRI the lesions usually appear iso- or hyperdense on CT and iso- or hyperintense on T1-weighted MRI. After the administration of contrast material or gadolinium, PCNSL has a dense and homogeneous enhancement pattern that is quite characteristic (Fig. 1). The lesions are periventricular and may be accompanied by peritumoral edema. Frequently the amount of edema is much less than expected for the size of the lesion, but this is an unreliable sign, and the presence of extensive edema does not exclude a PCNSL. Necrosis is not a prominent pathologic feature of PCNSL and is not seen radiographically. These typical radiologic features of PCNSL are present in more than 90 percent of patients with this tumor. Occasionally, ring-enhancing lesions, or areas of diffuse, patchy enhancement are seen in PCNSL and are indistinguishable from other types of intracranial lesions. However, the overwhelming majority of patients with PCNSL have a CT/MRI so characteristic that the diagnosis is often suggested by the radiographic appearance. The differential diagnosis includes metastases, glioma, infection, sarcoidosis, and multiple sclerosis.

Because PCNSL is frequently multifocal, patients are often suspected of having brain metastases. To further confuse this issue, in our series of non-AIDS patients with PCNSL at Memorial Sloan-Kettering Cancer Center, 13 percent of our patients had a prior history of a systemic cancer. Many of these patients had a remote history of a cured malignancy, such as Hodgkin's lymphoma treated 25 years previously or a colon cancer resected 21 years earlier, but the history of

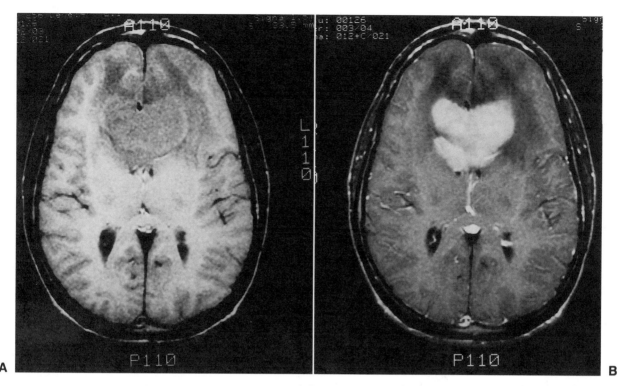

Figure 1 Pregadolinium (*A*) and postgadolinium (*B*) MRI of a primary central nervous system lymphoma (PCNSL). A large bilateral, periventricular, diffusely enhancing mass is evident. Note the absence of central necrosis and the moderate amount of peritumoral edema.

cancer often led to the presumptive diagnosis of brain metastases. Histologic diagnosis was not obtained, and inappropriate therapy, using rapid fractionation schedules for cranial RT, was instituted before the correct diagnosis was established. In addition, patients with or without a history of cancer often undergo an extensive series of tests searching for a systemic malignancy that is not there.

Patients with a single mass lesion are often presumed to have a malignant glioma, certainly a more common cause of a mass lesion, particularly in the older population. However, malignant gliomas should not be confused radiographically with a PCNSL. Malignant gliomas are usually ring-enhancing masses, always associated with surrounding edema. While both PCNSL and malignant gliomas require histologic confirmation to accurately establish the diagnosis, the surgical approach to the two tumor types is different. Stereotactic biopsy is the technique of choice to diagnose a PCNSL since surgery does not have an important therapeutic role in the management of this tumor. However, because the extent of surgical resection is directly related to survival in the treatment of malignant glioma, craniotomy with the intention of achieving a complete resection is the procedure of choice for a malignant glioma.

Early consideration of PCNSL on the basis of the CT/MRI appearance is also important regarding the use of corticosteroids prior to pathologic confirmation of the diagnosis. When an intracranial mass lesion is identified

on CT or MRI, corticosteroids are often employed immediately to control cerebral edema surrounding the lesion, reducing the overall mass effect and usually producing rapid neurologic improvement. This approach is effective for most brain tumors but can interfere with the histologic diagnosis of PCNSL. Steroids should not be administered to patients with suspected PCNSL until tissue has been obtained unless there is danger of immediate clinical herniation, a rare situation. In systemic and cerebral lymphoma alike, corticosteroid is an effective cytotoxic agent that is used as a chemotherapeutic drug. It causes direct cell lysis, resulting in regression, and in some cases complete disappearance, of the enhancing mass seen on CT/MRI (Fig. 2). Biopsy after corticosteroid administration often produces normal or nondiagnostic tissue, even if a contrast-enhancing mass is still seen on a preoperative CT/MRI. A significant tumor response is seen in at least 40 percent of patients, and the degree of tumor regression is related in part to the duration of corticosteroid administration. Disappearance of mass lesions may be appreciated after only a few days of standard-dose dexamethasone (16 mg per day), or weeks may be required to observe a response. There are reports of rare cures or patients with a durable remission lasting years after corticosteroid therapy alone, but the majority of patients have only a temporary response to steroid, and tumor regrowth usually occurs within a few months. Corticosteroid cannot be considered definitive treat-

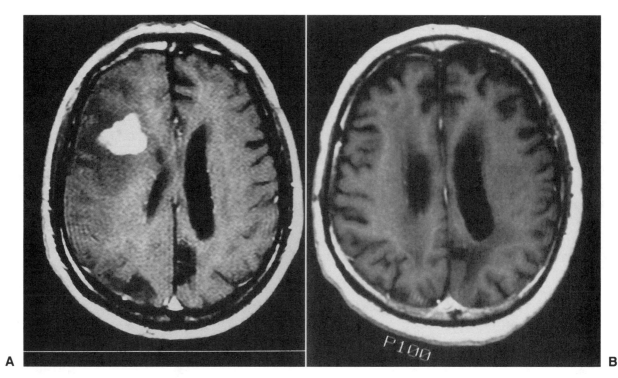

Figure 2 Resolution of PCNSL with corticosteroid. Postgadolinium MRIs of a patient with a recurrent right frontal PCNSL before (*A*) and 2 weeks after (*B*) corticosteroid administration. The patient refused all further therapy, and no tumor was evident in the brain at autopsy.

ment for PCNSL and should always be accompanied by chemotherapy and/or cranial irradiation.

It is important to note that not all patients with PCNSL have tumor regression with corticosteroid administration. In animal models of systemic lymphoma, a response to corticosteroid correlates with the presence of glucocorticoid receptors in the lymphoma cells. Animals whose tumor cells lack the receptor fail to respond to steroid. The absence of tumor regression to corticosteroid does not militate against the diagnosis of PCNSL, particularly if the lesion has the typical radiographic appearance of cerebral lymphoma. Occasionally a steroid response is used as a diagnostic test for PCNSL. This may yield a false-negative if the tumor does not respond but can also lead to a false-positive result. Other conditions can present as contrast-enhancing masses that resolve with corticosteroid, specifically multiple sclerosis and sarcoidosis. In the occasional patient it may also be difficult to differentiate these entities on clinical grounds since patients with indolent or relapsing-remitting courses of PCNSL have been reported, and CNS sarcoid can occur in the absence of systemic disease. For these reasons, the diagnosis of PCNSL should be based on pathologic material. A "steroid test" should be used only as a last resort.

The typical radiographic features of PCNSL are seen primarily in immunocompetent individuals. Immunodeficient patients, particularly those with AIDS, have a more variable appearance of PCNSL on CT or MRI.

While a densely and diffusely enhancing lesion may be seen, typically the lesions are ring-enhancing or have a patchy enhancement pattern, a result of the higher incidence of necrosis seen pathologically in PCNSL lesions in AIDS patients. The lesions are indistinguishable from other causes of intracranial mass lesions in these patients, specifically toxoplasmosis. Therefore, the radiographic appearance will not suggest a specific diagnosis in immunocompromised patients, and no lesion can be excluded as a possible PCNSL on the basis of the CT or MRI appearance. Immunocompromised patients can have a clinical and radiographic response to corticosteroids identical to that seen in normal patients, and therefore corticosteroids should be withheld while patients are receiving a therapeutic trial of antitoxoplasmosis therapy so that an accurate assessment can be made of the response to treatment. Institution of antitoxoplasmosis treatment is the appropriate first step in the management of AIDS patients with an intracranial mass lesion, but early stereotactic biopsy should be considered in patients with negative toxoplasmosis titers and in those patients who are clinically deteriorating during antibiotic therapy.

Cerebrospinal Fluid

Lumbar puncture is rarely necessary or appropriate in the diagnosis of a brain tumor. However, the CSF should be examined in every patient with presumed or

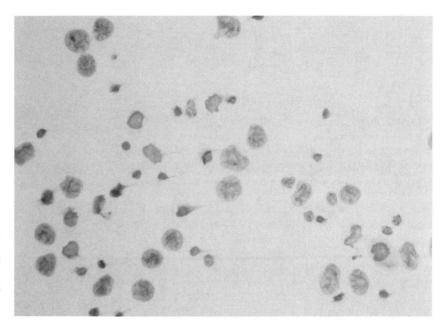

Figure 3 A positive cerebrospinal fluid cytologic specimen for lymphoma from a patient with PCNSL. The large anaplastic cells are malignant lymphocytes, while the smaller cells represent an accompanying reactive lymphocytosis.

established PCNSL. A lumbar puncture is particularly essential in immunocompromised patients to exclude other diagnoses that may be more common than or may coexist with PCNSL. Although most patients with PCNSL have substantial intracranial mass lesions, lumbar puncture can be performed safely in the overwhelming majority. A spinal tap should be deferred only in patients with large posterior fossa lesions or in those with prominent shift due to an inferior temporal mass. In the 95 patients seen with PCNSL at our institution, only one could not have a lumbar puncture due to a large cerebellar lesion. All others had a lumbar puncture without complication.

Because most PCNSL lesions are periventricular, tumor cells can gain easy access to the CSF. Despite the fact that microscopic leptomeningeal tumor is present in all patients at autopsy, and probably at diagnosis as well, the CSF chemistry profile is frequently unremarkable. The CSF protein concentration is elevated in 85 percent of patients. The majority have only a mildly increased protein concentration, rarely greater than 100 mg per deciliter. The CSF glucose concentration is normal except in the unusual patient who has florid leptomeningeal lymphoma, resulting in a low glucose concentration. A lymphocytosis is seen in approximately half of patients, frequently with white cell counts less than 20 per cubic millimeter.

While the routine chemistry and cell count analyses are rarely specific in PCNSL, the CSF cytologic examination affords the opportunity to establish a histologic diagnosis. In our series of 95 patients with non-AIDS PCNSL, 15 percent had the diagnosis made on the basis of CSF cytology alone, sparing the patient a brain biopsy. Although most patients still require a stereotactic biopsy for diagnosis, diagnosis by CSF examination may be particularly useful in the desperately ill patient or the AIDS patient who is at increased risk for the hemor-

rhagic complications of biopsy and whose treatment would be delayed awaiting a therapeutic trial of anti-toxoplasmosis therapy. Most series report a less than 25 percent incidence of a positive CSF cytologic examination in patients with PCNSL. However, only a minority of patients studied had a lumbar puncture. In our series, one-third of patients had malignant lymphocytes in their CSF, and another third had suspicious cells, indicating that at least two-thirds of patients had definite or probable leptomeningeal tumor at diagnosis. This high incidence of meningeal involvement not only offers a means of diagnosis, but also has therapeutic implications since tumor in the leptomeninges requires specific treatment.

A potential source of difficulty in the interpretation of the CSF specimens from patients with PCNSL is the frequent presence of an accompanying reactive lymphocytosis, a manifestation of the inflammatory response generated by some lymphomas. Reactive lymphocytes infiltrate tissue specimens from PCNSL as well as systemic NHL but rarely cause diagnostic confusion. In the CSF they may accompany malignant or suspicious cells or be the only identifiable cell (Fig. 3). Malignant cells can be differentiated from reactive lymphocytes on the basis of their cytologic features. However, most pathologists are reluctant to call a positive cytology when more than one population of cells is evident in the specimen, since reactive cells can occasionally appear atypical. However, reactive lymphocytes are always T cells, and lymphocyte markers will identify the cytologically malignant cells as B cells, demonstrating the distinct nature of the two cell types.

Like parenchymal brain PCNSL, leptomeningeal lymphoma can have a prompt and dramatic response to corticosteroids. CSF analyzed after the patient has received corticosteroid may be negative or normal. An accurate assessment of meningeal involvement is important for treatment decisions regarding the use and duration of intrathecal chemotherapy, and lumbar puncture should be performed prior to the start of corticosteroid.

Systemic Evaluation

Pathologic confirmation of a diagnosis of cerebral lymphoma often prompts an extensive systemic search for widespread lymphoma. There is no report of an occult systemic lymphoma presenting as an intracranial mass lesion. We have studied all our patients with PCNSL with abdominal and pelvic CT scans, chest x ray or CT scan, and bone marrow biopsy, and none had evidence of systemic lymphoma. Furthermore, only 7 to 8 percent of patients with PCNSL have evidence of systemic disease at autopsy, usually single sites of microscopic disease thought to be due to metastatic spread from uncontrolled cerebral lymphoma. Therefore, an extensive systemic evaluation is not necessary for apparently immunocompetent patients with PCNSL.

Immunodeficient patients, particularly those with AIDS, should have a systemic evaluation because of the high incidence of extranodal lymphomas in this population and their very high incidence of associated CNS involvement. However, even in this population, the identification of systemic lymphoma when a patient presents with an intracranial mass is decidedly uncommon. Nevertheless, a thorough assessment will guarantee administration of the best therapeutic regimen.

SUGGESTED READING

Balmaceda C, DeAngelis L. Leptomeningeal (LM) involvement in primary central nervous system lymphoma (PCNSL). Ann Neurol 1992; 32:286.

Ciricillo SF, Rosenblum ML. Use of CT and MR imaging to distinguish intracranial lesions and to define the need for biopsy in AIDS patients. J Neurosurg 1990; 73:720–724.

DeAngelis LM: Primary central nervous system lymphoma imitates multiple sclerosis. J Neurooncol 1990; 9:177–181.

DeAngelis LM. Primary central nervous system lymphoma as a secondary malignancy. Cancer 1991; 67:1431–1435.

DeAngelis LM. Primary central nervous system lymphoma. In: DeVita VT Jr, Hellman S, Rosenberg SA, eds. Principles and practice of oncology updates. Philadelphia: JB Lippincott, 1992; 6(11):1.

DeAngelis LM, Yahalom J, Thaler HT, Kher U. Combined modality therapy for primary CNS lymphoma. J Clin Oncol 1992; 10:635–643.

Hochberg FH, Miller DC. Primary central nervous system lymphoma. J Neurosurg 1988; 68:835–853.

Singh A, Strobos RJ, Singh BM, et al. Steroid-induced remissions in CNS lymphoma. Neurology 1982; 32:1267–1271.

RADIATION NEUROTOXICITY

MICHAEL J. GLANTZ, M.D.

Most cancer therapies are nonspecifically cytotoxic. This is certainly true of radiation therapy (RT). As a result, when RT is used to treat primary or metastatic nervous system cancers, or non-nervous system malignancies located close to neural structures, injury to the normal nervous system can occur and is often dose-limiting. Since individual tolerances vary, safe radiation thresholds are not precisely known and may be altered by concurrent chemotherapy or pre-existing disease. Intentional "overdoses" may be given with curative or long-term palliative intent. Thus, neurologic complications of RT continue to arise despite a heightened awareness of the risks. In fact, since conventional radiation therapy techniques are being applied more aggressively, new approaches such as brachytherapy and radiosurgery are becoming commonplace, and patients are surviving longer, the incidence of radiation-related nervous system injury appears to be increasing.

Radiation-related nervous system injury may be acute, subacute, or late (chronic) (Table 1). Acute toxicity, occurring within hours to weeks after treatment, is probably related to increased edema. Subacute damage, occurring within weeks to months after treatment, may reflect demyelination. Late injury, occurring months to decades after treatment, can be caused by neurovascular damage, progressive fibrosis, or disruption of cellular DNA. Accurate diagnosis is critical in order to exclude alternative, potentially treatable disorders, to prevent unnecessary diagnostic procedures and inappropriate antineoplastic therapy, and to allow meaningful prognostication.

ACUTE COMPLICATIONS

The most common and often debilitating consequence of cranial RT is progressive tiredness. Patients typically begin to notice increasing fatigue half to two-thirds of the way through conventional RT for primary brain tumors (between weeks 3 and 5) and near the end, or 1 to 2 weeks following completion of the shorter course of RT used for brain metastases. The effect of radiation on normal brain adjacent to tumor plays some part in the production of these symptoms, particularly when whole-brain or large-field radiation is used. The logistic challenge of obtaining treatment (dressing, driving, parking, walking to the treatment facility) is also important. Symptoms are more pronounced in older patients, and can be so severe that patients suspect that their treatment is not working. Symptoms often persist for several weeks after the

Table 1 Types, Timing, and Outcome of Radiation-Induced Nervous System Injury

Anatomic Location	Latency of Onset	Predisposing Factors	Outcome
Brain			
Acute encephalopathy	Hours to days	Increased ICP	Good
Subacute encephalopathy	8–16 weeks	Large tumor-edema	Good
Delayed radionecrosis	14 months (median)	Vascular disease, CTX	Poor
Atrophy and dementia	6–60 months	Pre-existing dementia	Poor
Cognitive and behavioral changes	6–60 months	Age <7 or > 60 years	Variable
Second primary tumors	15–30 years	VRD, AT	Poor
Neuroendocrine			
Hypothalamic and pituitary hypofunction	3 months–6 years	Young age	Good
Thyroid hypofunction	3–5 years	Thyroid irradiation	Good
Cranial nerves and eyes			
Retinopathy	18–36 months	Eye irradiation	Poor
Optic neuropathy	11 months (median)	Vascular disease	Poor
Cranial neuropathy	5.5 years (median)	Surgery, CTX, diabetes	Poor
Spinal cord			
Transient myelopathy	2–40 weeks	Cervical RT	Good
Chronic progressive myelopathy	14 months (median)		Poor
Brachial and lumbosacral plexopathy	14 months (median)		Poor
(See Table 2)			
Peripheral nerves			
Peripheral neuropathy	Years	Diabetes, CTX	Variable
Peripheral nerve sheath tumors	15.4 years (median)	VRD	Poor
Cerebral vasculature			
Intracranial arterial occlusion	9 mo–15.5 yr	VRD	Poor
Internal carotid artery thrombosis	3 mo–27 yr	High-dose RT	Variable
Accelerated atherosclerosis	1 to >30 yr	Vascular disease	Variable
Carotid artery rupture	4–52 wk	Perioperative infection	Poor
Cardioembolic TIA or stroke		Mediastinal irradiation	Good
Other			
Impaired taste, decreased appetite	During therapy		Good
Decreased hearing	During therapy		Good
Tiredness, easy fatigability	During therapy	Age >60 yr	Good
Hair loss	During therapy		Good
Erythema, itching, dryness of skin	During therapy		Good

ICP = intracranial pressure, CTX = chemotherapy, VRD = von Recklinghausen's disease, AT = ataxia telangiectasia, RT = radiation therapy, TIA = transient ischemic attack.

completion of therapy. In the typical case, necessary diagnostic studies are limited to a routine blood count and electrolyte determination and a review of medications. Anticonvulsants, especially phenobarbital, and analgesics frequently have a pronounced sedating effect on patients with brain tumors, particularly during radiation. No specific intervention beyond adequate rest and planning of activities is available. When concomitant tapering of corticosteroids has taken place, a return to higher doses may be beneficial.

Lethargy is also a feature of acute radiation encephalopathy. New or progressive focal deficits, headache, nausea, vomiting, fever, and seizures may develop. Onset is within the first 2 weeks of treatment. Increased edema is seen on a computed tomography (CT) or magnetic resonance imaging (MRI) scan, and increasing doses of corticosteroids usually ameliorate the symptoms. We have also observed acute symptom exacerbation within hours after the use of stereotactic radiosurgery in patients with high-grade primary, but not metastatic, brain tumors. Similar worsening of symptoms may occur during irradiation of epidural spinal cord tumors, and new weakness, sphincter dysfunction, or sensory disturbances may appear. When new symptoms develop over days to a few weeks, are mild, or improve over the weekend break from RT, we generally make a presumptive diagnosis and increase steroids empirically. Marked or abrupt deterioration or fluctuating symptoms raise the possibilities of tumor-associated hemorrhage, obstructive hydrocephalus, unrecognized seizures, or infection, intracranial or systemic. An urgent CT or MRI is among the appropriate first diagnostic steps.

The same exacerbation of symptoms may develop 1 to 4 months after the completion of RT and is termed as "early delayed encephalopathy." The CT or MRI again shows increased edema and sometimes enhancement. Spontaneous resolution occurs after several months. Corticosteroids hasten improvement. A biopsy is performed only if the severity of symptoms suggests the possibility of treatment failure and makes the need for additional therapy an urgent question.

SUBACUTE COMPLICATIONS

Subacute myelopathy is a common form of radiation neurotoxicity, which follows RT to the cervical spinal cord. Lhermitte's sign is the sole symptom. The neurologic exam is normal. Subacute myelopathy occurs in up to 15 percent of patients receiving mantle irradiation for Hodgkin's disease. Similar symptoms have been reported following high-dose chemotherapy with autologous bone marrow transplant, and with conventional doses of cisplatin chemotherapy. Symptom onset peaks at 4 to 6 months (range 1 to 30 months) after treatment, and symptoms resolve spontaneously over about 4 months. In the absence of a confounding neurologic disease such as multiple sclerosis, additional diagnostic investigations are unnecessary.

Transient brachial plexopathy, like subacute myelopathy, can develop weeks to a few months after the initiation of RT and is clinically identical to delayed radiation plexopathy. Unlike their late counterparts, no treatment is necessary for either subacute myelopathy or brachial plexopathy. The diagnostic concerns of metastases to the plexus, spinal cord, leptomeninges, or epidural space often require exclusion by lumbar puncture and appropriate radiographs.

LATE EFFECTS OF RADIATION

The delayed consequences of therapeutic radiation can affect every level of the nervous system (see Table 1). Their incidences vary with the radiation dose and fractionation scheme, age of the patient, underlying diseases, concomitant treatments, and length of survival after completion of radiation. As a rule, incidence increases and latency decreases with higher total doses, higher fraction size, and larger volumes of treated nervous system. These complications, though uncommon, are generally progressive and severe and are of particular concern in patients with potentially curable disease, such as childhood acute leukemias, intracranial germ cell tumors, oligodendrogliomas, and meningiomas, or tumors compatible with long survivals, such as low-grade gliomas or solitary brain metastases with well-controlled systemic disease.

Brain Injuries

Delayed cerebral radionecrosis is the best-described late complication of cranial radiation and occurs after intentional irradiation of the intracranial contents or inadvertent exposure of the brain to radiation, such as the temporal lobes in patients with head and neck cancer. An incidence of 5 percent has been estimated for patients receiving more than 5,000 cGy, although the actual incidence is dose and fraction size dependent. Typically, headache, personality change, focal deficits, and seizures develop insidiously 4 months to 4 years or more (median 14 months) after treatment. Papilledema and other signs of increased intracranial pressure may be present. Rarely, the presentation is fulminant. CT scanning reveals a low-density white matter lesion with heterogeneous enhancement, mass effect, and occasional calcification. Increased T2 signal is prominent on MRI scans. Angiography demonstrates an avascular

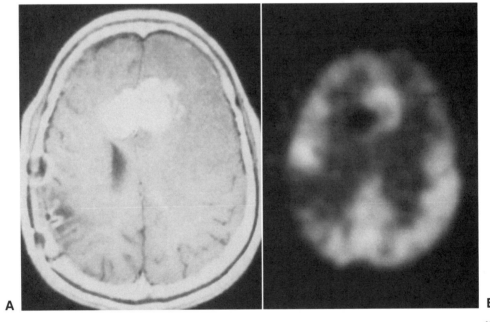

Figure 1 Enhanced magnetic resonance imaging (MRI) scan (*A*) and corresponding axial [^{18}F] fluorodeoxyglucose positron emission tomography (PET) scan (*B*) obtained 2 years after gross total resection of a right parietal breast metastasis in a 62-year-old woman, followed by whole brain radiotherapy with a boost to the right frontal and parietal regions. The MRI shows an enhancing corpus callosum mass extending into both frontal lobes. The right-sided lesion was hypometabolic, and the left-sided lesion hypermetabolic on PET scan. Subsequent stereotactic biopsies showed radiation necrosis on the right, and metastatic tumor on the left.

mass, which is hypometabolic on [^{18}F]fluorodeoxy-glucose or [^{11}C]methionine positron emission tomography (PET) scanning (Fig. 1), "cold" on thallium-201 scanning, and fails to enhance on "flash" MRI scans.

Nevertheless, an unequivocal diagnosis cannot be made radiographically or clinically. The diagnostic gold standard is histologic. However, tumor and radionecrosis often coexist, and biopsy specimens may result in misleading diagnoses because of sampling errors. In patients with a recurrent mass in the same location as the original tumor, which develops within 8 months after the completion of RT, the presumption of recurrent tumor can be made with good certainty. We obtain PET, single photon emission CT (SPECT), or flash MRI scans on such patients, and if further aggressive therapy is planned, we perform a second resection or stereotactic biopsy, if feasible, before initiating treatment. In cases where the "recurrence" develops late, particularly after 2 years, when the original tumor was low grade, when PET, SPECT, or flash MRI scanning is suggestive of radionecrosis, or when unconventional radiation and chemotherapy protocols were used in the initial treatment, a tissue diagnosis is mandatory. While tumor and radionecrosis are the leading diagnostic possibilities, abscess and stroke can occasionally be present. Hypertension, diabetes, and concurrent chemotherapy, particularly with methotrexate, may increase the incidence of radionecrosis and hence the index of suspicion.

A second, more diffuse form of late brain injury is manifested clinically by gradual intellectual decline, short-term memory loss, fatigue, and personality change,

culminating after one to several years in full-blown dementia. Occasionally, gait impairment, incontinence, and dysarthria occur. Significant declines in IQ, and deficits in memory, fine motor, and visual-spatial function are especially common in children under 7 and are more pronounced with decreasing age at the time of RT. Patients over 60 are also particularly susceptible to this type of late radiation toxicity. Diffuse cerebral atrophy, ventricular enlargement, and white matter abnormalities are seen on CT and MRI (Fig. 2), but focal lesions are absent clinically and radiographically. Radiographic abnormalities of this type are common, are seen in at least half of patients following conventional whole-brain or large-field cranial irradiation, and may be progressive, but do not necessarily correlate with symptoms. As many as 20 percent of radiographically affected patients developed radiation-induced dementia. The incidence is greatest in patients receiving whole-brain RT and in those surviving more than 1 year. Concurrent methotrexate or nitrosourea chemotherapy may increase the risk. Subtle, nonprogressive personality and cognitive changes are even more frequent and are more pronounced in children and in those over 60 years of age. Rarely, radiographic confusion with periventricular small vessel disease, multiple sclerosis, progressive multifocal leukoencephalopathy, or transependymal cerebrospinal fluid (CSF) resorption in the setting of hydrocephalus can occur. Clinically, leptomeningeal disease, encephalitis, concurrently administered drugs (anticonvulsants, steroids, analgesics), metabolic abnormalities, systemic infection, and malnutrition enter into

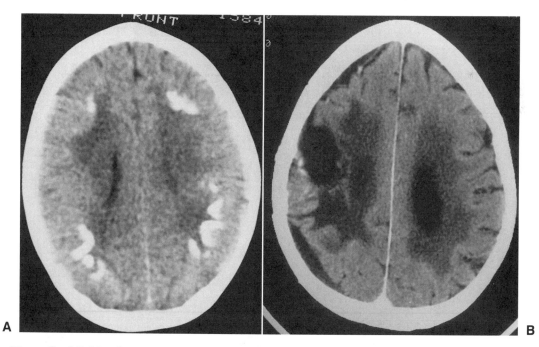

Figure 2 (*A*) Unenhanced computed tomography (CT) scan of a 12-year-old taken 5 years after prophylactic cranial irradiation and intrathecal methotrexate for ALL. Note the abundant calcifications and white matter hypodensity. (*B*) Enhanced CT scan of a 57-year-old taken 2 years after wide field irradiation of a large right frontotemporal glioblastoma multiforme. Cortical atrophy, ventricular enlargement, and white matter hypodensity are prominent.

the differential diagnosis. Practically, a diagnosis should not be made on radiographic grounds alone. A careful search for infection, review of concurrent medications, measurement of serum electrolytes, and a lumbar puncture for pressure, cytology, and cultures are generally indicated. Electroencephalograms are helpful only when seizures are suspected.

Spinal Cord Complications

Chronic progressive myelopathy is the delayed spinal cord syndrome corresponding to cerebral radionecrosis. It occurs most commonly after RT of tumors in the chest, mediastinum, cervical region, or head and neck. The syndrome frequently presents with ascending paresthesias, dysesthesias, or sensory loss in one or both lower extremities, followed by weakness and signs of myelopathy. A partial transverse myelitis or Brown-Séquard's syndrome is common, as is disturbance of sphincter function. Symptoms begin 3 to 30 months or more (median 14 months) after treatment, and progression is usually gradual over weeks to months. Estimates of incidence range from 1 to 12.5 percent of treated patients. Epidural metastases, intramedullary tumor or hemorrhage, leptomeningeal disease, and paraneoplastic subacute necrotizing myelopathy are competing diagnostic possibilities. Radiation-induced myelopathy is characteristically painless, while pain is usually prominent with epidural and intramedullary tumor. Rarely, spinal cord atrophy or fusiform enlargement of radiated segments of spinal cord may be seen on MRI or myelography in radiation myelopathy, but MRI will reliably demonstrate tumor from epidural, intramedullary, and leptomeningeal metastases. The CSF protein may be elevated in all four disorders, but a pleocytosis, hypoglycorrhachia, and positive cytology distinguish leptomeningeal spread of tumor. Radiation myelopathy is slowly progressive, while abrupt worsening often occurs in malignant cord disease, and paraneoplastic myelopathy is a fulminant process leading to death in weeks to a few months.

Brachial and Lumbar Plexus Injuries

The brachial and lumbar plexuses are damaged by radiation in 1 to 3 percent of conventionally treated patients, usually following treatment of head and neck, breast, lung, thyroid, testicular, gynecologic, prostate, or colorectal cancers or Hodgkin's and non-Hodgkin's lymphomas. Paresthesias or dysesthesias of the affected limb and gradually progressive weakness are characteristic (Table 2). Pain is unusual, in contrast to malignant plexopathy. In cases of radiation-induced brachial plexopathy, ipsilateral lymphedema is common. The upper plexus is almost always involved (75 percent of cases), while lower plexus involvement is common with malignant plexopathy. In radiation-induced lumbosacral plexopathy, bilateral, though often asymmetric, plexus involvement is the rule. Pain, sphincter dysfunction, unilateral or isolated upper (L2 to L4) plexus symptoms, bony erosion, and hydronephrosis suggest a malignant origin. Ischemic plexitis, brachial or lumbosacral neuritis, diabetic, compression, and chemotherapy-induced neuropathies, cervical arthritis, joint bursitis, myofascial pain, and intragluteal injection may complicate the differential diagnosis between radiation and malignant plexopathy. Electromyography, MRIs of the pertinent plexus and spinal cord levels (Fig. 3), and CSF cytologic

Table 2 Radiation versus Neoplastic Plexopathy

	Brachial Plexopathy		Lumbosacral Plexopathy	
	Radiation-Induced	*Neoplastic*	*Radiation-Induced*	*Neoplastic*
Latency (median)	5 yr	< 1 yr	5 yr	< 1 yr
Presenting symptom				
Pain	20%	80%	7%	91%
Weakness	13%	5%	58%	4%
Numbness	73%	19%	36%	4%
Anatomic distribution				
Upper plexus	42%	11%	17%	30%
Lower plexus	24%	62%	46%	49%
Entire plexus	30%	26%	38%	23%
Horner's syndrome	8%	47%	NA	NA
Bowel-bladder symptoms	NA	NA	0%	12%
Bilateral symptoms	0%	0%	79%	23%
CT scan				
Mass lesion	0%	92%	0%	91%
Loss of tissue planes	62%	12%	?	?
Myelogram positive	0%	35%	0%	21%
Myokymia on EMG	63%	4%	64%	0%
Usual outcome	Disability	Death	Disability	Death
Median survival	> 10 yr	18 mo	> 10 yr	18 mo

CT = computed tomography, EMG = electromyogram, NA = not applicable.
From Glantz M, Rottenberg D. Harmful effects of radiation on the nervous system. In: Asbury AK, McKhann GM, McDonald WI, eds. Diseases of the Nervous System: Clinical Neurobiology. 2nd ed. Philadelphia: WB Saunders, 1992:1136; with permission.

studies are usually necessary to exclude metastases to the plexus, epidural space, or leptomeninges, which may mimic or coexist with radiation-induced plexopathy. Failure to image tumor, particularly in the brachial plexus, does not exclude a malignant origin. In patients with no active disease, prolonged disease-free intervals, or medically intractable pain, we often resort to surgical exploration for both diagnosis and therapy.

Optic Neuropathy

Postradiation optic neuropathy can complicate RT to the optic apparatus for tumors involving the retina, optic nerve, chiasm, and pituitary region and can also occur after RT for intracranial tumors not directly contiguous with the visual system. Painless, progressive, monocular visual loss or constriction of visual fields is the typical presentation. Altitudinal field cuts are very common. "Dimming" of vision or "spotty" visual loss are typical patient descriptions. The presence of pain or homonymous field defects weigh strongly against the diagnosis. Retinal arteriolar narrowing, disk edema, and peripapillary hemorrhages are the early funduscopic correlates (Fig. 4). The disorder usually progresses to severe, bilateral visual loss in the setting of optic atrophy. Onset ranges from 3 months to 3 years after RT (median 11 months), and compromise of the local vascular supply (e.g., by pituitary region tumors) or concurrent vincristine, methotrexate, or 5-FU chemotherapy may increase the incidence of this complication. Widening the differential diagnosis are primary optic nerve tumors, including radiation-induced tumors; metastases to the orbit (breast cancer accounts for half of these), optic nerves or chiasm, pituitary, skull base, or leptomeninges; increased intracranial pressure; cerebrovascular disease (including treatment-induced types); chemotherapy effects (most importantly, tamoxifen, cisplatinum, and intra-arterial BCNU); venous sinus thrombosis; and paraneoplastic disease (retinopathy, optic neuritis, and encephalomyelitis). Careful imaging studies, medication review, and an examination of the CSF are necessary initial studies.

Cranial Neuropathy

Rarely, other cranial neuropathies can occur after exposure to therapeutic radiation. Radiation-induced cranial neuropathy develops 1 to 37 years (mean 5.5 years) after RT, generally for head and neck or orbital tumors, and is progressive and permanent. In order of frequency, cranial nerves XII, XI, X, V, and VI are affected. The recurrent laryngeal nerve can be injured after RT for breast or lung cancer, or iodine-131 treatment of thyroid cancer. Prominent fibrosis of the soft tissues of the neck precedes cranial nerve involvement by months or years. Disturbances of taste, gag, and salivation are also common, usually develop during RT, and are the result of damage to afferent receptors rather than the cranial nerves themselves. Decreased hearing secondary to cochlear (not eighth nerve) injury or serous otitis media is frequent, but vestibular dysfunction does not occur. The most common competing diagnosis is malignant disease at the base of the skull. A shorter latency following RT (2 to 27 months) and different frequency of cranial nerve involvement (V and VI are most common, followed by IX, X, and XII) help identify malignant disease. Pre-existing neuropathy (secondary to diabetes), ischemia (secondary to surgery), or chemotherapy (cisplatin, vincristine, bleomycin, adriamycin) may predispose to radiation-induced cranial neuropa-

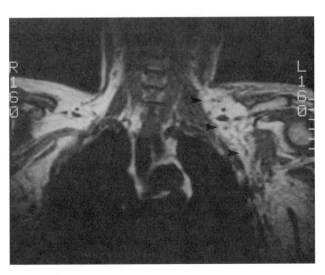

Figure 3 Unenhanced, intermediate-weighted (TR 666.7, TE 10) magnetic resonance image of the brachial plexus in a 48-year-old woman with recurrent breast cancer and a painful left brachial plexopathy. The neurovascular bundle on the right is well-defined; on the left it is engulfed by centrally necrotic tumor, and tumor-containing lymph nodes (*arrowheads*).

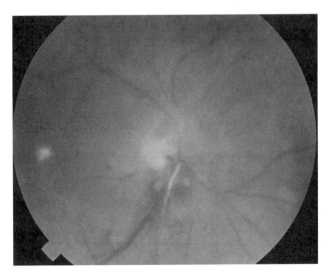

Figure 4 Left fundus of a 51-year-old complaining of progressive, binocular visual loss 3 years after irradiation of a large left frontal astrocytoma. Peripapillary hemorrhages, irregular retinal arteriolar narrowing, and mild disc edema are all present.

thy. CT scanning may be diagnostic of tumor recurrence at the skull base, although prolonged and careful observation is frequently required. Since leptomeningeal disease, sarcoidosis, Lyme disease, basilar meningitis, and paraneoplastic encephalomyelitis can also present with cranial neuropathies, a lumbar puncture and brain MRI are also required.

Endocrinopathies

The same types of RT that predispose to optic neuropathy can result in endocrine dysfunction, usually on a hypothalamic basis. Growth hormone (GH) is most frequently affected, followed by thyrotropin and corticotropin. Hyperprolactinemia is common and may resolve spontaneously. Diabetes insipidus is rare. Disturbances of sleep, libido, personality, appetite, thirst, and cognitive function occasionally result directly from hypothalamic dysfunction. Rarely, corticotropin deficiency may complicate the tapering of steroids. Hypothyroidism may account for symptoms of generalized weakness, easy fatiguability, weight gain, and cold intolerance attributed to corticosteroids, other medications, or to the underlying disease. Since hypothyroidism of this type is secondary to thyrotropin underproduction, measurement of triiodothyronine (T3) uptake, thyroxine (T4), and thyroid-stimulating hormone (TSH) is usually necessary for diagnosis. Occasionally, empiric treatment in the face of minimally abnormal values provides a diagnosis and produces a gratifying clinical response. Children appear to be more sensitive than adults to the endocrine effects of radiation, and increased activity of the hypothalamic-pituitary axis during RT may also predispose to late complications.

The symptoms of radiation-induced endocrinopathy may be subtle. The effects of steroids, chemotherapy, surgery, vertebral body irradiation, psychological disturbances, nutritional deficiencies, and the tumor itself may mask or be mistaken for endocrinopathy. Compensated or minimally symptomatic abnormalities may precede overt disease by years. We routinely obtain biochemical screening (T3 uptake, T4, TSH, follicle-stimulating hormone, luteinizing hormone, prolactin, and, in children, GH) before RT, 6 months after RT, and then yearly or when suggestive symptoms develop. In cases where compelling clinical evidence of hypothyroidism exists in the absence of diagnostic laboratory abnormalities, a therapeutic trial of synthroid is frequently given. Such an approach is not taken in growth-delayed children with normal biochemical GH studies.

Cerebrovascular Injuries

The cerebral vasculature itself may be damaged by radiation of the brain, sellar region, head and neck, and thorax. Depending on the portion of the vascular tree affected and the type of lesion, transient ischemic attacks (TIAs), strokes, or hemorrhage may occur (Table 3). TIAs and stroke can also occur after irradiation of the ascending aorta and proximal common carotid arteries, as for lymphoma or breast cancer. A syndrome consisting of multiple TIAs occurring months to years (median 2 years) after mantle irradiation for Hodgkin's disease has also been described. Pre-existing disease (including hypertension, hypercholesterolemia, and diabetes), von Reckinghausen's disease, and concurrent chemotherapy may predispose to these syndromes. In addition to standard causes of cerebrovascular disease, others that must be considered include chemotherapy-induced and paraneoplastic vasculopathy, compression of cerebral vessels by tumor, and parainfectious vasculitis (e.g., secondary to varicella zoster following ophthalmic shingles). CT or MRI scanning is used to document infarcts, and angiography helps select among potential causes. In patients with accelerated carotid atherosclerosis, segments of vessel within the radiation ports but *not* commonly involved by typical atherosclerosis (the proximal common carotid artery, internal carotid artery distal

Table 3 Radiation-Induced Vasculopathies

Syndrome	Age	Affected Vessels	Latency After Radiation	Frequency Dose (rad)	Associated Conditions
Intracranial vascular occlusive disease	Child	ICA, MCA, PCA moya moya pattern on angiogram	6 mo–20 yr (7 yr)	Rare >4,500	Usually after RT to optic glioma; VRD and young age predispose
Thrombotic occlusion	Adult	Internal carotid	3 mo–27 yr (>3 yr)	Rare >6,500	After neck irradiation (lymphoma, head and neck)
Accelerated atherosclerosis	Adult	EC or IC vessels within RT ports	6 mo–57 yr (19 yr)	>10% >5,000	Hypertension, hyperlipidemia, pre-existing vascular disease (diabetes) predispose
Carotid artery rupture	Adult	Common carotid	4–52 wk	Rare >5,500	Preceded by radical neck dissection and wound infection

ICA = internal carotid artery, MCA = middle cerebral artery, PCA = posterior cerebral artery, RT = radiation therapy, VRD = von Recklinghausen's disease, EC = extracranial, IC = intracranial.

From Glantz M, Rottenberg D. Harmful effects of radiation on the nervous system. In: Asbury AK, McKhann GM, McDonald WI, eds. Diseases of the Nervous System: Clinical Neurobiology. 2nd ed. Philadelphia: WB Saunders 1992:1138; with permission.

to the bifurcation, small and medium-sized intracranial arteries) are affected. Occlusion of one or more arteries of the circle of Willis and a moya moya pattern of collateral vessels (Fig. 5) are seen in cases of intracranial vascular occlusive disease. Because of the high incidence of hemodynamically significant carotid disease (17 percent by ultrasound), symptomatic carotid disease (12 percent) and stroke (6.9 percent) in patients surviving 5 years or more after cervical irradiation, prophylactic antiplatelet therapy, cholesterol lowering agents, and yearly carotid ultrasound screening are appropriate in selected patients.

Second Primary Brain Tumors

Second primary tumors may arise within the brain (meningiomas, gliomas), dura (fibrosarcoma), cranial bones (osteosarcoma), or peripheral nerves (malignant peripheral nerve sheath tumor, malignant schwannoma, neurofibrosarcoma) following therapeutic, prophylactic, or diagnostic irradiation. Latencies are long: 3 to 41 years (mean 15.4 years) for peripheral nerve sheath tumors and 5 to 26 years (median 15 years) for meningiomas. Even low-dose radiation used for acne, tinea capitis, or dental diagnosis has been associated with an increased incidence of tumors at an even longer latency (mean of 37 years for meningiomas). Peripheral nerve sheath tumors present as painful, enlarging masses within the field of previous radiation and produce

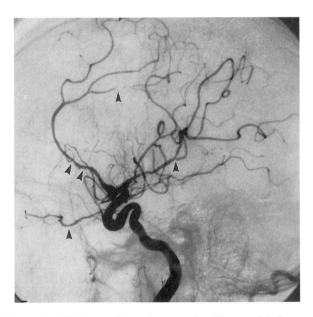

Figure 5 Right carotid angiogram of a 42-year-old, 7 years after resection of a right frontal astrocytoma followed by radiation therapy (4,000 cGy to the whole brain, 2,000 cGy to both frontal lobes). The patient suffered right and left frontal and right parietal strokes 5 years after completing radiotherapy. The angiogram demonstrates abnormal narrowing and dilatation of multiple branches of the middle cerebral artery (*arrowheads*), and prominent lenticulostriate vessels (moya moya pattern).

progressive neurologic dysfunction. The signs and symptoms of intracranial second primary tumors are indistinguishable from their spontaneously arising analogues. Scarring, atrophy, and keratoses in the overlying skin are clinical clues to the cause, even when the previous radiation has been forgotten. Most of these tumors are histologically and clinically aggressive, and treatment is rarely successful. Genetic susceptibility, in the form of von Recklinghausen's disease or ataxia-telangiectasia (even the heterozygous carrier state) are important predisposing factors, and recurrent cancer is the most pressing differential diagnostic consideration.

SUMMARY AND APPROACH TO THE PATIENT

Despite the potential for injury to all levels of the nervous system, radiation therapy remains an integral part of treatment for most patients with primary and metastatic brain tumors and for many other types of cancer that occur outside of but adjacent to the nervous system. As patients are followed more carefully, as more aggressive treatments are employed, and as therapeutic successes lead to longer survivals, the incidence of radiation-induced nervous system toxicity has increased. Recognition of the spectrum of potential symptoms and the multiple alternative causes for each symptom frequently falls to the neurologist. The superimposed effects of generalized debility, poor nutrition, intercurrent illness, medication side effects, and persistent or recurrent cancer are often difficult to differentiate from radiation-related symptoms, but treatment and prognosis differ greatly depending on cause. The neurologic complications of radiation, particularly the late onset ones, are typically progressive and may result in debilitating or life-threatening symptoms at a time when the tumor itself is stable or inapparent. We hold an initial bias in favor of recurrent cancer as the cause of symptoms, and in addition to careful physical examination and medication review, we depend heavily on neuroradiologic, CSF, and in many cases tissue diagnostic studies. Therapeutic trials, such as hormone replacement for suspected endocrine hypofunction, steroids for acute decompensation after the start of RT, or withdrawal of a potentially sedating analgesic or anticonvulsant frequently have a role. Often, meticulous and repeated investigations over time are required to establish a diagnosis. Even after the diagnosis of a radiation-induced complication is made, continued vigilance for additional sites or manifestations of injury or new cancer-related symptoms is obligatory.

SUGGESTED READING

Atkinson JLD, Sundt TM, Dale AJD, et al. Radiation-associated atheromatous disease of the cervical carotid artery: Report of seven cases and review of the literature. Neurosurgery 1989; 24:171–178.

Constine LS, Woolf PD, Cann D, et al. Hypothalamic-pituitary dysfunction after radiation for brain tumors. N Engl J Med 1993; 328:87–94.

DeAngelis LM, Delattre J-Y, Posner JB. Radiation-induced dementia in patients cured of brain metastases. Neurology 1989; 39:789–796.

Glantz MJ, Rottenberg DA. Harmful effects of radiation on the nervous system. In: Asbury AK, McKhann GM, McDonald WI, eds. Diseases of the nervous system: Clinical neurobiology. Philadelphia: WB Saunders, 1992:1130.

Graus F, Rogers LR, Posner JB. Cerebrovascular complications in patients with cancer. Medicine 1985; 64:16–35.

Murros KE, Toole JF. The effect of radiation on carotid arteries. Arch Neurol 1989; 46:449–455.

Ron E, Modan B, Boice JD, et al. Tumors of the brain and nervous system after radiotherapy in childhood. N Engl J Med 1988; 319:1,033–1,039.

Rottenberg DA, ed. Neurologic complications of cancer treatment. Boston: Butterworth-Heinemann, 1991.

Samaan NA, Vieto R, Schultz PN, et al. Hypothalamic, pituitary and thyroid dysfunction after radiotherapy to the head and neck. Int J Radiat Oncol Biol Phys 1982; 8:1,857–1,867.

NEUROLOGIC COMPLICATIONS OF CHEMOTHERAPY

RUSSELL W. WALKER, M.D.

Neurologic complications of chemotherapy, although not seen as frequently as other systemic complications, are usually far more disabling and cause severe morbidity, with a profound impact on a patient's quality of life. It is crucial that chemotherapy-related neurologic symptoms be accurately diagnosed and not attributed to infection, cerebrovascular disease, or underlying malignancy. The signs and symptoms of these problems are typically the same regardless of cause, and the diagnosis of a treatment-related disorder is made by clinical inference. Diagnosis is based on the temporal relation of the problem to treatment received and the knowledge that the presumed offending agent has been associated with such problems in the past. Those complications that are seen most frequently are those associated with drugs most commonly in use. Physicians often perform tests necessary to exclude the infectious, vascular, metabolic, and other complications of the malignancy itself in order to help confirm the diagnosis.

As chemotherapeutic agents have become established in the cancer armamentarium, the incidence, expected severity, and outcome of their neurologic side effects have become well recognized and the pathogenesis established in some cases. For newer drugs in less frequent use, patterns of neurologic toxicity are only now being recognized.

Chemotherapeutic agents may affect the nervous system at any level, causing encephalopathy, cerebellar dysfunction, myelopathy, and peripheral neuropathy. Some complications are the result of chemotherapy in conventional doses, while others are seen only with more intensive doses. Neurologic problems may be associated with a certain route of administration, such as intrathecal, or seen only when an agent is given in combination with another treatment modality. This chapter discusses the chemotherapeutic agents most commonly in use and the neurologic toxicity that may be seen. Less well-known agents with rarely encountered complications are noted in Table 1.

Table 1 Neurologic Complications of Chemotherapy

Encephalopathy – acute	*Encephalopathy – chronic*
Methotrexate (HD IV; IT)	Methotrexate (IV, IT, HD IV)
5-fluorouracil	5-fluorouracil & levamisole
Procarbazine	BCNU (HD IV, IA)
Hexamethylmelamine	Cytosine arabinoside
Vincristine	Fludarabine (HD)
Cytosine arabinoside	
L-asparaginase	*Cerebellar syndrome*
Ifosfamide	5-fluorouracil
Nitrosourea	Cytosine arabinoside
Tamoxifen	Procarbazine
Etoposide (HD)	Cisplatin
Spirogermanium	Spirogermanium
PALA	
	Myelopathy
Neuropathy	Methotrexate
Vinca alkaloids	Procarbazine
Cisplatin	Thiotepa
Cytosine arabinoside	Ara-C cytosine arabinoside
Taxol	
Podophyllotoxin	*Cerebral vasculopathy*
Suramin	Cisplatin (IA)
Misonidazole	L-asparaginase (IV)

HD = high dose, IA = intra-arterial, IT = intrathecal, IV = intravenous.

VINCA ALKALOIDS

The clinically important vinca alkaloids include vincristine, vinblastine, and vindesine. Because these compounds are in such frequent use, their neurotoxicity is well known. Vincristine (VCR) is the most commonly used, affecting the peripheral nervous system primarily, although it may affect the central nervous system (CNS), cranial nerves, and autonomic nervous system as well. It causes a dose- and dose frequency–related sensorimotor neuropathy in virtually all patients. Loss of ankle jerks is the earliest sign of VCR neuropathy, but with continued drug administration other reflexes are affected as well. The most common complaint of patients is tingling and paresthesias of the fingers and toes. Objective sensory loss is uncommon, but weakness, especially of the foot and wrist extensors, is to be expected. In patients receiving the drug frequently, foot drop may develop. The weakness seen with VCR is usually tolerable, but, rarely, patients may become nonambulatory or even quadriparetic. The sensory symptoms, weakness and lost reflexes are nearly always reversible, although recovery may require several months. No clinical intervention can hasten recovery. Certain clinical factors predispose to this condition. Adults are more severely affected than children, as are patients with pre-existing neuropathy (diabetic, familial, compression).

VCR occasionally causes cranial neuropathy, most commonly oculomotor nerve involvement with ptosis. Less frequently seen is ophthalmoplegia with diplopia. The recurrent laryngeal nerve may be affected with vocal cord paralysis, and, rarely, there is facial nerve involvement. Cranial nerve involvement is usually bilateral but may be unilateral.

Autonomic neuropathy is most commonly manifested by colicky abdominal pain and constipation, occurring in as many as one-third of patients. Rarely, paralytic ileus may develop. This is most often reported in children, and may be fatal. Metaclopromide may ameliorate VCR-induced ileus. All patients receiving VCR should be on a prophylactic bowel regimen of stool softeners. Other manifestations of autonomic neuropathy that occur only rarely include bladder atony, impotence, and postural hypotension.

CNS toxicity occurs only infrequently, the most common manifestation being seizures. This is usually seen in association with the syndrome of inappropriate secretion of antidiuretic hormone and low-serum sodium. Rarely, generalized seizures have been reported in patients with no other predisposing factors, approximately 5 days following a dose of VCR. Encephalopathy and delirium may occur, but so rarely that other causative factors in such patients should be sought.

METHOTREXATE

Neurotoxicity after oral, intravenous, or intrathecal injection of methotrexate (MTX) is a well-recognized complication of therapy. There are both acute and chronic forms of neurotoxicity. The type of toxicity seen depends on the dose, route of administration, and the addition of other treatment modalities, which may increase the incidence of side effects.

Acute and Subacute Toxicity

The most common form of acute MTX neurotoxicity is aseptic meningitis. This complicates intrathecal administration of the drug (more often by the lumbar than the intraventricular route) and is seen in at least 10 percent of patients. The clinical syndrome is marked by the abrupt onset of headache, stiff neck, nausea, vomiting, lethargy, and fever, usually occurring anywhere from 2 to 4 hours after MTX instillation and typically lasting for 12 to 72 hours. There is usually a CSF pleocytosis. Rarely, this may mimic bacterial meningitis, but it occurs too soon after drug instillation to be due to bacterial growth, and CSF cultures are negative. The syndrome resolves spontaneously and does not appear to have any long-term sequelae. Patients who are retreated usually do not experience difficulty with subsequent

injections. There are no known risk factors, and the pathogenesis is unknown. Some investigators advocate the instillation of hydrocortisone along with MTX in an attempt to prevent it.

Transverse myelopathy is a rare complication of intrathecal MTX that usually occurs after several treatments. It generally presents within 48 hours of injection, but the onset may be delayed for up to 2 weeks. The patient complains of pain in the back, with or without radiation into the legs. This is followed by loss of sensation, paraplegia, and bowel and bladder dysfunction. The degree of recovery, if any, is variable. The exact pathogenesis remains unknown but is thought to represent an idiosyncratic drug reaction. Pathology examination reveals necrosis of the spinal cord without striking inflammatory or vascular changes. There is no treatment, nor can one predict which patient will be affected, though the presence of active CNS leukemia or prior irradiation may be predisposing factors.

Following the administration of weekly intravenous high-dose MTX (HDMTX), a strokelike syndrome can occur in either adults or children. This disorder typically occurs following the second or third treatment by 5 or 6 days. Patients present with altered mental status (ranging from inappropriate laughter to lethargy), usually accompanied by hemiparesis and other focal findings, which may fluctuate from one side to the other. Patients generally recover spontaneously within 48 to 72 hours, usually without sequelae. They can be treated again without undue fear of recurrence, though a subsequent episode may, rarely, be observed. MTX levels are nontoxic at the time of the symptoms, and the CT scan and cerebrospinal fluid (CSF) are normal. The electroencephalogram (EEG), however, shows diffuse slowing without epileptiform discharges. The pathogenesis is unknown.

Delayed Toxicity

Diffuse leukoencephalopathy is the most devastating form of delayed MTX neurotoxicity. This disorder generally follows repeated doses of intravenous HD-MTX or intrathecal MTX but may occur after standard-dose intravenous MTX as well. This is especially true in the setting of cranial irradiation. The effects of MTX and irradiation are synergistic, leading to an increased risk of leukoencephalopathy. Altered CSF dynamics, causing prolonged MTX exposure due to delayed egress, also increase the risk of encephalopathy. This complication may appear months to years following therapy, beginning insidiously or abruptly with personality changes and learning disability. Seizures in this setting are not uncommon. The clinical picture may stabilize or progress to spasticity, hemi- or quadriparesis, dementia, and death. The CT scan reveals cerebral atrophy as well as bilateral and diffuse white matter hypodensity. Areas of focal enhancement may be seen in the early stages. These abnormalities are even more apparent on MRI and may also be seen in leukemia patients who are asymptomatic. CSF examination may demonstrate the presence of myelin basic protein. Pathology examination reveals disseminated foci of white matter degeneration characterized by demyelination, axonal swelling, and dystrophic mineralization of axonal debris. These necrotizing changes may occasionally be accompanied by fibrinoid necrosis of small blood vessels. The clinical course of the encephalopathy is variable. Patients may recover slowly over weeks or months, their symptoms may remain unchanged, or there may be a relentless progressive course ending in death.

CISPLATIN

Cisplatin is a heavy metal–containing compound, and it is therefore not surprising that peripheral neuropathy is a relatively common complication of therapy. Peripheral neuropathy is usually seen in patients receiving more than 400 mg per square meter and is characterized by bilateral symmetrical numbness and tingling of the hands and feet, which may be painful. Large sensory fibers are primarily affected, resulting in loss of vibratory and position sense, though all sensory modalities may be involved. Motor power is spared, but deep tendon reflexes are diminished or disappear altogether. Nerve conduction studies demonstrate decreased sensory nerve action potentials and prolonged sensory latencies compatible with a sensory axonopathy. Neuropathologic studies reveal a loss of large myelinated fibers with evidence of axonal degeneration. With cessation of the drug, patients may experience some improvement and occasionally a return to normal.

Cisplatin also causes vestibular and ototoxicity due to damage to the hair cells of the organ of Corti. This is initially subclinical, with only high-tone hearing loss detected by serial audiograms. Patients often complain of transient tinnitus following treatment, but with continued exposure they become deaf to a degree that is dose-dependent. The hearing impairment is usually bilateral and symmetrical. Older patients appear to be more susceptible to hearing loss, as do patients who have had cranial irradiation. Hearing loss is worsened by the administration of ototoxic antibiotics, which should be avoided in patients receiving platinum. There may be partial recovery following cessation of therapy, but this is probably modest.

Ocular toxicity has been reported with cisplatin in the form of retinopathy, papilledema, and retrobulbar neuritis, complications reported more commonly after intra-arterial infusion. Cortical blindness, encephalopathy, and vascular strokelike events are all rarely reported complications of cisplatin, again seen more often with intra-arterial administration.

CYTOSINE ARABINOSIDE

Cytosine arabinoside (Ara-C) is used systemically and intrathecally in conventional doses and intravenously in a high-dose regimen. Intravenous Ara-C does not usually produce neurotoxicity at conventional doses but at higher doses is associated with a cerebellar syndrome and encephalopathy. The clinical picture of Ara-C toxicity is dependent on the route of administration as well as patient age, drug dosage, and frequency of administration.

Intrathecal Ara-C is associated with aseptic meningitis and myelopathy. Meningeal irritation causing headache, stiff neck, and pleocytosis has been encountered in some 30 percent of patients given the drug intrathecally, but no direct relationship between this syndrome and the individual or cumulative dose has been established. The myelopathy seen with Ara-C, like the aseptic meningitis syndrome, is similar to that seen with MTX, though rarer. It presents with back pain, with or without leg pain, weakness, sensory alterations, and bowel or bladder dysfunction, occurring any time from a few days to a few weeks following treatment. CSF protein is usually elevated, with a modest pleocytosis. The pathologic picture of Ara-C myelopathy is one of demyelination with associated white matter vacuolization, histologically indistinguishable from MTX-induced myelopathy. Rarely, intrathecal administration of Ara-C is associated with seizures or an acute or subacute encephalopathy.

The administration of intravenous high-dose Ara-C (3 g per square meter every 12 hours for 8 to 12 doses) may result in encephalopathy and cerebellar dysfunction. This syndrome is dose-related, occurring more frequently with cumulative doses of at least 36 grams, although it has been reported with as little as 3 grams. Patients present with nystagmus and gait ataxia progressing over a few days to confusion, lethargy, somnolence, dysarthria, and severe ataxia. With cessation of the drug there is generally complete resolution of signs and symptoms within 2 weeks of onset. Predisposing factors are abnormal renal function, prior neurologic disorders, and age over 50. Lumbar puncture is normal, the EEG may show some slowing, and cerebellar atrophy may be seen on CT scan. Neuropathologic changes include widespread Purkinje cell loss, most pronounced in the deeper portion of the primary and secondary cerebellar sulci. Rarely, a Guillain-Barré syndrome or painful peripheral sensorimotor neuropathy is seen.

5-FLUOROURACIL

The primary neurotoxicity of 5-fluorouracil (5-FU) is a pancerebellar syndrome consisting of truncal and limb ataxia, dysmetria, nystagmus, and slurred speech. This syndrome is seen more frequently in patients receiving intensive regimens. It is reversible with cessation of the drug, usually within a week, but may recur with reintroduction of 5-FU. CT or MRI is usually normal, ruling out intracranial metastasis or meningeal infiltration as the cause of the cerebellar syndrome. Extraocular muscle abnormalities, optic neuropathy, and extrapyramidal syndromes are rarely seen. Encephalopathy with EEG changes but no cerebellar symptoms may be seen in patients given large single intravenous doses.

Doxifluridine, a new fluoropyrimidine, may cause a disorder similar to Wernicke-Korsakoff syndrome.

5-FU in combination with levamisole causes an encephalopathy with multiple demyelinating lesions in the brain. Symptoms are progressive encephalopathy and ataxia with or without focal weakness or dysarthria. MRI demonstrates multiple enhancing white matter lesions. 5-FU in combination with PALA or carmofur, rarely, produces a similar clinical picture. The neuropathologic substrate is one of demyelination.

L-ASPARAGINASE

L-asparaginase interferes with coagulation and may cause either thrombosis or hemorrhage. The onset of seizures, headache, or focal neurologic signs should alert the physician to the possibility of sagittal sinus thrombosis and venous infarction. Other cerebral sinuses may be involved as well. This typically occurs after a few weeks of therapy but may not appear until after it is completed. A definitive diagnosis is made by gradient echo sequences on MRI but may be suggested by an "empty delta sign" on CT scan. Treatment is controversial. Some investigators recommend anticoagulation, while others favor administration of fresh frozen plasma. We have found that steroids alleviate the headache, and low doses may be necessary for several days to weeks.

PROCARBAZINE

Procarbazine is currently given orally because prior experience with intravenous administration revealed unacceptable neurotoxicity. With the oral form, however, encephalopathy, from mild drowsiness to stupor, may still occur. Occasionally patients develop confusion, agitation, or even psychosis. Peripheral neuropathy occurs in 10 to 20 percent of patients with distal paresthesias, decreased deep tendon reflexes, and myalgias. This resolves spontaneously with discontinuation of the drug.

NITROSOUREAS

Of the nitrosoureas, BCNU is probably the most commonly employed. At usual dosages in conventional regimens, BCNU is not neurotoxic. This is true even in the large number of brain tumor patients with neurologic

disability who have been treated with this compound. Neurologic toxicity has been seen, however, in patients who have received very intensive intravenous dosages and in those who have received intra-arterial BCNU. This has consisted of necrotizing encephalopathy or encephalomyelopathy as well as strokes and seizures. Because of this, these regimens are no longer in clinical use.

IFOSFAMIDE

Ifosfamide is a relatively new alkylating agent, similar in many respects to cyclophosphamide. Unlike cyclophosphamide, which has negligible if any neurotoxicity, somnolence and encephalopathy occur with this compound in approximately 20 percent of patients. Disorientation, somnolence, confusion, and lethargy may occur within hours of the infusion and last for 24 to 48 hours. These symptoms generally resolve completely. Cases of severe encephalopathy have been reported in patients receiving the drug as a continuous intravenous infusion, and the incidence of severe encephalopathy ranges from 5 to 9 percent. This is accompanied by typical EEG findings of predominant delta activity, with or without sharp complex wave forms.

SUGGESTED READING

Bleyer WA. Neurological sequelae of methotrexate and ionizing radiation: A new classification. Cancer Treat Rep 1981; 65:89.

Delattre JY, Posner JB. Neurological complications of chemotherapy and radiation therapy. In: Aminoff MJ, ed. Neurology and general medicine. New York: Churchill Livingstone, 1989:365.

Feinberg WM, Swenson MR. Cerebrovascular complications of L-asparaginase therapy. Neurology 1988; 38:127–133.

Hildebrand J, ed. Neurological adverse reactions to anticancer drugs. Berlin: Springer-Verlag, 1990.

Hwang TL, Yung A, Estey EH, Fields WS. Central nervous system toxicity with high-dose Ara-C. Neurology 1985; 35:1475.

Kaplan RS, Wiernick PH. Neurotoxicity of antitumor agents. In: Perry MC, Yarbro JW, eds. Toxicity of chemotherapy. Orlando: Grune & Stratton, 1984:365.

MacDonald DR. Neurologic complications of chemotherapy. Neurol Clin 1991; 9:955–967.

Sandler SG, Tobin W, Henderson ES. Vincristine-induced neuropathy: A clinical study of fifty leukemic patients. Neurology 1969; 19: 367–374.

Weiss HD, Walker MD, Wiernick PH. Neurotoxicity of commonly used antineoplastic agents. N Engl J Med 1974; 291:75–81, 127–133.

Young DF, Posner JB. Nervous system toxicity of the chemotherapeutic agents. In: Vinken PJ, Bruyn GW, eds. Handbook of clinical neurology. Vol 39. Amsterdam: Elsevier, 1980:91.

DRUG-RELATED DISORDERS

L-TRYPTOPHAN EOSINOPHILIA MYALGIA SYNDROME

JEROME E. KURENT, M.D.
RICHARD M. SILVER, M.D.

Eosinophilia myalgia syndrome (EMS) was first described in October 1989. Three patients who had been taking L-tryptophan developed a constellation of signs and symptoms, consisting primarily of severe myalgia and peripheral eosinophilia. Since then, approximately 1,500 patients have been identified with EMS, but perhaps four times this number may have been affected. Scleroderma-like cutaneous manifestations occurred in the majority of patients, with contractures developing in those more severely affected. Neurologic manifestations were among the most severe and life-threatening features of EMS. The Centers for Disease Control criteria for the diagnosis of EMS include (1) severe incapacitating myalgia, (2) peripheral eosinophilia, and (3) exclusion of known causes of eosinophilia, such as neoplasm or parasitic infestations (Table 1).

L-tryptophan is a naturally occurring amino acid and serotonin precursor that has been in common usage in the United States since at least 1974. It has been considered a "natural" hypnotic and has been widely used for treatment of insomnia, depression, and premenstrual syndrome. It has also been used as an additive to health foods and body-building regimens.

THE CLINICAL SYNDROME

Patients with EMS typically presented with a several week history of severe myalgia. Many developed

Table 1 Diagnostic Criteria for Eosinophilia Myalgia Syndrome

Severe incapacitating myalgia
Peripheral eosinophilia
Exclusion of parasitic infestation and malignancy as causes of eosinophilia

scleroderma-like cutaneous manifestations, but unlike systemic sclerosis, the acral areas and face were generally spared. The majority of patients gave a clear history of L-tryptophan ingestion over the previous weeks to months, even up to several years. Some patients had latent periods of several weeks following cessation of L-tryptophan ingestion and development of clinical EMS. Following the identification of EMS as a specific syndrome, the Food and Drug Administration advised that L-tryptophan be removed from store shelves, essentially halting the epidemic. Although the epidemic of EMS has peaked, additional patients with EMS may still present. The differential diagnosis of L-tryptophan EMS includes scleroderma, eosinophilic fasciitis (Shulman's syndrome), parasitic infestation, and neoplasm. Table 2 lists distinguishing features of the clinical entities that may resemble EMS.

Neurologic manifestations of EMS include generalized peripheral neuropathy, mononeuritis multiplex, and a Guillain-Barré syndrome–like illness (Table 3). Proximal weakness may also occur but is often difficult to distinguish from pain-limited patient effort. Many patients experience painful muscle cramps in addition to

Table 2 Distinguishing Features of L-Tryptophan EMS, Eosinophilic Fasciitis (Shulman's Syndrome), and Scleroderma

	EMS	Eosinophilic Fasciitis	Scleroderma
Rash	+ +	±	−
Skin induration	+ +	+ +	+ + +
Acrosclerosis	−	−	+ + +
Raynaud phenomenon	−	−	+ + +
Myalgia	+ + +	+	+
Eosinophilia	+ + +	+ +	±
Pulmonary involvement	+ +	−	±
Antinuclear antibody positive	±	±	+ +
Anticentromere	−	−	±
Anti-Scl-70	−	−	±
Abnormal capillary microscopy	−	−	+ +

− = does not occur, ± = variable-uncommon, + = occurs in significant number of cases, + + = frequent but occasionally absent, + + + = frequent-characteristic finding

Modified from Bulpitt KJ, Verity MA, Clements PJ, Paulus HE. Association of L-tryptophan and an illness resembling eosinophilic fasciitis. Clinical and histopathologic findings in four patients with eosinophilia-myalgia syndrome. Arthritis Rheum 1990; 33:918–929; with permission.

Table 3 Neurologic Manifestations of Eosinophilia Myalgia Syndrome

Symptom	Cause or Pathogenetic Mechanism	Evidence
Myalgias	Inflammation of sensory nerve twigs	Chronic inflammation present on biopsy specimens
Generalized weakness, distal greater than proximal	1. Axonal peripheral neuropathy, possibly toxic	Neurotoxic products of eosinophil degranulation present on biopsy specimens Elevated quinolinic acid and kynurenine in serum and CSF
	2. Demyelinating peripheral neuropathy, possibly autoimmune	Sural nerve with perineural inflammation
	3. Possible myopathic component in some patients	Perimyositis on biopsy Elevated serum aldolase in some patients Some patients with myopathic motor unit potentials
Focal weakness	Mononeuritis multiplex	Electrophysiologic evidence of focal peripheral nerve injury
Neurocognitive impairment	Depression; encephalopathy possibly secondary to toxic or vasculitic mechanism	Some patients with reactive depression but others with organic impairment as supported by formal neuropsychiatric testing

CSF = cerebrospinal fluid

muscle aching, a symptom that persists despite resolution of other features of the disease. Peripheral neuropathy occurs in approximately 50 percent of patients. Neuropsychiatric manifestations of EMS are described, sometimes with magnetic resonance imaging (MRI) brain scan evidence of white matter lesions. Depression and encephalopathy have been seen as long-term sequelae, even after significant recovery from cutaneous and neuromuscular manifestations. The neuropsychiatric syndromes are incompletely characterized and the underlying pathogenesis is poorly understood. It has been suggested that a toxic or vasculitic mechanism may be involved.

LABORATORY EVALUATION

In patients with myalgia, the history of the present illness should include inquiries about possible L-tryptophan ingestion, average daily dosage, and duration of intake. The risk of developing EMS, and perhaps the severity of symptoms, correlate with the average daily dosage of L-tryptophan. However, some patients developed EMS even after minimal exposure. Specific host susceptibility factors remain to be identified.

Table 4 lists laboratory tests useful in evaluating patients with suspected EMS. Although the majority of EMS patients have peripheral eosinophilia, some patients do not. The median eosinophil count is 5×10^9 per liter. Serum creatine kinase levels are normal in EMS, but some patients had elevated serum aldolase during the active phase of the disease. The erythrocyte sedimentation rate is usually normal, but occasionally the antinuclear antibody is mildly positive. Rheumatoid factor, serum complement, and serum protein electrophoresis are normal in EMS.

A striking feature of EMS is the prompt and sustained reduction of the peripheral eosinophilia asso-

Table 4 Laboratory Testing in Eosinophilia Myalgia Syndrome

Test	Findings
CBC	Increased eosinophil count, which normalizes after prednisone therapy
ESR	Normal
Serum creatine kinase	Normal
Serum aldolase	Mild elevation in some patients
ANA	Positive in occasional patients
Rheumatoid factor, serum complement, serum protein electrophoresis	Normal
EMG, nerve conduction testing	Axonal or demyelinating peripheral neuropathy in symptomatic weak patients Denervation as shown by fibrillations and sharp waves in patients with weakness, atrophy, and axonal peripheral neuropathy Myopathic motor unit potentials present in proximal muscle groups in occasional patients

CBC = complete blood count, ESR = erythrocyte sedimentation rate, ANA = antinuclear antibody, EMG = electromyogram.

ciated with corticosteroid therapy. The eosinophil count normalizes after 1 to 2 days of prednisone therapy and usually remains normal even after steroids are discontinued. No uniform dosage schedule for corticosteroids has been developed for patients with EMS, and no controlled therapeutic trials have been conducted to assess the relative value of various immunosuppressive medical therapies, including plasmapheresis.

Skin biopsies demonstrate histopathologic features of fasciitis. There is increased collagen and chronic inflammation of a mild to moderate intensity, with lymphocytes and plasma cells predominating. Eosinophils are sparse, if present at all, in skin biopsies, even before corticosteroid therapy. The dermatopathologic changes, while characteristic of EMS, are not specific. Patients with scleroderma, eosinophilic fasciitis, toxic oil syndrome, and EMS share similar pathology. The pathologic changes may reflect a spectrum of abnormality with similar pathogenetic mechanisms causing inflammation and fibrosis characteristic of all these conditions.

Electromyography of EMS patients has demonstrated a variety of abnormalities. Peripheral neuropathy has been reported to be present in up to 65 percent of EMS patients, but its true prevalence is unknown. It usually reflects axonal damage, but patients with demyelinating neuropathy have also been described. EMG needle examination may show evidence of active denervation manifested by fibrillations and sharp waves. These are usually most prominent in severely affected patients with weakness and atrophy. Loss of motor units as shown by reduced recruitment during maximal effort is also present in more severely affected patients.

Muscle biopsies in patients with EMS demonstrate characteristic changes. Perimyositis with lymphocytes and occasional plasma cells is present. The inflammation is of mild to moderate intensity. Eosinophils are usually not present in muscle biopsies even in untreated patients but may be seen on rare occasions. Intramysial inflammation is conspicuously absent, with most inflammation being perimysial. Sural nerve biopsies demonstrate perineural round cell infiltrates, with only rare intraneural infiltrates. Eosinophils are only rarely present.

The pathogenesis of L-tryptophan EMS is speculative. Although peripheral eosinophilia is a hallmark of this condition, its specific role in causing myalgia, peripheral neuropathy, and other systemic manifestations is poorly understood. Eosinophilic cationic protein and neurotoxic products have been identified in biopsied tissues of EMS patients. This suggests an important, albeit undefined, role for the eosinophil in causing neurotoxicity. Products of L-tryptophan metabolism, such as quinolinic acid, have also been postulated to play a role in EMS pathogenesis. It has been suggested that the severe myalgia in EMS is due to cellular infiltration proximate to sensory nerve twigs.

DISCUSSION

Why was EMS first described in 1989, many years after L-tryptophan was in widespread use? It seems likely that the disease existed before 1989 but occurred only sporadically. In fact, a substantial percentage of patients diagnosed in the 1980s as having eosinophilic faciitis, in retrospect appeared to have a history of L-tryptophan ingestion. The association of L-tryptophan ingestion and EMS was made only after the disease assumed epidemic proportions. Large numbers of EMS patients were recognized in conjunction with changes made by one manufacturer in the production of L-tryptophan, and most cases of EMS have been traced to consumption of L-tryptophan manufactured by a single company. A number of trace contaminants have been found in implicated batches of L-tryptophan and linked epidemiologically to the epidemic. The first contaminant to be identified was 1,1-ethylidenebis (tryptophan) (EBT). Animal studies suggest that EBT may induce a syndrome resembling EMS. Phenyl-amino (alanine) (PAA) has recently also been found in implicated lots of L-tryptophan. It may also play a causative role. It may be significant that PAA resembles one of the putative contaminants of rapeseed oil associated with the toxic oil syndrome (TOS), which was described in 1981. This epidemic occurred in Spain and affected nearly 20,000 individuals. It bears a striking resemblance to EMS. The precise cause and pathogenesis of both EMS and TOS, which may share similar mechanisms, remain to be determined.

Establishing a diagnosis of EMS is relatively straightforward. A history of L-tryptophan ingestion in a patient with severe myalgia, peripheral eosinophilia, and scleroderma-like cutaneous changes is strong presumptive evidence for EMS. Rare patients have no known exposure to L-tryptophan. It is particularly important to rule out malignant disease and parasitic infestation in such patients. Clinical features and serologic testing should help distinguish EMS from scleroderma. Eosinophilic fasciitis is very similar to EMS, but the former generally spares the nervous system, except for carpal tunnel syndrome. On full-thickness skin biopsy, EMS is more pancutaneous, whereas eosinophilic fasciitis is usually confined to the subcutis. In obvious cases of EMS, biopsies of skin, muscle, and nerve are no longer considered necessary to confirm the diagnosis. However, they may be helpful in less certain circumstances.

SUGGESTED READING

Belongia EA, Hedberg SW, Gleich GJ, et al. An investigation of the cause of the eosinophilia-myalgia syndrome associated with tryptophan use. N Engl J Med 1990; 323:357–365.

Bulpitt KJ, Verity MA, Clements PJ, Paulus HE. Association of L-tryptophan and an illness resembling eosinophilic fasciitis: Clinical and histopathologic findings in four patients with eosinophilia-myalgia syndrome. Arthritis Rheum 1990; 33:918–929.

Culpepper RC, Williams RG, Mease PJ, et al. Natural history of the eosinophiolia-myalgia syndrome. Ann Intern Med 1991; 115:422–437.

Feldman SR, Silver RM, Maize JC. A histophathologic comparison of Shulman's syndrome (diffuse fasciitis with eosinophilia) and the fasciitis associated with the eosinophilia-myalgia syndrome. J Am Acad Dermatol 1992; 26:95–100.

Heiman-Patterson TD, Bird SJ, Parry GJ, et al. Peripheral neuropathy associated with eosinophilia-myalgia syndrome. Ann Neurol 1990; 28:522–528.

Kilbourne EM, Posada de la Paz M, Borda IA, et al. Toxic oil syndrome: A current clinical and epidemiologic summary, including comparisons with eosinophilia-myalgia syndrome. J Am Coll Cardiol 1991; 18:711–717.

Silver RM, Heyes MP, Maize JC, et al. Scleroderma, fasciitis, and eosinophilia associated with the ingestion of L-tryptophan. N Engl J Med 1990; 322:874–881.

Smith BE, Dyck PJ. Peripheral neuropathy in the eosinophilia-myalgia syndrome associated with L-tryptophan ingestion. Neurology 1990; 40:1035–1040.

Talpos D, Carstens S, Silverman J, Gladson C. Perimyositis with perineuritis and myofiber type grouping in the eosiniphilia myalgia syndrome associated with tryptophan ingestion. Am J Surg Pathol 1991; 15:222–226.

Tolander LM, Bamford CR, Yoshino MT, et al. Neurologic complications of the tryptophan-associated eosinophilia-myalgia syndrome. Arch Neurol 1991; 48:436–438.

COCAINE TOXICITY

JOHN C.M. BRUST, M.D.

Like amphetamine and related psychostimulants, cocaine is a sympathomimetic agent, and many of its central nervous system (CNS) effects are the result of indirect agonism at dopamine and norepinephrine receptors. Unlike amphetamine, cocaine is also a local anesthetic, and its procaine-like actions probably contribute to toxicity.

The current American cocaine epidemic involves two major forms of the drug. Cocaine hydrochloride is most often "snorted" intranasally; such use tends to be recreational and sporadic. It is also taken parenterally, usually intravenously; such use is more often compulsive and repetitive. Cocaine hydrochloride cannot be smoked. By contrast, alkaloidal cocaine—one form of which is "crack"—is nearly always smoked, and such use also tends to be compulsive and repetitive, sometimes in binges lasting hours or days. The increased mortality and morbidity that accompanied the spread of crack in the 1980s was the combined result of more users and higher doses.

Serious toxicity has also followed sublingual, rectal, vaginal, and intraurethral cocaine, as well as the swallowing of cocaine-filled packets for smuggling ("body-packing") or concealment. Small children have accidentally ingested cocaine, been deliberately poisoned, or become toxic from passive exposure to crack smoke or cocaine in breast milk. Cocaine intoxication also affects newborns of mothers who use cocaine shortly before delivery.

Injected or smoked cocaine produces a brief "rush," peaking at ½ to 2 minutes and followed by euphoria, excitement, garrulousness, and a sense of increased mental and physical powers. Such effects last about 20 to 40 minutes. Snorted cocaine produces similar effects, without a comparable rush, that last up to 90 minutes. Low doses slow the heart rate. Higher doses cause tachycardia, tachypnea, and hypertension. Skin pallor is secondary to vasoconstriction. Other symptoms include chest pain, palpitations, dyspnea, sweating, anxiety, dizziness, syncope, and headache (Table 1). Although cocaine causes coronary artery vasoconstriction, chest pain is most often noncardiac in origin. Syncope, which occurs frequently, is similarly of uncertain cause but should raise the possibility of cardiac arrhythmia.

Table 1 Symptoms of Acute Cocaine Toxicity

Psychiatric
  Anxiety, insomnia, agitation
  Paranoia, violence
  Psychosis, hallucinations
  Depression

Neurologic
  Dizziness, syncope
  Headache
  Tremor
  Stereotypic movements
  Bruxism, chorea, dystonia
  Myoclonus
  Seizures
  Coma
  Occlusive or hemorrhagic stroke

Cardiopulmonary
  Dyspnea, pulmonary edema
  Angina pectoris, myocardial infarction
  Palpitations, cardiac arrhythmia

Other
  Sweating
  Throat tightness
  Blurred vision (mydriasis)
  Nasal congestion
  Nausea, vomiting, abdominal pain
  Fever, chills
  Myalgia, back pain, noncardiac chest pain
  Rhabdomyolysis, myoglobinuria

Headaches may be secondary to surges of blood pressure but sometimes have a migraine-like pattern, including focal neurologic symptoms, and are sometimes relieved by additional cocaine.

With repeated cocaine use, neurologic symptoms become increasingly prominent, a phenomenon referred to as "sensitization" or "reverse tolerance" and considered analogous to electrical kindling. Irritability, hyperactivity, and disturbed eating and sleeping progress to anxiety and paranoia and then agitation (leading to violence), depression (leading to suicide), or psychosis (with visual, auditory, or tactile hallucinations), which occur regardless of predrug personality. Abnormal movements also emerge, beginning with tremor and stereotypy and progressing to bruxism, chorea, or dystonia. Seizures too are more common in chronic users, occurring either immediately or within a few hours of use, with or without other signs of toxicity. A single major motor seizure is usual, but some seizures are focal, and status epilepticus tends to be refractory to conventional treatment.

Acute cocaine overdose can be life-threatening, with psychosis or delirium progressing to stupor or coma, plus fever, hypertension, hyperreflexia, dyskinesias, muscular rigidity, myoclonus, or seizures. Fever can be severe, with muscular rigidity and myoglobinuria resembling heat stroke or the neuroleptic malignant syndrome. Marked hypertension also represents a medical emergency. Cardiac arrhythmia and pulmonary edema, in some instances possibly neurogenic, presage cardiac arrest. Disseminated intravascular coagulation occurs. The most striking laboratory abnormality is metabolic acidosis, which can be severe and require considerable amounts of bicarbonate therapy.

Cocaine snorters usually take 20 to 50 mg of cocaine hydrochloride at a time. Crack smokers, by contrast, sometimes smoke hundreds of milligrams over a few hours. In contrast to psychosis, dyskinesias, and seizures, there is tolerance for cardiac and other systemic effects, so the lethal dose varies widely among users. Among novices it is usually about 500 to 800 mg, but as much as 14 g of alkaloidal cocaine has been smoked daily without serious complication, and as little as 20 mg of cocaine hydrochloride intravenously has proven fatal. Sudden death may be from ventricular fibrillation or anaphylaxis related to impurities in the mixture.

Myoglobinuria sufficient to cause renal failure can occur without additional signs of toxicity. Other acute effects include angina pectoris and myocardial infarction, which are responsible for the acute chest pain of cocaine intoxication in about one-third of patients. Such subjects are often young and lack other evidence of coronary artery disease. Tobacco smoking provides additional risk. Cocaine has also been associated with aortic dissection and rupture; bowel, renal, and splenic infarction; limb gangrene; and ischemic and hemorrhagic stroke, which can accompany acute intoxication or occur hours or days after cocaine use. The basis of ischemic stroke is uncertain. In most instances cerebral vasospasm seems more likely than vasculitis. (The opposite appears to be the case with amphetamine.) Proposed mechanisms of hemorrhagic stroke include surges of high blood pressure and bleeding into infarcted brain as cerebral vasospasm clears. The management of cocaine-related strokes is no different than that of other strokes, but it is worth noting that of over 100 reported patients with cocaine-related hemorrhagic stroke who have received angiography or autopsy, more than half have had underlying saccular aneurysms or vascular malformations. Lumbar puncture, generally unrevealing in cocaine intoxication, becomes necessary when headache or other neurologic symptoms suggest subarachnoid hemorrhage and when head computed tomography (CT) is nondiagnostic. A spinal tap is also, of course, indicated when meningitis — another possible cause of delirium and fever — is a serious diagnostic consideration. Magnetic resonance imaging, magnetic resonance angiography, or radiographic cerebral angiography are performed in selected patients suspected of harboring vascular malformations or saccular aneurysms.

The major features of cocaine abstinence are hunger, fatigue, and dysphoria. Objective systemic or neurologic signs are difficult to identify, but depression may be severe enough to require hospitalization.

Cocaine is frequently taken with other drugs, confusing the clinical picture and complicating treatment. Cocaine and heroin are co-injected ("speedball"), crack and heroin are smoked together, and many patients receiving methadone maintenance therapy use cocaine. Compulsive cocaine users often take sedatives to induce sleep, and alcohol reportedly enhances cocaine toxicity. Abused drugs associated with delirium or psychosis, either from toxicity or withdrawal, include amphetamines, anticholinergics, ethanol, barbiturates and other sedatives, hallucinogens, phencyclidine, and marijuana. Clinicians should remember that a patient may be displaying additive or synergistic signs of drug toxicity or withdrawal or be simultaneously toxic from one agent while withdrawing from another.

Cocaine's plasma half-life is about 40 to 60 minutes. It is detectable in urine for up to 36 hours. Metabolites include benzoylecgonine, which is the substance identified in most toxicology screens. In novices, benzoylecgonine is usually present in plasma for a few days. In heavy users it can be detected for up to 3 weeks. Benzoylecgonine persists even longer in hair, but testing is costly and unavailable at most centers.

Diverse medical illnesses affect cocaine users, further complicating management. Parenteral users develop infection, including osteomyelitis, hepatitis, tetanus, and acquired immunodeficiency syndrome. Crack users are also at risk for human immunodeficiency virus infection. Sex is often traded for drugs, and other sexually transmitted diseases provide portals of viral entry. Nasal botulism has affected snorters. Cocaine is associated with contraction band myocardiopathy, further predisposing to arrhythmia, congestive heart failure, and embolism. Crack smokers develop tracheobronchitis, pneumomediastinum, bronchiolitis obliterans, and alveolar hemorrhage.

Anecdotal reports, including studies with CT, positron emission tomography, and single photon emission computerized tomography, suggest that chronic cocaine use causes cerebral atrophy, patchy decreases in cerebral blood flow, and cognitive impairment. Similarly anecdotal — and controversial — are reports implicating *in utero* cocaine exposure in developmental delay, congenital anomalies, and later cognitive or behavioral disturbance.

SUGGESTED READING

Brody SL, Slovis CM, Wrenn KD. Cocaine-related medical problems: Consecutive series of 233 patients. Am J Med 1990; 88:325–331.

Brust JCM. Neurological aspects of substance abuse. Stoneham, Mass: Butterworths, 1993.

Gawin FH. Cocaine addiction: Psychology and neurophysiology. Science 1991; 251:1580–1586.

Goldfrank LR, Hoffman RS. The cardiovascular effects of cocaine. Ann Emerg Med 1991; 20:165–175.

Levine SR, Brust JCM, Futrell N, et al. Cerebrovascular complications of the use of the "crack" form of alkaloidal cocaine. N Engl J Med 1990; 323:699–704.

Lowenstein DH, Massa SM, Rowbotham MC, et al. Acute neurologic and psychiatric complications associated with cocaine abuse. Am J Med 1987; 83:841–846.

Lutiger B, Graham K, Einarson TR, Koren G. Relationship between gestational cocaine use and pregnancy outcome: A meta-analysis. Teratology 1991; 44:405–414.

Pascual-Leone A, Dhuna A, Altafullah I, Anderson DC. Cocaine-induced seizures. Neurology 1990; 40:404–407.

Satel SL, Southwick SM, Gawin FH. Clinical features of cocaine-induced paranoia. Am J Psychiatry 1991; 148:495–498.

Weinrieb RM, O'Brien CP. Persistent cognitive deficits attributed to substance abuse. In: Brust JCM, ed. Neurologic complications of drug and alcohol abuse. Neurol Clin 1993 (in press).

DEMYELINATING DISEASES

LEUKO-ARAIOSIS

R. MICHAEL POOLE, M.D.
MARC I. CHIMOWITZ, M.B., Ch.B.

DEFINITION AND CLASSIFICATION

Leuko-araiosis is a term used to describe subcortical white matter lesions that are seen most clearly on magnetic resonance imaging (MRI) of the brain (Fig. 1). Leuko-araiosis derives from the Greek roots *leuko-,* meaning "white," and *araios-,* meaning "rarefied, with its units far apart."

Four morphologic types of subcortical lesions on T2 weighted MRI have been described: (1) rim, a thin line of hyperintensity surrounding the lateral ventricles; (2) caps, hyperintense signals around the poles of the lateral ventricles; (3) punctate lesions, dotlike hyperintense signals in the white matter or basal ganglia; and (4) patches, nonpunctate areas of hyperintensity in the white matter that may be discrete or confluent.

In this chapter we focus on the clinical approach to patients with leuko-araiosis and discuss briefly the epidemiology and pathology of these radiologic lesions.

CLINICAL APPROACH

Rims, small caps, and punctate lesions are found so commonly in normal subjects that many authors do not consider them to be pathologic. On the other hand, large caps and patches may be seen in several neurologic diseases. The radiologic features of large caps and patches have low diagnostic specificity; hence the diagnostic approach to patients with these lesions depends almost entirely on the associated clinical findings.

We classify patients with leuko-araiosis into four groups depending on the associated clinical findings: Group 1 consists of patients who are found to have leuko-araiosis incidentally as part of an evaluation for unrelated symptoms such as chronic headache or dizziness; Group 2 consists of patients with symptomatic ischemic cerebrovascular disease and leuko-araiosis; Group 3 consists of patients with dementia and leuko-araiosis; Group 4 comprises patients with multifocal signs and leuko-araiosis.

The pathologic correlates of leuko-araiosis depend on this clinical classification. A patch in a neurologically intact patient is usually associated with myelin pallor and dilated perivascular spaces. A patch in a patient with long-standing multiple sclerosis is associated with acellular fibroglial tissue, rare perivascular lymphocytes, and loss of axons. In a patient with pure motor hemiparesis, a well-circumscribed patch in the internal capsule is associated with infarction.

Patients with Leuko-Araiosis as an Incidental Finding

Rims, caps, and punctate lesions are seen in up to 92 percent of patients older than 60 years and in 22 percent of patients under the age of 40. Patches are seen less frequently, but not uncommonly, in neurologically intact patients.

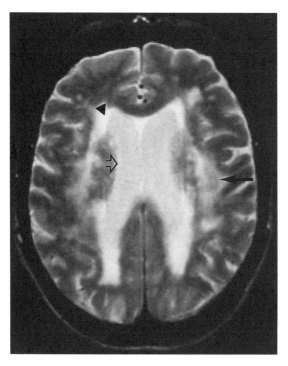

Figure 1 T2-weighted MRI scan of a 73-year-old woman seen for transient ischemic attacks showing caps (*arrowhead*), rims (*open arrow*), and patches. Some of the patches in the centrum semiovale are confluent (*arrow*).

Postmortem studies in neurologically intact patients show that each of these radiologic abnormalities has a distinct histologic correlate. Rims are characterized by subependymal gliosis. Caps are associated with myelin pallor, gliosis, and arteriosclerosis. Punctate lesions are characterized by dilated perivascular space. Patches are associated with myelin pallor and dilated perivascular spaces.

The cause of these lesions in neurologically intact patients is uncertain. Our opinion is that rims, small caps, and punctate lesions usually do not have a pathologic basis. Normal aging is probably the underlying cause.

Some authors believe that patches are also caused by normal aging. However, these lesions have consistently been associated with vascular risk factors, especially hypertension. We believe that asymptomatic subcortical ischemia is a common cause of patches in neurologically intact elderly patients. Therefore, in these patients we look carefully for evidence of hypertension and diabetes and inquire about other vascular risk factors. Apart from simple measurements of blood pressure, serum cholesterol, and glucose, we do not subject these patients to additional tests.

In neurologically intact younger patients with patches on MRI, we also rule out vascular risk factors and follow these patients closely for the development of focal neurologic deficits. Young patients with migraine headaches frequently have small subcortical patches on MRI that may resolve over time. We treat these patients with migraine prophylactic agents, including aspirin.

Patients with Ischemic Cerebrovascular Disease and Leuko-Araiosis

In our practice, we commonly see leuko-araiosis in patients with a history of transient ischemic attack (TIA) or stroke. Our approach to these patients is identical to our approach to patients with symptomatic ischemic cerebrovascular disease who do not have leuko-araiosis. We direct the investigation toward defining the underlying pathophysiology of the TIA or stroke.

We do not routinely order carotid ultrasound studies, echocardiography, or cerebral angiography in patients with leuko-araiosis and cerebrovascular symptoms unless these tests are clearly indicated by the clinical history and examination. For example, we would not order these studies in a patient with a typical lacunar syndrome whose MRI showed leuko-araiosis without cortical infarction. On the other hand, we would perform carotid ultrasound on a patient with the same MRI findings whose complaint was stereotypical episodes of hand weakness.

We manage all of these patients by identifying and aggressively treating vascular risk factors. In addition, we initiate appropriate secondary stroke preventive therapy. Depending on the underlying cause of cerebral ischemia, this might include carotid endarterectomy, antiplatelet agents (aspirin or ticlopidine), or anticoagulation with warfarin.

We also maintain a high index of suspicion for underlying coronary artery disease in patients with ischemic cerebrovascular disease (with or without leuko-araiosis). We sometimes suggest cardiac stress testing for these patients even if they have no symptoms of coronary artery disease. In patients with ischemic cerebrovascular disease and leuko-araiosis who are undergoing coronary artery bypass surgery, we suggest maintaining a mean arterial blood pressure of at least 60 mm Hg while on cardiopulmonary bypass, because the lower limit of mean arterial pressure at which autoregulation fails to protect cerebral blood flow may be higher in these patients.

Patients with Dementia and Leuko-Araiosis

In patients with a dementing illness, leuko-araiosis suggests a broad differential diagnosis. In the elderly, Alzheimer's disease (with or without amyloid angiopathy), ischemic vascular dementia, Binswanger's disease, and normal pressure hydrocephalus should be considered.

The clinical features are most useful for making the diagnosis. For example, ischemic vascular dementia typically presents with stepwise deterioration in cognitive function in a patient with a history of one or more strokes. Imaging may show multiple areas of cortical and subcortical infarction. Normal pressure hydrocephalus is readily suggested by the triad of ataxia, incontinence, and dementia. In this disease, transependymal migration of cerebrospinal fluid (CSF) can sometimes be seen as a smooth and diffuse periventricular high-signal abnormality.

Binswanger's disease, or subcortical arteriosclerotic encephalopathy, is characterized by slowly progressive cognitive abnormalities, with gradual deterioration in gait and progressive appearance of focal neurologic signs, usually in patients with hypertension. MRI images show confluent high-signal abnormalities that are extensive and symmetric across both hemispheres. Subcortical U-fibers are often spared. Alzheimer's disease is usually diagnosed when a patient has no other identifiable cause for progressive memory loss, visuospatial abnormalities, language disturbance, and apraxia. MRI findings may include cortical atrophy and leuko-araiosis. In this setting, leuko-araiosis may be caused by amyloid angiopathy or may reflect white matter changes secondary to cortical neuronal loss.

The most common causes of leuko-araiosis and dementia in young adult patients are multiple sclerosis, human immunodeficiency virus (HIV) dementia, progressive multifocal leukoencephalopathy, and toluene abuse. Multiple sclerosis is characterized by episodes of visual loss, paralysis, sensory disturbance, ataxia, incontinence, and cognitive abnormalities. CSF examination and MRI of the brain and spinal cord are useful confirmatory tests. Typical abnormalities in the CSF include oligoclonal bands, elevated IgG index, and elevated myelin basic protein. MRI images vary widely but typically show multiple high-signal lesions on T2-

weighted imaging adjacent and oriented perpendicularly to the lateral ventricles. There is often significant atrophy of the corpus callosum. Coexistent lesions in the brain stem, cerebellum, and spinal cord help to distinguish multiple sclerosis from other rare demyelinating diseases and vascular disorders.

Dementia and leuko-araiosis in a patient with a history of intravenous drug abuse or homosexuality should suggest the diagnosis of HIV dementia. Progressive multifocal leukoencephalopathy should also be considered in this setting and in patients who are immunocompromised for other reasons. Patients with progressive multifocal leukoencephalopathy often present with visual agnosia as the major clinical feature, with confluent high-signal lesions in the occipital lobes on T2 weighted images (Fig. 2).

Toluene abuse typically occurs in teenagers or very young adults and is suggested by a history of sniffing vapors from spray paint or paint thinners, progressive encephalopathy, and white matter abnormalities on neuroimaging.

Adrenoleukodystrophy and metachromatic leukodystrophy can also be associated with dementia and leuko-araiosis. These diseases are more common in children but can present rarely in adults. Adrenoleukodystrophy is an X-linked recessive disorder that typically manifests in young males. The usual presentation is visual agnosia, dementia, or myelopathy. MRI typically shows white matter lesions in the parieto-occipital regions that enhance with gadolinium contrast, suggesting breakdown of the blood-brain barrier. The diagnosis is confirmed by finding elevated very long-chain fatty acid levels in the serum. Metachromatic leukodystrophy, an autosomal recessive disorder, usually presents with peripheral neuropathy, upper motor neuron signs, and dementia. The white matter changes are more diffuse than in adrenoleukodystrophy, and there usually is no enhancement of the lesions with gadolinium. The diagnosis is established by finding slowed nerve conduction velocities and decreased arylsulfatase-A levels in the serum.

Patients with Multifocal Neurologic Signs and Leuko-Araiosis

Multiple sclerosis, systemic lupus erythematosus, Sjögren's syndrome, adrenoleukodystrophy, metachromatic leukodystrophy, and infections are the most common diagnoses in this group. Although the findings on MRI may help with the differential diagnosis, the clinical information is most important.

Systemic lupus erythematosus typically occurs in young women, with a broad range of symptoms and signs that include joint pains, malar rash, alopecia, and polyserositis. Neuropsychiatric manifestations include hallucinations, psychotic and affective disturbances (most common), delirium, seizures, or focal neurologic signs. MRI scans show lesions in cortical and subcortical regions and are much more likely to occur in patients with seizures or focal abnormalities on neurologic

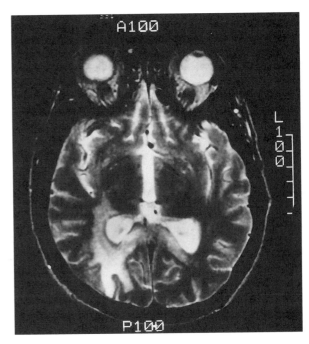

Figure 2 T2 weighted MRI scan of a 50-year-old man with biopsy-proven progressive multifocal leukoencephalopathy (PML). There is characteristic involvement of the deep occipital white matter, most pronounced on the left, which outlines the cortical margins. This case shows involvement of the corpus callosum and extension of signal changes out to the cortical surface, both of which are somewhat unusual in PML.

examination. The presence of serum antibodies directed at nuclear antigens helps to make the diagnosis. Sjögren's syndrome is characterized by failure of multiple exocrine organs (lacrimal, salivary, biliary, and pancreatic) and by the presence of anti-Ro (SS-A) and anti-La (SS-B) antibodies. The diagnosis is confirmed by finding lymphocytic infiltrates on a minor salivary gland biopsy. Central nervous system Sjögren's lesions are indistinguishable from those of multiple sclerosis on MRI images.

Other causes of leuko-araiosis and multifocal neurologic signs include the osmotic demyelination syndrome that occurs in children with diabetic ketoacidosis; central pontine myelinolysis as a consequence of overrapid correction of hyponatremia; radiation therapy for cerebral metastatic disease; and carbon monoxide poisoning. In each of these conditions the correct diagnosis is made by an awareness of the patient's history and current medical problems. Both the osmotic demyelination syndrome and central pontine myelinolysis are acute neurologic catastrophes. The osmotic demyelination syndrome is characterized by the sudden development of coma during rehydration therapy for ketoacidosis. White matter changes typically are diffuse, and there is evidence of increased intracranial pressure. Central pontine myelinolysis presents with quadriparesis and a locked-in state occurring during or soon after treatment for hyponatremia. As the name implies, central pontine myelinolysis affects white matter tracts in the pons primarily, but can also involve white matter in the cerebral hemispheres.

The clinical picture of radiation-induced white matter disease varies and includes subacute development of encephalopathy, cognitive disturbances, or long-tract signs that cannot be attributed to the underlying neoplastic process. Radiation-induced changes on MRI are usually diffuse and confluent and appear from months to years after radiation therapy.

The presentation of carbon monoxide poisoning depends on the duration and intensity of exposure. Coma and seizures occur in patients with sudden, rapid increases in carbon monoxide concentration. Headaches, ataxia, impaired vision, and dizziness occur in those with more protracted poisoning. Carbon monoxide poisoning is diagnosed by finding elevated carboxyhemoglobin levels in an arterial blood sample. These patients may have profound white matter abnormalities on MRI depending on the duration and intensity of exposure.

Leuko-araiosis is seen along with multifocal neurologic signs in several infectious diseases such as cytomegalovirus ventriculitis (with or without concomitant HIV infection), toxoplasmosis, or postinfectious demyelinating diseases such as acute disseminated encephalomyelitis. Cytomegalovirus ventriculitis is diagnosed by an abnormal spinal fluid profile and serologic evidence of recent infection, or direct culture of the virus from the buffy coat. Toxoplasmosis occurs in immunocompromised patients and is diagnosed both by serologic tests and by contrast-enhancing mass lesions that regress with appropriate therapy with pyrimethamine and sulfadiazine. Toxoplasmosis is the most common central nervous system infection in the acquired immunodeficiency syndrome. Acute disseminated encephalomyelitis, as the name implies, can affect many levels of the nervous system and present with multiple symptoms and signs. This diagnosis should be suspected when leuko-araiosis occurs in a patient with stupor, convulsions, hemiplegia, or spinal cord involvement and a history of recent upper respiratory infection, vaccination, or viral exanthem.

Isolated central nervous system vasculitis is often suggested as a cause of leuko-araiosis in patients with multifocal neurologic deficits. Our experience is that this diagnosis is usually incorrect. Cerebral vasculitis is rare and usually presents with headache, encephalopathy, and seizures. Focal neurologic deficits are less common. We rely on brain biopsy to make the diagnosis before instituting therapy with corticosteroids and cytotoxic drugs, since these agents can have serious side effects. We strongly disagree with the use of these agents solely on the basis of MRI or angiographic findings unless there are clear contraindications to performing a brain biopsy.

SUGGESTED READING

Awad IA, Johnson PC, Spetzler RF, et al. Incidental subcortical lesions identified on magnetic resonance imaging in the elderly, II: Postmortem pathological correlation. Stroke 1986; 17:1090–1097.
Chimowitz MI, Awad IA, Furlan AJ. Periventricular lesions on MRI: Facts and theories. Stroke 1989; 20:963–967.
Chimowitz MI, Estes ML, Furlan AJ, Awad IA. Further observations on the pathology of subcortical lesions identified on magnetic resonance imaging. Arch Neurol 1992; 49:747–752.
Fazekas F, Chawluk JB, Alavi A, et al. MR signal abnormalities at 1.5 T in Alzheimer's disease and normal aging. AJNR Am J Neuroradiol 1987; 8:421–426.
Filley CM, Heaton RK, Rosenburg NL. White matter dementia in chronic toluene abuse. Neurology 1990; 40:532–534.
Hachinski VC, Potter P, Merskey H. Leuko-araiosis. Arch Neurol 1987; 44:21–23.
Inzitari D, Diaz F, Fox A, et al. Vascular risk factors and leuko-araiosis. Arch Neurol 1987; 44:42–47.
Roman GC. Senile dementia of the Binswanger type: A vascular form of dementia in the elderly. JAMA 1987; 258:1782–1788.
Soges LJ, Cacayorin ED, Petro GR, Ramachandran TS. Migraine: Evaluation by MR. AJNR Am J Neuroradiol 1988; 9:425–429.
Sze G, DeArmond SJ, Brant-Zawadzki M, et al. Foci of MRI signal (pseudo lesions) anterior to the frontal horns: Histologic correlations of a normal finding. AJNR Am J Neuroradiol 1986; 7:381–387.

OPTIC NEURITIS

NEIL R. MILLER, M.D.

The term *optic neuritis* describes a set of clinical signs and symptoms that are assumed to be produced by inflammation of the optic nerve.

CLINICAL MANIFESTATIONS

Optic neuritis usually occurs in patients between 15 and 45 years of age, with women being affected about four times as often as men. Most patients present with blurred vision in one eye, preceded or accompanied by pain. The pain may be sharp or dull and is often exacerbated by movement of the affected eye. Visual acuity in an eye with optic neuritis varies considerably, from a minimal decrease in central vision to no perception of light in about 4 percent of patients. Color vision is almost always impaired, even when central vision is normal or nearly so. Almost all patients with optic neuritis have a defect in the central visual field of the affected eye, which occasionally may extend into the peripheral visual field. True central scotomas are rare, however, with many patients having arcuate, altitudinal, and even hemianopic defects in the central field. Patients with unilateral optic neuritis always have a relative afferent pupillary defect (Marcus Gunn pupil) on the affected side, as do many patients with asymmetric bilateral optic neuritis. However, some patients with bilateral optic neuritis may have no evidence of a relative afferent pupillary defect despite clinically asymmetric disease, indicating that pathologic damage to both optic nerves is more symmetric than the clinical picture would suggest.

The optic disc in an eye with optic neuritis may appear swollen, normal, or pale. If the disc is swollen, the optic neuritis is called *papillitis* or *anterior optic neuritis,* and it is assumed that the inflammation is occurring within the intraocular portion of the optic nerve. If the disc is normal in appearance, the disorder is called *retrobulbar optic neuritis* or simply *retrobulbar neuritis.* Retrobulbar neuritis occurs about twice as often as papillitis. However, whether the optic disc appears swollen or normal has no visual or systemic prognostic significance in a patient with optic neuritis. Optic atrophy in a patient with acute optic neuritis indicates previous damage to the optic nerve, since it takes at least 4 to 6 weeks to develop optic pallor after an acute optic neuropathy.

NATURAL HISTORY

The characteristic course for optic neuritis is one of maximum visual loss over about 2 weeks, followed by some degree of recovery over the subsequent 2 to 12 months. Recovery may be complete in some patients, but most patients complain that visual function is not as good as it was before the attack. Even patients without any visual symptoms after an attack of optic neuritis often have some degree of optic nerve dysfunction that can be demonstrated by clinical, electrophysiologic, or psychophysical testing.

DIAGNOSIS

Most patients who experience an attack of isolated optic neuritis will eventually develop multiple sclerosis, and it is thus believed that the majority of cases of optic neuritis are caused by demyelination. Although most patients with optic neuritis have no premonitory illness, some patients develop signs and symptoms indicative of a nonspecific viral illness several days or weeks before the onset of visual loss. Optic neuritis may also occur as the initial manifestation or in the setting of systemic inflammatory disorders other than multiple sclerosis, such as syphilis, sarcoidosis, systemic lupus erythematosus, and Lyme disease (Table 1). Some patients, particularly men, have no evidence of systemic or neurologic disease at the time the optic neuritis occurs, nor do they ultimately develop such disease. In such cases, the condition is considered to be idiopathic. Many physicians believe that idiopathic optic neuritis is actually a limited form of multiple sclerosis.

Pathologic processes other than inflammation may cause an acute optic neuropathy that mimics optic

Table 1 Causes of Optic Neuritis

Most Common	*Less Common*	*Least Common*
Multiple sclerosis	Idiopathic Postviral	Granulomatous inflammation, especially syphilis or sarcoidosis Collagen vascular (autoimmune) disorders Infectious mononucleosis Adjacent inflammation of paranasal sinuses or orbit

Table 2 Differential Diagnosis of Optic Neuritis

Other optic neuropathies
    Compressive
        Orbital
        Intracanalicular
        Intracranial
    Ischemic (e.g., migraine, diabetes, or other nonarteritic anterior ischemic optic neuropathy)
    Toxic (e.g., ethambutol toxicity)
    Nutritional deficiency (e.g., vitamin B_{12} or folic acid deficiency)
    Infiltrative
    Hereditary (particularly Leber's)
    Glaucoma
    Drusen of the optic disc

Intraocular disease
    Retinal disease
    Retinal vascular disease (e.g., arterial occlusion)
    Diseases of the ocular media
        Corneal disease
        Cataract

Nonorganic visual loss
    Conversion reaction
    Malingering

neuritis (Table 2). These processes include compression, ischemia, infiltration, and toxicity. In addition, Leber's hereditary optic neuropathy may present initially as a unilateral visual loss that mimics optic neuritis, although such patients never complain of ocular or orbital pain, and the second eye always becomes affected sooner or later.

Because the diagnosis of optic neuritis is based entirely on clinical grounds, the responsibility of the physician with a patient with presumed optic neuritis is to eliminate the possibility of a process that is causing an optic neuropathy that is mimicking optic neuritis and, if no such lesion is present, to determine if there is an underlying and potentially treatable cause for the optic neuritis. The minimum evaluation of such a patient includes a complete systemic and neurologic history. If there is no history suggesting an underlying inflammatory disorder such as syphilis, sarcoid, systemic lupus erythematosus, or Lyme disease, it is probably not necessary to obtain any serologic studies. If the history is unreliable or suggestive of a systemic inflammatory disease, however, the physician may wish to obtain some or all of the following, depending on the setting: a complete blood count, erythrocyte sedimentation rate, serum tests for syphilis, assay for antinuclear antibodies, assay for angiotensin converting enzyme, Lyme titers, assay for human immunodeficiency virus (HIV), and a chest x-ray. Patients with presumed optic neuritis that is painless, patients with bilateral presumed optic neuritis, and patients whose vision does not improve spontaneously or with treatment (see below) should undergo a blood test for the mitochondrial DNA mutations that are associated with Leber's hereditary optic neuropathy.

There are two schools of thought regarding neuroimaging in patients with presumed optic neuritis. Many experts believe that no imaging studies are needed in a "typical" case of optic neuritis and that neuroimaging should be performed only if the clinical presentation is atypical for optic neuritis (subacute, slowly progressive, painless) or if vision does not begin to improve spontaneously or with treatment within 3 to 6 weeks. Others, myself included, prefer to obtain magnetic resonance imaging (MRI) of the orbits and optic chiasmal region in patients with presumed retrobulbar neuritis to make certain that there is no evidence of a mass compressing the intracranial portion of the affected optic nerve, such as a pituitary adenoma, meningioma, or aneurysm. Given the significant amount of information obtained from MRI scanning, there would seem to be little or no justification for obtaining a plain skull x-ray or polytomogram in any patient with an acute optic neuropathy, and computed tomography scanning probably should be reserved for those patients who cannot for some reason undergo MRI. MRI is not necessary for patients who have presumed anterior optic neuritis. Such patients are unlikely to have an intracranial mass producing the visual loss. An orbital mass could be responsible for acute visual loss associated with optic disc swelling, but patients with such lesions generally have other evidence of an orbital process, such as proptosis, chemosis, and limitation of eye movement.

Patients with optic neuritis whose history and examination suggest the diagnosis of multiple sclerosis should undergo a complete neurologic evaluation. Other tests that may be considered in such patients include evoked potentials (visual, brain stem, somatosensory), MRI, and a lumbar puncture with cerebrospinal fluid analyzed for protein, glucose, cellular, and immunoglobulin G (IgG) content as well as for oligoclonal bands and myelin basic protein.

SUGGESTED READING

Beck RW, Cleary PA, Anderson MM Jr, et al. A randomized, controlled trial of corticosteroids in the treatment of acute optic neuritis. N Engl J Med 1992; 326:581–588.

Beck RW, Optic Neuritis Study Group. The Optic Neuritis Treatment Trial: Implications for clinical practice. Arch Ophthalmol 1992; 110:331–332.

Beck RW, Optic Neuritis Study Group: Corticosteroid treatment of optic neuritis: A need to change treatment practice. Neurology 1992; 42:1133–1135.

Optic Neuritis Study Group. The clinical profile of optic neuritis: Experience of the Optic Neuritis Treatment Trial. Arch Ophthalmol 1991; 109:1673–1678.

MULTIPLE SCLEROSIS

AARON E. MILLER, M.D.

Multiple sclerosis (MS) is an inflammatory, demyelinating disease of the central nervous system. It typically affects young adults and most often follows an exacerbating-remitting pattern, at least early in its course. Most regard MS as an autoimmune disorder occurring in genetically predisposed individuals. However, the factors triggering the pathologic changes and the resultant clinical manifestations remain enigmatic.

DIAGNOSTIC CRITERIA

The diagnosis of MS depends upon demonstration of lesions disseminated in time and space. These requirements were incorporated into criteria established by Schumacher, which form the framework for diagnosis. The specific features he required for the diagnosis of "clinically definite" MS were:

1. Age of onset 10 to 50 years
2. Signs and symptoms indicative of white matter disease
3. Objective neurologic signs
4. Two or more lesions, not anatomically contiguous
5. Two or more episodes in time or progression for more than 6 months
6. No better clinical explanation

Schumacher required at least five of these criteria, always including the last, to be met for a diagnosis of clinically definite MS.

In 1983, a committee chaired by Poser proposed criteria that incorporated modern techniques for demonstrating subclinical lesions (referred to as paraclinical evidence) and immunologic abnormalities in the cerebrospinal fluid (CSF), such as oligoclonal bands or abnormal synthesis of IgG.

The Poser criteria are as follows:

Clinically Definite Multiple Sclerosis

1. Two attacks and clinical evidence of two separate lesions
2. Two attacks, clinical evidence of one and para-clinical evidence of another separate lesion

Laboratory-Supported Definite Multiple Sclerosis

1. Two attacks, either clinical or paraclinical evidence of one lesion, and CSF immunologic abnormalities
2. One attack, clinical evidence of two separate lesions and CSF abnormalities
3. One attack, clinical evidence of one and para-clinical evidence of another separate lesion, and CSF abnormalities

Clinically Probable Multiple Sclerosis

1. Two attacks and clinical evidence of one lesion
2. One attack and clinical evidence of two separate lesions
3. One attack, clinical evidence of one lesion, and paraclinical evidence of another separate lesion

Laboratory-Supported Probable Multiple Sclerosis

1. Two attacks and CSF abnormalities

In each situation, an attack is defined as the occurrence of neurologic symptoms or signs lasting more than 24 hours. A second attack must be separated from the first by at least a month. Certain symptoms, such as Lhermitte's symptom (transient paresthesias following neck flexion) or tonic "seizures" (paroxymal dystonic posturing, usually of a limb), occur very briefly, but their recurrence over days or weeks may be regarded as an attack. In those categories described above in which only one attack is required, the two lesions, whether demonstrated by clinical or paraclinical evidence, must *not* both have been present at the time of initial examination and must be separated in time by at least 1 month. This temporal requirement minimizes the possibility of misdiagnosing acute disseminated encephalomyelitis as MS.

HISTORY

Diagnosis of MS is most challenging in the patient presenting with monosymptomatic disease. While the initial manifestations of MS are myriad, the most frequent presenting complaints are numbness, weakness, or visual disturbance. When the presentation is sensory, the patient may complain of paresthesias, burning, tight sensation, or diminished sensation in a body part. The distribution is often puzzling, not always conforming to well-recognized anatomic territories. Frequently, objective sensory loss is not demonstrable. When weakness predominates, it is most typically in one or both legs. Less commonly, a hemiparetic pattern may be evident or a brachial monoparesis may develop. Optic neuritis is a common presentation of MS, with the patient typically complaining of monocular visual acuity loss, usually accompanied by retro-orbital pain or pain on eye movement. The visual impairment may manifest as a central scotoma or, in more subtle cases, by desaturation of color.

Among the less frequent initial symptoms and signs are vertigo, gait ataxia, trigeminal neuralgia, incoordination or tremor of a limb, and sphincteric or sexual dysfunction. At any point in the illness, fatigue may be a prominent symptom. Although fatigue may result from certain specific situations such as overexertion or depression, the typical MS fatigue is an inexplicable sense of enervation, usually sufficient to interfere with everyday functions.

When the patient presents with one episode and symptoms or signs pointing to a solitary anatomic locus, the clinician must probe diligently for evidence of other "attacks," occurring at least a month before, as well as for other anatomic sites of involvement. Because previous symptoms may have been mild and self-limited, the patient may neglect to mention them. The physician must ask specific and often leading questions to elicit previous episodes of neurologic symptoms. Prior bouts of sensory symptoms are particularly likely to be omitted by the patient.

PHYSICAL EXAMINATION

Whether or not the history reveals prior episodes of neurologic dysfunction, physical examination and, if necessary, subsequent investigation must focus on the demonstration of a second lesion. A thorough neurologic exam may show abnormalities such as Babinski signs or impairment of vibratory sensation — in my experience an extremely common finding — indicative of dysfunction unassociated with clinical symptoms. If the neurologic examination, current or past, does not show evidence of involvement of a second anatomic site, subclinical lesions may be sought through other investigations. The highest yielding study is magnetic resonance imaging (MRI) of the brain, which reveals second lesions in approximately 50 to 60 percent of monosymptomatic patients. Most characteristic is the finding of multiple white matter lesions, mainly in periventricular locations. Very typical is an oval-shaped lesion with the long axis directed perpendicular to the anterior-posterior dimension of the lateral ventricle. Also helpful in diagnosis is the presence of lesions in the posterior fossa. Should MRI fail to demonstrate additional lesions, evoked potential testing may be performed. Thus, visual evoked responses may reveal a subclinical lesion in the optic nerves, useful in patients presenting with symptoms other than optic neuritis. Alternatively, abnormal somatosensory evoked potentials may indicate spinal cord lesions, helpful in patients whose clinical symptomatology indicated abnormality elsewhere. Abnormal brain stem auditory evoked responses are much less common.

LABORATORY EVALUATION

The role of CSF examination is more often corroborative than diagnostic. Immunologic abnormalities in the CSF may, however, allow patients to be classified as laboratory-supported definite MS (see above). Particularly in cases where the abnormalities on neurologic examination are subtle or equivocal, an abnormal CSF provides increased confidence in the diagnosis. In addition to routine spinal fluid cell count and chemistries, one should request determination of oligoclonal bands and IgG levels. I usually offer the possibility of lumbar puncture to the patient with the caveat that increasing our certainty of the diagnosis at that point will not change the management. Although some series indicate that as many as 90 percent of patients with clinically definite MS have abnormal CSF examinations, in my experience the figure is much lower for patients presenting with early symptoms and signs in whom the finding of a CSF abnormality would be helpful diagnostically.

DIFFERENTIAL DIAGNOSIS

When an otherwise healthy young adult presents with a clear history of multiple episodes of neurologic dysfunction and unequivocal signs of two or more lesions, the diagnosis is straightforward and there are few other considerations. However, under other circumstances, a variety of other neurologic conditions enter the differential diagnosis. Acute disseminated encephalomyelitis is a monophasic illness, usually following a viral infection. Multiple anatomic sites may be involved, and, occasionally, immunologic abnormalities similar to those in MS may be found in the CSF. Under such circumstances, when no antecedent episode has occurred, great caution should be exercised in offering a definitive diagnosis. Certain isolated neurologic syndromes, such as optic neuritis, carry a very high probability of ultimately proving to be a presentation of MS. However, acute transverse myelitis, in contrast, is usually a monophasic illness and is seldom followed by subsequent attacks of neurologic disease.

As the age of the patient increases, the differential diagnosis tends to become more difficult. Multifocal vascular disease may be confused with MS, especially small vessel disease producing multiple white matter lesions on MRI.

A fairly common problem is the middle-aged (or older) patient who presents with progressive spastic paraparesis. Although the differential diagnosis for this syndrome is extensive, probably the most common

causes are cervical spondylosis and MS. Cranial MRI can be particularly helpful, and the finding of lesions typical of MS should make one very suspicious of that diagnosis, even in the presence of cervical spondylosis. The radiographic changes and clinical status of the patient with cervical spondylosis do not always correlate reliably.

Another consideration in patients with progressive spastic paraparesis is HTLV-1–associated myelopathy, or tropical spastic paraparesis. This retroviral illness, endemic in parts of the Caribbean, parts of Japan, and elsewhere, appears occasionally in the United States. The symptoms usually develop insidiously, but the onset may be more rapid. Occasionally, signs referable to sites outside the spinal cord may occur, increasing the difficulty of distinguishing it from MS. Cranial MRI, while occasionally showing lesions in tropical spastic paraparesis, is generally normal and thus makes MS a less likely diagnosis. Definitive diagnosis depends on serologic evidence of HTLV-1 infection.

Systemic lupus erythematosus (SLE) or central nervous system (CNS) vasculitides may present a challenging diagnostic problem because of their multifocal and, at times, episodic manifestations. In SLE, seizures, psychiatric disturbances, and aseptic meningitis are more common than white matter lesions. Serologic indication of SLE should facilitate the correct diagnosis. In the vasculitides, with the exception of isolated CNS angiitis, systemic manifestations should rule out MS. At times, CSF examination, cerebral angiography, or leptomeningeal biopsy may lead to the correct diagnosis of CNS vasculitis.

Spinocerebellar degenerations appearing in adolescence or young adulthood, or olivopontocerebellar degenerations may pose difficult diagnostic dilemmas because of the progressive course, comparable age of onset, and occasionally multifocal signs. Careful family history must be sought, though additional cases are not always present. A lack of hemispheric white matter lesions on MRI and normal CSF will favor these diagnoses rather than MS.

RECOMMENDATIONS

The diagnosis of MS is usually made without difficulty when the patient presents with multiple episodes of neurologic dysfunction referable to multiple sites within the CNS. In such patients, costly investigations are unnecessary. Where less certainty exists about the reliability of the historical data or the neurologic signs, studies should be undertaken to increase the confidence in the diagnosis. Similarly, in patients with monosymptomatic disease, the investigation should be directed toward identifying a second lesion and should be performed in sequential fashion designed to obtain the critical information at the lowest cost and least inconvenience to the patient.

Finally, I emphasize the importance of sharing one's diagnostic opinion with the patient in a direct and easily comprehensible manner. If the diagnosis is certain, the patient should be told that he or she has multiple sclerosis and not offered euphemistic terms in substitution. If the diagnosis is likely but not certain, the nature of that doubt should be explained. A reasonable discussion of the disease should be offered, and the patient should arrive at an understanding of the neurologist's inability to predict the future course with reliability.

SUGGESTED READING

Fazekas F, Offenbacher H, Fuchs S, et al. Criteria for an increased specificity of MRI interpretation in elderly subjects with suspected multiple sclerosis. Neurology 1988; 38:1822–1825.

McDonald WI, Silberberg DH. The diagnosis of multiple sclerosis. In: McDonald WI, Silberberg DH, eds. Multiple sclerosis. London: Butterworths, 1986.

Miller AE. Clinical features. In: Cook SD, ed. Handbook of multiple sclerosis. New York: Marcel Dekker, 1990.

Ormerod JEC, Miller DH, McDonald WI, et al. The role of NMR imaging in the assessment of multiple sclerosis and isolated neurological lesions. Brain 1987; 110:1579–1616.

Poser CM, Paty DW, Scheinberg L, et al. New diagnostic criteria for multiple sclerosis: Guidelines for research protocols. Ann Neurol 1983; 13:227–231.

Schumacher GA, Beebe G, Kubler RF, et al. Problems of experimental trials of therapy in multiple sclerosis: Report by the panel on the evaluation of experimental trials of therapy in multiple sclerosis. Ann NY Acad Sci 1965; 122:522–568.

DEGENERATIVE DISEASES

ALZHEIMER'S DISEASE

BRIAN R. OTT, M.D.

Since Alzheimer's clinical and pathologic description of a 55-year-old woman with dementia in 1907, the diagnosis of dementia remains a common challenge facing physicians in many fields of practice. In the 1960s, recognition that senile and presenile onset cases share a common pathology resulted in application of the diagnostic term *Alzheimer's disease* to cases of primary degenerative dementia, regardless of age.

The clinical diagnosis of Alzheimer's disease is one of both inclusion and exclusion. Accuracy of diagnosis has been improved by the use of standardized guidelines such as those of the NINCDS-ADRDA Work Group developed in 1984. This approach defines patients as having possible, probable, or definite Alzheimer's disease. Definite diagnosis of Alzheimer's disease is reserved for those cases in which the characteristic neuritic plaques and neurofibrillary tangles are seen in large numbers in the cortex of biopsy or postmortem brain specimens.

Using such criteria, accuracy of the premortem diagnosis of probable Alzheimer's disease approaches 85 to 90 percent in dementia referral clinics. Diagnostic dilemmas still arise from heterogeneity within the disease as well as overlap with other, coexistent causes of dementia.

INCLUSION CRITERIA

The first step in the evaluation of a patient who presents with an apparent memory disorder is to determine whether dementia exists (Table 1). Dementia is primarily a behavioral syndrome in which acquired impairment of memory is typically an early and prominent feature. There are many causes for dementia. It is usually a chronic syndrome spanning months to years that is often, though not always, progressive. The number and type of cognitive impairment may vary with the patient and the cause. However, there must be

Table 1 Clinical Features of Alzheimer's Disease

Dementia:
  Impaired activities of daily living
  Altered behavior patterns
  Cognitive deficits in two or more areas, including memory
  Apraxia, aphasia, agnosia, and visuospatial impairment are
    common
Delusions, hallucinations, and depression may occur.
Progressive course; plateaus may occur.
Normal level of consciousness
Insidious onset between 40 and 90 years of age; usually after age 65
Family history may be positive.

impairments in other areas besides memory, involving cognition, judgment, or personality. Level of consciousness is preserved, however. The impairments are of sufficient severity to interfere with occupational or social function. Finally, a primary psychiatric disorder such as major depression must be excluded, if an organic explanation for the impairments is not apparent from the clinical evaluation.

Dementia may not be recognized by physicians when social propriety is relatively preserved early in the course and when the patient lacks insight into his or her own deficits. These are features often seen in patients with Alzheimer's disease. It is usually necessary to obtain corroborative history from a friend or relative regarding the presence of dementia.

The most common cause for incorrectly diagnosing a patient as having dementia is depression. The patient with depression may lack concentration and motivation, producing an apparent memory disorder. Therefore it is very important to inquire about such factors as mood, energy, sleep, appetite, and thought content when examining the patient with presumed dementia.

Depressive features related to partial awareness of dementia early in the course of true Alzheimer's disease and to vegetative features late in the course may also occur. The diagnoses of depression and dementia should not be regarded as mutually exclusive. In my experience, the presence of constructional apraxia is often a helpful indicator that a depressed patient with amnesia has true dementia. A therapeutic trial of antidepressant medication may be indicated in ambiguous cases.

In the earliest stage of Alzheimer's disease, forgetfulness occurs as the sole or primary feature. Amnesia is greatest for recent memories compared to remote memories. At this point, a probable diagnosis of Alzheimer's disease is often deferred until a progressive decline and development of other cognitive deficits can be documented. Attention deficit and mild disorientation for time may be seen.

Anomia also occurs early in the disease, eventually developing into a fluent aphasia with impaired comprehension, repetition, and writing. Geographic disorientation and constructional apraxia are important features to note, since they suggest visuospatial dysfunction, probably on the basis of right parietal involvement. Deficits in language and visuospatial function can usually be demonstrated in the first several years.

As the disease progresses, judgment and social function are lost. Sleep disorder with multiple awakenings and nocturnal confusion develops. Many patients develop delusions with paranoid ideation and compulsions as well as frank hallucinations. Psychiatric symptoms may occur in 30 to 50 percent of patients with Alzheimer's disease.

In late stages of the disease, seizures, myoclonus, gait disorder, rigidity, and other extrapyramidal features occur. Loss of personal hygiene, apraxia, and incontinence often lead to institutional care. At this point the clinical distinction of Alzheimer's disease from other progressive dementing illnesses is impossible without knowledge of the patient's prior history.

Heterogeneity

Although the features I have described are fairly consistent for most cases of Alzheimer's disease, there exists considerable variability in the clinical expression of the disease.

Asymmetry. Greater involvement of one cerebral hemisphere has been documented in some patients, despite comparable degrees of overall dementia severity. Asymmetry is illustrated by functional brain imaging studies such as positron emission tomography (PET) and single photon emission computed tomography (SPECT). Clinically, left hemisphere predominant cases have greater language and verbal memory deficits, which may lead to earlier recognition. Right hemisphere predominant cases have greater visuospatial deficits and impairments in nonverbal memory. In similar fashion, greater involvement of frontal association cortex in some patients can lead to more prominent personality disturbance, loss of insight, and impaired executive functions such as planning and changing set.

Age of Onset. The distinction between early and late onset cases is still controversial. Although age of onset is no longer used as a diagnostic marker, evidence exists that those patients with onset prior to age 65, the so-called presenile cases, may experience more severe language dysfunction, a more rapidly progressive course, and have more widespread and severe neurochemical deficits. Misdiagnosis of Alzheimer's disease may also be higher in these cases, possibly due to lower prevalence of Alzheimer's disease in younger persons with dementia.

Duration of Disease. The usual duration of disease is 5 to 10 years. However, some cases may follow a rapid progressive course over 2 to 3 years or a prolonged course of greater than 12 years. Identification of prognostic factors for rate of decline is an area of active research. Severity of illness at any one point in time does not appear to predict rate of decline.

Familial Disease. A dominant family history of dementia secondary to Alzheimer's disease is uncommon, occurring most often in early onset cases. About one-third of cases report a first degree relative with dementia.

A genetic link between the twenty-first chromosome, beta amyloid protein, and Alzheimer's disease is present in patients with Down's syndrome in whom the neuropathologic changes of Alzheimer's disease occur in virtually everyone who reaches the age of 40. About 20 to 30 percent of these patients develop clinical evidence of dementia.

Extrapyramidal Signs and Myoclonus. The presence of extrapyramidal signs and myoclonus require the neurologist to consider the diagnoses of Parkinson's or Creutzfeldt-Jacob disease. Extrapyramidal signs have been reported to occur in patients with Alzheimer's disease. Bradykinesia and rigidity are most common. The presence of tremor is rare and should suggest concurrent Parkinson's disease. About 10 percent of patients develop myoclonus. The subgroup of patients with myoclonus and extrapyramidal signs appear to have more severe disruption of dopaminergic and serotonergic ascending systems than their counterparts without these physical features.

EXCLUSION CRITERIA

Alzheimer's disease is the most common disease causing dementia, accounting for approximately 50 to 65 percent of all cases. Since approximately 10 to 20 percent of dementias may be specifically treatable, it is important that all patients undergo a careful evaluation to rule out such disorders before making a final diagnosis of probable Alzheimer's disease.

A full discussion of the many other causes of dementia that must be excluded is beyond the scope of this section. The differential diagnosis of Alzheimer's disease includes vascular dementia, drug intoxication, hypothyroidism, pernicious anemia, general paresis, chronic subdural hematoma, normal pressure hydrocephalus, Creutzfeldt-Jacob disease, brain neoplasm, and other degenerative diseases. A few of the more common pitfalls in diagnosis will be discussed. The following features, if present, should suggest an alternative cause for dementia.

Sudden Onset. Although occasionally patients with Alzheimer's disease or their relatives may date the onset of their memory impairment to specific life events, such as retirement or the death of a spouse, Alzheimer's disease should be regarded as a disease with slow, insidious onset. Sudden onset of dementia should prompt an investigation for such disorders as stroke, subdural hematoma, or infection of the central nervous system (CNS). Subacute progression over days to weeks suggests infection, neoplasm, metabolic disorders, and depression.

Gait Disorder Early in the Course. As mentioned previously, gait disorder may occur late in the course of Alzheimer's disease. Gait disorder as an early feature of a dementing illness is seen commonly in the multi-infarct state and in subcortical diseases such as multiple sclerosis, acquired immunodeficiency syndrome encephalopathy, hydrocephalus, progressive supranuclear palsy, and Huntington's and Parkinson's disease.

Seizures Early in the Course. Seizures occur in approximately 10 percent of patients with Alzheimer's disease, late in their course. Early onset of seizures suggests stroke, head trauma, or neoplasm as more likely causes of dementia.

Focal Neurologic Signs and Symptoms. Focal neurologic signs, including aphasia out of proportion to the degree of dementia, suggest the presence of focal brain lesions such as stroke or neoplasm in most cases. Lobar degeneration syndromes must also be considered.

OVERLAP SYNDROMES

Not infrequently one encounters patients with clinical features of more than one type of dementing illness. Such cases may result from the co-occurrence of two different pathologies (Fig. 1).

Lobar Degenerations

A full discussion of this group of progressive disorders is presented in the section in this text on focal cortical degeneration. The syndromes of primary progressive aphasia and posterior cortical atrophy probably represent a heterogeneous group of disorders, which may appear to be Alzheimer's disease due to the insidious onset of cognitive deficits and progressive course. Postmortem examinations have revealed pathologic features of Alzheimer's or Pick's disease in some cases, as well as severe gliosis and spongiform changes in others. Therefore, it may be appropriate to refer to such patients with progressive circumscribed cognitive deficits as having possible Alzheimer's disease, particularly if dementia develops during follow-up.

Pick's disease results from degeneration of frontal and temporal lobes, whereas Alzheimer's disease most severely affects the parietal and temporal lobes. Though having different pathologies, the two disorders share many clinical features, such as insidious onset and tempo of progression. In moderate to advanced cases, the two disorders cannot be reliably distinguished.

Features that favor a diagnosis of Pick's disease over Alzheimer's disease during the early stages include prominent loss of social propriety and behavioral restraint, insight, judgment, and occupational function, as well as the Kluver-Bucy syndrome. Also notable is

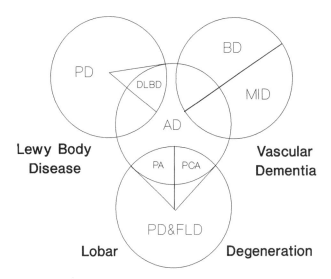

Figure 1 Syndromes that overlap with Alzheimer's disease. PD = Parkinson's disease; DLBD = diffuse Lewy body disease; MID = multi-infarct dementia; BD = Binswanger's disease; AD = Alzheimer's disease; PA = progressive aphasia syndrome; PCA = posterior cortical atrophy syndrome; PD&FLD = Pick's disease and frontal lobe dementia.

relative sparing of memory, visuospatial function, and language at onset. Neuropsychometric tests and functional brain imaging studies may help to separate Pick's disease and other frontal lobe dementias from Alzheimer's disease. The relationship of Pick's disease to frontal lobe dementia (without Pick's bodies and ballooned cells) remains to be fully elucidated.

Vascular Dementia

Vascular dementia is the second most common cause of dementia, representing about 10 to 25 percent of cases. Because the prevalence of stroke and Alzheimer's disease both rise with advancing age, it is not surprising that co-occurrence of the two diseases is common. Such cases may be referred to as "mixed" dementia, and account for another 10 to 15 percent of dementia cases.

Clinically, patients with vascular dementia are likely to have dysarthria, rigidity, gait disturbance, and incontinence, as well as focal signs and symptoms. Deep white matter abnormalities, referred to as leuko-ariosis, are often seen on computed tomography (CT) and magnetic resonance imaging (MRI) scans, as well as more focal and well-defined areas of infarction. The exact contribution of stroke to dementia in the individual patient may be indeterminate, particularly if there is only one documentable stroke or the strokes are in locations such as cerebellum that do not explain the observed cognitive impairments.

Vascular dementia may arise as the result of multiple hemorrhagic, embolic, or thrombotic strokes. Ischemic vascular dementia may result from multiple lacunar infarcts, multiple cortical infarcts, or a combination of the two. Chronic ischemia of the periventricular territories of deep penetrating vessels may cause a gradual rather than stepwise progressive dementia referred to as Binswanger's disease. This condition occurs typically in patients with long-standing hypertension who have extensive periventricular abnormalities on CT or MRI studies.

Parkinson's Disease

Approximately 15 to 30 percent of patients with idiopathic Parkinson's disease develop dementia. Although relatively mild or isolated cognitive deficits such as amnesia and bradyphrenia probably occur as part of the disease, a large number of such patients have concurrent Alzheimer's disease. The reason for a higher than expected frequency of Alzheimer's disease pathology in patients with Parkinson's disease has not been explained.

An even less well-understood disorder is diffuse Lewy body disease. These patients share pathologic features of both Alzheimer's and Parkinson's disease, such as neuritic plaques and Lewy bodies. Lewy bodies are found in high numbers in cerebral cortex, unlike either disorder, leading to its recent distinction as a separate entity. The clinical presentation at onset may be one of primarily extrapyramidal features or dementia. Patients tend to have hallucinations and delusions early in their disease, unlike Alzheimer's disease in which hallucinations usually occur late.

DIAGNOSTIC TESTS

Because the diagnosis of Alzheimer's disease remains a clinical one, the most important part of the diagnostic evaluation is a thorough history and physical examination. Key features of the evaluation for dementia are listed in Table 2. The use of standard mental status screening tests such as the Mini-Mental Status Examination and the Blessed Information-Memory-Concentration Test is recommended. Neuropsychological tests may provide further information in cases where the diagnosis of dementia is uncertain or where a specific pattern of cognitive impairment, such as frontal lobe dementia, is suspected. Such tests are also useful for documentation and measurement of progression over time.

Computed tomography without contrast injection is a safe and usually well tolerated procedure for the exclusion of stroke, hydrocephalus, tumor, and chronic subdural hematoma and is recommended as a routine screening procedure. In specific cases where tumor is suspected, contrast-enhanced CT or MRI should be performed instead. MRI is more sensitive than CT for the detection of small infarcts and demyelination. However, interpretation of the significance of hyperintensities in periventricular and subcortical regions on T2 weighted images may be difficult in the absence of clinical correlation with the history and physical exam-

Table 2 Evaluation of Dementia

History	*Tests*
Psychiatric/social	Laboratory:
Drug and alcohol use	Chemistry profile, B_{12},
HIV and stroke risk factors	RPR, T4, TSH, blood
Family history of dementia	count, ESR
Medications	Radiologic:
	Chest radiograph
Physical Examination	Brain computed tomography
Mental status	Ancillary:
Neurologic:	Neuropsychometric tests
Extrapyramidal features	Electroencephalogram
Gait	Magnetic resonance imaging
Focal signs	Functional imaging
	(SPECT/PET)
	Lumbar puncture
	HIV

HIV = human immunodeficiency virus; RPR = rapid plasma reagin; T_4 = thyroxine; TSH = thyroid-stimulating hormone; ESR = erythrocyte sedimentation rate; SPECT = single photon emission computed tomography; PET = positron emission tomography.

ination. Abnormalities of this type have been reported in patients with Alzheimer's disease as well as in those with normal aging.

Routine blood studies including complete chemistry profile and blood count, sedimentation rate, thyroid function tests, vitamin B_{12} level, and RPR will help detect most commonly encountered treatable causes of dementia. Electroencephalogram may be useful in distinguishing depression from organic dementia, as well as in evaluating rapidly progressive dementia suspected to be Creutzfeldt-Jakob disease. Lumbar puncture may be indicated in the evaluation of hydrocephalus or chronic CNS infection. A human immunodeficiency virus (HIV) test should be strongly considered in any patient with risk factors who is relatively young and sexually active or who presents with features of a subacute subcortical dementia, including abulia, social withdrawal, gait disorder, and tremor.

If available, functional brain imaging studies may provide supportive evidence for the diagnosis of Alzheimer's disease. A pattern of diminished metabolism (PET) or perfusion (SPECT) is seen in the temporal and parietal cortices bilaterally. In cases where this characteristic pattern is seen, other lesions such as infarction must be ruled out by CT or MRI studies. Because of its lower expense and wider availability, SPECT scanning shows promise in this regard. However, false-negative studies are common.

To date, there is no single biologic test to confirm the clinical diagnosis of Alzheimer's disease. Assays for specific proteins in CSF are presently in development and hold promise for the future. Due to improved accuracy of clinical diagnosis, brain biopsy is no longer performed or recommended for cases of Alzheimer's disease. Families should be encouraged to consent to autopsy to determine the definite diagnosis of Alzheimer's disease. Knowledge gained from autopsy is also needed to produce reliable clinical and epidemiologic research studies.

EARLY DIAGNOSIS

Because amnesia is central to the disease, tests of delayed memory recall are most sensitive in identifying patients with early Alzheimer's disease. Misdiagnosis is a risk since cognitive effects of aging may be the cause of failure to perform adequately on memory tests.

Distinguishing normal age-related changes in memory from early Alzheimer's disease may not be possible. Serial observations of function and cognition over time remain the most important means of making this determination. Treatment of concurrent medical illnesses and adjustment of medications, particularly in the elderly, may also be necessary before reaching a diagnosis of Alzheimer's disease.

SUGGESTED READING

Brust JC. Vascular dementia is overdiagnosed. Arch Neurol 1988; 45:799–801.

Chui HC, Victoroff JI, Margolin D, et al. Criteria for the diagnosis of ischemic vascular dementia proposed by the State of California Alzheimer's Disease Diagnostic and Treatment Centers. Neurology 1992; 42:473–480.
Cummings JL, Benson DF. Dementia: A clinical approach. Boston: Butterworths, 1983.
Friedland RP, Koss E, Haxby JV, et al. Alzheimer's disease: Clinical and biological heterogeneity. Ann Intern Med 1988; 109:298–311.
Kukull WA, Larson EB, Reifler BV, et al. The validity of three clinical diagnostic criteria for Alzheimer's disease. Neurology 1990; 40: 1364–1369.
McKhann G, Drachman D, Folstein M, et al. Clinical diagnosis of Alzheimer's disease: Report of the NINCDS-ADRDA Work Group under the auspices of the Department of Health and Human Services Task Force on Alzheimer's disease. Neurology 1984; 34:939–944.
NIH Consensus Development Conference Statement. The differential diagnosis of Alzheimer's disease and other dementias. JAMA 1988; 258:3411–3416.
O'Brien MD. Vascular dementia is underdiagnosed. Arch Neurol 1988; 45:797–798.

FOCAL CORTICAL DEGENERATION

RICHARD J. CASELLI, M.D.

Degenerative diseases that are asymmetrically distributed in the cerebral cortex result in slowly progressive, complex, but relatively focal neurologic syndromes. For example, Pick's disease has a predilection for the frontal and temporal lobes and is often worse on one side. Pick's disease affecting the left temporal lobe, therefore, can produce slowly progressive aphasia.

Several clinical presentations of focal cerebral degenerative diseases have been described, including progressive aphasia, progressive perceptual-motor disorders (including apraxia and visual agnosia), and progressive neuropsychiatric syndromes (Table 1). Not surprisingly, the clinical presentation is determined by the location of the lesion. The lesion in such cases may be a sharply demarcated focus of cortical degeneration or, more commonly, a widespread degenerative process that is highly accentuated focally. It is the focally severe area that determines the predominant clinical manifestations. I prefer the term *asymmetric cortical degeneration syndrome* (ACDS) rather than *focal cortical degeneration* to reflect both the focal and diffuse aspects of the clinical and pathologic manifestations of these conditions. However, the term *focal* better portrays the clinical presentation in most patients.

Several histopathologic patterns may underlie ACDS, including nonspecific degenerative changes (neuronal loss, gliosis, vacuolar changes, increased neuronal lipofuscin), senile plaques and neurofibrillary tangles (as are typically seen in Alzheimer's disease), a spectrum of neuronal morphologic alterations that are either suggestive (achromatic neurons) or typical of Pick's bodies, and combinations of the above. The histology, however, does not correlate with a specific clinical pattern. Progressive aphasia, for example, has been associated with each of the histologic patterns listed. One interpretation of these findings is that multiple degenerative diseases can all produce the same pattern of symptoms. A second theory is that a single pathophysiologic insult produces asymmetric cortical

Table 1 Clinical Classification of Asymmetric Cortical Degeneration Syndromes

Syndrome	Brain Topography
Progressive aphasia	
Nonfluent	Frontal operculum
Fluent	Posterior temporal
Anomic	Anterior temporal
Progressive perceptual-motor syndrome	
Visual disorientation	Parietal occipital
Visual agnosia	Temporal occipital
Apraxia	Parietal frontal
Progressive neuropsychiatric syndrome	Frontal
Neuropsychiatric alone	
Neuropsychiatric and spasticity	
Spasticity alone	

degeneration, but the histologic expression of this insult is multifactorial and therefore variable.

Patients presenting with a particular clinical subtype of ACDS do *not* revert to another subtype or to a more common pattern of dementia such as clinically typical Alzheimer's dementia. However, as ACDS worsens, cognitive and other neurologic functions that were initially less affected become increasingly impaired with progressive disability. For example, a patient presenting with apraxia and visual disorientation may ultimately develop aphasia, even though the apraxia and visual disorder continue to be far more severe. The clinical course is variable, but a typical patient will be severely disabled within 5 to 10 years. Mean age of onset of ACDS is 60 years, which is younger than for typical Alzheimer's dementia. A wide range has been observed, however, from 42 to 80. Almost twice as many women as men have been diagnosed with ACDS to date. Handedness and educational and occupational backgrounds seem to play no role. Heredity may play a role, but most patients have no family history of ACDS or dementia in general.

No specific treatment is available for these degenerative conditions. We have employed various rehabilitative strategies in physical, speech, and occupational therapy with minimal, short-lived benefit. Nonetheless, recognition of this pattern of degenerative brain disease is important for counseling patients and their families, to aid in clinicopathologic correlations, and for focussing selection criteria in experimental drug trials for Alzheimer's disease. ACDS is sometimes equated with Alzheimer's disease because of a failure to appreciate the clinical distinctions between the two. There remains much to be learned about ACDS, and it is premature to infer such relationships.

HISTORICAL CONSIDERATIONS

The Historian

Anosognosia and anosodiaphoria are common in patients with Alzheimer's dementia and necessitate that a responsible relative or friend convey the details of the illness. This is not the case in ACDS, save for patients with a neuropsychiatric syndrome due to frontal lobe degeneration. Aphasia may preclude patients with the progressive aphasia variant from communicating the details of their illness, but they are visibly upset and indicate in every way they can that they have a big problem. Patients with perceptual-motor syndromes can generally convey their problem quite well. Late in the clinical course, however, their motor impairment may preclude communication either verbally or nonverbally. Some severely affected patients can answer simple yes-no questions with eye movement, although ocular motility disturbances and eyelid apraxia may also be present in preterminal stages, confounding even this simple form of communication.

The History

As with all degenerative diseases, onset of symptoms is insidious, progression is gradual, and apart from minor day-to-day fluctuations, progression is relentless over several years. Patients initially consult a physician within 1 or 2 years following onset.

Fears and Misdiagnoses

Patients with aphasia often fear they have Alzheimer's dementia or that they have had a stroke. Patients with progressive perceptual-motor syndromes often fear they have Parkinson's disease, Alzheimer's disease, or a stroke. Patients with neuropsychiatric symptoms occasionally express their fear that something is wrong with their mind but most of the time seem not to be thinking about it at all. They are commonly misdiagnosed as having atypical depression and later on as having either Alzheimer's or Parkinson's disease.

Specific Symptoms

No single classification system can account for the myriad variations of ACDS, but three predominant clinical patterns have emerged. The unifying theme is that neural topography dictates clinical manifestations.

Progressive Aphasia. Progressive aphasia may have one of three patterns: nonfluent, fluent, and anomic.

Nonfluent Aphasia. Patients with nonfluent speech (Broca's aphasia) are generally easily recognized. Dysfluent aphasia may affect speech more than writing in some patients, so patients should be asked to write at least some of their concerns, especially if their speech is unintelligible. Most patients with progressive, nonfluent aphasia have no other cognitive or neurologic deficits. Occasionally, however, concurrent involvement of motor cortices may lead to progressive spasticity affecting speech alone (spastic dysarthria) or limb control as well, so the patient should be asked about activities such as writing, dressing, eating, driving, and walking. Concurrent involvement of the anterior frontal lobe may cause neuropsychiatric dysfunction, including abulia, emotional lability, and perseveration. Rarely, patients presenting with a progressive spastic dysarthria and dysfluent aphasia develop increasing difficulty swallowing, with signs of widespread motor neuron disease including fasciculations and limb weakness, which may be mild, and actually suffer rapidly progressive aphasic dementia associated with motor neuron disease. Therefore, patients should be asked about swallowing, muscle twitches, and limb weakness as well.

Fluent Aphasia. Paraphasic, effortless speech (Wernicke's aphasia) can be confused with typical Alzheimer's dementia, but progressive fluent aphasia is not accompanied by disabling degrees of generalized cognitive impairment. Nonetheless, some patients have concomitant inferior parietal atrophy with parietal lobe signs such as acalculia and apraxia and should be questioned regarding such nonlinguistic cognitive functions as arithmetic skills, writing ability, dressing, sense of direction, and driving in particular. Maurice Ravel, as described by Alajouanine, had progressive impairment of musical performance and progressive fluent aphasia and may have had such a temporal-parietal variant of ACDS.

Anomic Aphasia. Naming is impaired in most forms of aphasia, but anomia occurring in isolation is rare. Pure anomic aphasia is easily overlooked because fluency and comprehension are normal. Patients generally complain of memory loss, but clues may be provided by asking for specific examples. Verbal memory is commonly impaired in the setting of anomic aphasia since both naming and verbal recall are subserved by contiguously situated regions of the left temporal lobe. Pathologic processes, including degenerative diseases, affecting one usually affect the other. Nonetheless, exemplary patients with pure anomia without amnesia and pure amnesia without anomia support the distinction of the two functions.

Perceptual-Motor Syndromes. ACDS centered in the parietal lobe usually involves contiguous cortices subserving vision posteriorly and motor control anteriorly. In most cases, however, either visuospatial or motor dysfunction predominates. Somesthetic function, subserved by parietal cortices, is commonly impaired in either setting but is rarely the most disabling feature.

Perceptual Disorders. Multiple cortical areas are dedicated to vision and are broadly divisible into dorsal (occipitoparietal) and ventral (occipitotemporal) streams. Involvement of dorsal visual cortices causes visual disorientation syndromes, and patients may complain of difficulty finding an object that is one of many on a table, though it is right in front of them (asimultanagnosia). They may also complain of difficulty driving due to difficulty estimating distance and depth. Involvement of ventral visual cortices impairs object recognition (visual agnosia) that may be specific for certain categories of objects such as familiar faces (prosopagnosia) or places (atopographagnosia) so that they become lost in familiar parts of town. Some with either type of visual dysfunction find map reading nearly impossible.

Motor Disorders. Patients are typically apraxic. They describe difficulty using eating utensils, writing or drawing, playing a musical instrument, using tools to make mechanical repairs, and dressing. They usually have much greater difficulty on one side and may state that they are losing control of one arm. In patients with corticobasal degeneration, the affected limb may become progressively more rigid and akinetic until it is virtually useless. Patients may describe an occasional myoclonic jerk in the affected limb. Gait impairment is generally mild early on, but as the disease progresses some patients describe losing their balance, falling, dragging their leg, and eventually become wheelchair bound.

Other Cognitive and Neurologic Deficits. Patients with this form of ACDS commonly complain of impaired arithmetic skills. Memory complaints are also typical but

are generally less severe and not as disabling as in Alzheimer's dementia. Most patients with ACDS lateralized to the dominant hemisphere have a mild fluent aphasia, but this is less severe than the progressive aphasia variety. Somesthetic impairment, as noted above, is common. Few patients admit to numbness, but testing may reveal astereognosis or tactile agnosia.

Progressive Neuropsychiatric Syndromes. These patients are abulic and anosodiaphoric and complain very little about their problems, so the history is best obtained from a close relative or friend. When asked what the patient does all day, the answer is typically "nothing." Patients often state they feel fine, and sit quietly while their spouse relates the disturbing history of their cognitive decline. They rarely offer a rebuttal and generally agree that their spouse has offered an accurate account. In contrast, many patients with Alzheimer's dementia vehemently deny their deficits and become accusatory or frankly abusive toward their spouse, whom they perceive to be condemning them with their history.

Occasionally neuropsychiatric patients become clingy and dependent and may appear superficially to be depressed. They do not admit to feelings of depression and have no vegetative features of depression. Some patients have outbursts of crying or laughing due to pseudobulbar affect. A subset of patients develop more prominent symptoms of spasticity affecting speech (spastic dysarthria) or limb control and may ultimately become anarthric and wheelchair bound.

Progressive Amnesia. It is uncertain whether this represents a form of focal cortical degeneration, but some patients complain of isolated, slowly progressive memory loss without any other features of dementia. Whether this is a forme fruste of Alzheimer's disease that ultimately evolves into dementia in all patients, or a form of ACDS that maintains the same pattern over the years is presently unknown.

CLINICAL COGNITIVE ASSESSMENT AND NEUROLOGIC EXAMINATION

Focal cortical degeneration should produce a focal neurologic syndrome, but since these disorders are asymmetric rather than truly focal in most patients, there can be additional milder deficits reflecting other, less involved regions of the cerebrum. The goal of the cognitive and neurologic examination, therefore, is to identify the specific pattern of impairment that should reflect the asymmetric pattern of involvement. The tests mentioned below are those I frequently use during my initial office evaluation of patients with cognitive complaints.

Mental Status Test

Several brief tests of mental status are available. The one I use (Kokmen Short Test of Mental Status) includes eight subtests: orientation, attention, learning, arithmetic, construction, abstraction, information, and recall. Simple reliance on the cutoff score of a brief mental status tool is inadequate for this group of patients. Aphasic patients may do poorly on everything, or they may have certain islands of preservation such as constructional praxis. Perceptual-motor patients have particular difficulty with constructional praxis and arithmetic. Neuropsychiatric patients may be normal, grossly impaired, or selectively impaired on tests requiring a sustained mental effort such as attention (digit span), mental arithmetic, and abstraction. Amnesics may perform well on everything except tests of memory, which include the recall, learning, information, and orientation subtests, and care must be taken to note whether a patient's failed responses reflect a single problem, such as amnesia or aphasia, or a more widespread pattern of dementia.

Temporal Orientation

In addition to the orientation subtest of a mental status test, a very brief but handy tool is the Benton Orientation Questionnaire, which asks the year (minus 10 points for each year off, up to minus 60), month (minus 5 for each month off, up to minus 30), date (minus 1 for each day off, up to minus 15), day of the week (minus 1 for each day off, up to minus 3), and time (minus 1 for each half-hour off, up to minus 5). Minus 3 is the cutoff. Aphasic patients may mis-state any portion of the date due to language impairment rather than actual temporal disorientation. Perceptual-motor patients usually perform normally. Neuropsychiatric patients are temporally disoriented more often than the other subgroups, as are patients with Alzheimer's dementia. Amnesic patients may not remember the year or month but can be surprisingly accurate regarding the time.

Complex Figure Test

This is an extremely useful and clinically adaptable neuropsychological tool that provides a quantitative measure of constructional praxis and visual memory. Observing the patient copy the figure also provides qualitative insight into organization and planning. There are two parallel forms (Rey-Osterrieth and Taylor versions). Aphasics and some frontal lobe patients may perform normally on this test, but the perceptual-motor group have severe difficulty. In mildly affected patients, or those with visual complaints, this may be the only test in the clinician's repertoire that is abnormal. Amnesics perform normally, but patients with dementia often do not.

Controlled Oral Word Association Test

A test of "verbal associative fluency," the Controlled Oral Word Association Test (COWAT) is another easily administered neuropsychological test that is sensitive to both language and some aspects of frontal lobe function. There are different versions, but all employ the notion of timed verbal output. "Tell me all the words you can think of that begin with the letter _____ in 60 seconds" is the general idea. In the absence of aphasia, this test is particularly useful for neuropsychiatric patients, whose spontaneous word list generation is usually very poor, even when other clinical indicators such as mental status tests appear normal.

Writing Sample

As a screening test, I give patients two sentences ("Today is a beautiful day" and Geschwind's "No ifs, ands, or buts"), which they may write in cursive. I also ask patients to print some common graphemically complex spelling words (such as *idea, people,* and *enough*). Aphasic patients may make paragraphic errors and have great difficulty with syntax. Perceptual-motor patients often have striking apraxic agraphia in addition to milder language-related errors. Neuropsychiatric patients often perform normally.

Visual Naming

The Boston Naming Test, developed by Goodglass and Kaplan, is easily adapted to the clinical setting. The examiner can give several stimuli as a screening test, and if felt to be relevant, the neuropsychological examination can incorporate more comprehensive testing of visual naming. Anomia is prevalent in Alzheimer's disease but is also present in asymmetric atrophy involving the left temporal pole, as may occur in patients with progressive aphasia and some with neuropsychiatric syndromes. Naming, as noted earlier, is commonly abnormal in most aphasics, but isolated anomia is not always apparent without formal testing.

Other Tests

Patients with primarily visual complaints may perform poorly on routinely administered tests of constructional praxis and reading, but these tests are generally insufficient for concluding that the patient has a disorder of visual association cortices. Two tests developed by Benton and collaborators may be helpful, though they may be better administered by the neuropsychologist: the Judgement of Line Orientation Test, which is particularly affected by occipitoparietal dysfunction, and the Facial Recognition Test, which is particularly affected by occipitotemporal cortical dysfunction. Amnesia, aphasia, and neuropsychiatric syndromes do not generally interfere with performance on these measures.

Some neuropsychiatric patients are inattentive, and a simple means of quantitating their lack of vigilance is a target cancellation task, of which several versions are available. A target cancellation task may also be performed abnormally in perceptual-motor patients, although frank hemineglect is distinctly uncommon in this setting.

Neurologic Examination

Patients with progressive aphasia rarely have any somatic abnormalities, but exceptional cases include patients with dysfluent aphasia associated with progressive frontal lobe and basal ganglia degeneration. Such patients may have corticobasal degeneration with an asymmetric akinetic-rigid syndrome and myoclonus.

Perceptual-motor patients typically have prominent somatic abnormalities. Motor dysfunction includes not only apraxia but hyperactive deep tendon reflexes that are generally asymmetric and occasionally may be accompanied by Babinski's sign. Gait is often unsteady. Rarely, patients may have greater involvement of the lower than the upper limb with frank spastic circumduction when walking. Somatosensory function is commonly impaired, especially in the more apraxic or spastic upper limb. Tactile object recognition is most commonly affected, and less often, more basic submodalities such as proprioception and two-point discrimination are also impaired. Visual impairments are alluded to above and are difficult to elicit on neurologic examination. Some severely affected patients may be presented with a wide array of objects on a desk top and asked to find a specific one. Such patients are slow and may fail altogether, reflecting asimultanagnosia or another aspect of disturbed spatial perception.

Neuropsychiatric patients usually have primitive "frontal release" reflexes such as palmomental and snout reflexes. These are entirely nonspecific and can be seen in any of the patients described in this chapter as well as in normal elderly individuals, but they may be diagnostically helpful when present in a young patient. Some have pronounced spasticity, which may involve speech (spastic dysarthria) as well as limbs. This may be asymmetric. Some patients may have subtle signs more commonly seen in extrapyramidal syndromes due to the intimate anatomic relationships between the frontal cortices, basal ganglia, and ascending dopaminergic pathways, which together comprise an integrated "frontostriatal system." Such signs may include hypomimia (reduced facial expression) and a mild hypokinetic dysarthria. Patients with motor neuron disease and dementia may present with a neuropsychiatric syndrome, so care should be taken to look for fasciculations and muscle weakness.

TESTS

Neuropsychology

Neuropsychological assessment needs to be tailored to the patient and to the severity of the disease. Patients who are evaluated late in their clinical course may not be suitable for detailed neuropsychological testing. Further, many clinical features are shared by different degenerative cortical diseases in their terminal stages.

Progressive Aphasia

Language must be carefully surveyed to confirm the presence and type of aphasia. Secondly, tests that do not depend on language must be utilized to document the relative preservation of nonlanguage skills.

Perceptual-Motor Syndrome

Unusual visual disorders such as visual disorientation, asimultanagnosia, prosopagnosia, and other complex visual disturbances may preserve visual acuity yet render the patient visually disabled. Some available tests include the Judgement of Line Orientation and Facial Recognition Tests developed by Benton and collaborators. Timed motor tasks provide quantitative measurement of motor dysfunction and may be used to gauge future disease progression.

Neuropsychiatric Syndrome

Frontal lobe degeneration may produce subtle clinical signs early in the course so that detailed neuropsychological testing is essential. In such patients with normal intelligence quotients, memory, and language, tests of executive control may be very helpful. The Wisconsin Card Sorting Test invites perseveration, and frontal lobe patients make many perseverative errors. A second useful test is the Booklet Category Test, which assesses abstraction abilities.

Neuroimaging

Structural

Computed tomography (CT) and magnetic resonance imaging (MRI) are the most important diagnostic tests to obtain in any patient with a progressive focal neurologic syndrome, particularly because a tumor or other structural lesion may be the underlying cause. If no structural lesion is found, however, the area of clinical interest should be carefully scrutinized for focal atrophy. Focal atrophy is subtle, but it supports the clinical impression of ACDS. It is also nonspecific, however, and patients with focal atrophy serendipitously discovered on CT-MRI performed for problems unrelated to ACDS should not be inferred to have ACDS.

Physiologic

Single photon emission CT (SPECT) and positron emission tomography (PET) are generally far more sensitive than CT and MRI for demonstrating a focal cortical abnormality in patients with ACDS, although

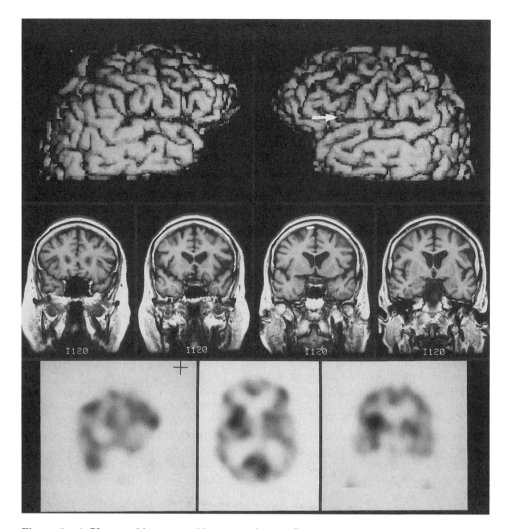

Figure 1 A 73-year-old woman with progressive nonfluent aphasia of 5 years duration. *Top row,* Magnetic resonance imaging (MRI)–based surface rendered lateral views of right and left hemispheres. Note normal contour of pars triangularis of the frontal operculum on the right, and compare it to focally atrophic pars triangularis on the left (*arrow*). *Middle row,* Coronal MRI demonstrating atrophy of left frontal operculum. *Bottom row,* Left sagittal, transaxial, and coronal single photon emission computed tomography (SPECT) images demonstrating (*from left to right*) hypoperfusion of the left frontal operculum, anterior temporal lobe, and basal ganglia. (From Caselli RJ, Jack CR Jr, Peterson RC, et al. Asymmetric cortical degenerative syndromes: Clinical and radiologic correlations. Neurology 1992; 42:1462–1468; with permission.)

SPECT and PET are more nonspecific. Areas of hyometabolism on SPECT and PET are generally larger than areas of atrophy on CT and MRI, although some patients may have normal physiologic studies early in their course. Patients with metabolic abnormalities of unknown significance should not be inferred to have ACDS. As with focal atrophy on CT and MRI, focal metabolic abnormalities on SPECT and PET support the clinically suspected diagnosis of ACDS but do not necessarily imply ACDS in a patient who does not have the appropriate clinical syndrome.

Neuroimaging studies, including surface rendered MRI, planar MRI, and SPECT from patients represent-

ing each of the three main categories of ACDS are shown in Figures 1, 2, and 3.

Electroencephalography

Electroencephalography (EEG) usually serves little purpose in the diagnostic evaluation of a patient suspected of having ACDS. However, exceptional patients presenting with a rapidly progressive course of several months duration should have an EEG to look for the periodic complexes of Creutzfeldt-Jakob disease, which can, rarely, present in a fashion similar to ACDS.

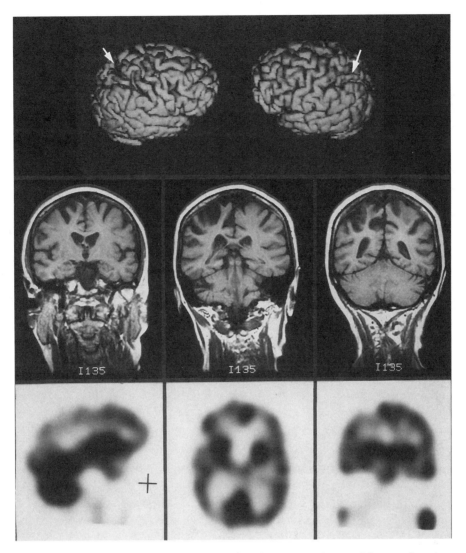

Figure 2 A 64-year-old woman with perceptual-motor syndrome of 2 years duration, particularly affecting left upper limb. *Top row,* MRI-based surface rendered lateral views of right and left hemispheres demonstrating atrophy of the right and, to a lesser degree, the left superior parietal lobules (*arrows*). *Middle row*, Coronal MRI demonstrating severe right parietal and mild left posterior parietal lobe atrophy. *Bottom row,* Right sagittal, transaxial, and coronal SPECT images demonstrating (*from left to right*) severe right parietal and mild left parietal lobe hypoperfusion. (From Caselli RJ, Jack CR Jr, Peterson RC, et al. Asymmetric cortical degenerative syndromes: Clinical and radiologic correlations. Neurology 1992; 42:1462–1468; with permission.)

Cerebral Angiography

I do not generally perform angiograms on these patients, and in the few who have undergone angiography, no causative cerebrovascular lesion was discovered. Nonetheless, if a patient has a suggestive cerebrovascular history, angiography is reasonable. Patients with a stuttering, progressive hemiparesis may have a tightly stenotic, surgically correctable carotid artery. None of the full, slowly progressive ACDS syndromes as described earlier, however, have ever been shown to result from such a vascular lesion. The recent advent of magnetic resonance angiography may provide a nonin-

vasive alternative to intra-arterial cerebral angiography in patients suspected of having ACDS.

Brain Biopsy

Because the presentations of ACDS are generally so characteristic and the differential diagnosis (following noninvasive testing) entirely degenerative, it is hard to justify a brain biopsy, particularly in an elderly individual. However, in young patients, after full discussion with patient and family, brain biopsy is reasonable if just to secure the suspected diagnosis. In patients who undergo

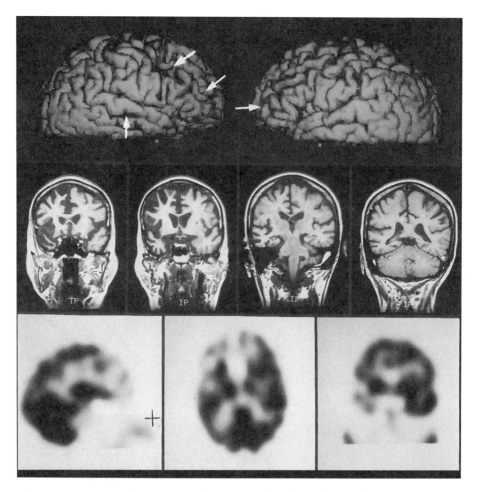

Figure 3 A 71-year-old woman with a neuropsychiatric syndrome of 2 years duration. *Top row,* MRI-based surface rendered lateral views of right and left hemispheres demonstrating bilateral frontal lobe atrophy (worse on the right), and atrophy of right temporal lobe. Note widening of the superior and middle temporal gyri (*arrows*). Inferior aspects of the temporal lobes could not be reproduced in this patient due to a failure of data acquisition. *Middle row,* Coronal MRI demonstrating bifrontal and severe right temporal atrophy. *Bottom row,* Right sagittal, transaxial, and coronal SPECT images demonstrating (*from left to right*) bifrontal (worse on the right) and right temporal hypoperfusion. (From Caselli RJ, Jack CR Jr, Peterson RC, et al. Asymmetric cortical degenerative syndromes: Clinical and radiologic correlations. Neurology 1992; 42: 1462–1468; with permission.)

biopsy, SPECT or PET may be useful for selecting a biopsy site. The area selected should be involved by the disease process (judged clinically and radiologically) but should be chosen to cause the least further neurologic dysfunction to the patient. Attendant risks, including that of a nondiagnostic biopsy, must be understood by all concerned before proceeding.

Other Tests

Cerebrospinal Fluid Examination

I usually perform this in any patient with cerebral dysfunction of less than 1 year's duration if noninvasive testing provides no definitive diagnosis, even if the diagnosis suspected is degenerative. It should be performed in all patients in whom brain biopsy is contemplated.

Blood Tests and General Laboratory Studies

An adequate general survey of routine, general medical tests is reasonable in any patient who has not undergone similar testing for over a year. Unlike global dementias, however, which resemble chronic encephalopathies that may complicate some systemic illnesses, ACDS is not a recognized complication of a systemic disorder.

SUGGESTED READING

Alajouanine T. Aphasia and artistic realization. Brain 1948; 71: 229–241.

Brun A. Frontal lobe degeneration of the non-Alzheimer type: I. Neuropathology. Arch Gerontol Geriatr 1987; 6:193–208.

Caselli RJ, Jack CR Jr. Asymmetric cortical degeneration syndromes: A proposed clinical classification. Arch Neurol 1992; 49:770–780.

Caselli RJ, Jack CR Jr, Petersen RC, Wahner HW, Yanagihara T. Asymmetric cortical degeneration syndromes: Clinical and radiologic correlations. Neurology 1992; 42:1462–1468.

Green J, Morris JC, Sandson J, McKeel DW Jr, Miller JW. Progressive aphasia: A precursor of global dementia? Neurology 1990; 40: 423–429.

Jagust WJ, Davies P, Tiller-Borcich JK, Reed BR. Focal Alzheimer's disease. Neurology 1990; 40:14–19.

Lezak MD. Neuropsychological assessment: A compendium of neuropsychological tests. 2nd ed. New York: Oxford University Press, 1983.

Mesulam MM. Slowly progressive aphasia without generalized dementia. Ann Neurol 1982; 11:592–598.

Neary D, Snowden JS, Northen B, Goulding P. Dementia of frontal lobe type. J Neurol Neurosurg Psychiatry 1988; 51:353–361.

Sawle GV, Brooks DJ, Marsden CD, Frackowiak RSJ. Corticobasal degeneration. Brain 1991; 114:541–556.

PARKINSON'S DISEASE AND OTHER AKINETIC RIGID SYNDROMES

JOSEPH H. FRIEDMAN, M.D.

The advantages which have been derived from the caution with which hypothetical statements are admitted, are in no instance more obvious than in those sciences which more particularly belong to the healing art. It therefore is necessary that some conciliatory explanation should be offered for the present publication: in which, it is acknowledged, that mere conjecture takes the place of experiment; and, that analogy is the substitute for anatomical examination, the only sure foundation for pathological knowledge.

Preface to James Parkinson's *Essay on the Shaking Palsy*

The diagnosis of Parkinson's disease (PD), as in James Parkinson's day, rests purely on clinical criteria. Laboratory studies, when obtained, are useful only in excluding other diagnoses and cannot be used, as of this writing, to confirm a diagnosis. There is no way to be certain of the diagnosis of PD in life, as autopsy studies have shown. My own practice is to obtain no neurologic studies in cases that I believe are straightforward and lack atypical features.

The cardinal features of PD are tremor at rest, rigidity, akinesia, bradykinesia, and postural abnormalities. Disease onset is always insidious and often unilateral. Tremor typically affects the fingers (pill rolling tremor) or hands but may involve the feet, legs, jaw, or tongue. The tremor resolves with movement but may return with sustained posture. Tremor rarely involves the head or voice. Reinforcement maneuvers sometimes bring out a mild tremor, and the typical rest tremor of PD is often seen best while the patient is walking, hands hanging at the sides.

Increased tone is appreciated through passive movements of a limb at rest. Cogwheeling may or may not be present, but hypertonia should be. Tone may be increased on both flexion and extension and is not rate related, unlike spasticity, which is rate dependent. Reinforcement maneuvers such as having the patient tap or repetitively move the limb *not* being assessed often increase tone or produce cogwheeling. This also distracts the patient from actively moving the tested limb. Not only may tone be markedly asymmetric, but it may be markedly different at different joints in the same limb. Hence a wrist may be extremely rigid while the ipsilateral elbow may be only mildly affected. The neck should be checked since some patients suffer from greater axial than appendicular rigidity.

Akinesia is obvious to the trained eye yet often missed by the less experienced. Parkinson's patients move less, blink less, and swallow less than normal people. They also move more slowly and display problems with both rhythmicity and amplitude on performing repetitive tasks. Testing should involve a variety of simple maneuvers since abnormalities may be apparent on one test only, whereas other maneuvers may reveal borderline or possibly normal movements. I have patients perform rapid finger tapping, hand opening, alternating hand movements, heel tapping, and toe tapping.

The postural abnormalities of PD refer to the abnormal flexion that is present to some degree in all joints, as well as to the common tilt to one side that may result in scoliosis. Combined with this problem are the postural instability and impaired postural reflexes that result in falls. Balance should be tested by pulling patients backwards. This should be done forcefully if mild pulls do not cause the patient to step backward. Obviously the subject must be warned in advance and the physician must be prepared to catch the patient. Responses vary from the normal single step backward to multiple steps, persistent festination, or no righting response at all, with the patient falling like a stiff board.

Some authorities consider a positive response to levodopa a cardinal feature of PD. While this is certainly supportive evidence of PD, there have been pathologically documented, albeit rare, cases of PD without a response to levodopa. In addition, patients with akinetic rigid states other than PD may benefit from this drug, although usually not to a great extent. Hence a positive response to levodopa may be misleading. A negative response should prompt trials of higher doses to a ceiling of about 1 g daily. Lack of response to 1 g generally predicts a lack of response at higher doses.

Asymmetry of onset is common in PD and is taken as a supportive sign of the diagnosis. Early in the course of the disease, especially if the patient is young, asymmetric hypokinesia and rigidity may simulate a corticospinal tract lesion and trigger a very appropriate concern for a mass or demyelination in the brain. When the brain magnetic resonance imaging (MRI) is normal in a patient with unilateral slowness and stiffness, with only a slight degree of tremor, the differential diagnosis should include PD. It should be kept in mind that drug-induced parkinsonism can also be asymmetric.

My own approach to the diagnosis rests more on the neurologic exam than on the history, although the history is clearly important. The history must exclude recent use of dopamine blocking or depleting drugs. These drugs never cause irreversible parkinsonism, but their parkinsonian side effects may persist for up to 18 months. Family history is useful. While most cases of PD are not familial, some are, the genetics of which are not clear. Multiple traumatic injuries to the brain may result in a progressive neurologic degenerative state, dementia pugilistica, but should be rare outside of former boxers. Typically this simulates a multisystem atrophy more than PD. Postencephalitic parkinsonism is exceedingly rare but may occur. A history of strokes and stroke risk factors suggest a possible multi-infarct state.

The neurologic exam should, of course, be complete and should be particularly detailed with respect to motor control. The mental status exam may reveal speech abnormalities that include low amplitude, breathy speech, and, occasionally, slurring, stuttering, and hesitancy. Rare patients become mute. Cranial nerves are normal except for visual pursuit, which is often saccadic instead of smooth. When the parkinsonism is asymmetric, there is often facial asymmetry that can easily be mistaken for facial weakness.

DIFFERENTIAL DIAGNOSIS

While PD is by far the most common akinetic rigid syndrome, many other parkinsonian syndromes should be considered when making a diagnosis. Lack of tremor, balance problems out of proportion to gait dysfunction, and prominent dementia should always signal a cautious approach. Probably the most common syndrome to mimic PD, at least early in the course, is progressive supranuclear palsy (PSP). These patients constitute about 5 percent of the total number of patients seen at PD referral centers. Interestingly, although PSP is clearly distinguishable from PD in advanced cases and is relatively common, this was not a recognized entity until 1960. PSP is manifest primarily by akinesia, postural instability, and eye movement abnormalities. The clinical diagnosis cannot be made until impairment of voluntary

eye movements in the vertical plane occurs. Tremor is rare, and axial dystonia is common. The voice changes may be quite different from PD in that nasal, slow, labored speech is common. The early features of PSP that frequently predate the eye movement abnormality are falling due to poor balance with a surprisingly intact gait; a dystonic facial appearance that looks more like a fixed smile than the "masked" facial expression of PD; and inappropriate visual orienting, with the patient turning the head before moving the eyes to look at visual stimuli. Optokinetic nystagmus abnormalities and difficulty with visual fixation, which causes "macro square wave jerks" (sudden horizontal saccades to either side), predate the limitation in voluntary eye movements. Patients frequently complain of visual dysfunction despite having normal acuity and fields. Commonly patients complain of having recently had changes in their eyeglasses without improvement in their vision. This history alone is highly suggestive of PSP.

The "dolls' eyes" test is performed to prove that the gaze palsy is supranuclear. If a patient cannot voluntarily move the eyes, but the eyes move on reflex testing, then clearly the brain stem nuclei are intact and the lesion must be higher, hence *supranuclear*. Unfortunately, patients with vertical palsies may have extremely rigid necks, making flexion and extension impossible. Since the brain stem reflexes should be intact, one can use warm or cold caloric stimulation in the ear canals, giving both simultaneously, to force the eyes conjugately up or down. Since this can be uncomfortable, only small amounts of water should be used. The patient should be positioned so that the ears are at about 30 degrees to the horizontal.

Drug-induced parkinsonism is impossible to distinguish from idiopathic PD. It may even be asymmetric, so that any patient with parkinsonism who has been taking a dopamine blocking drug can at most be considered a PD "suspect" but cannot be diagnosed as having PD until the syndrome worsens after the drug has been discontinued.

Aside from drug-induced parkinsonism and PSP, the other akinetic rigid syndromes, excluding perhaps striatonigral degeneration (SND), are considerably less common. SND is an illness that may present exactly like PD. Some experts think it is the most common disorder to mimic PD, but there is little data to support this. SND is one of the multisystem atrophies that include Shy-Drager syndrome (SDS) and olivopontocerebellar atrophy (OPCA). Clinically, SND may manifest as PD, or PD without tremor. Other signs such as cerebellar ataxia, autonomic dysfunction, or corticospinal tract signs may clearly distinguish SND from PD. Typically the response to levodopa is poor. SDS is, like normal pressure hydrocephalus (see below), more talked about than seen. SDS is a rare syndrome that is clinically defined by severe orthostatic hypotension, to the point of difficulty maintaining a vertical posture, bladder and bowel dysfunction, sweating and heart rate abnormalities, coupled with an akinetic rigid syndrome plus cerebellar and corticospinal tract signs. This is such an uncommon syndrome that I am reluctant to diagnose it unless autonomic failure is the central, overwhelming clinical problem. It is fairly common for PD patients to suffer from mild to moderate autonomic problems due to the side effects of PD medications plus the occasional degeneration in central (and rarely peripheral) sympathetic nervous system sites. If the patient first develops PD, responds well to levodopa, and then suffers orthostatic hypotension, PD is a much more likely diagnosis than SDS.

OPCA is another rare syndrome in which cerebellar findings are prominent features in addition to the akinetic rigid state. OPCA may be either hereditary or sporadic. Brain imaging may be helpful in making this diagnosis, as olivary and pontine atrophy should be present.

Normal pressure hydrocephalus (NPH) is an exceedingly difficult entity to diagnose. If a patient has a known cause for the hydrocephalus, such as meningitis or a subarachnoid hemorrhage, then a progressive gait problem with dementia, incontinence, and hydrocephalus under normal pressure, coupled with an appropriate computed tomography scan makes the diagnosis. For patients without a known cause for the hydrocephalus, there is no diagnostic test that increases the chance of a positive shunt response other than perhaps a transient response to withdrawal of large amounts of cerebrospinal fluid (CSF) (30 cc daily for 3 days). My own approach to NPH is to consider the diagnosis in patients with a gait disorder that looks like PD from the waist down but with relatively intact arm swing and little in the way of dementia. I will accept minor parkinsonian features in the arms as well.

Urinary urgency and frequency are supportive symptoms. In this setting, I will obtain a brain magnetic resonance image (MRI) to look at ventricular size, check for the presence of periventricular edema, and ascertain whether the patient has suffered multiple small, subclinical strokes. Unfortunately, the diagnosis of NPH can be made only if the patient responds to shunting. For patients whom I am unsure whether to shunt, I perform serial CSF withdrawals. Since the sensitivity of this test is unknown, I do not withdraw CSF in patients I will shunt anyway. Although NPH has been clinically defined as a triad of gait disturbance, urinary incontinence, and dementia, patients with prominent dementia are less likely to respond to shunting, thereby, a posteriori, making the diagnosis difficult to confirm.

Multi-infarct state, or *atherosclerotic parkinsonism,* a term that has found some resurgence since the advent of MRI, usually produces an akinetic rigid state without tremor. Corticospinal signs, often asymmetric, are present along with dementia and frontal release signs. The presence of stroke risk factors, previous clinical strokes, and weakness makes the diagnosis more certain, but frequently one sees patients without a stepwise progression, presumably reflecting the cumulative effects of multiple tiny infarcts.

There are other "Parkinson plus" disorders—that is, syndromes of parkinsonism plus other abnormalities—to consider. Diffuse Lewy body disease has been receiving attention recently due to advances in neuropathology. In this disorder there is degeneration in the pigmented brain stem nuclei plus the cortex, with Lewy bodies present in both. This produces a parkinsonian condition with a "cortical dementia"—that is, involving aphasia or apraxia. The clinical spectrum appears to be quite broad, with pathologically verified cases presenting as typical PD, typical Alzheimer's type dementia, combinations of the two, and atypical parkinsonism or dementia.

Corticobasalganglionic degeneration is unusual for a cerebral degeneration in that it is generally quite asymmetric, producing rigidity and slowness either on one side or in one arm and the opposite leg. Mental status changes are prominent, with progressive aphasia or apraxia without memory dysfunction. Early on, this condition is frequently misdiagnosed as a stroke. Only with insidious progression does the error become apparent. Resting tremor does not occur. Corticospinal tract signs and limb dystonia are common. Supranuclear gaze palsies may occur.

Dementia pugilistica is a neurodegenerative process resulting from multiple concussive or subconcussive blows to the head and may develop years after the last trauma. Patients are usually demented but not always, with progressive parkinsonian features along with cerebellar or corticospinal tract signs. The history of boxing is obviously crucial.

Creutzfeldt-Jakob disease can mimic PD but should not be confused with it, because of the prominent dementia and rapid progression.

Depression in the elderly can simulate PD, just as PD may simulate depression. Distinction is sometimes complicated by the normal slowness that comes with aging. Obviously depressed patients have an abnormal affect and should not have rigidity or resting tremors. Gait, balance, and posture assessments can be hard to interpret, especially in the frail elderly.

In assessing a patient, one can usually decide immediately if the syndrome is typical or atypical for PD. When dealing with akinetic rigid syndromes that are atypical for Parkinson's disease, one must try to decide whether two distinct syndromes are occurring concurrently or there is one unifying illness. For example, when dementia develops in an elderly PD patient, is it the PD alone, diffuse Lewy body disease, PD plus Alzheimer's disease, or PD plus depression with pseudodementia? In this common scenario I use the presence of so-called cortical features such as language and praxis disorders to determine the presence of cortical degeneration. If it is not present and the progression is slow, I assume that the dementia is part of the PD. If it is present, I cannot reliably distinguish diffuse Lewy body disease from PD plus Alzheimer's disease. Neuropsychological testing may be helpful in diagnosing pseudodementia.

When the PD suspect has corticospinal tract features, one must be alert for the presence of strokes or cervical myelopathy. Since certain strokes can ameliorate tremor, the atypical features of focal reflex changes, absent tremor, and mild weakness in a patient with otherwise typical PD should prompt a concern for dual diagnoses.

COMMENTS

In the best of hands the clinical diagnosis of PD is incorrect 20 percent of the time. There are seemingly typical cases that are found at autopsy to be something else. However, other akinetic rigid syndromes are treated with the same drugs used to treat PD. Typically the response is disappointing and the prognosis poorer, but rarely is harm done to the patient through an incorrect diagnosis.

SUGGESTED READING

Calne DB, Snow BJ, Lee C. Criteria for diagnosing Parkinson's disease. Ann Neurol 1992; 32(suppl):125–127.
Hughes AJ, Daniel SE, Kilford L, Lees AS. Parkinson's disease: A clinico-pathological study. J Neurol Neurosurg Psychiatry 1991; 54:181–184.
Jankovic J, Tolosa E, eds. Parkinson's disease and movement disorders. Baltimore: Urban & Schwarzenberg, 1988.
Koller WC, ed. Handbook of Parkinson's disease. 2nd ed. New York: Marcel Dekker, 1992.
Koller WC, Stern MB, eds. Parkinsonian syndromes. New York: Marcel Dekker, 1993.
Lang AE, Weiner WJ, eds. Drug induced movement disorders. Mt Kisco, NY: Futura, 1992.

AMYOTROPHIC LATERAL SCLEROSIS

RICHARD K. OLNEY, M.D.

Amyotrophic lateral sclerosis (ALS) is an adult onset, idiopathic form of motor neuron disease. By definition, the disease affects both upper and lower motor neurons, with sparing of sensory, autonomic, cerebellar, extrapyramidal, and higher cortical functions. ALS is typically sporadic in its occurrence, but roughly 5 percent of cases are familial, usually with autosomal dominant inheritance. ALS is the most common, but not the only, form of motor neuron disease. I use the term *motor neuron disease* broadly, to include many other diagnostic entities, from hereditary lower motor neuron syndromes (spinal muscular atrophies) to motor neuron syndromes that have recognized causes (e.g., infection with poliovirus or intoxication with lead). With regard to

a motor neuron syndrome that may have a recognizable cause (but may not have been fully evaluated yet) or a remediable cause (e.g., a laboratory abnormality has been recognized, but the benefit of treatment has not yet been determined), I also use the term *an ALS-like syndrome,* if unequivocal signs of upper and lower motor neuron involvement are present.

ALS is a syndrome clinically characterized by weakness, muscular wasting, incoordination, and spasticity that affects two or more levels of the neuraxis and is progressive over months to years (Table 1). The levels to which I refer are bulbar, cervical, and lumbosacral, with thoracic being useful as an additional potential level of lower motor neuron involvement in distinguishing spondylitic polyradiculopathy from motor neuron disease. Fasciculations and cramping occur in many patients with ALS and other motor neuron diseases. These symptoms may precede the recognition of weakness by the patient. However, neither fasciculations nor cramping need be present to diagnose ALS. I base the diagnosis of ALS or an ALS-like syndrome first and foremost on *unequivocal* signs of upper motor neuron disease affecting two or more levels of the neuraxis, and

Table 1 Primary Clinical Signs of Amyotrophic Lateral Sclerosis

Level	Upper Motor Neuron	Lower Motor Neuron
Bulbar	Weakness of the soft palate with hyperactive gag reflex Spastic dysarthria	Weakness, wasting, and fasciculations of tongue (and possibly facial) muscles
Cervical	Weakness with slow movements Spastic tone in flexors Hyperactive tendon reflexes with intersegmental spread or clonus	Weakness and wasting (or EMG signs of acute and chronic partial denervation) in 2 or more muscles innervated by different nerves and different roots
Lumbosacral	Weakness with slow movements Spastic tone in extensors Hyperactive tendon reflexes with intersegmental spread or clonus Extensor plantar response	Weakness and wasting (or EMG signs of acute and chronic partial denervation) in 2 or more muscles innervated by different nerves and different roots

EMG = electromyogram.

of lower motor neuron disease affecting two or more levels of the neuraxis. Whereas I conclude that either ALS or an ALS-like syndrome is present by the extent of motor neuron involvement, I render the diagnosis of ALS only if full clinical and laboratory evaluation has disclosed no abnormality that may explain the motor neuron disease, or if the condition identified by the laboratory abnormality has been treated effectively and significant progression continues. In the remainder of this chapter, I will describe first the signs that I accept as unequivocal documentation of upper and lower motor neuron involvement for each level of neuraxis. Then I will summarize my diagnostic approach to the various presentations of ALS based on these definitions, and include my differential diagnosis and laboratory evaluation for each of these presentations. In each of these sections, I will also discuss the point in the evaluation or evolution of the disease at which I tell the patient that he or she has ALS.

CLINICAL SIGNS OF UPPER AND LOWER MOTOR NEURON INVOLVEMENT FOR EACH LEVEL OF THE NEURAXIS

Bulbar, Lower Motor Neuron

The primary signs of lower motor neuron involvement of bulbar musculature are weakness, wasting, and fasciculations of the tongue. Weakness precedes wasting and usually begins asymmetrically. The tongue protrudes less fully and often off midline; it is also pushed less forcefully into the cheeks. Weakness of the tongue may produce lingual dysarthria, which is most easily detected during repetitive pronunciation of a consonant such as *t*. However, weakness of the tongue may be due to either upper or lower motor neuron disease. Thus, the unequivocal sign of lower motor neuron involvement is significant wasting. This is manifest as scalloping of one or both edges before an obvious loss of tongue thickness. If wasting is associated with frequent fasciculations while the tongue is relaxed within the mouth, lower motor neuron involvement is unequivocal. I do not consider lower motor neuron involvement definite if I see only subtle scolloping without fasciculations at rest. Weakness of facial and palatal muscles is commonly associated with lower motor weakness of the tongue but may be seen also with purely upper motor neuron diseases. Wasting is more difficult to see in facial and palatal, than in tongue, muscles until the lower motor disease is advanced. Fasciculations without wasting are not alone diagnostic of lower motor neuron degeneration.

Bulbar, Upper Motor Neuron

The primary signs of upper motor neuron involvement of the bulbar musculature are spastic weakness of the soft palate and spastic dysarthria. To have unequivocal clinical signs of spastic weakness, the soft palate must be obviously weak, with clearly decreased speed and amplitude of voluntary movement when saying "Ahhhh" and must be obviously spastic by having much brisker and greater amplitude of movement precipitated by the gag reflex than was seen with voluntary effort. Spastic speech is dysarthric with slow, indistinct articulation of labial ("m,m,m"), lingual ("t,t,t") and guttural ("k,k,k") consonants, and has a characteristic strained and nasal quality. Whereas the preceding signs are usually the most objective and early signs of unequivocal upper motor neuron disease, several other signs are often present to a mild extent early. Alternating movements of the tongue are slower than normal and disproportionately so relative to the extent of any associated lower motor neuron weakness. The jaw jerk may be brisk, and rarely even exhibits clonus. Facial movements may demonstrate mildly delayed relaxation; for example, a delay may be seen during rapid alternation of smiling and relaxation. Pseudobulbar affect may be present.

Cervical or Lumbosacral, Lower Motor Neuron

The primary clinical signs for lower motor neuron involvement of limb musculature are weakness and wasting. To unequivocally document lower motor neuron disease in a limb, the weakness and wasting must affect two or more muscles whose innervation does not share the same nerve root or the same peripheral nerve structure. Within the rubric of the same peripheral nerve structure, I include any portion of a plexus, a branch of a plexus, or a limb nerve. If I have even the slightest question with regard to the distribution of significant weakness and wasting within a limb, I perform electromyographic (EMG) studies. For EMG studies to provide evidence of lower motor neuron disease affecting any one muscle, I require reduced recruitment of motor unit action potentials (that is, recruitment of fewer motor units than is appropriate for the firing frequency), an increased incidence of long-duration or large-amplitude motor unit action potentials than is appropriate for age in that muscle, *and* fibrillation potentials in two or more areas of the muscle. For EMG studies to document unequivocal lower motor neuron disease in the limb, the preceding EMG signs must be recorded in two or more muscles whose innervation does not share the same nerve root or the same peripheral nerve structure. The presence of fasciculations is supportive but by itself not diagnostic of lower motor neuron disease.

Cervical or Lumbosacral, Upper Motor Neuron

The signs of upper motor neuron involvement of limb muscles are weakness, slowness of movement, loss of dexterity of movements, spastic resistance to passive stretch, and pathologically hyperactive tendon reflexes and extensor plantar responses. Of these signs, weakness is the least specific because it may be explained by associated lower motor neuron disease. Slowness and loss of dexterity of movement develop early in the course of upper motor neuron disease. Mild amounts of such incoordination may be due to lower motor neuron weakness, arthritis, or even poor effort from depression. Thus, to confidently document upper motor neuron disease, I require at least one of three additional signs. The first of these is spastic resistance to passive stretch (that is, a catch followed by a release) of the biceps brachii, forearm pronators, or quadriceps muscle groups. The second is a pathologically hyperactive reflex, either one with clonus or one that produces intersegmental spread (for example, a biceps tendon reflex that spreads ipsilaterally to finger flexors, or a quadriceps tendon reflex that spreads contralaterally to the adductor). The third sign is an unequivocal extensor plantar response. I define this as one in which I elicit a slow dystonic extension of the great toe and a fanning flexion-abduction of the lateral toes.

DIAGNOSTIC EVALUATION

Amyotrophic Lateral Sclerosis–Like Syndrome

Patients occasionally present for evaluation after their motor neuron disease has become sufficiently widespread to have unequivocal signs of upper motor neuron disease affecting two or more levels of the neuraxis, and of lower motor neuron disease affecting two or more levels of the neuraxis. Usually these patients have been evaluated and followed by other physicians earlier in their course and are referred for confirmation of the diagnosis of ALS. With this presentation, the focus of the diagnostic evaluation is to identify secondary forms of motor neuron disease, for which treatment may be available (Table 2). Labeling any form of a fully developed ALS-like syndrome as potentially treatable is controversial, but there are four possible secondary forms of motor neuron disease that I routinely evaluate (or ensure have been previously evaluated) in this clinical context: a monoclonal protein disorder, a reticuloendothelial cell neoplasia, an immune-mediated disorder, and lead intoxication. I believe that the incidence of ALS-like syndromes may be increased in association with these diseases, but that treatment of the non-neurological disorder infrequently results in meaningful improvement in the motor neuron disease. Thus, if one of these diseases is identified, I do not change the diagnosis from an ALS-like syndrome to ALS, at least initially. I acknowledge to the patient and the other treating physicians that the association of the two diseases may be coincidental rather than causative, and that aggressive treatment of the non-neurological disease has only a low probability of reversing the motor neuron disease. Yet, given the alternative of no treatment and the high probability of progression to respiratory failure without treatment, therapy is usually initiated with the patient's informed consent. If neurological progression continues for 3 to 6 months after effective therapy has been instituted, I then change the diagnosis to ALS.

Table 2 Laboratory Findings in Classic Amyotrophic Lateral Sclerosis

Normal results for:
Complete blood count with differential and platelet count
Serum protein electrophoresis
Serum immunofixation (or immunoelectrophoresis)
Urinalysis, including a test for light chains
Cerebrospinal fluid analysis, including protein, glucose, cells, cytology
Bone marrow biopsy, if abnormalities above suggest need
Erythrocyte sedimentation rate
Antinuclear antibody and rheumatoid factor
Anti-GM1–ganglioside antibody
Blood lead
Free erythrocyte protoporphyrin, or 24 hour urine for lead, delta-aminolevulinic acid, and porphobilinogen

With regard to the possibility of a monoclonal protein disorder or reticuloendothelial cell neoplasia, I obtain (or review) complete blood count (CBC) with differential, platelet count, serum protein electrophoresis, serum immunofixation, urinalysis, and cerebrospinal fluid (CSF) analysis. If a monoclonal protein is identified, the CBC has unexplained abnormalities, or the CSF protein is 75 mg per deciliter or higher, I obtain a bone marrow biopsy. If a monoclonal protein disorder, plasma cell dyscrasia, lymphoma, or leukemia is identified, I then recommend chemotherapy for 3 to 6 months.

With regard to the possibility of an immune-mediated disorder causing the motor neuron disease, I obtain an erythrocyte sedimentation rate, antinuclear antibody titer, rheumatoid factor titer, and anti-GM1–ganglioside antibody titer. I raise the possibility of an immune-mediated mechanism primarily if the titer of anti-GM1–ganglioside antibody is markedly elevated, and recommend immunosuppressive therapy for 3 to 6 months. Abnormalities of the other three tests heighten suspicion of immune-mediated disease but confound the interpretation of a modestly high titer of anti-GM1–ganglioside antibody, because this titer is commonly elevated in connective tissue diseases without motor neuron disease.

With regard to the possibility of lead intoxication, I obtain a blood lead level and one additional test on all patients. The additional test is either a free erythrocyte protoporphyrin or a 24 hour urine study for lead, delta-aminolevulinic acid, and porphobilinogen. If the history of exposure is extensive and the clinical syndrome predominantly a lower motor neuron one, a 24 hour urine study for quantitative lead excretion immediately before and after one dosage of chelation therapy is indicated. Only if chelation significantly increases lead excretion do I strongly consider that lead intoxication is the cause for the ALS-like syndrome.

Asymmetrical Lower Motor Neuron Weakness of a Hand

Progressive weakness of a hand is the single most common presentation for ALS. However, if objective signs are limited to those of lower motor neuron involvement of the one symptomatic limb, the diagnosis of ALS cannot be made. The initial differential diagnosis is quite broad and includes focal neuropathies, brachial plexopathy, cervical radiculopathy, cervical spinal cord disease, and segmental anterior horn cell disease. Detailed EMG and nerve conduction studies are almost always necessary to narrow these diagnostic possibilities. Electrodiagnostic signs of asymmetrical sensory axonal loss redirects attention to a peripheral nerve disease process distal to the dorsal root ganglion. Whereas objective sensory involvement is apparent clinically in most focal peripheral nerve disease processes, three with insidious onset require special consideration because of the absence or subtlety of sensory impairment. Patients over the age of 60 years with carpal tunnel syndrome occasionally present with severe thenar weakness and wasting, with minimal clinical or electrophysiological evidence for sensory involvement. Patients of any age with ulnar neuropathy at or distal to the wrist often present with weakness and wasting of ulnar intrinsic hand muscles without sensory involvement. These focal neuropathies cannot be excluded if electrodiagnostic signs of lower motor neuron degeneration are limited to the single peripheral nerve distribution. Furthermore, surgical decompression may be beneficial. The third focal peripheral nerve disease process is the true neurogenic thoracic outlet syndrome, in which patients develop weakness and wasting of both thenar and hypothenar muscles (and often C8-innervated forearm muscles too), but may not have objective sensory loss clinically. A reduction in the amplitude of the ulnar sensory nerve action potential then suggests the correct diagnosis.

A final peripheral nerve disease, multifocal motor neuropathy, has been the subject of much recent literature because of the similarity of its presentation to that of early ALS. Patients with multifocal motor neuropathy insidiously develop weakness and fasciculations, usually in one hand, which are not associated with clinical or electrophysiologic evidence of sensory involvement. However, weakness is limited to the distribution of one or more named peripheral nerves, and wasting is usually minimal for the degree of weakness and duration of the disease. The patient is usually young (two-thirds are less than 45 years old) and twice as likely to be male as female. Although highly elevated titers of anti-GM1-ganglioside antibody occur in 80 to 90 percent of these patients, the hallmark of the disease is multifocal conduction block. I confidently diagnose the presence of conduction block if the amplitude is reduced 50 percent and the area is reduced 40 percent (with an increase in duration less than 20 percent) when comparing the compound muscle action potential elicited by distal compared with proximal stimulation at the ends of a 20 cm or less nerve segment. I most often find such evidence for conduction block in the forearm or arm segments of the median or ulnar nerves. Even if weakness is limited to the distribution of a single nerve, the possibility of an early motor neuron disease is often raised by the referring physician. When two or more

nerves are affected, the diagnostic challenge becomes greater. Recognition of this syndrome is important because disabling weakness can usually be reversed by treatment with immunosuppressive drugs or intravenous immunoglobulins.

Cervical spondylitic polyradiculopathy can be a difficult differential diagnostic possibility in patients over the age of 60 years. Radiating cervical pain and dermatomal sensory loss may not be apparent in spondylitic polyradiculopathy. The electrodiagnostic signs of lower motor neuron degeneration must extend beyond a single root distribution to exclude C8 or T1 radiculopathy. The greater degree of tendon reflex depression, and abnormalities on imaging studies such as magnetic resonance imaging (MRI) are most useful in distinguishing cervical spondylitic polyradiculopathy from motor neuron disease. Cervical MRI is also important to evaluate the possibility of syringomyelia and other focal cervical spinal cord pathology with secondary involvement of the anterior horn cells.

After carefully considering the preceding possibilities with electrodiagnostic studies and cervical MRI, the entities remaining in the differential diagnosis are forms of motor neuron disease. ALS cannot be distinguished from idiopathic segmental forms of lower motor neuron disease unless generalization and upper motor neuron involvement develop over time. The probability of weakness remaining restricted to segmental involvement is increased if the patient is young (less than 40 years) and male. In a syndrome variously called juvenile muscular atrophy of unilateral upper extremity, benign focal amyotrophy, or monomelic amyotrophy, weakness and wasting of the hand and forearm develop predominantly over several months to 3 years, usually in males from 15 to 25 years. In a minority, similar symptoms and signs later affect the contralateral upper limb. However, generalization of the lower motor neuron weakness beyond the cervical segment does not occur. In a different syndrome called chronic asymmetrical spinal muscular atrophy, distal or proximal weakness and wasting of first one, and then often the other upper limb develops insidiously between the ages of 20 and 40 years. About one-third of those affected are female. Whatever the age of the patient, I do not diagnose ALS unless the distribution of involvement extends over time to that necessary for an ALS-like syndrome, as previously described. In these patients, immune-mediated disease and lead intoxication warrant evaluation. A syndrome of lower motor neuron disease without conduction block has been described that commonly affects the upper limbs distally and is associated with elevated titers of anti-GM1–ganglioside antibody. However, in contrast to multifocal motor neuropathy, the benefits of immunosuppressive treatment are less clearly established.

Asymmetrical Lower Motor Neuron Weakness of a Leg

The considerations for this clinical presentation are similar to those for asymmetrical upper limb weakness, but the differential diagnostic possibilities are fewer. Peripheral nerve disease processes are usually easily distinguished from lower motor neuron disease. Rarely, multifocal motor neuropathy with conduction block or diabetic amyotrophy may create confusion if they are not considered. L5 radiculopathy or lumbosacral polyradiculopathy is the most common confounding diagnosis. Electrodiagnostic and imaging studies are usually the first steps in the evaluation.

Although the peripheral nerve and nerve root diseases can be distinguished by ancillary studies at presentation, the various forms of motor neuron disease generally cannot be. Chronic asymmetrical spinal muscular atrophy can present with asymmetrical leg weakness. I do not make the diagnosis ALS unless generalization occurs and I have excluded monoclonal protein disorder, reticuloendothelial cell neoplasia, an immune-mediated disorder, and lead intoxication. The syndrome of lower motor neuron disease without conduction block that is associated with elevated titers of anti-GM1-ganglioside antibody affects one or both legs distally in one-third or more of these patients.

Spasticity of Limbs

Progressive upper motor neuron weakness and spasticity of limbs without bulbar or lower motor neuron signs is a presentation of motor neuron disease that usually evolves into ALS, but infrequently remains limited to an upper motor neuron disease referred to as primary lateral sclerosis. The initial differential diagnostic possibilities are primarily those for progressive myelopathy. These include other common disorders, such as compressive cervical myelopathy and multiple sclerosis, and less common diagnoses such as dural arteriovenous fistula and foramen magnum meningioma. The presence of sensory and sphincter symptoms and signs suggests a diagnosis other than motor neuron disease. The evaluation usually starts with EMG studies (to look for subclinical lower motor neuron abnormalities), MRI at and above the highest level of spinal cord involvement, and CSF examination (to include IgG index and oligoclonal bands). Less common considerations may include systemic lupus erythematosus, B_{12} deficiency, HTLV-1 myelopathy, and familial spastic paraplegia. When ALS presents in this manner, lower motor neuron involvement usually develops within 2 years.

Dysarthria or Dysphagia

Bulbar weakness may be the presenting symptom and sign for neuromuscular junction disorders (including myasthenia gravis), muscle diseases (including polymyositis), and various diseases with involvement of upper or lower motor neurons. A small number of patients who eventually prove to have ALS are included in this latter category. Thus, the first step in the diagnostic evaluation of patients who present with dysarthria or dysphagia is to clarify the pathophysiology of the bulbar weakness.

On neurologic examination, patients with diminished voluntary movement of the soft palate, a hyperactive gag reflex, slow weak voluntary movements of the tongue, but normal muscular bulk have upper motor weakness, or pseudobulbar palsy. This is discussed further in the subsequent section. Patients with diminished voluntary movement of the soft palate, a blunted gag reflex, weak voluntary movements of the tongue, but nearly normal speed for these movements have neuromuscular junction, muscle or lower motor neuron weakness. If the tongue has normal bulk and no fasciculations, neuromuscular junction or muscle diseases are more likely. The dysarthria usually has a nasal, breathy sound. If fatigability of the nasal dysarthria is observable, myasthenia gravis or another neuromuscular junction disease is likely. If the tongue has diminished bulk with scalloped edges and fasciculations, lower motor neuron weakness is present.

Electrodiagnostic studies are helpful in clarifying the pathophysiology of bulbar weakness and in assessing the pathophysiology of possibly associated subclinical limb weakness. Needle EMG studies are often performed on facial and tongue muscles but not on the soft palate. EMG examination of the tongue may be less sensitive than EMGs on other muscles but sometimes provides specific information on the cause for tongue weakness. The finding of signs of myopathic lower motor neuron or upper motor neuron weakness in facial and limb muscles suggests the same cause for bulbar weakness. Repetitive stimulation studies on the facial, spinal accessory, and limb nerves can be quite helpful in identifying the presence of neuromuscular junction diseases and in distinguishing myasthenia gravis from the Lambert-Eaton myasthenic syndrome.

If the pathophysiology of the bulbar weakness is ambiguous clinically, and the electrodiagnostic studies suggest neuromuscular junction or muscle disease, muscle enzyme levels (creatine kinase levels in particular) and anti-acetylcholine receptor antibody titers are ordered. If lower motor neuron weakness is identified, metastatic disease (including to the base of the skull), carcinomatous and other forms of basilar meningitis, granulomatous disease (such as sarcoidosis), vasculitis, and other infiltrating and vascular diseases remain in the differential diagnosis.

Pseudobulbar Palsy

Patients with pseudobulbar palsy may present with spastic dysarthria and dysphagia or with labile affect. The differential diagnosis includes many diseases, such as primary and metastatic brain tumors, cerebrovascular disorders, demyelinating disease, and, less commonly, infectious diseases. The evaluation usually starts with an MRI scan of the brain. If this is normal, or at least reveals no signs of mass effect, a CSF examination is usually the next diagnostic step. Subsequent diagnostic steps are dependent upon the differential diagnosis and, if this includes primary CNS involvement from vasculitis, may involve cerebral angiography or other studies.

However, after normal MRI and CSF examinations, the possibility of motor neuron disease may be highest in the differential. Then EMG studies may be the next test ordered, to look for subclinical evidence of lower motor neuron disease. Among the motor neuron diseases, the distinction of primary lateral sclerosis from amyotrophic lateral sclerosis may be suggested if no clinical or electromyographic signs of lower motor neuron involvement develop within 2 years.

SUGGESTED READING

Boothby JA, deJesus PV, Rowland LP. Reversible forms of motor neuron disease: Lead "neuritis." Arch Neurol 1974; 31:18–23.

Li T-M, Alberman E, Swash M. Comparison of sporadic and familial disease amongst 580 cases of motor neuron disease. J Neurol Neurosurg Psychiatry 1988; 51:778–784.

Parry GJ, Clarke S. Multifocal acquired demyelinating neuropathy masquerading as motor neuron disease. Muscle Nerve 1988; 11:103–107.

Pestronk A, Adams RN, Cornblath D, et al. Patterns of serum IgM antibodies to GM1 and GD1a gangliosides in amyotrophic lateral sclerosis. Ann Neurol 1989; 25:98–102.

Pestronk A, Cornblath DR, Ilyas AA, et al. A treatable multifocal motor neuropathy with antibodies to GM1 ganglioside. Ann Neurol 1988; 24:73–78.

Rowland LP, Sherman WH, Latov N, et al. Amyotrophic lateral sclerosis and lymphoma: Bone marrow examination and other diagnostic tests. Neurology 1992; 42:1101–1102.

Shy ME, Rowland LP, Smith T, et al. Motor neuron disease and plasma cell dyscrasia. Neurology 1986; 36:1429–1436.

Williams DB, Windebank AJ. Motor neuron disease (amyotrophic lateral sclerosis). Mayo Clin Proc 1991; 66:54–82.

Younger DS, Chou S, Hays AP, et al. Primary lateral sclerosis: A clinical diagnosis reemerges. Arch Neurol 1988; 45:1304–1307.

Younger DS, Rowland LP, Latov N, et al. Lymphoma, motor neuron diseases, and amyotrophic lateral sclerosis. Ann Neurol 1991; 29:78–86.

INFLAMMATORY DISEASES

CENTRAL NERVOUS SYSTEM VASCULITIS

PATRICIA M. MOORE, M.D.

Vasculitis is a clinicopathologic process of inflammation and necrosis of the blood vessel wall resulting in tissue ischemia. Vasculitis may be the central process in a variety of primary and secondary disorders. The vasculitides affecting the nervous system are a diverse and interesting subgroup. Central nervous system (CNS) vasculitis, in particular, may be (1) a cell-mediated process that appears to affect only the CNS vasculature (isolated CNS angiitis), (2) part of a systemic vasculitis, (3) secondary to certain infections, toxins, or neoplasias, or (4) a component of another inflammatory disease not primarily vascular (such as Sjögren's syndrome).

Immunologically mediated diseases result from a variety of mechanisms. Knowledge of the predominant pathogenic mechanism in specific diseases aids the physician in appropriate diagnosis and treatment. Antibody-mediated disorders may result from direct interaction of antibody with the target tissue or the more common indirect mechanisms of immune complex deposition with secondary inflammation. Cell-mediated diseases typically result from interaction of antigen-specific lymphocytes with the target and secondary recruitment of nonspecific cells via cytokines.

SPECIFIC DISEASES (TABLE 1)

Isolated angiitis of the CNS (IAC) is a vasculitis restricted to the CNS. Alternate names, including granulomatosis angiitis of the CNS, may be misnomers because granulomas are often absent. Isolated angiitis of the CNS is unusual but not rare. Typical clinical features include headaches, changes in cognition, and, if medium-sized vessels are involved, focal neurologic abnormalities. Other neurologic abnormalities also occur, including seizures, subarachnoid hemorrhage, cranial neuropathies, myelopathies, and radiculopathies. Patients do not have symptoms or signs of systemic

Table 1 Vasculitides that Potentially Affect the Nervous System

Isolated angiitis of the central nervous system (IAC)
Temporal arteritis (TA)
Polyarteritis nodosa (PAN)
Churg-Strauss angiitis (CS)
Wegener's granulomatosis (WEG)
Lymphomatoid granulomatosis (LG)
Hypersensitivity vasculitis (HS)
Vasculitis secondary to infection, malignancy, and toxins ($V^{i, m, t}$)
Vasculitis associated with connective tissue diseases (V^{ctd})

inflammation. The diagnosis may be missed early in the course of the disease, or the headaches may be erroneously attributable to a process such as migraine. Angiography and biopsy are the mainstays of diagnosis.

Temporal arteritis (giant cell arteritis) is a systemic vasculitis clinically affecting the extracranial vessels, most often in patients over the age of 50. Headaches, visual loss, ophthalmoplegia, and jaw claudication are the most typical presenting features. Because the vascular inflammation also affects the posterior circulation, vertigo, syncope, and cranial neuropathies may occur. Strokes and encephalopathies are less frequent. An elevation of the sedimentation rate is the classic serologic abnormality. Liver function tests may also be elevated, reflecting the systemic nature of the vasculitis. Diagnosis by temporal artery biopsy must be pursued promptly. Delay in the diagnosis and treatment may result in irreversible visual loss.

The systemic necrotizing vasculitides are a group of diseases sharing certain features, including widespread inflammation and necrosis of blood vessels. Distinguishing these disorders from one another depends upon characteristic clinical and histologic features.

Polyarteritis nodosa (PAN) is a multisystem disease of small and medium-sized muscular arteries. Typically the lungs are spared. Hypertension occurs in more than half the patients. Neurologically, abnormalities of the peripheral nervous system, present in 50 to 60 percent of patients, appear early, while CNS abnormalities usually occur later in the course of disease. The diagnosis is most often established by renal or peripheral nerve biopsy. When CNS complications occur, the physician must determine whether the abnormalities result from persistent vasculitis or from a complication of treatment.

The iatrogenic complications include infections, as a complication of immunosuppression; encephalopathies, as a complication of medications such as corticosteroids or antihypertensives; and metabolic abnormalities from renal disease. The physician must thus remain vigilant for treatable causes other than vasculitis.

Churg-Strauss angiitis, distinctive for pulmonary involvement and peripheral eosinophilia, produces a predominance of small vessel inflammation. Clinically, peripheral neuropathies and encephalopathies in association with an allergic diathesis and cutaneous and pulmonary lesions suggest the disease. As with PAN, the diagnosis is most often established by biopsy.

Wegener's granulomatosis is characterized by granulomatous vasculitis of the respiratory tract, with or without glomerulonephritis. Initial symptoms are commonly related to the upper respiratory tract. Neurologic abnormalities result from both contiguous extension of the necrotizing granulomas and from the systemic vasculitis. Contiguous extension of the granulomas results in cranial neuropathies in the middle and posterior fossa. Diabetes insipidus also appears to result from local spread of disease. The peripheral neuropathies result from systemic vasculitis. Computed tomographic (CT) and magnetic resonance imaging (MRI) scans have been exceptionally useful in the diagnosis of Wegener's, enabling the physician to distinguish between, for example, optic neuropathies from compression by granulomas (requiring surgery) and those of ischemia secondary to vasculitis (requiring adjustment of immunosuppression).

Lymphomatoid granulomatosis is an unusual vasculitis affecting the skin, lungs, and nervous system. A destructive, pleomorphic mononuclear infiltrate involves both arteries and veins. These infiltrating lymphocytoid and plasmacytoid cells transform to neoplasia in up to 50 percent of patients. Both the central and peripheral segments of the nervous system are affected. Rarely, neurologic abnormalities may be the only antemortem manifestation of disease. MRI abnormalities often appear as mass lesions.

Hypersensitivity vasculitis is the most common vasculitis. Primarily a venulitis of the skin, this group of disorders includes drug-induced allergic vasculitis, Henoch-Schönlein purpura (HSP), cutaneous vasculitis, postinfectious vasculitis, and some cases of mixed cryoglobulinemia. Neurologic abnormalities are not common (<10 percent) with the hypersensitivity vasculitides, with the exception of serum sickness, which has a higher incidence of brachial plexopathy, encephalopathy, and seizures. Subarachnoid hemorrhage and stroke have been reported with HSP. Although there are serologic abnormalities associated with individual diseases such as HSP (increased circulating IgA levels) and serum sickness (circulating immune complexes and reduced complement levels), the diagnoses are made by skin biopsy. The typical leucocytoclasia in the venules refers to phagocytosis of nuclear debris.

Vasculitis associated with malignancy, infection, and toxins may result in neurologic abnormalities. Care in diagnosis is important to avoid immunosuppressing a patient with an underlying infection that is eliciting the inflammatory vascular disease. Treatment of vasculitis secondary to neoplasia or toxins should also be directed at removing the underlying cause. The clinical manifestations of these secondary vasculitides are similar to those of isolated angiitis of the CNS: headache, encephalopathies, seizures, and focal neurologic abnormalities. Clues to the correct diagnosis reside firmly in the history and cerebrospinal fluid (CSF) analysis. A careful history will usually provide information on drug abuse (amphetamines, heroin, cocaine, prescription stimulants) or over-the-counter sympathomimetic agents. Family members may provide useful information. Drug screens are also appropriate. If the history reveals weight loss, fever, malaise, and myalgias, a malignancy should be strongly considered. The neoplasm classically associated with CNS vasculitis is Hodgkin's disease, but other lymphomas occur as well. Alternately, the cause of stroke or diffuse ischemia in patients with malignancy may be vascular occlusions by infiltration of blood vessels with tumor rather than inflammatory cells.

Although numerous infections result in vascular inflammation, the diagnosis of an underlying infection is most elusive with the indolent, opportunistic infections. At least two lumbar punctures should be performed if a fungal infection is considered. Occasionally the diagnosis is made by leptomeningeal-cortical biopsy. Because these are potentially treatable conditions, the physician should not hesitate to perform a brain biopsy in a patient with a progressive encephalopathy of uncertain cause. The risks of the procedure are quite low.

Vasculitis may be associated with connective tissue diseases. Neurologic abnormalities are frequent in systemic lupus erythematotsis, but vasculitis is rarely the pathogenesis. In other disorders, such as systemic sclerosis and rheumatoid arthritis, CNS abnormalities are very unusual, but when they do occur there may be a vasculitis. In Sjögren's syndrome, neurologic abnormalities are being reported with increased frequency. Trigeminal neuropathy, a common abnormality in the connective tissue diseases, does appear to be due to a vasculitis. A venulitis has been suggested, as have other CNS abnormalities, but is not proven. Diagnosis is made on the basis of serologic abnormalities and histologic changes associated with the individual diseases. The features observed with CSF, electroencephalogram, and MRI studies are nonspecific and do not yet help us to delineate the mechanisms of the neurologic disease.

DIAGNOSTIC STUDIES (TABLE 2)

Angiography. Angiography identifies abnormalities of blood vessels in a variety of disorders, although it does not disclose the pathogenesis. Vascular disease is revealed by (1) irregularities of the vessel, frequently segemental narrowings as in the vasculitides, (2) abnormalities of caliber, including stenoses and occlusions, and (3) absence, diminution, or reversal of flow, as well

Table 2 Utility of Diagnostic Studies in the Nervous System Vasculitides

Study	*IAC*	*TA*	*PAN*	*Weg*	*CS*	*LG*	*HS*	$V^{i, m, t}$	V^{ctd}
Angiography	+ +	+	+	+	+	+	−	+ +	+/−
Brain biopsy	+ +	+ +	+ +	+ +	+ +	+ +	+ +	+ +	+
MRI	+	−	+	+ +	+	+ +	+/−	+ +	+
CSF	+/−	−	+/−	+/−	+/−	+/−	+ −	+ +	+
CT	+/−	−	+/−	+	+/−	+/−	+ −	+	+/−
EEG	+	−	+/−	+/−	+	+/−	−	+/−	+
Serologic studies	−	+	+/−	+	+/−	−	+	+	+ +

as opening of collaterals. The likelihood of a vasculitis producing abnormalities on angiogram depends on the caliber of the vessel involved in the disease. Smaller vessel vasculitides may elude detection by angiography, even with magnification and subtraction studies to enhance the image.

Brain Biopsy. Biopsy is the most specific of the diagnostic studies. Biopsy is crucial to demonstrate vascular inflammation and to exclude secondary processes such as infection and malignancy. Leptomeningeal-cortical biopsy has few side effects and is potentially life-saving. A major limitation of the study is the false-negatives associated with sampling error, particularly early in the course of disease. Biopsies of the brain cortex are more likely to be diagnostic with small rather than large vessel vasculitides. Biopsy of the temporal artery or occasionally the occipital artery is central to the diagnosis of temporal arteritis but is not useful in the other vasculitides. Biopsy of tissue for investigation of myelopathies and radiculopathies possibly secondary to vasculitis remains difficult, although arachnoidal tissue obtained at laminectomy has occasionally yielded the diagnosis.

Magnetic Resonance Imaging. Lesions on MRI result from increased water proton density typically associated with edema, gliosis, and tissue infarction. Vasculitis is evident on MRI when the parenchyma is involved by ischemia or infarction. When present, MRI lesions are more evident in the white matter and are occasionally mistaken for those of multiple sclerosis. The MRI may be normal in patients with angiographically and biopsy-evident vasculitis when induration of the blood vessel is prominent but ischemic changes are scanty.

Magnetic Resonance Angiography. MRA is a newer technique that visualizes medium and large cerebral blood vessels. Although useful for some vascular diseases, the resolution is insufficient for delineation of vessel wall abnormalities in the vasculitides. A normal MRA does not indicate that cerebral angiography will also be normal. The latter procedure is still recommended in the evaluation of CNS vasculitis.

Cerebrospinal Fluid. CSF in patients with CNS vasculitis is usually normal. It may show a mild, nonspecific pleocytosis or several hundred to several thousand red blood cells. Nonetheless, CSF analysis is critically important because it may be the only diagnostic study to reveal evidence of infection, particularly with indolent fungal and some bacterial, treponemal, or mycobacterial organisms.

Computed Tomography. The CT scan is less sensitive than the MRI but may be useful in identifying multifocal vascular disease and differentiating it from tumor.

Electroencephalogram. Both encephalopathies and seizures occur in the vasculitides and have accompanying abnormalities on the electroencephalogram (EEG). Although these changes are not specific for the vasculitides, the EEG may nonetheless be useful in following patients with primarily small-vessel vasculitis. The slow waves on the EEG usually improve with treatment of the vasculitis.

Single Photon Emission Computed Tomography. This is a promising diagnostic study in cerebrovascular disease. In some patients with cocaine abuse, focal brain perfusion defects have been observed. In my experience with vasculitis, SPECT is currently insufficiently sensitive to discern regions of vascular inflammation prior to infarction and insufficiently specific to be diagnostically useful.

Serologic Studies. Humorally mediated vasculitides typically produce some serologic manifestations of disease. These include immune complexes, decreased complement levels, elevated sedimentation rate, and occasionally, specific autoantibodies such as antineutrophil cytoplasmic antibodies, as in Wegener's granulomatosis. Cell-mediated processes occurring in diseases such as isolated angiitis of the CNS demonstrate no serologic changes. In temporal arteritis, an elevated sedimentation rate is often the sole, albeit extremely prevalent, marker. Autoantibodies, immune complexes, and immunoglobulins identify those patients with associated connective tissue diseases. Antibody titers to infectious agents may be pertinent. However, vasculitis may occur and progress with no serologic abnormalities. Thus, it is important to remember that there are no serologic studies that definitively diagnose or exclude a diagnosis of vasculitis.

ACUTE CARE CONSIDERATIONS

Acute neurologic abnormalities may occur as the primary manifestations of disease, thus presenting a diagnostic challenge, or they may occur after a diagnosis

Table 3 CNS Vasculitides and Diseases That Mimic Them

CNS Vasculitis	CNS Vasculopathy Not Vasculitis	CNS Vascular Occlusion 2° Coagulopathy
Isolated angiitis of CNS	Neoplasia (lymphoma)	Thrombotic thrombocytopenic purpura
Drug-associated	Degenerative	Hyperviscosity syndromes
Infection-associated	Radiation	Sticky platelet syndrome
Neoplasia-associated	Amyloid	Factor VIII deficiency
Polyarteritis nodosa	Atrial myxoma	Protein S deficiency
Churg-Strauss	Vasospasm	Antiphospholipid antibodies
Wegener's granulomatosis		
Lymphomatoid granulomatosis		
Temporal arteritis		
Behçet's disease		
Cryoglobulinemia-associated		
Hypersensitivity vasculitis (serum sickness)		

has been made. In the first case, the physician may encounter an encephalopathy, seizures, or subarachnoid hemorrhage and question whether there is an underlying and potentially treatable disease. Clues to an associated vasculitis or connective tissue disease reside in the presence of clinical or subclinical visceral disease. The presence of abnormal renal function, casts or sediment in the urine, or an abnormal creatinine clearance provides a clue to a multisystemic disease. The physician then determines if the processes are associated with autoantibodies or cellular infiltration. With autoantibodies, there are serologic clues to the diagnosis, but with cellular infiltration, possibly none. Histologic information is invaluable, both to confirm antibody-mediated changes and to diagnosis cell-mediated injury. Histology may be the only definitive study.

The vasculitides are appropriately included in the differential diagnosis of acute or subacute neurologic abnormalities because their diagnoses would require specific therapy. Despite the wide variety of individual vasculitic diseases, noninflammatory vascular diseases are even more common (Table 3) and may mimic the vasculatides. A diagnosis of a nonvasculitic vasculopathy may limit therapeutic options but will spare the patient the serious potential side effects of corticosteroids and immunosuppression.

SUGGESTED READING

Allison MC, Gallagher PJ. Temporal artery biopsy and corticosteroid treatment. Ann Rheum Dis 1984; 43:416–417.

Caselli RJ, Hunder GG, Whisnant JP. Neurologic disease in biopsy-proven giant cell (temporal) arteritis. Neurology 1988; 38:352–359.

Delecoeuillerie G, Poly P, Delara AC, Paolaggi JB. Polymyalgia rheumatica and temporal arteritis: a retrospective analysis of prognostic features and different corticosteroid regiments. Ann Rheum Dis 1988; 47:733–739.

Drachman DA. Neurological complications of Wegener's granulomatosis. Arch Neurol 1963; 8:145–153.

Feasby TE, Ferguson GG, Kaufman JCE. Isolated spinal cord arteritis. Can J Neurol Sci 1975; 2:143–146.

Ferris EJ, Levine HL. Cerebral arteritis: classification. Radiology 1973; 109:327–341.

Hoffman GS, Kerr GS, Leavitt RY. Wegener Granulomatosis: An analysis of 158 patients. Ann Intern Med 1992; 116:488–498.

Lanham JG, Elkon KB, Pusey CD, Hughes GR. Systemic vasculitis with asthma and eosinophilia: a clinical approach to the Churg-Strauss syndrome. Medicine 1984; 63:65–81.

Leonhardt ETG, Jakobson H, Ringqvist OT. Angiographic and clinicophysiologic investigation of a case of polyarteritis nodosa. Am J Med 1972; 53:242–256.

Miller DH, Ormerod IEC, Gibson A, et al. MR brain scanning in patients with vasculitis: differentiation from multiple sclerosis. Neuroradiology 1987; 29:226–231.

Moore PM. Diagnosis and management of isolated angiitis of the central nervous system. Neurology 1989; 39:167–173.

Moore PM. Immune mechanisms in the primary and secondary vasculitides. Neurolog Sci 1989; 93:129–145.

Moore PM, Cupps TR. Neurological complications of vasculitis. Ann Neurol 1983; 14:155–167.

Patton WF, Lynch JP III. Lymphomatoid granulomatosis: Clinicopathologic study of four cases and literature review. Medicine 1982; 61:1–12.

Schwartz RA, Churg J. Churg-Strauss syndrome. Br J Dermatol 1992; 127:191–204.

Wees SJ, Sunwoo IN, Oh SJ. Sural nerve biopsy in systemic necrotizing vasculitis. Am J Med 1981; 71:525–532.

Zax RH, Hodge SJ, Callen JP. Cutaneous leukocytoclastic vasculitis. Arch Dermatol 1990; 126:69–72.

SARCOIDOSIS

BARNEY J. STERN, M.D.

Sarcoidosis is a disease of unknown cause characterized by noncaseating granulomatous inflammation. The diagnosis is most secure if inflammation is demonstrated in multiple organ systems and other causes of granuloma formation are excluded.

The pathophysiology of sarcoidosis involves the activation of CD4 (helper) lymphocytes, which aggregate at sites of disease activity. Various cytokines are released and promote inflammation as well as antibody secretion. Monocytes and macrophages gather and form granulomas. With time, fibrosis can develop.

The most constant pathologic feature of central nervous system (CNS) sarcoidosis is meningeal inflammation. The cranial nerves can be affected. Inflammation can impede cerebrospinal fluid (CSF) circulation. The brain or spinal cord can be involved, perhaps as inflammation penetrates the parenchyma via the Virchow-Robin spaces. Parenchymal inflammation can take the form of a focal or widespread encephalopathy/vasculopathy or a discrete mass. Peripheral nerves and muscle can also host the inflammatory process.

The diagnosis of neurosarcoidosis should be entertained in the patient with known sarcoidosis who develops neurologic symptoms and the individual without documented sarcoidosis who presents with symptoms compatible with neurosarcoidosis. The neurologic manifestations of sarcoidosis can be categorized, and their relative frequencies approximated, as shown in Table 1. It is helpful to approach patients from the perspective that they have "possible" or "probable" neurosarcoidosis, remembering that even patients with "definite" neurosarcoidosis can ultimately prove to have another diagnosis or develop an intercurrent illness.

Some 5 percent of sarcoidosis patients develop neurosarcoidosis. Patients are typically in their 20s or 30s, though individuals of any age can become ill. Approximately three-quarters of patients destined to have neurologic complications do so within 2 years of presenting with sarcoidosis. Neurologic symptoms are the presenting complaint in one-half of patients with neurosarcoidosis. Nearly one-third of patients have more than one neurologic manifestation.

NEUROLOGIC ILLNESS IN PATIENTS WITH SARCOIDOSIS

If a patient with known systemic sarcoidosis develops a neurologic problem consistent with the commonly encountered neurologic manifestations of sarcoidosis, the possibility of neurosarcoidosis should be entertained. Care should be taken to exclude an intercurrent infectious or neoplastic process. Biopsy of the CNS is rarely indicated if the patient presents in a relatively

Table 1 Neurologic Manifestations of Sarcoidosis

Clinical Manifestation	Approximate Frequency (%)
Cranial neuropathy	50–75
Any nerve can be affected, especially	
2: disk edema, papillitis, retrobulbar optic neuritis, optic atrophy	
5: sensory loss, neuralgia	
7: unilateral or bilateral; simultaneous or sequential; recurrent	25–50
8: auditory, vestibular	
Meningeal disease	10–20
Aseptic meningitis	
Mass	
Hydrocephalus	10
Parenchymal disease	
Brain	
Neuroendocrinopathy	10–15
Vegetative dysfunction	
Vasculopathy-encephalopathy	5–10
Mass	5–10
Seizures	5–10
Spinal canal	
Extramedullary or intramedullary disease	
Cauda equina syndrome	
Peripheral neuropathy	5–10
Axonal neuropathy	
Mononeuropathy	
Mononeuropathy multiplex	
Sensorimotor	
Sensory	
Motor	
Demyelinating neuropathy	
Guillain-Barré syndrome	
Myopathy	10
Asymptomatic	
Nodule	
Polymyositis	
Atrophy	

Adapted from Stern BJ, Schonfeld SA. Neurosarcoidosis. In: Arieff AI, Griggs RC, eds. Metabolic brain dysfunction in systemic disorders. Boston: Little, Brown, 1992; and Stern BJ. Neurosarcoidosis. Neurol Chron 1992; 2:1–6; with permission.

straightforward manner and responds readily to corticosteroid therapy.

Patients with a CNS mass lesion can be a particularly vexing group since the need for surgery must be considered. In general, if the patient is relatively stable, a course of corticosteroid therapy can be pursued. If the patient's neurologic status deteriorates or the mass persists in spite of adequate anti-inflammatory medication, diagnoses other than neurosarcoidosis should be aggressively pursued.

PATIENTS WITHOUT KNOWN SARCOIDOSIS

The patient without known systemic sarcoidosis who develops an illness suggestive of neurosarcoidosis can

Table 2 Frequency of Organ Involvement in Sarcoidosis

Manifestation	Frequency (%)
Intrathoracic	87
Hilar nodes	72
Lung parenchyma	46
Upper respiratory tract	6
Peripheral lymphadenopathy	28
Dermatologic	
Skin	18
Erythema nodosum	15
Ocular	15
Uveitis	
Conjunctival nodule	
Periphlebitis	
Hepatomegaly	10
Splenomegaly	10
Parotid	6
Lacrimal	3
Bone	3
Cardiac	3
Hematologic, endocrinologic, gastrointestinal, and genitourinary	rare
Hypercalcemia	13

Adapted from Stern BJ, Schonfeld SA. Neurosarcoidosis. In: Arieff AI, Griggs RC, eds. Metabolic brain dysfunction in systemic disorders. Boston: Little, Brown, 1992; with permission.

Table 3 The Search for Systemic Sarcoidosis

Chest x ray
Serum calcium
Serum angiotensin-converting enzyme
Pulmonary function tests including diffusion capacity
Ophthalmologic examination
Endoscopic nasal examination
Whole body gallium scan
24-hour urinary calcium excretion
Anergy screen
Muscle MRI

From Stern BJ. Neurosarcoidosis. Neurol Chron 1992; 2:1–6; with permission.

present a diagnostic challenge. The goal in this situation is to demonstrate multisystem inflammation, though in 5 to 10 percent of patients, disease will be limited to the nervous system. Sarcoidosis can involve any organ system, as listed in Table 2 along with the approximate frequencies of occurrence. If possible, corticosteroid therapy should be withheld until a diagnosis is made since treatment can eliminate evidence of systemic disease.

Clues to the existence of systemic sarcoidosis can be pursued as outlined in Table 3 . Patients can be asked if they have difficulty smelling or tasting, which would suggest nasal or olfactory nerve disease, or dry eyes or mouth, suggestive of lacrimal, parotid, or salivary gland disease. Evidence of skin lesions or enlarged lymph nodes should be sought. A whole body gallium scan can be especially helpful in difficult cases since otherwise-occult lacrimal, parotid, or salivary gland inflammation can be detected as well as intra-abdominal lymphadenopathy or organomegaly.

The diagnosis of sarcoidosis is most secure if noncaseating granulomas are documented in multiple organ systems and neoplasia and fungal and mycobacterial infection can be excluded. Readily accessible sites such as a palpable lymph node, skin or mucosal lesion, or conjunctival nodule should be preferentially biopsied. Transbronchial biopsy can be pursued if there is evidence of pulmonary disease. The Kveim-Siltzbach test is not readily available but can be helpful in the diagnosis of sarcoidosis. Some patients may not need biopsy confirmation of their diagnosis. The individual with symmetric bilateral hilar lymphadenopathy and erythema nodosum almost certainly has sarcoidosis. Patients with sarcoidosis can also demonstrate several nonspecific findings that raise the possibility of a systemic disorder: anemia, leukopenia, thrombocytopenia, hypergammaglobulinemia, and hepatic or renal dysfunction.

THE NEUROLOGIC EVALUATION

When evaluating neurologic symptoms, it is helpful to look for disease at more than one site in the nervous system. Although inquiries should be guided by the nature of the patient's complaints, it is especially important to ask about abnormal smell and taste and altered hypothalamic and pituitary function as reflected in disordered thirst, sleep, appetite, body temperature, libido, potency, menses, and micturition. Women should be asked about galactorrhea. There are reports of unusual presentations of neurosarcoidosis (Table 4), which emphasizes the need to consider the diagnosis in many circumstances.

Neurodiagnostic testing should be customized to the individual patient. If systemic disease is documented, rarely is biopsy of the CNS indicated. However, if systemic disease is not found, examination of CNS tissue is indicated for mass lesions and probably for the encephalopathy/vasculopathy of CNS sarcoidosis. Occasional patients with progressive optic nerve disease, multiple cranial neuropathies, and chronic meningitis are also biopsied. The diagnosis of neurosarcoidosis should always remain suspect unless there is pathologic examination of tissue from a site of neurologic disease. Systemic sarcoidosis may develop in patients presenting with isolated neurosarcoidosis, especially as the intensity of immunosuppressive therapy is moderated.

Examination of the CSF in patients with CNS sarcoidosis can reveal an elevated pressure, raised total protein, low glucose level, or a predominantly mononuclear pleocytosis, in varying combinations. The CSF, which should be sterile, can also exhibit an elevated IgG index and oligoclonal bands. The CSF angiotensin converting enzyme activity can be elevated, especially if the patient is not immunosuppressed. None of these CSF tests is pathognomonic for CNS sarcoidosis. They must be viewed within the context of the clinical setting.

A brain computed tomography scan can detect hydrocephalus, a mass lesion or multiple nodules, diffuse inflammation, or areas of periventricular hypodensity.

Focal or diffuse meningeal inflammation can be documented, as can orbital disease. The typical granulomatous mass is slightly hyperdense and enhances dramatically with contrast administration.

Brain magnetic resonance imaging (MRI) is the imaging procedure of choice to evaluate a patient for brain or spinal cord sarcoidosis. On T1 weighted images, a granulomatous mass is usually slightly hyperintense, as compared to the cerebral cortical signal. Optic nerve or chiasm enlargement is readily seen. T2 weighted images can demonstrate abnormal signal secondary to focal or diffuse disease, including periventricular foci. MRI with contrast enhancement is particularly sensitive in detecting meningeal or ependymal inflammation. The spinal cord and cauda equina images can reveal enlargement or enhancement. Spinal cord atrophy can be documented. A normal enhanced MRI does not exclude CNS sarcoidosis, especially if the patient's findings are limited to cranial neuropathies or the patient is intensely immunosuppressed.

Patients with a diffuse or multifocal encephalopathy or strokelike events may occasionally demonstrate small vessel "beading" or large artery occlusive disease on cerebral angiography. In general, the information supplied by angiography is limited.

Visual, brain stem auditory, or somatosensory evoked potentials can document disease in patients with appropriate symptoms. The findings, however, are diagnostically nonspecific. Occasional patients with CNS disease, but without symptoms referrable to the visual, auditory, or sensory pathways, will have abnormal evoked potentials.

Nerve conduction velocities can document the more usual axonal neuropathy as well as the occasional demyelinating neuropathy. A mononeuropathy or mononeuropathy multiplex can also occur. Electromyography can detect a myopathy or the denervation pattern associated with a neuropathy. Nerve or muscle biopsy can demonstrate granulomatous inflammation and can be performed if the diagnosis is unclear. Muscle MRI can highlight foci of inflammation to increase the yield of a biopsy.

Tests to evaluate the integrity of hypothalamic-pituitary function include serum sodium and osmolality, urinary osmolality, thyroid hormone and thyroid-stimulating hormone assays, and prolactin, cortisol, and, as appropriate, testosterone or estradiol levels.

Table 4 Sarcoidosis Presenting as Selected Clinical Oddities

Light-near pupillary dissociation
Ocular flutter
Akinetic rigid syndrome
Sleep apnea syndrome
Hiccups
Sudden hearing loss
Benign intracranial hypertension
Superior sagittal sinus thrombosis
Lumbosacral plexopathy
Muscle cramps or myalgia

OTHER DIAGNOSTIC CONSIDERATIONS

Many disorders can mimic sarcoidosis. Several diseases are particularly important to consider in the differential diagnosis of sarcoidosis (Table 5). Multiple sclerosis and sarcoidosis can occasionally present in a similar fashion. However, except for optic nerve disease, extra-axial cranial neuropathies are unusual in multiple sclerosis. Also, leptomeningeal enhancement is much more common in sarcoidosis. Sjögren's syndrome, in turn, can mimic multiple sclerosis, and can be associated with peripheral neuropathy or myopathy, also mimicking sarcoidosis. Sjögren's syndrome, like sarcoidosis, can cause a sicca syndrome.

Rare conditions such as Wegener's granulomatosis, lymphomatoid granulomatosis, and dysgerminoma need to be considered on occasion. An element of doubt should always exist when evaluating a patient with "definite" neurosarcoidosis if the patient is not responding as expected to immunosuppressive therapy. This statement is relevant even when CNS tissue has been examined.

Finally, complications of sarcoidosis and immunosuppressive treatment need to be sought if the patient is not doing well. Some of these conditions include corticosteroid-induced myopathy, spinal epidural lipomatosis, cryptococcal or tuberculous meningitis, progressive multifocal leukoencephalopathy, herpes simplex encephalitis, and inclusion body myositis.

In summary, neurosarcoidosis is a disorder with protean manifestations. The patient with known systemic sarcoidosis who develops a neurologic illness is often found to have neurosarcoidosis. Patients without a known systemic illness can present with neurosarcoido-

Table 5 Other Selected Diagnostic Considerations in Patients with Suspected Neurosarcoidosis

---

Infection
  Neurosyphilis
  Neuroborreliosis
  Tuberculosis
  Human immunodeficiency virus complications
  Brucellosis
  Listeria monocytogenes
  Whipple's disease

Neoplasia
  Meningeal carcinomatosis
  Lymphoma
  Germ cell tumors
  Craniopharyngioma

Inflammatory disorders
  Multiple sclerosis
  Sjögren's syndrome
  Systemic lupus erythematosus
  Behçet's disease
  Vogt-Koyanagi-Harada disease
  Isolated angiitis of the central nervous system
  Wegener's granulomatosis
  Lymphomatoid granulomatosis
  Cogan's syndrome
  Fibrosclerosis/hypertrophic pachymeningitis

---

sis. A thorough evaluation will often allow a diagnosis to be made with a reasonable degree of certainty, but the clinician should always be alert to the possibility that another disorder has masqueraded as sarcoidosis.

SUGGESTED READING

Peeples DM, Stern BJ, Violet J, Sahni KS. Germ cell tumors masquerading as central nervous system sarcoidosis. Arch Neurol 1991; 48:554–556.

Sherman JL, Stern BJ. Sarcoidosis of the CNS: Comparison of unenhanced and enhanced MR images. AJNR Am J Neuroradiol 1990; 11:915–923.

Stern BJ, Krumholz A, Johns C, et al. Sarcoidosis and its neurological manifestations. Arch Neurol 1985; 42:909–917.

Stern BJ, Schonfeld SA. Neurosarcoidosis. In: Arieff AI, Griggs RC, eds. Metabolic brain dysfunction in systemic disorders. Boston: Little, Brown, 1992.

METABOLIC DISORDERS

VITAMIN B₁₂ DEFICIENCY

EDWARD B. HEALTON, M.D.
JOHN LINDENBAUM, M.D.

DEFINITION

Vitamin B_{12} (cobalamin [Cbl]) deficiency is a chronic, progressive disorder characterized clinically by abnormalities of the hematopoietic and nervous systems and the tongue. Deficiency usually develops because of a disorder of absorption of the vitamin. Approximately 80 percent of patients have the adult onset type of pernicious anemia in which impaired absorption results from lack of intrinsic factor caused by chronic atrophic gastritis. In others, the malabsorption of Cbl results from jejunal diverticulosis, tropical sprue, or resection of the stomach or ileum. Approximately 2 percent of patients have the newly recognized syndrome of food Cbl malabsorption in which Cbl cannot be liberated from animal proteins because of impaired acid-peptic digestion of food. The Schilling test is normal in this disorder. Finally, in a small group of dentists and anesthetists who abuse nitrous oxide, Cbl is inactivated by the anesthetic. Very rarely, strict vegetarianism for many years leads to Cbl deficiency.

In the late nineteenth and early twentieth centuries, initial reports of the nervous system disorder associated with Cbl deficiency emphasized severe spinal cord disease in anemic patients. The term *subacute combined degeneration* was introduced to refer to patients with simultaneous involvement of the posterior and lateral columns. In the modern era, since the introduction of more specific diagnostic and therapeutic measures, the clinician must consider Cbl deficiency in patients with varied and frequently less advanced neurologic disease, with and without anemia. Because the neurologic abnormalities are highly responsive to treatment in patients with less advanced damage, early diagnosis is very important. The long-standing debate regarding the relative contributions of spinal cord and peripheral nerve damage to the clinical syndromes seen in Cbl deficiency has not been resolved. Considerable evidence indicates the importance of both. Most patients appear to have features consistent with both myelopathy and neuropathy.

In this chapter we review the diverse neurologic presentations of Cbl deficiency, the range of hematologic abnormalities, the role of serum Cbl and Cbl-related metabolites and therapeutic trials in diagnosis, and considerations in differential diagnosis.

NEUROLOGIC FINDINGS

Cbl deficiency of the nervous system produces a diverse group of neurologic abnormalities with a high degree of variability among patients. Approximately 40 percent of patients with Cbl deficiency seen in current practice exhibit neurologic symptoms or signs. Neurologic symptoms usually precede other manifestations of deficiency and are often the predominant complaints. The onset of symptoms typically occurs in the seventh decade or later, but 20 percent develop symptoms before the age of 50 years. By far the most common complaints are paresthesias, alone or together with ataxia. The paresthesias usually involve the feet or the feet and hands in a symmetrical fashion and are often severe and disabling. In a minority, however, paresthesias are reported only in the hands or hands and arms, although they may occur later in the feet and legs. Severe gluteal and genital region paresthesias may occur associated with similar symptoms in the lower limbs.

Gait ataxia is the second most common initial symptom. It usually accompanies paresthesias but may be the only complaint. Weakness occasionally is reported first but almost always with paresthesias or ataxia. A small number of patients report a variety of other initial symptoms, including impaired manual dexterity or coin recognition, diminished visual acuity, memory impairment, personality change, psychosis, orthostatic lightheadedness, anosmia and impaired taste, urinary or fecal incontinence, and impotence. Non-neurologic symptoms such as sore tongue, anorexia, vomiting, diarrhea, weight loss, and syncope associated with severe anemia are the first complaints in about one-fourth of patients who have neurologic abnormalities at diagnosis. Occasionally, patients without neurologic symptoms but findings on neurologic examination are diagnosed when anemia and Cbl deficiency are found as a result of a routine complete blood count.

Sensory abnormalities are the most common finding on examination. Diminished vibratory sensation is present in nearly 90 percent of patients. Usually this modality is impaired in the feet or may extend to the knees. In more severely affected patients, vibratory sensation may be reduced up to a segmental level in the thoracic area and in the arms up to the elbows or shoulders. Decreased proprioception in the toes or ankles and occasionally in the fingers or wrists is the next most common abnormality. We have never seen proprioceptive loss in patients with normal vibratory sensation. The Romberg sign is frequently positive.

Cutaneous touch and pain sensation is diminished in up to 30 percent of patients and is occasionally the only neurologic abnormality. It is usually impaired in a "stocking" distribution in the feet or feet and legs up to the knees, and occasionally in the hands and arms. Rarely, there may be a lumbar or thoracic cutaneous sensory level.

Corticospinal tract or motor nerve involvement is seen only in advanced cases. Motor and reflex abnormalities are always associated with sensory deficits. Weakness affects the legs or legs and arms in a bilateral, symmetrical fashion. Rarely, it may predominate on one side. Tendon reflexes are absent or diminished in the majority of patients. Hyper-reflexia, spasticity, or extensor plantar responses are less common. Lhermitte's sign is also occasionally found. For some reason it is particularly common in abusers of nitrous oxide.

Autonomic disorders such as impotence and urinary incontinence are always accompanied by sensory or sensory and motor abnormalities. Postural hypotension and syncope, without other autonomic symptoms, may be the most salient manifestation, even in the absence of severe anemia.

Cognitive disorders are the most difficult neurologic abnormalities to evaluate in patients with Cbl deficiency. When more common causes of abnormal mental function are carefully excluded, marked mental impairment attributable to Cbl deficiency is relatively infrequent. Nonetheless, reduced intellectual function and psychiatric symptoms occurred in 14 percent of our patients. Global dementia or a predominantly amnestic syndrome are the most frequent cognitive disorders. A wide variety of psychiatric symptoms such as depression, hypomania, severe agitation, and even fully developed psychosis may be seen. In some patients the psychiatric symptoms are predominant, but almost always they are accompanied by reduced intellectual function. Although dementia alone, or other forms of altered mental status with no other abnormalities, has been reported, we have never seen mental impairment attributable to Cbl deficiency in the absence of other neurologic findings when an adequate examination could be performed. When it occurs, however, mental impairment frequently is the dominant and most disabling neurologic problem, and other findings may be slight.

Although there are numerous case reports of optic nerve disease in patients with Cbl deficiency (in men much more commonly than in women), decreased vision with or without optic atrophy is seen in less than 1 percent of patients.

Rare neurologic findings reported in the literature include positional vertigo, paralysis of upward gaze, downbeat nystagmus, and coma. In infants and in the first years of childhood, remarkable abnormal involuntary movements have been described.

FACTORS AFFECTING THE SEVERITY OF NEUROLOGIC ABNORMALITIES

When diagnosis is delayed, progression beyond the initial neurologic symptoms often occurs, usually over weeks to months. The rate of progression varies markedly from patient to patient and is not always relentless. Initial symptoms may worsen or extend proximally in the extremities, or new symptoms may be added. Patients can become bed or wheelchair bound under observation before the diagnosis of Cbl deficiency is made. In current practice, however, only a mild to moderate disability is noted by the time of diagnosis in most patients, despite prominent symptoms or well-defined abnormalities on neurologic examination. Nearly two-thirds are functionally independent, with little or no reduction in their ability to carry out activities of daily living, and only 10 percent are severely disabled and wheelchair or bed bound. The duration of symptoms prior to diagnosis directly correlates with the degree of neurologic disability. There is also a striking inverse correlation between the hematocrit and the severity of neurologic abnormalities. The higher the hematocrit, the worse the neurologic disorder. It is likely that in some persons, the manifestations of Cbl deficiency are predominantly neurologic and in others, predominantly hematologic. This represents all the more reason not to wait for the development of megaloblastic anemia before making the diagnosis.

NEUROLOGIC DIAGNOSTIC TESTS

The frequency and type of electrophysiologic abnormalities in a large population of Cbl-deficient patients with and without neurologic findings have not been determined. In patients with sensory or sensory and motor abnormalities consistent with peripheral nerve disease, electromyographic studies may be normal or consistent with demyelinating or axonal neuropathy or, not infrequently, both. Pure axonal neuropathy has been reported. When abnormal, nerve conduction velocities are usually mildly to moderately reduced.

Somatosensory evoked response testing may be normal or show delayed cervical conduction in patients with sensory abnormalities. Similarly, there may be delayed conduction or normal studies in visual evoked response testing in patients with impaired vision. Brain stem auditory evoked response testing has usually been normal in the few patients tested. Electrophysiologic tests do not distinguish the neurologic abnormalities caused by Cbl deficiency from other disorders.

Computerized tomography may be normal or show

signs of generalized atrophy in patients with mental impairment. Magnetic resonance imaging of the brain and spinal cord has been normal in the few patients studied. The cerebrospinal fluid is usually normal, although the protein concentration may be slightly elevated.

HEMATOLOGIC ABNORMALITIES

It must be emphasized that hematologic changes are often modest or minimal, even in patients with severe neurologic disease. In fact, either the hematocrit or the mean corpuscular volume (MCV) is normal in as many as 25 percent of patients. In our series only 19 percent were severely anemic (hematocrit less than 20 percent). Both the hematocrit and the MCV are normal in approximately 15 percent. In some patients the initially normal MCV falls after treatment, indicating an elevated value over baseline for the patient. The clinician cannot rely on the presence of anemia or an elevated MCV before making the diagnosis of Cbl deficiency.

Careful examination of the blood smear usually shows hypersegmentation of neutrophils and oval macrocytes, although not invariably. However, these findings must be carefully sought and are often missed in routine hospital laboratory examinations. In our experience, examination of the bone marrow always shows megaloblastic changes in patients with Cbl deficiency of the nervous system. However, the alterations are often subtle.

ESTABLISHING THE DIAGNOSIS

In most patients the serum Cbl level will be low, less than 200 pg per milliliter. However, the Cbl concentration is often only mildly depressed, in the range of 160 to 200 pg per milliliter. There are problems with both the sensitivity and specificity of this test. The level may be low normal (200 to 350 pg per milliliter) in 5 to 10 percent of patients with neurologic abnormalities caused by Cbl deficiency that will improve after Cbl therapy. Second, since by definition the normal range for a laboratory test excludes the 2.5 percent of the normal population who fall below the lower limit of normal, many patients with a low serum Cbl value are not deficient in the vitamin. Consequently, measurement of two metabolites that accumulate in the serum when Cbl-dependent reactions are impaired, methylmalonic acid and total homocysteine, is useful in establishing the presence of deficiency. Methylmalonic acid or homocysteine are uniformly elevated in more than 99 percent of patients with true deficiency of Cbl. These laboratory tests, which are now available in several national commercial laboratories, should be used when there is uncertainty about the diagnosis. We currently obtain them in any patient with neuropsychiatric abnormalities compatible with Cbl deficiency in whom the serum Cbl level is 350 pg per milliliter or less. If the metabolites are normal, the diagnosis of deficiency is virtually excluded. Lacking availability of these tests, a trial of Cbl therapy and observation for neurologic or hematologic improvement may be necessary to confirm the diagnosis in some patients.

The Schilling test is less reliable than the serum metabolite levels in excluding Cbl deficiency, since it is normal in certain deficient patients such as those with food Cbl malabsorption, vegetarians, and nitrous oxide abusers.

TREATMENT RESPONSES

Consideration of treatment response is appropriate here because establishing the relationship between Cbl deficiency and the observed neurologic abnormalities depends on the response to treatment in some patients. This is especially true when other disorders may explain the neurologic abnormalities, even if the patient is simultaneously deficient in Cbl. For example, if a patient with diabetes and a peripheral neuropathy also develops a megaloblastic anemia, a therapeutic trial may be the only means of establishing whether the neurologic findings are caused by lack of Cbl.

The promptness and degree of response depend on the specific neurologic disorder. Paresthesias commonly show substantial improvement in the first 2 weeks of therapy, while corticospinal tract abnormalities respond much more slowly. Even patients with paresthesias may show no amelioration or even worsen transiently during the first 4 to 6 weeks of treatment only to improve later. Overall, if there is no response after 3 months of therapy, the neurologic disorder is unlikely to be caused by Cbl deficiency. It is quite unusual in current practice to see no improvement whatsoever by 3 months in a patient with Cbl deficiency of the nervous system. When symptoms are unchanged at 3 months, another underlying diagnosis should be strongly considered. Although virtually every patient shows some response to therapy, about half are left with variable residual neurologic disability or abnormal findings. The degree of disability directly correlates with the duration of symptoms and the severity of neurologic abnormalities prior to treatment, again emphasizing the importance of early diagnosis.

DIFFERENTIAL DIAGNOSIS

Because of the wide variety of neurologic findings, Cbl deficiency must be considered when sensory, motor, and reflex abnormalities suggest peripheral neuropathy, myelopathy, or both, or in the differential diagnosis of optic nerve disease, intellectual or psychiatric impairment, and autonomic dysfunction. The principal disorders that must be distinguished from Cbl deficiency of the nervous system are diabetic neuropathy; alcoholic neuropathy; the paraneoplastic syndromes associated with carcinoma, multiple myeloma, and other malignancies; hypothyroidism; multiple sclerosis; human immunodeficiency virus (HIV)–related neurologic disease; neurosyphilis; cervical spondylosis; Alzheimer's disease; and psychiatric disorders. The following findings favor Cbl deficiency: a subacute to chronic progression of symptoms, symmetry of neurologic findings, lack of pain, and multiple simultaneous neurologic syndromes. Once deficiency is considered, the diagnosis can usually be made in most patients by a careful search for the typical hematologic abnormalities and measurement of the serum Cbl level, although metabolite determinations and a therapeutic trial may be necessary. It is important to remember that a low serum Cbl level can occur coincidentally in other disorders under consideration in the differential diagnosis, such as multiple sclerosis, HIV infection, and Alzheimer's disease. When the causative role of Cbl is uncertain, measurement of methylmalonic acid and homocysteine as well as a carefully monitored trial of therapy are in order.

In patients with myelopathy, very few disorders present with severe sensory loss before corticospinal tract abnormalities occur, especially if the sensory loss includes vibratory impairment and diminished proprioception together with reduced cutaneous pain and touch sensation. Cervical spondylosis is often considered in the differential diagnosis of Cbl-related myelopathy. Cervical spondylosis usually has significant cervical and sometimes radicular pain. Prominent corticospinal tract signs usually precede substantial sensory impairment, and peripheral nerve signs are confined to the territory of one or two nerve roots.

Multiple sclerosis may resemble various presentations of Cbl deficiency. When it involves the spinal cord and optic nerve, it may be difficult to distinguish from Cbl deficiency. The symptoms of multiple sclerosis often are rapidly progressive, unlike those of Cbl deficiency. Multiple sclerosis never affects peripheral nerves and is often highly asymmetrical. It also does not involve both eyes simultaneously when it is the cause of optic neuropathy, unlike Cbl deficiency, which almost always causes bilateral optic nerve disease, although one eye may be more severely affected than the other. If dementia or other types of mental impairment are present, this favors deficiency over multiple sclerosis.

The peripheral neuropathy caused by Cbl deficiency may be difficult to distinguish from other disorders in which vibratory sensation, proprioception, and cutaneous sensation may be impaired, such as diabetes mellitus, chronic alcoholism, or a paraneoplastic syndrome. When corticospinal tract abnormalities, autonomic disturbance, visual abnormalities, or mental impairment and macrocytic anemia or other characteristic hematologic abnormalities are also present, Cbl deficiency is the likely diagnosis. In some patients with evidence of only peripheral neuropathy, measurement of serum Cbl and metabolite levels or a response to Cbl therapy will be required to make the diagnosis.

In patients with dementia or behavioral disorders, those with Alzheimer's disease and psychiatric syndromes do not usually have other accompanying neurologic abnormalities. One exception is chronic alcoholism associated with psychiatric disorders. In elderly patients the type of mental impairment in Alzheimer's disease is similar to that found in Cbl deficiency. The presence of additional sensory, motor, or autonomic abnormalities, which are virtually always associated with mental impairment in Cbl deficiency, and do not occur in Alzheimer's disease, should distinguish the two disorders. This assumes that adequate assessment of sensory deficits is possible.

The neurologic syndromes accompanying HIV infection that may resemble Cbl deficiency include the acquired immunodeficiency syndrome dementia complex and vacuolar myelopathy, which often occur together, as well as the distal symmetrical, predominantly sensory polyneuropathy associated with advanced immunodeficiency.

None of the guidelines discussed above is absolutely reliable in differential diagnosis. If there is any doubt, Cbl deficiency should be ruled out. We prefer to err on the side of a low threshold for obtaining serum Cbl determinations because of the importance of early diagnosis in preventing residual damage to the nervous system and the availability of inexpensive and highly effective therapy for this disorder compared to most of the conditions that are part of its differential diagnosis.

SUGGESTED READING

Dawson DW, Sawers AH, Sharma RK. Malabsorption of protein bound vitamin B₁₂. BMJ 1984; 288:675–678.

Hamilton HE, Ellis PP, Sheets RF. Visual impairment due to optic neuropathy in pernicious anemia: Report of a case and review of the literature. Blood 1959; 14:378–385.

Healton EH, Savage DG, Brust JCM, et al. Neurologic aspects of cobalamin deficiency. Medicine 1991; 70:229–245.

Layzer RB. Myeloneuropathy after prolonged exposure to nitrous oxide. Lancet 1978; 2:1227–1230.

Lindenbaum J, Healton EB, Savage DG, et al. Neuropsychiatric disorders caused by cobalamin deficiency in the absence of anemia or macrocytosis. N Engl J Med 1988; 318:1720–1728.

Lindenbaum J, Savage DG, Stabler SP, Allen RH. Diagnosis of cobalamin deficiency: II. Relative sensitivities of serum cobalamin, methylmalonic acid, and total homocysteine concentrations. Am J Hematol 1990; 34:99–107.

Victor M, Lear AA. Subacute combined degeneration of the spinal cord. Am J Med 1956; 20:896–911.

Zucker DK, Livingston RL, Nakra R, Clayton PJ. B₁₂ deficiency and psychiatric disorders: Case report and literature review. Biol Psychiatry 1981; 16:197–205.

LEAD POISONING

PHILIP J. LANDRIGAN, M.D., M.Sc.

Lead is an ancient metal, and toxicity of lead to the nervous system has been recognized since antiquity. The following verse by Nikander, a Greek poet and physician of the second century BC, details the adverse consequences of exposure to cerussa (lead carbonate). This stanza notes specifically the occurrence of colic, paralysis, visual disturbance, and encephalopathy in lead workers:

The harmful cerussa that most noxious thing
Which foams like the milk in the earliest spring
With rough force it falls and the pail beneath fills
This fluid astringes and causes grave ills.
The mouth it inflames and makes cold from within
The gums dry and wrinkled, are parch'd like the skin
The rough tongue feels harsher; the neck muscles grip
He soon cannot swallow, foam runs from his lip
A feeble cough tries, it in vain to expel
He belches so much, and his belly does swell
His sluggish eyes sway, then he totters to bed
Phantastic forms flit now in front of his eyes
While deep from his breast there soon issue sad cries
Meanwhile there comes a stuporous chill
His feeble limbs droop and all motion is still
His strength is now spent and unless one soon aids
The sick man descends to the Stygian shades.

Ramazzini, the father of modern occupational medicine, described industrial lead poisoning including neurotoxicity in potters and portrait painters in his classic study *De Morbis Artificum Diatriba*:

In almost all cities there are other workers who habitually incur serious maladies from the deadly fumes of metals. Among these are the potters .... When they need roasted or calcined lead for glazing their pots, they grind the lead in marble vessels ... During this process, their mouths, nostrils, and the whole body take in the lead poison .... First their hands become palsied, then they become paralytic, splenetic, lethargic, and toothless.

In Victorian England, Charles Turner Thackrah, an early occupational physician, described chronic occupational lead poisoning in plumbers and white lead manufacturers:

Plumbers are exposed to the volatilized oxide of lead which rises during the process of casting. Men soon complain of headache, drowsiness, sickness, vomiting, griping, obstinate constipation, and to these succeed colic or inflammation of the bowels, disorders of the urinary organs, and finally, the most marked of the diseases from lead, palsy. We observed the muscles of the fore-arm, more frequently and sooner to suffer than other parts.

Despite this long recognition of the neurologic and other organ system injury caused by lead, intense interest continues to surround research into lead neurotoxicity. Moreover, the understanding has become widespread that lead can cause toxic injuries to the human nervous system at levels of exposure that only a decade ago were thought to be safe. Lead has thus become the paradigmatic subclinical neurotoxin.

Subclinical Toxicity of Lead. The term *subclinical toxicity* denotes the concept that relatively low-dose exposure to certain chemicals, lead among them, may cause harmful effects in various organ systems that are not evident in the standard clinical examination. The underlying premise is that there exists a continuum of toxicity in which clinically apparent effects have their asymptomatic, subclinical counterparts. Thus clinically obvious manifestations of the toxicity of lead such as anemia, peripheral neuropathy, and encephalopathy lie at the upper end of the range of toxicity, whereas such covert effects as slowed nerve conduction, impaired biosynthesis of heme, diminished intelligence, and altered behavior are their subclinical correlates. It is important to note that these subclinical changes represent truly harmful outcomes and are not merely homeostatic or physiological "adjustments" to the presence of lead.

Lead in the Environment. Although lead has been used for millennia, the quantity of lead used in the last five decades surpasses the cumulative total consumed in all previous centuries. This heavy recent use reflects industrial applications since World War II and the consumption of lead as a fuel additive in gasoline. In the mid-1970s, nearly 200,000 tons of lead were consumed annually in gasoline in the United States, and more was used abroad. Virtually all of this lead was emitted into the environment from vehicle exhaust in finely particulate form and caused widespread contamination of air, dust, and soil. Since 1976 the use of leaded gasoline has decreased sharply in the United States and will end entirely in the mid-1990s. However, the use of leaded gasoline in other nations remains extensive.

Adult Exposure to Lead. Most adult lead exposure occurs in the workplace. A wide variety of industrial populations are at risk of occupational exposure to lead, and virtually all industrial exposure to lead is by inhalation. The National Institute for Occupational Safety and Health estimates that more than three million workers in the United States have potential exposure to lead in their work. Lead exposure is also widespread in the general population but at lower levels than in the industrial setting. Persons of all ages encounter lead in air, dust, soil, and drinking water. Lead in drinking water is due principally to the use of lead solder to join pipes in home service lines.

Pediatric Exposure to Lead. Children, because of their normal oral exploratory behavior, are at high risk of ingesting lead from lead-based paint as well as from dust and soil. The mean blood lead level in children in the United States is about 5 μg per deciliter, a level significantly higher than that found in preindustrial populations living in remote areas but substantially less than that of American children in the mid-1970s, reflecting decreases in the use of lead in gasoline. An estimated 8.4 million American preschool children have blood lead levels above 15 μg per deciliter, a level that in children is associated with subclinical neurologic impairment (see below). Among poor, minority, inner-city preschool children, the prevalence of blood lead levels above 15 μg per deciliter is estimated by the Centers for Disease Control to be 68 percent.

LEAD POISONING

Inorganic Lead, Acute Toxicity

Intense, acute exposure to lead, either by inhalation in the workplace or by ingestion of paint chips among children, can cause a syndrome of acute lead poisoning. Characteristics of this life-threatening syndrome are abdominal colic, constipation, fatigue, anemia, peripheral neuropathy, and, in some cases, alteration of central nervous system (CNS) function. In profound cases, a full-blown acute encephalopathy with coma, convulsions, and papilledema may occur. In milder cases of acute lead encephalopathy, only headache or personality changes may be evident. In many instances, persons who have suffered from acute lead encephalopathy are left with permanent neurologic and behavioral sequelae.

Inorganic Lead, Chronic Neurologic Toxicity in Adults

In the peripheral nervous system, the motor axons are the principal target of lead toxicity. Lead-induced pathologic changes in these fibers include segmental demyelination and axonal degeneration. Extensor muscle palsy with "wrist drop" or "ankle drop" has, since the time of Hippocrates, been recognized as the classic clinical manifestation of the peripheral motor neurologic toxicity of lead.

Recent studies of the peripheral nerves in persons exposed to lead have used electrophysiologic probes to determine whether lower level exposures, insufficient to produce clinically evident signs and symptoms, cause covert subclinical abnormalities in function. With the development of increasingly sensitive test methodologies, these studies have identified neurologic toxicity at progressively lower blood lead levels. In one of the earliest studies, in the early 1970s, evidence was found for asymptomatic slowing of motor nerve conduction velocity in workers whose blood lead levels had never exceeded 70 μg per deciliter. Then in the late 1970s, in studies focusing on conduction in the small motor fibers of the ulnar nerve, conduction velocity was found to be slowed at blood lead levels below 50 μg per deciliter. Most recently, in a prospective study of new entrants to the lead industry, slowing of ulnar nerve conduction velocity has been reported at blood lead levels as low as 30 to 40 μg per deciliter.

In the CNS, extensive research has sought to determine whether lead causes asymptomatic impairment of function in adults at doses insufficient to produce clinical encephalopathy. In one investigation, a correlation was observed between lead exposure and diminished neuropsychologic performance in a group of asymptomatic adult workers, all of whom had blood lead levels below 70 μg per deciliter. The functions most severely impaired were those dependent on visual intelligence and visual-motor coordination. Also, an increased prevalence of fatigue and short-term memory loss was seen in smelter workers exposed to lead. The prevalence of these abnormalities increased with blood lead levels. Further clinical and epidemiologic studies will be required in adults to establish more precisely the dose-response relationships between lower levels of exposure to lead and asymptomatic neurologic dysfunction.

Does Lead Cause Dementia or Amyotrophic Lateral Sclerosis?

An unexplored implication of the finding that lead causes insidious asymptomatic injury to the CNS is the possibility that some as yet unknown fraction of cases of presenile dementia, motoneuron disease, or other chronic neurologic and psychiatric conditions may be caused by chronic exposure to lead. Such chronic exposure may result in an accelerated attrition of neurons that becomes clinically evident as persons age. Epidemiologic and clinical studies to assess prior lead exposure in persons with chronic neurologic disease will be needed to assess this possibility.

Chronic Pediatric Neurotoxicity

Recent prospective epidemiologic studies in children have linked blood lead levels as low as 10 to 15 μg per deciliter with subclinical but apparently irreversible decrements in CNS function. This dysfunction is characterized by diminished intelligence, shortened attention span, and slowed reaction time. These findings are highly credible and have been accepted by the Centers for Disease Control. Additionally, follow-up studies of young adults who had increased lead absorption and subclinical neurologic toxicity in early childhood have documented that these persons are at high risk for persistent learning deficits, reading difficulties, failing to graduate from school, and developing aberrant behavior patterns. These findings have stimulated major efforts in the pediatric and public health communities to reduce childhood lead exposure.

Organic Lead Toxicity

One organic compound of lead, tetraethyl lead (TEL), has been widely used as an antiknock agent in gasoline. Producers, blenders, and persons who clean and maintain tanks are at risk for poisoning by TEL. It is a volatile liquid that, unlike inorganic lead, is absorbed readily through the skin.

Exposure to TEL produces a syndrome very different from inorganic lead poisoning. TEL poisoning is limited largely to acute or subacute CNS signs and symptoms. Early symptoms of insomnia and anorexia are followed by muscle irritability. Agitated encephalopathy resembling delirium tremens occurs in cases of severe poisoning. Increased deep tendon reflexes, tremors, and ataxia are characteristic in severe cases.

CLINICAL EVALUATION STRATEGY

Inorganic Lead

The diagnosis of inorganic lead intoxication requires (1) demonstration of excess lead absorption, (2) documentation of impairment in an organ system consistent with the effects of lead, and (3) exclusion of other causes of impairment.

Increased lead absorption is most easily proven by demonstrating an increased level of lead in whole blood. Normal adult levels of lead in blood are less than 20 µg per deciliter. Symptoms may occur at blood lead levels of less than 40 µg per deciliter and become more frequent and profound as levels increase. At blood lead levels over 80 µg per deciliter, many workers show signs and symptoms of clinical lead poisoning.

The blood lead level is a good indicator of recent lead absorption but is less adequate as a measure of chronic absorption of lead. The half-life of lead in blood is approximately 36 days. Thus, in persons with relatively brief exposure, such as new entrants to the lead industry or children who have recently eaten paint chips, the blood lead level is a good indicator of exposure. However, in persons with long-term, heavy exposure to lead, such as workers with many years of employment in the lead industry, the blood lead level appears principally to reflect the release of stored lead from bone and other deep tissue compartments. For that reason, the blood lead level is of only limited value in assessing dose-response relationships for the long-term consequences of lead exposure, such as renal disease, hypertension, and chronic neurologic impairment.

A new technology that holds promise for accurate, noninvasive assessment of chronic lead exposure is measurement of the bone lead burden by x-ray fluorescence (XRF) analysis. In chronically exposed persons, over 95 percent of the body lead burden is contained in bone, and the half-life of lead in bone is approximately 10,000 days (25 years). The measurement of bone lead burden by XRF analysis offers a relatively rapid approach to the individualized assessment of body lead burden. Moreover, the radiation dose is minimal, amounting to only about one-tenth the radiation contained in a dental x-ray. Future use of XRF analysis in workers chronically exposed to lead will refine the dose-response relationships between cumulative lead exposure and chronic toxic effects on the nervous system.

Zinc protoporphyrin (ZPP) or free erythrocyte protoporphyrin (FEP) levels reflect the toxic effect of lead on the erythrocytic enzyme ferrochelatase, the final enzyme in heme synthesis. FEP levels rise abruptly in children when blood lead levels exceed 15 to 20 µg per deciliter and in adults when blood lead levels exceed 30 to 40 µg per deciliter. Once elevated, FEP levels tend to stay above background for several months. ZPP and FEP levels are easily and inexpensively measured. However, a disadvantage in use of the ZPP level as a screening test for increased lead absorption in children at current low levels of ambient exposure is the relative insensitivity of ZPP to blood lead levels below 25 µg per deciliter. For this reason ZPP is not an adequate screen for lead exposure in children today. In adults chronically exposed to lead, a problem with the use of ZPP is that it remains elevated long after the blood lead level has fallen. It thus provides only an imperfect picture of recent exposure and does not distinguish recent from past lead exposure. Iron deficiency also elevates FEP and must therefore be excluded.

At present, the reference standard for determination of body lead burden is measurement of urinary lead after intramuscular injection of 1 g of calcium EDTA. Urinary excretion of over 600 µg of lead in a 72-hour urine collection proves past excessive exposure resulting in an elevated body burden. In patients with normal renal function, a 24-hour urine collection is sufficient. In the future, XRF analysis of the lead content of bone may replace EDTA chelation as the reference standard of cumulative lead absorption.

No other test or finding is either very sensitive or specific for lead poisoning. Basophilic stippling in the red blood cells is seen in most patients with acute hemolysis and occasionally in patients with chronic syndromes but is not specific to lead poisoning. Lead lines on the gums are uncommon except in cases of severe poisoning and may be difficult to recognize in patients with poor dental hygiene. Hair lead levels are not reliable.

Complete blood counts and routine blood chemistry determinations should be performed as baseline measurements in asymptomatic workers exposed to lead. Other baseline tests that may be of value include creatinine clearance, uric acid, thyroid function tests, sperm counts, and some psychometric tests, as well as measurement of motor conduction velocity in the peripheral nerves. Blood lead levels are required by federal law to be obtained on a periodic basis in lead workers.

In pediatric practice, a blood lead determination should be performed on every child between the ages of 1 and 2 years and more frequently in children judged to be at high risk of lead absorption. If the whole blood lead level in a child exceeds 15 µg per deciliter, or if in an adult worker it exceeds 40 µg per deciliter, or if the FEP or ZPP level rises, these tests should be repeated monthly. Blood lead levels over 25 µg per deciliter in children and over 50 µg per deciliter in adults require immediate removal from exposure.

Organic Lead

Organic lead (TEL) intoxication is difficult to diagnose without a history of exposure. Blood or urine lead levels and EP levels are not predictably elevated in TEL poisoning. Increased values are useful, but normal or borderline values may be seen in mild poisoning. Cerebrospinal fluid examination is usually normal.

COMMENTS

The tragedy of the continuing epidemic of lead poisoning in the United States and internationally is that certain consequences, particularly the subclinical neurologic sequelae, appear to be irreversible. No therapy can replace neurons destroyed by lead. Thus the major effort of physicians and policy makers must focus on prevention.

Prevention of lead poisoning can be achieved through a series of steps, including the following: removing all lead from gasoline; banning lead from all pigments, including ink and paint; abating lead paint in dwellings across the nation; developing a safe alternative to the lead storage battery; stringently enforcing existing standards or instituting new standards based on recent understanding of the toxicity of lead at low doses; and more strictly regulating lead levels in soil, surface dust, and drinking water.

Finally, new sources of environmental lead exposure must not be allowed to develop. Of particular concern is incineration, rapidly emerging as a leading means of municipal solid waste disposal. Municipal waste contains substantial amounts of lead and other metals. Incineration may disseminate these materials into air and dust, creating a major source of environmental lead. This technology needs to be carefully evaluated before it is disseminated throughout the United States.

SUGGESTED READING

Bellinger D, Leviton A, Waternaux C, et al. Longitudinal analyses of prenatal and postnatal lead exposure and early cognitive development. N Engl J Med 1987; 316:1037–1043.

Cullen MR, Robins JM, Eskanazi B. Adult inorganic lead intoxication: Presentation of 31 new cases and review of recent advances in the literature. Medicine 1983; 62:2321–2347.

Feldman RG, Haddow J, Kopito L, Schwachman H. Altered peripheral nerve conduction velocity, chronic lead intoxication in children. Am J Dis Child 1973; 125:39–41.

Landrigan PJ. Strategies for epidemiologic studies of lead in bone in occupationally exposed populations. Environ Health Perspect 1991; 91:81–86.

Mahaffey KR. Health consequences of dietary and environmental exposure to lead. Amsterdam: Elsevier, 1985.

National Academy of Sciences. Environmental neurotoxicology. Washington, DC: National Academic Press, 1992.

Needleman HL, Schell A, Bellinger D, et al. The long-term effects of exposure to low doses of lead in childhood: An 11-year follow-up report. N Engl J Med 1990; 322:83–88.

Rutter M. Low level lead exposure: Sources, effects and implications. In: Rutter M, Jones RR, eds. Lead versus health. London: John Wiley, 1983.

DIALYSIS ENCEPHALOPATHY

BRIAN HAINLINE, M.D.

Maintenance dialysis and kidney transplantation have changed the natural course of renal failure. Formerly, uremic encephalopathy developed in patients with renal failure and progressed to coma or other systemic complications prior to death. Maintenance dialysis prevents untimely deaths in renal failure patients but causes other neurologic problems from metabolic, nutritional, or hematologic derangements or from complications of dialysis. Neurologic illnesses well described in dialysis patients include metabolic and hypertensive encephalopathy, dysequilibrium syndrome, subdural hematoma, Wernicke's encephalopathy, and drug intoxication.

Renal transplantation potentially cures renal failure, but graft versus host reactions usually necessitate the use of immunosuppressant medications. Neurologic complications of renal transplant include brain tumors (especially primary central nervous system lymphoma) and central nervous system infections secondary to immunosuppression.

The neurologic complications of dialysis and renal transplantation have been described under other clinical circumstances. Dialysis encephalopathy is the first new neurologic disorder described in patients with uremia undergoing hemodialysis.

HISTORICAL BACKGROUND

I have devoted several pages to the historical background of dialysis encephalopathy since, as a disease, it has been virtually completely eradicated. An understanding of pertinent historical developments in the understanding of causes and treatment will help the neurologist in properly diagnosing the rare patient who may present with symptoms and signs of dialysis encephalopathy.

In 1972 a unique neurologic disorder developed among several patients undergoing hemodialysis in Denver. Patients manifested a spectrum of clinical features: mixed dysarthric-dyspraxic speech, asterixis, multifocal myoclonus, progressive dementia, partial and generalized convulsive seizures, and a typical electroencephalogram (EEG) showing frontal bursts of delta waves with associated spike and wave complexes.

This unique syndrome was clearly distinct from other metabolic complications of renal failure. For example, the EEG showed frontal bursts rather than a diffuse slowing. Furthermore, patients with mild to moderate dialysis encephalopathy improved following low-dose diazepam. Myoclonus dissipated, speech cleared, and the EEG normalized. This led some investigators to speculate that dialysis encephalopathy was a seizure disorder. However, dialysis encephalopathy was refractory to treatment with other classes of anticonvulsants and typically progressed despite transient improvement following benzodiazepine administration.

Dialysis centers worldwide began reporting outbreaks of this curious illness among hemodialysis patients shortly after the initial report. Most patients developed progressive symptoms over a period of months, culminating in death. Patients typically worsened acutely during and immediately following dialysis treatment. Renal transplantation was usually not successful in reversing or even halting disease progression. Benzodiazepines appeared to have a short-acting beneficial effect, but no other attempted treatment modalities successfully treated this devastating illness.

Various causes were proposed, including atypical virus infection, unknown metabolic derangements resulting from chronic hemodialysis treatment, and metal intoxication, but all initial attempts at defining a cause were unsuccessful. Brain examinations postmortem were unremarkable, and the disease was not transmittable to primates. Not until 1976 was aluminum defined as the cause of dialysis encephalopathy.

Aluminum is ubiquitous in the environment, making up 8 percent of the earth's crust. Therefore, attempts to accurately and precisely measure body aluminum were initially flawed because of contamination. In 1976, through a technique of extracting tissue aluminum with disodium ethylenediaminetetraacetic acid and measuring this element with a flameless atomic absorption spectrophotometer, accurate and precise aluminum measurements became possible. Utilizing this technique, researchers demonstrated that dialysis encephalopathy patients have significantly more brain aluminum in the frontal cortex than nondialyzed controls and dialysis patients without dialysis encephalopathy. For the first time researchers uncovered the probable cause of dialysis encephalopathy.

Researchers initially postulated that aluminum accumulation developed in dialysis patients because these patients consumed large amounts of aluminum-containing phosphate binding gels to control serum phosphorus levels. The demonstration of statistically significant increased brain aluminum seemed to be explained by the fact that virtually all dialysis patients consumed aluminum antacids. However, epidemiologic studies showed that dialysis encephalopathy tended to occur as an epidemic in certain dialysis centers but not others. Since virtually all dialysis patients consumed aluminum antacids, and since the disease often presented in a fulminant manner, aluminum toxicity via orally consumed antacids was an inadequate explanation of the epidemiology of this disease.

Researchers then measured aluminum content in the dialysate used for dialyzing patients and discovered an enormous discrepancy among various dialysis centers, ranging from 1 to 1,600 μg per liter. Aluminum is easily transferred from the dialysate into the body. Once in the body, it is removed only minimally in dialysis patients since renal excretion is not possible and protein bound aluminum is not dialyzable. Epidemiologic studies demonstrated that outbreaks of dialysis encephalopathy occurred in centers with a large amount of aluminum in the dialysate.

When proper water purification was utilized and dialysate aluminum was consistently decreased to less than 10 μg per liter (preferably less than 1 μg per liter), dialysis encephalopathy epidemics were eliminated. However, sporadic cases became more prevalent over the years, with aluminum still looming as the culprit. Uremic patients continued to depend on oral aluminum ingestion to control serum phosphorus levels, and this element was demonstrated to accumulate significantly in long-term dialysis patients. Once a critical threshold of brain aluminum developed, so did symptoms and signs of dialysis encephalopathy.

Proper water purification was the most effective way to completely eliminate epidemics of dialysis encephalopathy. However, long-term dialysis patients continued to develop the disease, especially when they became ill from other causes. During illness-related catabolism, it was discovered that aluminum was shunted from bone to serum, thereby explaining this clinical relationship. In essence, all dialysis patients became vulnerable to developing this disease as long as total body aluminum continued to increase. Aluminum is strongly protein bound, and under ideal circumstances of zero aluminum in the dialysate, only small amounts of aluminum (100 μg per hour) are dialyzable.

Deferoxamine, a metal chelating agent, was traditionally used to treat patients with iron overload. Deferoxamine also strongly binds aluminum, and clinical studies convincingly demonstrated that deferoxamine-aluminum is dialyzable. Therefore, patients with aluminum overload can receive deferoxamine during dialysis, and the deferoxamine-aluminum complex is dialyzed. Serum aluminum can increase over tenfold following deferoxamine administration. With repeat treatment and dialysis, the acute rise diminishes and the baseline aluminum level eventually decreases. We demonstrated that deferoxamine crosses the blood-brain barrier and that cerebrospinal fluid aluminum significantly increases following deferoxamine treatment.

Since patients with dialysis encephalopathy improve after receiving deferoxamine treatment for many months, one can conclude that removal of aluminum from the body is beneficial. It is not known whether deferoxamine binds brain aluminum, but clinical experience and intuition suggest this must be so. However, patients with acute dialysis encephalopathy may deteriorate following deferoxamine treatment, and this correlates with an acute rise in cerebrospinal fluid aluminum. Presumably, aluminum is acutely shunted from other tissues to the brain as serum aluminum rises, and a clinical deterioration occurs that is similar to what had occurred in patients being dialyzed with a high aluminum content in the dialysate. It is unlikely that deferoxamine alone is neurotoxic, since patients treated with deferoxamine for other conditions do not develop such neurologic symptoms and signs. The deterioration that can occur in dialysis encephalopathy patients is an extension of their disease.

DIALYSIS ENCEPHALOPATHY TODAY

Sporadic cases of dialysis encephalopathy still surface, and the clinician must be aware of its unique clinical features so that proper treatment may begin.

The neurologist is often called to evaluate patients with renal failure who have become confused or who have developed some other alteration in mental status. Most often, the physical examination is nonfocal, and the patient appears encephalopathic. Although dialysis encephalopathy remains a diagnostic possibility, other reasons for a change in mental status must be vigorously pursued before accepting a diagnosis of dialysis encephalopathy. Figure 1 outlines the approach the neurologist may take when confronted with a newly confused dialysis patient. Careful history taking is essential. Some patients may have recently begun a new medication that causes confusion. Others may have changed their dialysis schedule, making them vulnerable to metabolic changes. Other patients may be harboring a systemic infection. Any focality in the neurologic exam warrants a brain computed tomography (CT) or magnetic resonance imaging (MRI) scan to rule out an underlying mass lesion such as a subdural hematoma or a brain abscess.

If the physical examination is nonfocal, the neurologist must vigorously search for an infectious or metabolic cause of the change in mental status. Careful attention should be directed to the dialysis shunt or fistula, common sources of infection. If there is no evidence of systemic infection, other metabolic causes of the change in mental status should be pursued. If an infectious cause is identified, appropriate treatment must begin.

The neurologist confronted with the dialysis patient must understand that these patients constantly live with metabolic derangements to which their brain has adapted. Therefore we are more concerned with a change from baseline metabolic parameters than with the absolute figures at the time of examination. Initial blood tests should include SMA-20 and liver enzymes. An acute derangement in serum sodium, calcium, or magnesium can result in a change in mental status, and if this becomes apparent after laboratory tests, appro-

priate treatment should begin. Blood urea nitrogen and creatinine are chronically elevated in these patients, but an acute change from baseline causes encephalopathy. In this case, the dialysis schedule may need to be changed. Dialysis patients are vulnerable to hepatitis, and an acute change in liver enzymes can also render these patients encephalopathic. It is reasonable to measure thyroid function, folic acid, and vitamin B_{12} levels. Be certain the patient is not thiamine deficient. Partial and nonconvulsive seizures should be ruled out. If a metabolic change is discovered, appropriate treatment of the underlying condition should begin.

If there is no evidence of systemic infection and no evident metabolic cause for the patient's change in mental status, then further neurodiagnostic tests are warranted. Brain CT or MRI scan should be performed. If this reveals a lesion consistent with the patient's clinical profile, begin appropriate treatment. If the brain imaging study is unremarkable, obtain an EEG. If the EEG shows characteristic frontal bursts with sharp waves, begin a more focused evaluation for dialysis encephalopathy (Fig. 2). If the EEG is normal, shows baseline slowing, or shows triphasic waves consistent with a metabolic encephalopathy, a further search for a metabolic or infectious cause of the patient's altered mental status should proceed. Cryptic central nervous system infections should be ruled out by careful examination of the cerebrospinal fluid.

The neurologist should be aware that dialysis encephalopathy is an extremely rare disease nowadays, and other diseases must be carefully excluded as outlined above. In patients with suspected dialysis encephalopathy, the first question that must be answered is whether the patient has been significantly exposed to aluminum. Nowadays, most patients take calcium carbonate supplements to reduce serum phosphorus. However, some patients have been undergoing dialysis for many years, and it is likely that they consumed large quantities of aluminum-containing antacids before beginning calcium carbonate supplements.

If the neurologist uncovers a history of significant prior or present aluminum exposure, careful consideration should be given to any signs of dialysis encephalopathy. Often these signs are subtle, and a careful history may be necessary to uncover symptoms that suggest dialysis encephalopathy. The most characteristic early manifestation is a subtle slurring of speech—often a combination of a dyspraxic and dysarthric speech—without classic aphasia. This may be coupled with multifocal myoclonus and memory impairment. If there is no suggestion of dialysis encephalopathy by way of speech signs, myoclonus, or EEG, the neurologist may consider pursuing this matter further. Perhaps there have been unexplained mild signs, which family members or even the patient may recollect. Serial EEGs may reveal subtle evidence of dialysis encephalopathy, with intermittent frontal sharp bursts. If diagnostic testing indicates that the patient may have dialysis encephalopathy, a deferoxamine infusion test should be performed.

Most long-term hemodialysis patients who have had

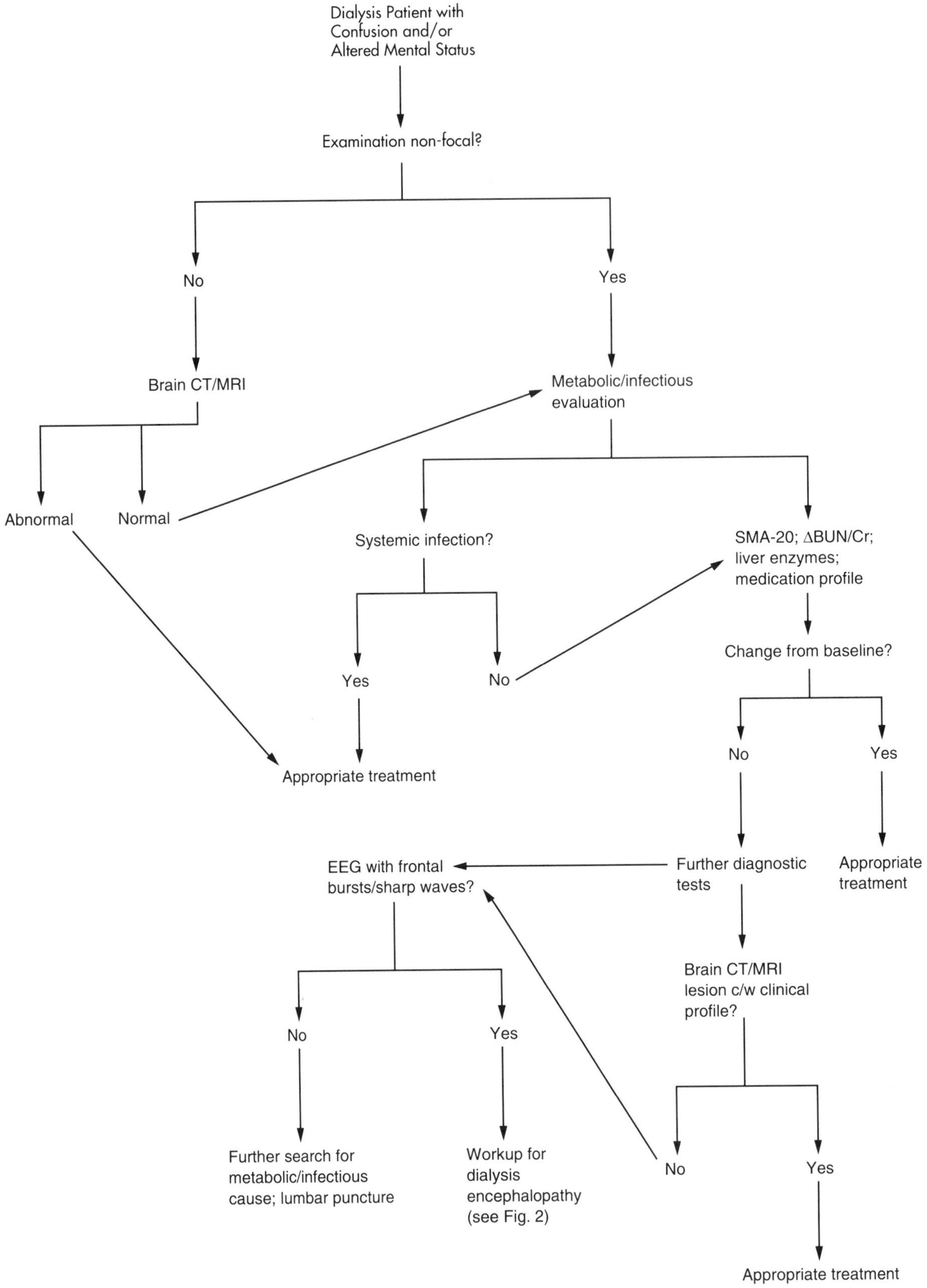

Figure 1 Algorithm for the evaluation of dialysis patients with an altered mental status. CT = computed tomography, MRI = magnetic resonance imaging, BUN/Cr = blood urea nitrogen/creatinine, EEG = electroencephalogram.

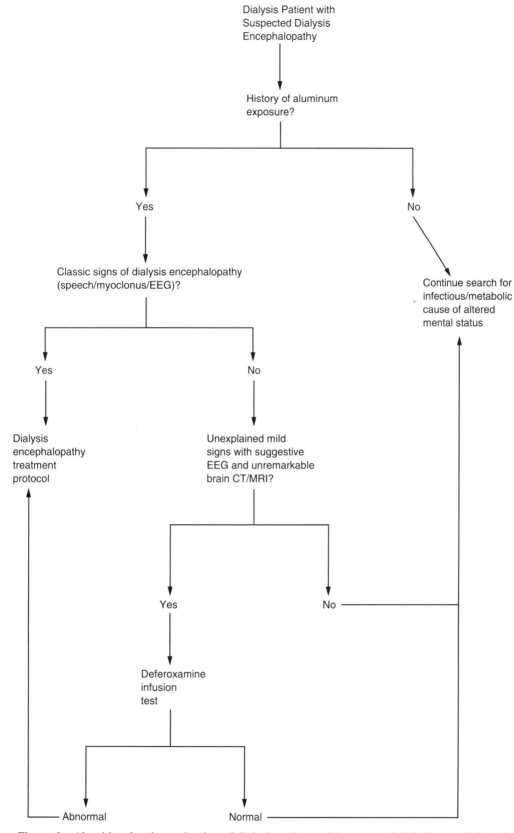

Figure 2 Algorithm for the evaluation of dialysis patients with suspected dialysis encephalopathy.

significant exposure to aluminum do not have elevated baseline serum aluminum levels, because most of the aluminum has been stored in various tissues such as bone and spleen. During catabolic states, serum aluminum increases as bone aluminum stores are released into the serum. A deferoxamine infusion test is based on the principle that deferoxamine will chelate aluminum from tissue stores and will circulate in the serum. The amount of deferoxamine used for the infusion test should be coordinated with the patient's nephrologist. In cases of dialysis encephalopathy, the serum aluminum should at least double after a deferoxamine infusion test.

If there is no significant rise in serum aluminum, return to analyzing other possible causes of the patient's altered mental status, such as human immunodeficiency virus (acquired immunodeficiency syndrome dementia), Lyme disease, herpes simplex encephalitis, and other cryptic infections. In addition, partial seizures and nonconvulsive status epilepticus should be ruled out. If the deferoxamine infusion test is positive and if all other causes have been reasonably excluded, the patient should be definitively treated for dialysis encephalopathy.

Unlike in earlier times, when dialysis encephalopathy presented in an epidemic and fulminant manner, the neurologist is usually not faced with a situation of emergently treating the patient. This means that treatment can be well thought out, and the patient should not deteriorate as a result of treatment. Large doses of deferoxamine may mobilize considerable amounts of aluminum and may cause a clinical deterioration. This is unnecessary, since patients are no longer exposed to a significant ongoing positive aluminum balance.

I prefer first treating dialysis encephalopathy patients with a low-dose benzodiazepine such as clonazepam (1 mg twice daily). Benzodiazepines are both therapeutic and diagnostic. Unlike patients with meta-bolic and infectious encephalopathies, who usually experience clinical deterioration after benzodiazepine administration, dialysis encephalopathy patients often improve dramatically after benzodiazepine treatment. Clonazepam, however, is not a definitive treatment. It simply protects the patient from the neurotoxic effects of aluminum. Once clonazepam has begun, deferoxamine treatment should be started. A reasonable dose is 500 mg given at the beginning of dialysis, and this may be repeated between once and three times weekly. Pre- and postserum aluminum levels should be measured once or twice monthly, and serial EEGs should be performed once or twice monthly. The end point of treatment is generally obtained in a few months' time, and aside from a clinical improvement, there should be no significant incremental increase in serum aluminum after deferoxamine administration.

SUGGESTED READING

Ackrill P, Ralston AJ, Day JP. Role of desferrioxamine in the treatment of dialysis encephalopathy. Kidney Int Suppl 1986; 29(Suppl 18):104–107.

Alfrey AC. Aluminum intoxication. N Engl J Med 1984; 310: 1118–1119.

Alfrey AC, LeGendre GR, Kaehny WD. The dialysis encephalopathy syndrome: Possible aluminum intoxication. N Engl J Med 1976; 294:184–188.

Hughes JR, Schreeder MT. EEG in dialysis encephalopathy. Neurology 1980; 30:1148–1154.

Nadel AM, Wilson WP. Dialysis encephalopathy: A possible seizure disorder. Neurology 1976; 26:1130–1134.

Schreeder MT, Favero MS, Hughes JR, et al. Dialysis encephalopathy and aluminum exposure: An epidemiologic analysis. J Chron Dis 1983; 36:581–593.

Sweeney VP, Perry TL, Price JDE, et al. Brain gamma-aminobutyric acid deficiency in dialysis encephalopathy. Neurology 1985; 35: 180–184.

HYPOGLYCEMIA

ALAN H. LOCKWOOD, M.D.

Hypoglycemia is a common problem that may be encountered in virtually every clinical setting ranging from the emergency room to the general medical ward and outpatient department. All age groups are affected and all social and ethnic groups. Since prolonged or severe hypoglycemia carries the risk of permanent neurologic injury, it is imperative to diagnose and treat hypoglycemia promptly.

Neurologists are likely to encounter these patients since the symptoms and signs of hypoglycemia are due to nervous system dysfunction. It is caused by depriving the brain of its needed substrate and the effects of the adrenergic discharge that occurs as the glucose homeostatic mechanisms attempt to stimulate gluconeogenesis.

CLINICAL ASPECTS OF HYPOGLYCEMIA

The diagnosis of hypoglycemia is difficult to make on the basis of clinical symptomatology alone. The duration and severity of the hypoglycemia interact to determine the manifestations of the disorder. Although the majority of symptoms are attributable to nervous system dysfunction, they are extremely varied, often nonspecific, or may not be present at all, even when blood glucose levels are extremely low. Because of the close link between the symptoms of hypoglycemia and the brain, Marks and Rose use the term *neuroglycopenia* to refer to symptomatic hypoglycemia.

They describe acute, subacute, and chronic hypoglycemic syndromes.

The acute syndrome occurs in a setting of euglycemia and follows a sudden reduction in the blood glucose concentration. It develops commonly because of the action of short-acting insulin preparations or sulfonylureas, or other oral hypoglycemic agents. It often begins with vague symptoms of malaise, environmental detachment, and restlessness, which are associated with hunger, nervousness, and diaphoresis that may lead to severe anxiety and panic. Ataxia, slurred speech, slight blunting of consciousness, disorientation, and ataxia are common. These symptoms are frequently recognized by the patient, family members, or other observers and respond quickly to oral or parenteral glucose. Electroencephalograms performed during this period may reveal nonspecific abnormalities. These episodes may terminate spontaneously if glucose homeostatic mechanisms are successful and the offending agent is cleared from the body. The attack may also increase in severity and proceed rapidly to generalized seizures and coma, with the attendant risk of permanent brain injury. These patients may arrive in the emergency room in coma with no history.

In a recent study of acute hypoglycemia in patients with insulin-dependent diabetes, Hepburn and co-workers evaluated the symptoms of hypoglycemia using the statistical technique of factor analysis. They induced hypoglycemia under controlled conditions and evaluated the symptoms. They attributed the symptoms of sweating, tremor, and warmth to autonomic nervous system activity and the symptoms of inability to concentrate, weakness, and drowsiness to neuronal glucose deprivation and cerebral dysfunction. Other common symptoms such as hunger, weakness, blurred vision, and drowsiness could not be grouped clearly in the autonomic or brain categories.

The subacute syndrome is the most common form observed in individuals with spontaneous hypoglycemia occurring in the fasting state. Most of the symptoms listed above are absent. In their place, there is a slowing of thought processes and a gradual blunting of consciousness. Although patients are conscious, subsequent amnesia for the episode is common. The diagnosis may be very difficult to establish until the possibility of hypoglycemia is considered or, commonly, routine testing uncovers the abnormality. Hypothermia is common in this form of the disorder, and unexplained low body temperatures should always be followed by a blood glucose measurement.

Chronic hypoglycemia is rare and, if confirmed, suggests a probable insulin-secreting tumor or obsessive behavior on the part of a diabetic who is preoccupied with keeping the blood glucose level low. Marks and Rose characterize this syndrome by insidious changes in personality, memory, and behavior that may be misconstrued as dementia. Unlike the acute and subacute forms of hypoglycemia, the symptoms are not promptly relieved by the administration of glucose, suggesting the presence of neuronal injury. Clinical improvement after

removal of the source of the exogenous insulin is very gradual, extending over periods as long as a year.

Many patients are unaware of any symptoms that indicate the development of hypoglycemia. This condition is termed *hypoglycemia unawareness* and poses additional risks to these patients because of delays in diagnosis and treatment. The cause of this condition is not clear and is likely to involve multiple factors. Most of these patients exhibit a reduced sensitivity to plasma epinephrine, norepinephrine, or both. This is not likely to be the consequence of a diabetic autonomic neuropathy, since these patients have an increase in sensitivity to catecholamines, a form of denervation hypersensitivity. These patients also appear to have an increase in the threshold (i.e., lower blood glucose levels are required) for the activation of normal glucose homeostatic mechanisms. Patients with hypoglycemia unawareness appear to have had multiple episodes of hypoglycemia. The prior episodes may contribute to the development of unawareness.

There are special problems associated with detecting hypoglycemia in neonates and children, which center on the variety and nonspecificity of the symptoms themselves, including pallor, irritability, feeding difficulties, and variability in the sensitivity of individual children to a given plasma glucose concentration. As with adults, the diagnosis is most likely to be made when the index of suspicion is consciously kept high by the physician and when glucose measurement is performed routinely when there is any doubt about a diagnosis. The risk of failing to establish the diagnosis and the development of irreversible neuronal injury justifies the liberal use of screening measures and, in some cases, presumptive treatment with parenteral glucose.

PATHOPHYSIOLOGIC CONSIDERATIONS

Because of the complexity of glucose homeostasis, the causes of hypoglycemia are many, and a detailed discussion is beyond the scope of this chapter. In general, most authors present a physiologic classification that segregates causes in terms of hyper- versus hypoinsulinism and whether glucose turnover is high, as in hyperinsulinism, or low, as in metabolic defects that impair glycogenolysis or gluconeogenesis. In the former group, insulinomas, insulin overdose, and the accidental or purposeful ingestion of drugs that lower glucose require consideration. Decreases in glucose turnover may be due to liver disease, alcohol, starvation, and various endocrine disorders. In neonates, hypoxia, sepsis, starvation, the small-for-gestational-age syndrome, and inheritable diseases of metabolism are important causes of hypoglycemia.

Drugs are an important cause of hypoglycemia. Selzer gathered almost 800 cases from personal experience and the literature. Sulfonylureas caused the vast majority of the episodes. In most instances, some restriction of food intake, varying from missing a single meal to severe starvation, potentiated the action of the drugs. Age-dependent causes were also identified and should aid in diagnosis. In the newborn period, the administration of sulfonylureas to the mother dominated. From 0 to 2 years, salicylate administration (ingestion) dominated. Surprisingly, alcohol was important in the 2- to 7-year age group. In this group, ingestion of alcohol-containing cough syrups occurred along with the ingestion of beer, wine, and liquor. Sulfonylureas dominated in the 11- to 30-year and 50-plus age groups. Alcohol was an important predisposing factor between the age of 30 and 50. Because of rising alcohol use among teenagers, alcohol-related hypoglycemia may be increasing in importance.

Beta-blocking agents mask the development of symptoms in many patients. These agents eliminate the symptoms and signs of the autonomic nervous system hyperactivity that may herald the onset of hypoglycemia. In spite of widespread knowledge about this potentially serious problem, it is not rare to find diabetics who have been instructed to take beta blockers. These agents have gained wide acceptance for the treatment of many disorders, ranging from the prophylaxis of migraine headaches to the treatment of hypertension and other cardiovascular diseases. This may be more of a problem when patients see one physician for the care of their diabetes and another for the hypertension and heart disease that are common complications of diabetes. The use of beta blockers in patients receiving insulin or oral hypoglycemic agents should be avoided.

Under normal circumstances, the brain has an absolute requirement for both glucose and oxygen. Since only small amounts of glucose are stored in the brain as glycogen, and since the brain glucose concentration is usually lower than the blood glucose concentration, glucose must be supplied to the brain at a rate that equals its use. The most efficient metabolism of glucose also requires oxygen. Although hypoxia stimulates glycolysis in the brain, this compensatory increase is never sufficient to maintain cerebral activity during severe hypoxia. The mechanisms by which reductions in the availability of glucose to the brain lead to the development of symptoms is not clear. Studies of energy metabolism have shown that the cerebral content of adenosine triphosphate is normal, or nearly normal, in animals with severe hypoglycemia. This implies the existence of mechanisms that reduce neural activity in response to a reduction in the availability of glucose.

Although hypoglycemia alone is sufficient to cause cerebral injury, this stress is often augmented by the presence of epileptic seizures caused by hypoglycemia. These seizures appear to be the result of the uncontrolled release of excitatory neurotransmitters. The excessively high concentration of excitatory neurotransmitters causes further neural injury, which can be prevented, in part, by treating animals with agents that prevent the binding of excitatory neurotransmitters to postsynaptic sites in the brain.

Hypothermia is common in patients with hypoglycemia. Animal studies have shown that hypothermia can be induced by intrahypothalamic injections of deoxyglucose, an agent that blocks glucose metabolism. This may explain, in part, some of the perceptions of altered body temperature reported by patients with hypoglycemia. All patients with unexplained hypothermia should be screened for hypoglycemia.

EMPIRIC TREATMENT

Hypoglycemia is a medical emergency that should be treated with an intravenous injection of glucose. Prompt treatment is essential to avoid potential complications, and continued monitoring of the plasma glucose concentration is necessary to detect repeated episodes. Patients should not be discharged until a working diagnosis has been established to assure patient safety and to minimize the risk of recurrent episodes.

In a recent study of 301 consecutive patients with an altered mental state identified by emergency medical technicians, 25 (7.4 percent) experienced complete resolution of all symptoms after empiric treatment with 50 percent glucose. This relatively high rate of response justifies empiric treatment of all patients suspected of being hypoglycemic, including all patients with coma of unknown cause. Empiric use may not be necessary if immediate screening for hypoglycemia can be performed in the field by emergency medical personnel. It is prudent, when practical, to draw extra blood so that insulin levels can be measured, if indicated by the subsequent course of the patient. This is particularly important in patients with obscure histories or where factitious hypoglycemia may be present.

Potential risks posed to the patient by the unnecessary administration of glucose, even in hyperglycemic states, is small. The amount of glucose administered is small compared to the amount present under these conditions, and the potential benefits are substantial.

Patients with hypoglycemia may require other medical investigations to determine the cause and plan the appropriate therapy of underlying conditions that cause hypoglycemia. These measures are beyond the scope of this chapter.

SUGGESTED READING

Auer RN. Progress review: Hypoglycemic brain damage. Stroke 1986; 17:699–708.

Aynsley-Green A, Soltesz G. Hypoglycemia in infancy and childhood. Edinburgh: Churchill Livingstone, 1985.

Gajar JBG, Plum F, Duffy TE. Cerebral oxidative metabolism and blood flow during acute hypoglycemia and recovery in unanesthetized rats. J Neurochem 1982; 38:397–409.

Gerich JE, Mokan M, Venman T, et al. Hypoglycemia unawareness. Endocr Rev 1991; 12:356–371.

Hepburn DA, Deary IJ, Frier BM, et al. Symptoms of acute insulin-induced hypoglycemia in humans with and without IDDM: Factor-analysis approach. Diabetes Care 1991; 14:949–957.

Marks V, Rose FC. Hypoglycemia. Oxford: Blackwell, 1981.

Seltzer HS. Severe drug-induced hypoglycemia: A review. Compr Ther 1979; 5:21–29.

Service FJ. Hypoglycemic disorders: Pathogenesis, diagnosis, and treatment. Boston: GK Hall, 1983.

WILSON'S DISEASE

GEORGE J. BREWER, M.D.

Wilson's disease is an autosomal recessive disorder resulting in copper accumulation. The basic defect is in the liver, which fails to regulate copper balance by appropriate excretion of excess copper in the bile. As a result, copper builds up in the liver over a period of years, and toxicity from the excess copper ultimately results in liver disease. Thus one mode of clinical presentation, involving about one-third of patients, is with various manifestations of liver disease. Alternatively, the liver damage may be clinically silent. However, the copper storage capacity of the liver has been exceeded, and copper levels have increased in the blood and other organs of the body. The brain appears to be the next most sensitive organ, and about two-thirds of patients present clinically with neurologic or psychiatric signs and symptoms. Diagnosis is particularly important in this disease because of the availability of effective treatment.

Patients may be identified in any one of four settings. One is the patient who develops a typical neurologic picture and is referred to a neurology clinic. Second is the patient who manifests behavioral or psychiatric symptoms for several years preceding neurologic manifestations and has been seen by behavioral health care workers. Third is the patient who presents with liver disease. Fourth is the presymptomatic patient who should be diagnosed in the course of working up the siblings of a newly diagnosed symptomatic patient.

PATIENTS WITH NEUROLOGIC DISEASE

Patients with neurologic disease typically present in the late teenage years or early 20s, with a peak at about age 21, but occasional patients may present at almost any age later in life. Factors influencing age of presentation no doubt include diet, the capacity of the liver in a particular person to detoxify or store copper, and a host of possible unidentified factors. Early symptoms may be quite subtle and involve mild speech abnormality, mild tremor, or abnormal handwriting, particularly with micrographia. Very commonly these symptoms are accompanied by a decline in school or work performance, and this may be one of the most significant factors bringing the patient to the physician. In other cases the neurologic presentation may be more florid and involve a variety of signs and symptoms, which are listed in Table 1. Approximately half the patients who ultimately present with neurologic disease have a rather extended history of psychiatric or behavioral problems, which antedated the neurologic symptoms by several years.

Because of the tangible nature of neurologic signs

Table 1 Neurologic Signs at First Evaluation in 31 Patients Presenting with Neurologic Disease

Sign	% of Patients
Dysarthria	97
Dystonia	65
Dysdiadochokinesia	58
Rigidity	52
Posture abnormality	42
Gait abnormality	42
Facial expression abnormality	39
Tremor	32
Abnormal eye movement	32
Increased deep tendon reflexes	29
Drooling	23
Bradykinesia	19
Motor impersistence	19
Frontal release signs	19
Paresis	16
Athetosis	10
Babinski's sign	10
Sensory deficit	3

Adapted from Starosta-Rubinstein S, Young AB, Kluin K, et al. Clinical assessment of 31 patients with Wilson's disease: Correlations with structural changes on magnetic resonance imaging. Arch Neurol 1987; 44:365–370; with permission.

and symptoms, the patient is usually referred to a neurologist. Thus, patients presenting early with neurologic signs and symptoms have the best chance of early diagnosis. Most neurologists, seeing the types of signs and symptoms described, would include Wilson's disease in their differential diagnosis and proceed to the next step of ruling the disease in or out by various laboratory and other examinations. The slightest hint of concomitant liver disease should further solidify the position of Wilson's disease as the condition to rule out. There are very few other disorders that affect both the brain and the liver in the absence of liver failure and hepatic encephalopathy. Indications of liver disease can include anything from mildly abnormal serum liver-derived enzymes, to abnormalities of bilirubin and other liver function tests, to evidence of hypersplenism, such as thrombocytopenia or leukopenia.

A list of the diagnostic steps used to evaluate the possibility of Wilson's disease is shown in Table 2, along with their difficulty, whether or not they are invasive, and their degree of utility in various types of patients. Table 3 provides numbers for the copper-related variables in normals, heterozygotes, symptomatic Wilson's disease patients, and presymptomatic Wilson's disease patients. The measurement of serum ceruloplasmin is easy to do and helps with index of suspicion but is not diagnostic. Values are quite low in 80 percent of patients with Wilson's disease, but the remainder of the patients have intermediate to normal values. Further, heterozygous carriers of the gene for Wilson's disease may also have low or normal values. On the other hand, a very useful diagnostic procedure is assay of 24 hour urine copper. All symptomatic patients will have an elevation of this value over 100 μg per 24 hours (see Table 3). While inexperienced technicians, poor procedures, or inade-

Table 2 Diagnostic Steps in Wilson's Disease

Procedure	Difficulty	Invasive	Utility
Serum ceruloplasmin assay	Easy	No	Some: 80% of patients have very low values, but 20% are intermediate to normal; 20% of carriers have low to intermediate values; all infants to age 6 months have low values.
24 hour urine copper	Fairly easy	No	High utility in symptomatic patients: May give false negative in presymptomatic patients. Obstructive liver disease can give false positive. Avoid contamination problem.
Slit-lamp examination for Kayser-Fleischer rings	Easy	No	Some: Very good in neurologic-psychiatric cases; only occasionally positive in other patients; may give false-positive in obstructive liver disease.
Magnetic resonance or computed tomography of brain	Easy	No	Some: Usually typical (although nonspecific) abnormalities are seen in patients presenting with neurologic disease but not with other presentations.
Hepatic copper determination from liver biopsy	Fairly hard	Yes	Excellent: False-negatives very rare if ever; only false-positives are patients with obstructive liver disease.
24 or 48 hour copper-64 incorporation into ceruloplasmin	Hard	No	Some: Considerable overlap between affected patients and heterozygotes.
DNA analysis for linkage	A specialized procedure at present	No	Excellent for the siblings of an affected patient.

Modified from Brewer GJ, Yuzbasiyan-Gurkan V. Wilson disease. Medicine 1992; 71:139–164; with permission.

Table 3 Copper-related Variables Useful for the Diagnosis of Wilson's Disease

Variables	Normal	Heterozygotes	Symptomatic Wilson's Disease	Presymptomatic Wilson's Disease
Serum ceruloplasmin, mg/dl	20–35	0–35, 20% have low or intermediate values	Typically 0–10; 20% have intermediate or normal values	Same as symptomatic
24–hour urine copper, μg	20–50	20–75	Over 100	Normal to high
Hepatic copper, μg/g dry weight	20–50	20–150	Over 200	Over 200 in adolescents and adults. Not well characterized in very young children although probably usually high.
Incorporation of copper-64 into ceruloplasmin at 24 or 48 hour				
Oral ratio of 24 hour peak to initial peak	0.6–1.3	0.3–1.2	0.1–0.5	Same as symptomatic
Intravenous, % of dose	Over 4%	2–5%	Less than 1%	Same as symptomatic

Adapted from Brewer GJ, Yuzbasiyan-Gurkan V. Wilson disease. Medicine 1992; 71:139–164; with permission.

quate equipment, may lead to contamination or other problems with the assay, if the urine is collected reliably in trace element–free containers and assayed accurately, this procedure is remarkably useful.

Another procedure that is extremely effective in the diagnosis of neurologically affected patients is the slit-lamp examination for Kayser-Fleischer rings. These copper deposits in the cornea are almost invariably present in patients who present with neurologic disease. In addition, imaging of the brain, with either magnetic resonance imaging (MRI) or computed tomography (CT), is almost invariably positive for typical lesions in patients with neurologic disease. All of our neurologic patients who have had MRI (22 patients) have shown lesions. A list of typical lesions is shown in Table 4. Of course these lesions are not specific for Wilson's disease, so their presence does not prove the diagnosis.

The gold standard for diagnosis is the determination of hepatic copper in liver tissue obtained by percutaneous needle biopsy. The hepatic copper *must* be quantitatively assayed. Histochemical hepatic copper stains are very unreliable in the diagnosis of Wilson's disease because a positive stain depends on the copper being sequestered in cell organelles as opposed to being diffusely cytoplasmic. Often in the early stages of Wilson's disease, the copper is diffusely cytoplasmic, and the copper stain will be negative in the face of very high liver copper values. The quantitative assay of hepatic copper is completely diagnostic for Wilson's disease patients presenting with neurologic symptoms (see Table 3).

Table 4 Frequency of Lesions Shown by Brain Magnetic Resonance Imaging in 22 Patients with Wilson's Disease Presenting with Neurologic Symptoms

Location	% of Patients with Lesions
Caudate	46
Putamen	41
Atrophy	36
Midbrain	
Any location	27
Substantia nigra region	23
Periaqueductal gray matter	9
Midbrain tectum	5
Red nucleus	5
Subcortical white matter	23
Pons	23
Thalamus	9
Vermis	9
Dentate	5
Globus pallidus	5

Adapted from Starosta-Rubinstein S, Young AB, Kluin K, et al. Clinical assessment of 31 patients with Wilson's disease: Correlations with structural changes on magnetic resonance imaging. Arch Neurol 1987; 44:365–370; with permission.

At this time I do not recommend routine use of the copper-64 incorporation procedures listed in Tables 2 and 3 and recommended by other authorities. The main difficulty, in my experience, is the overlap between affected patients and heterozygotes. Thus it is possible to get false-positive results with this procedure. Some people so diagnosed have been treated for several years with anticopper agents before being determined to be heterozygotes. The DNA linkage analysis approach is available in some research laboratories, but it is a specialized procedure and is currently applicable only in a research setting.

A practical question that often arises in the laboratory workup is whether a patient requires a liver biopsy for diagnosis. For example, if a patient presents with typical neurologic signs and symptoms, has a low ceruloplasmin, a high urinary copper excretion, and a positive slit-lamp examination, is a liver biopsy required for diagnosis? The answer is, probably not, assuming that the Kayser-Fleischer rings have been seen by an opthalmologist who is certain of their presence, and assuming that the 24 hour urine copper examination has been replicated at least once and has been done with reliable collecting materials in a reliable laboratory.

PATIENTS WITH BEHAVIORAL OR PSYCHIATRIC SYMPTOMS

Patients in the second category have experienced behavioral abnormalities and psychiatric disease for a long period before the onset of neurologic signs and symptoms. These patients are very likely to remain undiagnosed until neurologic symptoms appear, and they are therefore likely to sustain irreversible damage. In my experience, about half the patients who were

Table 5 Presenting Psychiatric Symptoms in 24 Neurologically Symptomatic Patients

	% of Patients with Presenting Psychiatric Symptoms
Personality changes*	71
Depression	42
Cognitive changes	17
Anxiety	13
Psychosis	8
Catatonia	8
Others	21

*Personality changes include irritability, emotionality, extreme anger, decreased threshold to anger and ability to control it, and, occasionally, agression.

Adapted from Akil M, Schwartz JA, Dutchak D, et al. The psychiatric presentations of Wilson's disease. J Neuropsychiatry 1991; 3:377–382; with permission.

ultimately diagnosed as a result of neurologic symptoms had seen a psychiatrist or other behavioral health care workers during the preceding years. The behavioral abnormalities can include a wide spectrum of problems, as illustrated in Table 5. It is important for the physician seeing these patients to consider the possibility of Wilson's disease because, as emphasized before, the disease is so treatable. One approach to identifying the occasional patient with Wilson's disease hidden in the large clinic population with psychiatric disorders would be to routinely screen psychiatric patients by ceruloplasmin and/or 24 hour urine copper assay.

These screening procedures are not ideal. A low ceruloplasmin level is not specific and is found in only 80 percent of affected patients, and a 24 hour urine copper evaluation is far from a routine procedure. Once the gene for Wilson's disease is cloned and a direct DNA test becomes available, the ease of screening such clinical populations may change.

Until a better screening approach emerges, the Wilson's patient presenting with psychiatric symptoms is most dependent upon the physician's considering the possibility of Wilson's disease and undertaking screening tests. Perhaps one helpful way of suspecting Wilson's disease in these patients is to recognize that they have a new onset of psychiatric disease in the absence of obvious causative factors. The behavioral symptoms of Wilson's disease occur in patients who have previously been psychiatrically normal and in the absence of severe life trauma. Thus, the presentation will be akin to that of patients with substance abuse. In both conditions there is a fall-off in school or work performance. Thus in any patient suspected of recent onset of substance abuse, in the absence of definitive evidence or admission of that abuse, the physician should consider the possibility of Wilson's disease. Of course the slightest indication of concomitant liver disease, such as elevated enzymes, abnormalities of liver function, or evidence of hypersplenism such as thrombocytopenia or leukopenia, should immediately trigger a Wilson's disease workup. Any indication of neurologic signs or symptoms should prompt an immediate referral to a neurologist.

Once the diagnosis is considered, the same battery of tests discussed under the neurologic presentation is available and should be used in generally the same sequence. The comments regarding ceruloplasmin, the 24 hour urine copper assay, and the slit-lamp examination, which were made with respect to neurologic disease patients, are also valid for psychiatric patients. Patients presenting with psychiatric disease almost invariable have Kayser-Fleischer rings present. Again, the liver biopsy is diagnostic when quantitative copper is measured but may be unnecessary in a patient with a low ceruloplasmin, high urinary copper, and positive Kayser-Fleischer rings.

PATIENTS WITH LIVER DISEASE

Patients who present with liver disease are younger than those who present with neurologic disease and are typically teenagers. However, an occasional patient will present in almost any older age group. Some of these patients have florid hepatic failure, with a disease so severe and progressive that only hepatic transplantation will save them. Other patients may present with hepatic failure that is more mild, and medical therapy is indicated that can save the patient and the liver. A prognostic index has been developed by Nazer et al, which helps in identifying those patients who present in hepatic failure who probably will not survive without transplantation. This prognostic index depends upon the level of bilirubin, the level of SGPT, and the prolongation of the prothrombin time.

Many of the patients who present with hepatic failure have hemolysis. During hepatic necrosis, liver cells are releasing large amounts of copper into the blood. If copper levels reach a high enough level in the plasma, red blood cell destruction will occur. The combined presence of hemolysis and liver disease in a patient should always trigger the suspicion of Wilson's disease.

Patients with liver disease may be a heterogeneous and confusing group. A common presentation is one of chronic hepatitis, which can be confused with viral hepatitis and chronic active hepatitis. Clinically, there are no distinguishing features between antigen-negative chronic active hepatitis and Wilson's disease hepatitis. An appropriate diagnosis of Wilson's disease will only be made if further screening is performed on this group of patients. The same can be said for patients who have chronic cirrhosis. If the patient drinks alcoholic beverages at all, the patient may be diagnosed with alcoholic cirrhosis when in fact the cirrhosis is due to Wilson's disease. Again, the only way of identifying the patient with Wilson's disease is through appropriate screening and testing.

Testing for Wilson's disease in this setting is similar to that described earlier for neurologic and psychiatric disease. However, one needs to be aware that Kayser-Fleischer rings are not as uniformly seen in patients with a hepatic presentation. Further, if the patient has an obstructive component to the liver disease, the urinary copper and hepatic copper can become falsely elevated in the absence of Wilson's disease. Patients with a significant obstructive component to their liver disease are, indeed, the hardest patients to diagnosis. In this setting the radio-copper tests described earlier are sometimes useful. A DNA test, when it becomes available, will also be very useful in this setting.

PRESYMPTOMATIC PATIENTS

The fourth and final type of patient is diagnosed from a family study because an affected symptomatic patient has been diagnosed. The disease is autosomal recessive, which means that every full sibling has a 25 percent risk for harboring the homozygous genotype that will produce Wilson's disease. Currently, the penetrance of the disease in persons homozygous for the Wilson's disease gene is thought to be 100 percent. It has been clearly shown that prophylactic therapy, with either a chelator-type drug or zinc, will prevent the onset of disease in these presymptomatic patients. Thus it is extremely important to work up the brothers and sisters of a newly diagnosed patient to see whether they also have the disorder. This often means aggressive pursuit of relatives who may live some distance from the index case. The workup of siblings should ignore their age or relative position in the sibling-ship. We have found that older brothers and sisters are almost as often diagnosed in the presymptomatic stage as are younger brothers and sisters.

The workup of siblings should include, at least, a blood ceruloplasmin and two 24 hour urine copper studies. The ceruloplasmin should not be the sole test because of the lack of complete sensitivity and specificity mentioned earlier. The ceruloplasmin value should be used to adjust one's index of suspicion, in conjunction with the urine test. The 24 hour urine copper, in this setting, can be interpreted as follows: if a replicated 24 hour urine copper is over 100 μg, it is virtually diagnostic of the disease. However, in this setting (presymptomatic siblings) we would recommend a liver biopsy for further final proof. A valid, replicated urine copper value below 50 μg in a sibling 15 years of age or older excludes Wilson's disease. A urine copper value between 50 and 100 μg is compatible with Wilson's disease or the heterozygous state and is therefore indeterminant. Our data indicate that some presymptomatic affected siblings can have values as low as 65 μg, and some heterozygous carriers of the gene can have values up in this range. Thus, we think patients who have urine copper values in this area should have a liver biopsy and liver copper assay.

If the sibling being evaluated with ceruloplasmin and 24 hour urine copper is between the ages of 5 and 15, we recommend, in the face of normal urine copper excretion, another 24 hour urine copper test carried out at about age 15, in order to exclude the possibility that the patient had not accumulated enough copper at the time of the first test to show a positive urine excretion test. We generally do not screen siblings before age 5 because of the difficulty in obtaining valid 24 hour urine collections, and because the likelihood of clinical presentation before that age is exceedingly small. However, a blood ceruloplasmin can be done any time after the age of 1 year. All infants up to 6 months have low values. In the face of a very low ceruloplasmin in a young child, workup should perhaps be done earlier and more aggressively. In fact, in all of the situations discussed above, an extremely low ceruloplasmin should increase suspicion and prompt a more complete workup to rule out the disease.

The screening of other relatives of patients with Wilson's disease can be performed in the same manner as described above. Some of the genetic risks (assuming a patient frequency of one in 40,000 and a carrier frequency of one in 100) are one in 200 in children or half-siblings of a patient, one in 600 for niece or nephew, and one in 800 for first cousins. These risks are small relative to those of full siblings but large relative to the population risk. In our opinion, it is worthwhile screening these types of relatives.

COMMENTS

In summary, the key to the diagnosis of Wilson's disease is recognizing the possibility of that diagnosis in certain patients. These are patients with liver disease (liver failure, chronic active hepatitis, or cirrhosis), patients with new psychiatric or behavioral abnormalities, and patients with classical, although often subtle, neurologic signs and symptoms. Once the diagnosis is under consideration, a series of laboratory studies and clinical procedures can be undertaken to establish the diagnosis. It is important not to forget a diagnostic workup on siblings of newly diagnosed patients, since 25 percent will have the disease in a presymptomatic form and should be treated prophylactically.

SUGGESTED READING

Akil M, Schwartz JA, Dutchak D, et al. The psychiatric presentations of Wilson's disease. J Neuropsychiatry 1991; 3:377–382.

Brewer GJ, Yuzbasiyan-Gurkan V. Wilson disease. Medicine 1992; 71:139–164.

Danks DM. Disorders of copper transport. In: Scriver CR, Beaudet AL, Sly WS, Valle D, eds. Metabolic basis of inherited diseases. 6th ed. Vol 1. New York: McGraw-Hill, 1989:1411.

Scheinberg IH, Sternlieb I. Wilson's disease. In: Smith LH Jr, ed. Major problems in internal medicine. Vol 23. Philadelphia: WB Saunders, 1984.

Starosta-Rubinstein S, Young AB, Kluin K, et al. Clinical assessment of 31 patients with Wilson's disease: Correlations with structural changes on magnetic resonance imaging. Arch Neurol 1987; 44:365–370.

Yuzbasiyan-Gurkan V, Johnson V, Brewer GJ. Diagnosis and characterizations of presymptomatic patients with Wilson's disease and the use of molecular genetics to aid in the diagnosis. J Lab Clin Med 1991; 118:458–465.

HEPATIC ENCEPHALOPATHY

KEVIN D. MULLEN, M.B., F.R.C.P.I.
MONROE COLE, M.D.

Hepatic encephalopathy (HE) is a term used to describe a spectrum of neuropsychiatric disturbances occurring in patients with significant liver dysfunction. Its manifestations can be subtle or overt, and in the vast majority of patients the syndrome is reversible. Based on years of clinical observation, it is thought that HE is caused by a substance or substances that arise from gastrointestinal metabolism of nitrogenous compounds. It has been proposed that in the presence of significant loss of hepatic function or portosystemic shunting of blood, these substances escape hepatic metabolism, accumulate in the systemic circulation, traverse the blood-brain barrier, and cause HE. Although the gastrointestinal tract produces many neuroactive compounds, ammonia has long been thought the most probable "toxin" arising from the gut to cause HE. However, only circumstantial evidence supports this hypothesis, which forms the framework for our understanding of the precipitation of HE and its response to current therapy. This chapter focuses on strategies to diagnose HE.

CLINICAL PRESENTATIONS

Two broad clinical settings are described for HE: acute catastrophic liver injury, which is rare, and HE in patients with chronic liver disease, which is common (Table 1). Although these two types of HE share some features, there are enough differences to suggest they be considered separate entities until more information is available (Table 2). Because of its rarity, HE in acute liver failure is not discussed here. Interested readers are directed to the excellent discussion of this topic by Schafer and Jones. Patients with chronic liver disease most commonly present with subtle subclinical encephalopathy only detectable by psychometric testing. The next most common manifestations of HE are single or recurrent episodes of overt encephalopathy. Formerly fairly common, chronic overt HE and HE associated with cerebral degeneration are rarely seen these days, presumably because of the infrequency of portacaval shunt surgery.

Table 1 Presentations of Hepatic Encephalopathy (HE)

Acute liver disease
  Fulminant hepatic failure

Chronic liver disease
  Subclinical HE
  Single or recurrent episodes of overt HE (neurologic status normal between episodes)
  Chronic HE (episodes of overt HE on background of mild chronic HE)
  Chronic overt HE
  Acquired hepatocerebral degeneration

Table 2 Comparison of Hepatic Encephalopathy in Acute and Chronic Liver Disease

	Acute Liver Disease	Chronic Liver Disease
Precipitating factors	Often none	Frequent
Seizures, delirium	20–30%	Very rare
Response to treatment	Poor	Good
Cerebral edema	Common	Very rare
Response to flumazenil	Possible	Probable

DIAGNOSIS

Subclinical Hepatic Encephalopathy

Diagnosis of subclinical HE requires the use of psychometric testing. Because of preservation of speech, memory, and gross intellectual function, this entity is usually not detected unless specifically sought. Apart from a relatively small number of enthusiastic investigators, most physicians ignore subclinical HE completely. The attitude is: if one must look so hard for alterations in brain function, the problem must be inconsequential. The growing evidence indicates that subclinical HE is not only common but potentially of clinical importance. Even in well-compensated cirrhotics, 70 to 80 percent have evidence of impaired speed of response to sensory stimuli and accuracy of performance. Patients might find it disturbing to hear that clinicians are not looking for this subtle HE, especially since it appears to be easily reversible.

Since the real impact of subclinical HE on the quality of life in patients with liver disease is uncertain, it can be argued that psychometric testing is unnecessary. Until further data are published, we tend to agree with this position. In the hands of experienced investigators, a combination of digit symbol, block design, and trail-making tests detect subclinical HE. The trail-making (Reitan) test is currently available to clinicians. We hope that in the near future a simple, widely available technique will be proven useful in the diagnosis of subclinical HE. P-300 evoked response and auditory reaction time hold the most promise. Until subclinical HE is proven to be of clinical significance, however, the detection of subclinical HE will be of little interest to clinicians.

Table 3 Diagnosis of Hepatic Encephalopathy

Clinical suspicion
Rule out other causes of encephalopathy
Identify precipitating factors
Observe response to empirical treatment:
  Low-protein diet
  Correction of precipitating factors
  Bowel cleansing
  Lactulose

Overt Hepatic Encephalopathy

Despite lacking a gold standard for its diagnosis, most experienced clinicians can make a confident diagnosis of typical HE (Table 3). Suspecting or knowing that the patient has significant liver disease is a prerequisite for the diagnosis. The history, physical examination, or standard laboratory testing indicates whether the patient has significant liver disease. If liver disease is suspected, a change in mental status is attributed to HE. Once HE is considered a possibility, treatment should be instituted while concurrently (1) ruling out other causes of encephalopathy and (2) identifying precipitating factors. The more severe the encephalopathy, the greater the urgency in evaluating the patient, especially if sepsis is suspected.

Clinical Suspicion

Classic neurologic features raise the clinical suspicion of HE, but virtually all the so-called typical features of HE can be seen in other causes of encephalopathy. Nonetheless, asterixis and a lack of lateralizing neurologic signs suggest the diagnosis of HE in the correct setting. As stated previously, a prerequisite for most clinicians to consider HE as a diagnosis is knowing or suspecting the patient has liver disease. This is simply based on prior medical history or signs of liver disease on physical examination. In such patients, the question is not "Does the patient have HE?" but rather "What precipitated this attack?" and "Is there something else going on?" Both of these points will be discussed.

Diagnosing HE in a patient with inapparent liver disease can be a challenge. Table 4 lists some conditions that are associated with major portosystemic shunting of blood with virtually normal standard liver function tests. In our experience, long-standing chronic hepatitis C is the commonest cause of cirrhosis with normal or near normal liver tests and portosystemic collateral formation. Most patients with portosystemic collaterals and normal synthetic hepatic function (i.e., normal serum albumin and prothrombin time) do not have frequent attacks of overt HE. However, when they do, the diagnosis is usually missed because of the occult nature of their liver problem. Moreover, when they do develop HE it presents with psychiatric rather than neurologic manifestations. Many psychiatric drugs tend to further aggravate the problem because they induce constipation. Exactly how frequently psychiatric problems and varying degrees of "dementia" are due to occult liver disease and

Table 4 Causes of Portosystemic Shunt and "Normal" Liver Tests

Long-standing, well-compensated inactive cirrhosis
Noncirrhotic portal hypertension
    Schistosomiasis
    Portal, splenic vein thrombosis
    Congenital hepatic fibrosis
    Nodular regenerative hyperplasia
    Idiopathic
Congenital intra- and extrahepatic portosystemic shunts
Postsurgical creation of portosystemic shunt

Table 5 Some Clues to Occult Portosystemic Shunts

Clinical examination
    Fetor hepaticus
    Spider nevi
    Splenomegaly
    Gynecomastia

Laboratory tests
    Hyperammonemia
    Thrombocytopenia, leukopenia
    Hypergammaglobulinemia

HE is unknown. Major reviews of dementia discuss evaluation of patients for change in mental status but do not mention occult liver disease as a potential diagnosis. Clues to identifying HE as a cause for change in mental status are shown in Table 5.

The major reason for the formation of portosystemic shunts is portal hypertension due to cirrhosis. This leads to splenomegaly in many patients, which, unfortunately, may not be detected on clinical examination. However, the hypersplenism associated with portal hypertension–induced splenomegaly frequently leads to mild to moderate thrombocytopenia. For example, a patient with a history of a blood transfusion in her 20s, seen 40 years later for a change in mental status, who has thrombocytopenia (e.g., 120,000 platelets per cubic millimeter compared to the normal 150,000 or greater) should be suspected of HE, even if her liver tests are normal. Of course, there may be other reasons for thrombocytopenia, but occult portal hypertension due to chronic hepatitis C–induced cirrhosis is an important differential diagnosis. Leukopenia is less prevalent but has the same implications. Another laboratory feature that may indicate portosystemic shunting of blood is hypergammaglobulinemia, calculated by subtracting serum albumin from total protein. More subtle laboratory data can also indicate cirrhosis, such as an AST to ALT ratio greater than 1 in a nonalcoholic patient whose transaminases are elevated. However, no laboratory test is superior to a full history and physical examination if it is performed well. Mild fetor hepaticus, spider nevi, ascites, loss of body hair, or a history of hepatitis, blood transfusion, or prior alcoholism can shed new light on the clinical situation. These suggestions are particularly important for clinicians whose levels of suspicion for HE may not be high.

Table 6 Blood Ammonia Measurement in Diagnosis of Hepatic Encephalopathy (HE)

Arterial blood sample is optimum.
Blood sample must be placed in ice and assayed promptly.
Elevated level supports diagnosis of HE.
Normal level does not rule out HE, especially in fasted state.
Main utility is in aiding diagnosis of occult liver diseases or
    shunting.

Utility of Ammonia Measurements. Ammonia is a high-extraction compound extensively metabolized by the liver. In the presence of shunts or poor hepatic function, ammonia escapes hepatic metabolism and can accumulate in the systemic circulation. Since it is actively taken up by muscle, the most reliable way to determine if ammonia is escaping into the systemic circulation is to measure an arterial plasma ammonia concentration (Table 6). Alternatively, an arterialized ammonia level can be obtained by sampling a forearm vein after heating the arm in a heating blanket or water bath. An elevated random (fasting or nonfasting) plasma arterial ammonia in a properly collected and handled specimen is good evidence of an abnormality in hepatic handling of ammonia. Loss of hepatic function or shunting are by far the commonest causes for altered hepatic ammonia metabolism. Rarely, an adult with congenital or acquired urea cycle defects will be discovered because of a raised blood ammonia level. However, the important caveat in ammonia measurement is that the test is worse than useless if the specimen is not promptly placed in ice and assayed quickly (within 15 to 30 minutes). Failure to do this will almost universally result in a falsely elevated result. Obtaining a venous plasma ammonia is not nearly as helpful but can be sufficient in patients with substantial loss of muscle mass. Extending blood ammonia estimations from fasting to 1 and 2 hours after a protein meal can increase the yield in detecting patients with portosystemic shunts. However, because of the variation in gastric emptying and the effects of different food on portal hemodynamics, it is difficult to standardize this test.

We only use the plasma ammonia test when we do not know if a patient has liver disease as a cause for mental status change. We never use sequential testing to tell us if the patient is improving on therapy. Instead, we use clinical evaluation with the grading system of HE described by Conn and Leiberthal. In more severe HE, we use the Glasgow Coma Scale. Physicians disagree on the role of ammonia in HE. Some believe it predicts patients at risk for HE, whereas others feel ammonia causes HE. Regardless, selected measurement of plasma ammonia levels has a role to play in the diagnosis of HE.

Rule Out Other Causes of Encephalopathy

Even when it is known that a patient has liver disease, it is not always easy to determine whether the patient's change in mental status is due to HE or to some other problem (Table 7). Visual hallucinations, diaphoresis, and tachycardia are typical of delirium tremens and are distinctly unusual in HE. Cranial trauma is a constant concern in liver patients, who not only tend to fall (if alcoholic), but also have underlying hemostatic and coagulation problems. Computed tomography scan of the head is routine for all patients to rule out subdural and extradural hematomas. The wide availability of drug screens makes it easy to rule out drug-induced encephalopathy in most cases. Sepsis is a particularly difficult problem. Cirrhotics tend to get infections frequently. This may present with precipitation of HE, septic encephalopathy, or a combination of both. We feel that ruling out sepsis is one of the most important aspects of caring for liver patients with a change in mental status. Chest X ray should be performed on all patients. Blood, ascitic fluid, urine, and sputum should all be cultured routinely. There is no coagulopathy that contraindicates diagnostic paracentesis. However, a lumbar puncture should be approached with more caution. It should be performed by an experienced person and, besides culture, cell counts, protein, glucose, and serology, the opening pressure should be measured and recorded. This is usually omitted by the non-neurologist and can be useful information.

Patients found after seizure episodes can be diagnostic puzzles if their recovery from the postictal state is protracted. Often these patients have suffered from alcoholic withdrawal seizures and, because of their alcohol history, can be mistaken initially for patients with HE. Having seen substantial elevations in venous plasma ammonia levels in these patients, presumably due to massive ictal muscle activity, we are aware of the limitations of blood ammonia measurements in diagnosing encephalopathy.

The advent of rapidly available laboratory testing generally makes identification of other causes of encephalopathy in liver patients fairly easy. Hypoglycemia, severe hypomagnesemia, and other conditions are usually quickly identified. It must be stressed that most liver patients have serum sodiums in the 125 mEq per liter range, and, even when lower than this, they should virtually never be given hypertonic saline. Restriction of free water administration is enough to raise serum sodium levels. Hypoxia or respiratory failure will not be missed if arterial blood gases are measured. It is worth remembering to perform a blood ammonia at the time of blood gases, if this test is desired, to avoid a second arterial puncture.

Table 7 Other Causes for "Encephalopathy" in Liver Disease Patients

Central nervous system trauma	Delirium tremens
Severe sepsis	Respiratory failure
Hypoglycemia*	Alcoholic ketoacidosis
Drug ingestion	Postictal confusion
Uremia	Alcohol intoxication
Severe hyponatremia	Wernicke's syndrome
Hypernatremia	Hypomagnesemia

*May indicate sepsis or hepatoma.

Identify Precipitating Factors

Ascertaining the precipitating cause of HE is part and parcel of making the diagnosis. Despite older reports that HE is spontaneous, we believe that 40 percent of cases in our hospital are precipitated by another problem. Table 8 lists precipitating factors. The commonest are gastrointestinal hemorrhage and sepsis. Identifying and correcting these precipitating factors is often sufficient to return patients to their baseline neurologic status. Failure to identify infection and treat it is the commonest reason patients fail to respond to empirical treatment in the usual 24 to 72 hour time period for severe stage IV HE. Thus, if one has made a tentative diagnosis of HE and treated the patient aggressively for 2 to 3 days without apparent improvement, two issues need to be considered: (1) Is the diagnosis incorrect? (2) Have we failed to identify and treat a precipitating factor? The one factor that repeatedly occurs is sepsis. Biliary, intra-abdominal, and worrisome central nervous system infections can be difficult to detect in some patients. The enthusiasm for treating patients with severe alcoholic hepatitis and HE with steroids, fostered by some recent publications, can lead to catastrophic results if tuberculosis is present. We have had experience in caring for some of these patients whose "HE" failed to improve. Possible tuberculosis meningitis dampens considerably our enthusiasm for steroid therapy of severe alcoholic hepatitis.

Empirical Treatment

Perhaps more than in other neurologic conditions, the diagnosis of HE often depends on observation of the response to empirical therapy (see Table 3). Improvement in neuropsychiatric status within 1 to 3 days of starting empirical treatment for HE allows a post hoc diagnosis of this condition. Failure to respond may indicate that the original diagnosis is incorrect or that an unidentified precipitating factor has not been adequately treated or has arisen as a nosocomial infection. Getting lactulose into the small intestine is far superior to enema therapy but sometimes cannot be achieved because of possible bowel obstruction (ileus or mechanical). Identifying the reason for the bowel obstruction is usually important in pinpointing the cause of encephalopathy, such as intra-abdominal sepsis.

Benzodiazepine Antagonists. It has been suggested that if a patient has HE, the diagnosis can be "confirmed" by significant improvement in mental status after administration of the benzodiazepine antagonist

Table 8 Precipitating Factors in Hepatic Encephalopathy

Gastrointestinal bleeding	Infection
Constipation	Poor compliance with lactulose
Dehydration	Excessive protein intake
Hypokalemia	Uremia
Drug ingestion	Superimposed hepatic injury
Electrolyte disturbances	Hepatocellular carcinoma

flumazenil. Benzodiazepines have been reported to be elevated in blood and even brain tissue (autopsy) in patients and animals with HE. However, at least in the human studies, it is uncertain whether prior intake of prescription benzodiazepine drugs is the explanation. Indeed, diazepam and its metabolite desmethyldiazepam have been definitely identified in the brains of patients with HE. The situation is confusing, however, because both these compounds and other benzodiazepines thought to be exclusively synthesized by industry have recently been shown to be present in the food cycle in trace amounts.

Thus, a cirrhotic patient "awakening" with flumazenil administration (0.5 to 1 mg IV slowly) could indicate either undetected prescription benzodiazepine intake or HE. At present it is not possible to distinguish one from the other. Alternatively, a failure to respond may indicate inadequate dosing, HE without benzodiazepine accumulation (at least 30 percent of patients are reported not to have elevated levels), or other causes of

encephalopathy. For these reasons, we do not recommend flumazenil administration as part of the diagnostic strategy in HE.

COMMENTS

The diagnosis of HE depends on clinical suspicion, excluding other causes of encephalopathy, identification and treatment of precipitating factors, and observation of the response to empirical treatment. Major diagnostic challenges arise when liver disease is occult, multiple causes of encephalopathy are present concurrently, or a precipitating factor is not detected. We have outlined a flow chart of our approach in Figure 1. We have touched on some of the issues we observe in clinical practice that fall outside the usually described situations in reviews of HE. Readers are encouraged to investigate the reviews cited below for a broader perspective on this syndrome.

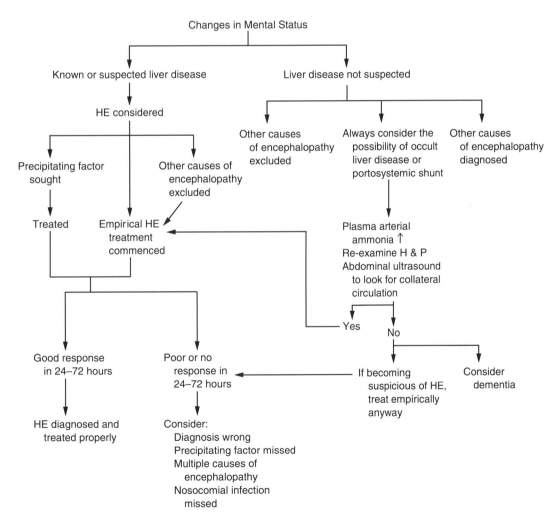

Figure 1 Algorithm for an approach to the diagnosis of hepatic encephalopathy (HE). (H & P = History and physical examination.)

SUGGESTED READING

Conn HO, Lieberthal MM. The hepatic coma syndrome and lactulose. Baltimore: Williams & Wilkins, 1979.

Gitlin N, Lewis DC, Hinkley L. The diagnosis and prevalence of subclinical hepatic encephalopathy in apparently healthy, ambulant, non-shunted patients with cirrhosis. J Hepatol 1986; 3:75–82.

Jones EA, Schafer DF. Fulminant hepatic failure. In: Zakin DI, Boyer TD, eds. Hepatology. 2nd ed. Philadelphia: WB Saunders, 1990:460.

Mullen KD. Hepatic encephalopathy. In: Rector WG Jr, ed. Complications of chronic liver disease. St. Louis: Mosby–Year Book, 1992:127.

Plum F, Posner JB. Diagnosis of stupor and coma. 3rd ed. Philadelphia: Davis, 1984.

Schafer DF, Jones EA. Hepatic encephalopathy. In: Zakin DI, Boyer TD, eds. Hepatology. 2nd ed. Philadelphia: WB Saunders, 1990:447.

HYPOXIC ENCEPHALOPATHY

JOHN J. CARONNA, M.D.

The brain does not store oxygen and, therefore, functions only for seconds and survives only for minutes after its oxygen supply is reduced below critical levels. A spectrum of clinical disorders can result, depending on the severity of cerebral anoxia. Patients who suffer mild degrees of cerebral anoxia have a reversible metabolic encephalopathy that lasts only a few hours to a few days. Patients who suffer severe or prolonged hypotension are usually comatose for a variable duration and on awakening have lasting motor, sensory, and intellectual defects. Finally, a third group of resuscitated patients who have widespread damage to the brain, less severe than that required to cause brain death, survive in the vegetative state only to die later from neurologic and systemic complications.

MILD HYPOXIC ENCEPHALOPATHY WITH TRANSIENT NEUROLOGIC DEFICITS

Brief episodes of cerebral anoxia, such as occur from uncomplicated syncope, are generally well tolerated, and patients awaken promptly. Patients with slightly longer episodes of circulatory arrest have a reversible metabolic encephalopathy. Coma in these patients, if present, lasts only a few hours, usually less than 12. Residual signs of confusion or amnesia may persist for hours to days. In general, recovery is rapid and complete, and these patients are able to resume their previous occupations.

An amnestic syndrome may follow a brief period of postanoxic confusion or may occur as an isolated phenomenon. Finklestein and I followed 16 patients after cardiac arrest. None remained in coma after resuscitation. All developed an amnestic syndrome as their only neurologic sequel. All had severe antegrade amnesia and variable retrograde memory loss with preservation of immediate and remote memory, resembling Korsakoff's psychosis, and a bland, unconcerned affect and confabulation. In 12 of the 16 patients, recovery was complete within 7 to 10 days. In the other

four, amnesia persisted for a month or longer, but all later recovered. The time required for recovery and the occasional instances of incomplete recovery distinguished this syndrome from transient global amnesia and the postictal state, from which recovery is rapid and complete. In view of the vulnerability of the hippocampal regions to anoxia, transient postcardiac arrest amnesia is thought to represent reversible bilateral damage to the hippocampi. Subtle but more permanent cognitive impairment may also follow cardiac arrest. Individuals with anoxic-ischemic coma of more than 6 hours duration but with unremarkable brain magnetic resonance imaging (MRI) and computed tomography (CT) have demonstrated persistent poor learning and recall of paired associations when compared with age- and IQ-matched controls. Impaired neurotransmitter synthesis may be responsible for these mild amnestic syndromes of anoxic amnesia, possibly through impairment of cholinergic memory circuits.

After apparently recovering from the immediate effects of an anoxic insult to the brain, rare patients develop a progressive cerebral disorder and relapse into unconsciousness. In fatal cases, pathologic lesions have been primarily restricted to the deep white matter of the parietal and occipital lobes. The clinical syndrome of this delayed anoxic leukoencephalopathy is distinctive: days to weeks after a period of improvement or recovery from global anoxia, patients suffer progressive neurologic deterioration and either die or remain comatose. Delayed neurologic deterioration has been reported after all types of anoxic insult but follows no more than one or two of each thousand arrests and is not predictable by the type of insult, the duration of anoxia, the period of coma, or any identifiable clinical feature.

HYPOXIC ENCEPHALOPATHY WITH PERSISTENT CENTRAL NERVOUS SYSTEM DAMAGE

Focal Cerebral Syndromes

Several types of strokelike focal brain lesions can occur after severe or prolonged hypotension. Patients in this group usually remain in coma for 12 hours or more and on awakening have lasting neurologic deficits. Among the focal signs clinically manifest in this group of patients are partial or complete cortical blindness, bibrachial paresis, and quadriparesis. Cortical blindness, usually transient but rarely a permanent sequel of systemic circulatory arrest, probably results from disproportionate ischemia of both occipital poles as a result of their location in an arterial border zone. Bilateral infarction of the cerebral motor cortex in the border zone between the anterior and middle cerebral arteries appears to be responsible for the syndrome of bibrachial paresis sparing the face and legs after arrest. Recovery is often delayed over a period of weeks to months and incomplete. Some of these patients are eventually able to lead a relatively independent existence at home, whereas others remain in nursing homes, severely disabled and dependent.

Spinal Cord Syndromes

The spinal cord is generally considered to be more resistant to transient ischemia than more rostral parts of the central nervous system (CNS). Nevertheless, cases of isolated spinal cord infarction occur without evidence of cerebral injury. Necrosis of central structures of the spinal cord can occur in the border zones of the territory supplied by a main contributory artery. These "watersheds" in the upper thoracic and lumbar regions of the spinal cord are at risk from any profound drop in perfusion pressure. The syndrome of spinal stroke from hypotension is characterized by flaccid paralysis of the lower limbs, urinary retention, and a sensory level in the thoracic region, with pain and temperature more affected than light touch or position sense.

HYPOXIC ENCEPHALOPATHY WITH DIFFUSE CEREBRAL DAMAGE

Some patients with severe, irreversible brain damage who survive more than 1 week after resuscitation regain eye opening, sleep-wake cycles, spontaneous roving eye movements, and other reflex activities at brain stem and spinal cord levels but remain in a functionally decorticate state of wakefulness without awareness. This state, distinct from the sleeplike condition of coma, has been named the *vegetative state*. In rare instances, recovery of cognition has occurred after prolonged periods in the vegetative state.

Extrapyramidal tract dysfunction after anoxia can produce a clinical syndrome identical to parkinsonism. It has been reported particularly after carbon monoxide poisoning but may follow an episode of anoxia or ischemia.

Myoclonic jerks and convulsions may follow episodes of acute cerebral ischemia, especially when they are severe enough to cause coma. Myoclonus refers to irregular, asynchronous shocklike jerks of one or more limbs and is a relatively common manifestation of disturbance in function of diverse regions of the CNS. The "action myoclonus" syndrome has been recognized after recovery from coma secondary to cerebral anoxia.

Although myoclonic jerks may be spontaneous, the action myoclonus jerks are frequently stimulus-activated and may be brought on by light, sound, or initiation of movement. Thus, these involuntary jerks can incapacitate the patient in walking, eating, and using the upper limbs for carrying out other activities of daily living.

Cerebellar ataxia is an infrequent postanoxic syndrome related to the selective vulnerability of Purkinje cells to ischemia.

DIAGNOSTIC APPROACH TO HYPOXIC ENCEPHALOPATHY

Patients in coma initially require intensive care to support life and prevent complications. In most cases of coma, sequential observation of physical signs is paramount because they may indicate the degree of reversibility of CNS damage and predict likely outcome, or detect a loss of neurologic function that precedes deterioration in cardiorespiratory function. The neurologic examination of the comatose patient consists of an assessment of the level of consciousness as determined by eye opening, verbal responses, and reflex or purposeful movements in response to noxious stimulation of the face, arms, and legs. Neuro-ophthalmologic function is indicated by pupillary size and response to light, spontaneous eye movements, oculocephalic ("doll's eyes") and oculovestibular (ice water caloric) responses. Vegetative function is reflected mainly by the respiratory pattern. Neurologic signs can be correlated with specific anatomic sites to establish the severity and extent of CNS dysfunction (Table 1).

Levels of Consciousness

Level of consciousness is best determined by the ease and degree, if any, of behavioral arousal. Attempts should be made to elicit a behavioral motor response by verbal stimulation alone. If no response follows even shouted commands, noxious stimulation can be applied to the face by digital supraorbital pressure and individually to the arms and legs by compression of distal interphalangeal joints with a tongue blade or pen. Eye opening indicates activity of the reticular activating system. Verbal responses indicate hemispheric function.

Motor Response

The absence of motor responses, especially with flaccidity and areflexia, indicates severe brain stem depression and is frequently found in terminal coma destined to become brain death or in severe sedative intoxication. Decerebrate or extensor responses correlate with destructive lesions of the midbrain and upper pons but may also be present in reversible metabolic states such as anoxic encephalopathy. Decorticate or flexor responses occur after damage to the hemispheres, as well as in metabolic depression of brain function. Withdrawal and localizing responses imply purposeful or

Table 1 Correlation Between Brain Anatomy and Clinical Signs

Structure	Clinical Sign

Cerebral cortex	Speech (including any sounds)
	Purposeful movement
	    Spontaneous
	    To command
	    To pain

Brain stem sensory pathways, reticular activating system	Eye opening
	    Spontaneous
	    To command
	    To pain

Brain stem motor pathways	Flexor posturing (decorticate) Extensor posturing (decerebrate)
Midbrain CN III	Pupillary reactivity

Upper pons
    CN V
    CN VII
	
	Corneal reflex – sensory
	Corneal reflex – motor response
	    Blink
	    Grimace

Lower pons CN VIII (vestibular portion) connects by brain stem pathways with CN III, IV, VI	 Doll's eyes Caloric responses
Medulla	Breathing and blood pressure do not require mechanical support
Spinal cord	Deep tendon reflexes Babinski's reflex

CN = cranial nerve.

voluntary behavior. Obeying commands is obviously the best response and marks the return of consciousness. Generalized or focal repetitive movements not affected by stimuli usually represent seizure activity. These sometimes take the form of repetitive eyelid twitching or several clonic jerks of a limb, but all of these movements are difficult to distinguish from myoclonus. Focal seizures usually indicate a focal cortical lesion but may also occur in hypoglycemia, hyperosmolarity, and in some drug intoxications, such as with aminophylline and tricyclic antidepressants.

Neuro-ophthalmologic Examination

The fundus of each eye should be examined for signs of increased intracranial pressure (ICP) (papilledema and hemorrhage), and the size, equality, and light reactivity of the pupils should be noted. Deeply comatose patients may have no spontaneous eye movements. In such cases, doll's eyes (oculocephalic) responses and the ice water caloric test can be used to determine the integrity of the eighth, sixth, and third cranial nerves and their interconnecting brain stem pathways.

When the cortical influences are depressed with intact brain stem mechanisms, the head can be rotated horizontally to one side and the eyes will deviate conjugately to the opposite side. Brisk back and forth eye movements, like those of a doll in response to rocking the head to and fro, are characteristic of metabolic coma. Doll's eyes indicate the integrity of proprioceptive fibers from the neck structures, the vestibular nuclei, and the nuclei of the third and sixth cranial nerves. When doll's eyes are absent, it becomes necessary to perform the ice water caloric test. In deep coma, the doll's eyes will disappear before the ice water caloric responses because the latter are produced by a stronger stimulus. The caloric response is elicited in comatose patients by irrigating the tympanum with 30 to 50 ml of ice water. When the patient is supine with the head elevated 30 degrees, cold water produces convection currents in the lateral semicircular canal that inhibit the firing of the ipsilateral vestibular nerve. In the absence of cortical influences on the oculovestibular pathways, cold water produces tonic deviation of the eyes to the side of irrigation. Metabolic factors, such as sedative-hypnotic coma or phenytoin overdosage, and structural brain stem lesions eliminate the caloric response, as does labyrinthine disease. The absence of elicited eye movements in anoxic coma is a grave prognostic sign.

Spontaneous, roving, horizontal eye movements in comatose subjects indicate only that the midbrain and pontine tegmentum are intact. They do not imply preservation of the frontal or occipital cerebral cortex. These movements, and those described below, appear to be release phenomena, namely, spontaneous movements generated by brain stem gaze mechanisms released from cortical or other suprasegmental control. Persistent downward deviation of the eyes is characteristic of tectal compression by a thalamic hemorrhage or pineal tumor but also occurs in anoxic coma and other metabolic encephalopathies. Upward deviation may indicate nonconvulsive epileptic activity. Ocular bobbing, a movement disorder usually associated with damage to the lateral gaze center in the pons, has been observed in postcardiac arrest patients, some of whom recovered. Bobbing is characterized by spontaneous downward deviation of the eyes and less rapid upward movement. By contrast, ocular dipping after global brain anoxia consists of slow downward deviations followed by rapid upward movement.

Further Diagnostic Assessment

Neuroimaging

In acute anoxic coma, CT scan usually fails to show any abnormalities unless the damage is catastrophic. Approximately 48 hours after a prolonged anoxic episode, hypodensities in the cerebral and cerebellar cortices and in the caudate and lenticular nuclei can occur. Days later, focal infarcts, edema, and diffuse and focal atrophy may be evident. In cases of persistent cerebral dysfunction, neuropsychological assessment combined with positron emission tomography (PET) scanning can define the extent of damage.

Electroencephalography

The electroencephalogram (EEG) is a sensitive indicator of cerebral function. In animal studies, EEG activity slows markedly when cerebral blood flow (CBF) falls below 16 ml per 100 g per minute, and becomes isoelectric with CBF below 12 ml per 100 g per minute. Several groups have correlated the pattern and frequency spectra of the postresuscitation EEG with neurologic outcome, but the absolute predictive value of the EEG has not been established. In general, the EEG is useful in assessing the degree of cortical dysfunction and identifying the presence of epileptic activity.

Evoked Potentials

Evoked potentials (EPs) provide information regarding the locus and severity of dysfunction in certain sensory systems and, unlike the EEG, are not influenced by the level of consciousness. If somatosensory cortical responses are bilaterally absent after global brain ischemia, mortality rate has been as high as 98 percent in most series. Patients who maintain normal responses throughout their illness have a better prognosis but may suffer permanent neurologic sequelae. Sensory EPs remain superior to motor EPs in assessing outcome of comatose individuals.

Brain stem auditory EPs (BAEPs) can correlate with brain stem dysfunction during coma but are not as useful as somatosensory potentials in anoxic coma. Simultaneous latency increase of all components is consistent with progressive ischemia of the posterior fossa and a decrease in cerebral perfusion pressure. Although BAEPs are not usually modified by exogenous factors, BAEPs can be altered and even abolished by hypothermia, anesthetics, and barbiturates.

OUTCOME OF POSTCARDIAC ARREST COMA

The clinical management of patients in coma after cardiac arrest involves the restoration of adequate cardiopulmonary function to prevent further cerebral injury, but no effective delayed therapy yet exists that can reverse anoxic damage. Recent evidence suggests, however, that neuropathologic abnormalities continue to evolve for hours to days after ischemic anoxia has occurred. In addition, certain factors that determine the extent of cerebral injury have been identified. States of reduced cerebral energy requirement, such as deep anesthesia and hypothermia, prevent or reduce brain damage from anoxic insults, particularly if administered before the ictus. By contrast, hyperglycemia, cerebral lactic acidosis, loss of calcium homeostasis, raised ICP, and excessive release of excitatory neurotransmitters, as occurs with seizures, increase ischemic cerebral damage.

The Cornell Multicenter Study

Population

As part of an international study to establish guidelines to predict outcome in comatose patients, my colleagues and I examined 310 patients in coma after cardiac arrest. Roughly equal numbers of patients had an anoxic insult in an intensive care setting (26 percent), general hospital ward (31 percent), or out of the hospital (34 percent). Patients were considered to be in coma who failed to open their eyes spontaneously or in response to noise, expressed no comprehensible words, and neither obeyed commands nor moved their extremities appropriately to localize or resist painful stimuli. To avoid including subjects with an obviously good prognosis, only those in coma for at least 6 hours were included. Patients who awakened after the initial examination but before 6 hours had elapsed were excluded.

Definition of Outcome

At predetermined intervals (initial examination and then 1, 3, 7, and 14 days after arrest), patients underwent neurologic examinations. Functional state was categorized at 1, 3, 6, and 12 months into one of five grades: (1) no recovery (coma until death), (2) the vegetative state (wakefulness without awareness), (3) severe disability (conscious but dependent on others for aspects of daily living), (4) moderate disability (independent but with residual neurologic deficits), (5) good recovery, that is, able to resume prior level of function. Data were subjected to univariate and multivariate analyses to relate the early clinical picture to functional outcome.

Outcome

Most patients destined to recover awakened within a short time. By 3 days, 25 patients had regained consciousness. By 2 weeks, the number of conscious patients had risen only to 28, with 21 recovering independence. The vegetative state also developed rapidly in many patients: 47 patients appeared vegetative within the first day. Of the surviving 33 vegetative patients at 1 week, only three ever improved to an independent state. Improvement after 1 month was rare. None of 15 patients vegetative at 1 month ever regained independent function, and only three of 16 patients severely disabled at 1 month did so.

The death rate associated with anoxic coma of 6 hours or more was high: 20 percent within the first 24 hours, 41 percent by the end of 3 days, and 64 percent by the end of the first week. Only 10 percent survived 1 year after arrest. Of the 191 patients who died within 1 year, approximately half died from non-neurologic causes. Because of the frequency with which non-neurologic factors interfered with full recovery, the ultimate status of the patient was not always a reflection of potential recovery from cerebral damage. Therefore, the best functional neurologic state attained within the first year was analyzed.

In terms of outcome, more than three-quarters of the patients either died without opening their eyes (121 patients) or, although they opened their eyes, showed no evidence of cognitive interaction with the environment and were considered to be vegetative (43 patients). The remaining 46 patients regained consciousness, but 20 of them remained severely disabled. At some point within the first year, more than 26 patients (13 percent) achieved a moderate disability or a good recovery and could be considered as having recovered.

Factors Not Related to Recovery

Patient age and sex, site of the initial insult (out-of-hospital, intensive care, operating room, or general ward), cause of the coma (cardiac arrest, respiratory arrest, or hypotension), and the presence of postanoxic seizures in 53 patients (20 percent) did not influence the degree of recovery in this study.

Individual Signs Related to Recovery

The absence of certain brain stem reflexes at the initial examination identified patients with little or no likelihood of meaningful recovery. None of the 52 patients without pupillary light reflexes ever recovered, and only three regained consciousness. Three of 71 patients without corneal reflexes when first examined recovered within 1 year, but no patient who lacked corneal reflexes after the first day ever regained consciousness. Although the pattern of motor responses eventually correlated with recovery, neither their initial absence nor the presence of extensor or flexor posturing ruled out recovery. After 3 days, however, absent or posturing motor responses were incompatible with future independent living. Five patients with motor responses poorer than withdrawal at 3 days and four patients in that condition at 7 days regained consciousness, but all remained severely disabled.

Certain early signs were associated with relatively good chances of recovery. At the initial examination, the most favorable sign was incomprehensible speech (moaning), but this was rare. At 1 day, the following signs were each associated with at least a 50 percent chance of regaining independent function: speech, even if confused or inappropriate, orienting spontaneous eye movements, normal oculocephalic or oculovestibular responses, obeying commands, and normal skeletal muscle tone.

Multivariate Analysis of Prognostic Variables

Reliance on individual signs can be misleading. For example, the likely outcome of a patient with intact pupillary light reflexes (a favorable prognostic sign) but absent corneal reflexes (an unfavorable prognostic sign) is uncertain. Therefore, a multivariate analysis was used to classify patients by likely outcome. For example, at initial examination, the presence of pupillary light reflexes, spontaneous eye movements, and a reflex or purposeful response to pain identified a group of 27 patients, 41 percent of whom regained independence in their daily lives. One day after cardiac arrest, 93 patients with a poor prognosis were identified by motor responses that were either absent or reflex only and by spontaneous extraocular movements that were absent. Only one of the 93 recovered. By contrast, the rate of recovery was 63 percent of 30 patients who at 1 day showed improvement in their eye opening responses and obeyed commands or had motor responses that were better than reflex only. Similarly, simple rules distinguished between good and poor prognosis patients on postarrest days 3, 7, and 14.

The Cornell study found that careful analysis of early clinical information distinguished between patients with good and poor prognosis. Evidence of brain dysfunction at brain stem levels or in a multifocal pattern implied a grave prognosis. Patients with the best chance of recovery had intact brain stem function at the time of initial examination postarrest (reactive pupils and motor responses), as well as spontaneous roving eye movements. At 1 day and beyond, evidence of intact cortical function (motor responses including withdrawal or better and orienting eye movements) indicated those who would recover. Any prognostic classification should be applied with caution. The clinician must be certain that the evaluation of clinical signs is accurate and must exclude the effects of drugs on these responses, such as anticholinergics on pupillary reactivity or paralytic agents on motor responses.

The ability to predict outcome in postanoxic coma can offer a major benefit to the physicians, patients, and their families. In addition, identification of patients with poor and good prognosis early after an arrest may facilitate the design and interpretation of appropriately stratified treatment trials and increase the likelihood that effective therapy will soon be available.

SUGGESTED READING

Caronna JJ. Diagnosis, prognosis and treatment of hypoxic coma. Adv Neurol 1979; 26:11–19.

Caronna JJ, Finklestein S. Neurological syndromes after cardiac arrest. Stroke 1978; 9:517–521.

Finklestein S, Caronna JJ. Amnestic syndrome following cardiac arrest. Neurology 1978; 28:389.

Levy DE, Bates D, Caronna JJ, et al. Prognosis in nontraumatic coma. Ann Intern Med 1981; 94:293–301.

Levy DE, Caronna JJ, Singer BH, et al. Predicting outcome from hypoxic-ischemic coma. JAMA 1985; 253:1420–1426.

Maiese K, Caronna JJ. Coma after cardiac arrest. In: Ropper AH, ed. Neurological and neurosurgical intensive care. 3rd ed. New York: Raven Press, 1993.

Plum F, Posner JB. The diagnosis of stupor and coma. 3rd ed. Philadelphia: FA Davis, 1980.

Plum F, Posner JB, Hain RF. Delayed neurological deterioration after anoxia. Arch Intern Med 1962; 110:56–63.

Silver JR, Buxton PH. Spinal stroke. Brain 1974; 97:539–550.

Simon RP, Aminoff MJ. Electrographic status epilepticus in fatal anoxic coma. Ann Neurol 1986; 20:351–355.

PAIN AND TRAUMA

BEHAVIORAL AND COGNITIVE SEQUELAE OF HEAD INJURY

DAVID L. BACHMAN, M.D.

Closed head injury is one of the most common causes of neurologic dysfunction, with an estimated annual incidence of approximately 150 per 100,000 population. Of particular concern is the fact that most head injuries occur in young people, especially those in their mid-teens to late 20s. Because most head injury survivors can expect a near normal life expectancy, the prevalence of affected individuals is very high, by some estimates 800 per 100,000 population. Although many head injury patients, especially those with severe injury, sustain some degree of motor dysfunction, the most common and disabling sequelae of closed head injury are behavioral and cognitive deficits. In this chapter I will address the problems physicians face in assessing patients with closed head injury during the recuperative or chronic phase of recovery. I will not address the assessment or management of the acutely head injured patient.

PATHOLOGY OF CLOSED HEAD INJURY

The patterns of cognitive and behavioral deficits exhibited by patients are directly correlated with the patterns of brain pathology. The most common pathology of closed head injury is diffuse axonal injury (DAI), the result of shearing strain forces following rapid deacceleration injuries such as motor vehicle accidents. Currently there does not exist a way to directly measure the amount of DAI suffered by a patient, although the degree of late "hydrocephalus ex-vacuo" on computed tomography (CT) scan or magnetic resonance imaging (MRI) does correlate somewhat with the degree of DAI. In severe DAI, scattered petechial hemorrhages in the deep white matter or hemorrhage of the corpus callosum or midbrain may be visualized. The diagnostician may estimate the degree of DAI from the clinical history. DAI is greatest in those who (1) are unconscious immediately at the time of injury, (2) have lengthy periods of unconsciousness, (3) have lengthy periods of retrograde amnesia (period of time prior to the accident during which patient is unable to recall events), and (4) have lengthy periods of post-traumatic amnesia (period of time from injury until patient is able to reliably recall new memories). In addition, the Glasgow Coma Scale score at the time the patient arrives at the emergency room (Table 1) inversely correlates with the degree of DAI. Glasgow Coma Scale scores of 13 to 15 correspond to mild injury, scores of 8 or less with severe injury. Even when a Glasgow Coma Scale score has not been given at the time of injury, the clinician may estimate the score from the medical records.

The acute confusional behavior of closed head injury is most likely secondary to DAI. Long-term neurobehavioral consequences of DAI probably include cognitive slowness, impaired attention, distractability, and fatigue.

The next most common pathology of closed head injury is cerebral contusion. Cerebral contusions, or direct bruising of the brain, occur in characteristic locations in adults: frontal polar, orbitofrontal, and anterior temporal regions. CT scans are especially good at visualizing contusions in the first 24 hours after injury

Table 1 Glasgow Coma Scale

Examination	Points
Eye opening	
Opens eyes spontaneously	4
Opens eyes to verbal command	3
Opens eyes to painful stimuli	2
Does not open eyes	1
Best motor response	
Follows simple commands	6
Resists painful stimuli	5
Withdraws to painful stimuli	4
Decorticate posturing to painful stimuli	3
Decerebrate posturing to painful stimuli	2
No motor response to painful stimuli	1
Best verbal response	
Fully oriented	5
Speech understandable but confused	4
Speaks but makes no sense	3
Makes unintelligible sounds	2
Makes no noise	1

but underestimate the degree of contusion after that. MRI scans are useful for visualizing cerebral contusion even years after an injury. As in DAI, historical information from the patient or the medical record may aid in establishing the likelihood of significant cerebral contusions. Patients more likely to have significant contusions include those who (1) sustained low-velocity injuries such as falls or blunt trauma, (2) were conscious briefly before lapsing into unconsciousness, (3) sustained a skull fracture, especially an orbital fracture, and (4) required the evacuation of an acute subdural hematoma.

Inferior orbitofrontal and anterior temporal contusions are usually bilateral and associated with emotional, behavioral, and personality changes. Basal forebrain contusions and posterior extension of temporal lobe contusions may be associated with memory loss.

Anoxic or hypotensive brain injuries frequently contribute to the behavioral and cognitive pathology of head injury patients. Not infrequently, I have encountered patients whose direct head injuries were in fact trivial in whom the residual neurologic deficits were the result of anoxia or hypotension. Anoxic injury may result in significant cortical damage, especially to the hippocampal formation and cerebellum. Hypotensive injury may result in watershed area infarction and/or basal ganglia damage. The clinician should inspect the medical record for evidence of (1) cardiorespiratory arrest, (2) shock, (3) urgent intubation, (4) crush chest injuries, (5) massive abdominal injuries or bleeding, and (6) abnormal arterial blood gases. CT scan or MRI is generally not helpful in assessing the degree of anoxic or hypotensive injury unless one detects a specific pattern of watershed infarction. The neurobehavioral effects of diffuse anoxic injury may be similar to DAI.

PATIENT SYMPTOMS

Patients with head injury often complain of symptoms classically associated with "postconcussive" injury. Such symptoms include headache, dizziness, memory loss, difficulty concentrating, slowness, irritability, sleep disturbance, depression, and fatigue. Head injury patients may exhibit subtle behavioral problems that cause them significant social difficulty. It has been suggested that head injury patients have particular difficulty interpreting the subtle verbal and body language of co-workers and family in work and social situations. These patients often have similar problems in romantic relationships.

It is especially important to obtain additional history from a reliable care giver for patients with head injury. Problems reported by care givers may include irritability with outbursts of anger, socially inappropriate behavior including sexually inappropriate behavior, distractability, loss of initiative, poor memory, word-finding difficulty, and significant physical limitations unreported by the patient. Many patients with severe head injury have limited insight into the significance of their deficits.

GENERAL CLINICAL EXAMINATION

Patients who have recovered from severe head injury often exhibit a variety of physical and sensory deficits on general neurologic examination. These findings will not be reviewed in detail except as they relate to the cognitive and behavioral deficits.

The clinician should examine the patient for evidence of craniotomy defects. Evidence of prior fractures, especially facial and orbital fractures, should be recorded. Impaired olfactory function suggests damage to the olfactory nerves, often associated with orbitofrontal contusion. Hemianopic field cuts may suggest damage to the optic chiasm or, perhaps, posterior cerebral artery stroke. A pattern of proximal motor weakness may suggest watershed infarction secondary to hypotension. Bilateral spasticity is often associated with DAI. Significant cerebellar tremor or ataxia may be associated with midbrain damage due to severe DAI or cerebellar damage secondary to anoxia. Evidence of parkinsonism may suggest basal ganglia damage secondary to hypotension. Focal motor and sensory deficits may correspond to left or right cerebral hemisphere damage. So-called frontal release signs are rarely seen except in patients with extremely severe injury.

MENTAL STATUS EXAMINATION

Deficits in attention are the hallmark of closed head injury. Attentional abilities may be tested with the digit span and mental control tasks such as spelling *world* backward or doing serial 7 subtractions. Obvious behavioral manifestations of diminished attention should also be sought. Patients often have difficulty getting set to do a task. Once set, they may demonstrate distractability and perseveration. Tasks may be done slowly and inefficiently or quickly and impulsively. Impaired attention and reduced performance speed are most likely secondary to DAI.

Memory may be assessed in a number of ways. Orientation provides some information about memory but is also dependent on motivation and opportunity. More important is the patient's ability to learn new information. Lists of words, single sentences, or brief stories can be given to the patient to be recalled after a delay. Examiners must assure themselves that impaired attention has not prevented the patient from encoding the test stimuli. Nonverbal memory can be tested by giving the patient simple figures to draw and redraw after a delay, or objects can be hidden around the room to be located after a delay. Impaired memory after closed head injury is more often a function of impaired attention and encoding rather than impaired memory storage and retrieval. Patients with severe memory problems after head injury, not due to attention, probably have suffered anoxic injury or, less commonly, severe temporal lobe or basal forebrain contusion.

Patients uncommonly exhibit classic aphasic syndromes after closed head injury. More often, language problems are a combination of anomia, impaired attention, and frontal lobe dysfunction. If speech is not slowed by dysarthria, patients may talk at length, rambling between topics or obsessively talking about a single topic. They may use stereotyped or overlearned phrases in a perseverative fashion. They may have difficulty with turn-taking in conversation and use socially inappropriate language. Word-finding can be assessed by having patients name common objects in the room, body parts, colors, and numbers.

Higher reasoning skills are often impaired in patients with moderate to severe head injury. This can be demonstrated by asking the patient to interpret proverbs or idioms, play games, or solve simple problems. A useful technique is to ask the patient to explain how to do something he or she already knows how to do, such as change a flat tire or bake a pie. This tests the patient's ability to identify the most important elements of a task, set them in correct temporal relationship, and organize a simple narrative. Especially valid is listening to patients discuss the way their deficits impact on their daily lives. Impaired problem solving and reasoning skills are usually the result of significant prefrontal lobe injury.

Behavior and personality may be the most important realms of higher cognitive function affected by head injury. Unfortunately, they are also the most difficult to test in an objective fashion. Patients with moderate and severe head injury often demonstrate poor self-critical monitoring, impaired insight, irritability, diminished motivation, inappropriate behavior, and emotional lability. Classic psychiatric syndromes such as mania, psychosis, and obsessive/compulsive disorder have been reported after head injury but are uncommon. Depression is relatively common after head injury. Depressed head injury patients may exhibit atypical depressive symptoms, such as unexplained urinary incontinence. For that reason, clinicians must maintain a high degree of clinical suspicion for depression. Work with stroke patients suggests that patients with anterior left cerebral injury may be at especially high risk for depression. Other specific neurobehavioral syndromes such as Kluver-Bucy syndrome, right cerebral parietal syndrome, extraordinary confabulation, and reduplicative paramnesia may be seen following closed head injury.

ASSOCIATED PROBLEMS

As mentioned above, depression may contribute significantly to the behavioral and cognitive deficits following head injury. Post-traumatic stress disorder may also be encountered, especially after mild head injury. Clinicians should be especially attuned to this syndrome. Litigation also has an impact on patient function. During litigation, patients are often forced to endure continued retelling of their accident and subsequent deficits. In addition, the lengthy time course of litigation and the associated financial uncertainties result in significant stress. For these reasons, litigation often results in an exacerbation of symptoms. However, in my experience it is uncommon for patients to purposefully fabricate symptoms.

Other stressors that should be considered include loss of job and financial security, diminished self-esteem, loss of autonomy and increased dependence, loss of self-confidence, diminished sense of self-worth because of cognitive or physical impairments, and marital and social conflicts. These psychological problems, indirectly caused by the accident, may cause more true disability in some patients than deficits due to direct brain injury.

Premorbid personality and intellectual function are also important variables to address in assessing patients following brain injury. Individuals especially likely to sustain head injury are young males, often abusing drugs and/or alcohol, who are antiauthority risk takers. Many of these patients have a strong premorbid history of attention deficit disorder and/or learning disability. Although an understanding of these issues is important, the clinician should be cautious about dismissing behavioral or cognitive problems after head injury as due simply to premorbid tendencies.

LATE NEUROLOGIC SEQUELAE OF HEAD INJURY

Although most cognitive and behavioral deficits following head injury are due to the brain damage occurring immediately or soon after the injury, it is important to remember that delayed neurologic sequelae of head injury may also be important. About 5 percent of patients with closed head injury develop late epilepsy (i.e., seizure occurring more than 7 days after injury). Interictal or peri-ictal behavioral and personality changes may occur in these patients. Normal pressure hydrocephalus or chronic subdural hematoma may occur in a small percentage of patients as late sequelae of head injury. Cognitive decline and, rarely, behavioral dysfunction may occur as the sole symptom of these disorders. For this reason, we recommend that any patient exhibiting an unexplained cognitive or behavioral decline following head injury undergo a follow-up CT scan or MRI.

ADDITIONAL TESTING

Neuropsychological testing may be extremely helpful in assessing patients after head injury. Neuropsychological testing enables the clinician to compare the patient's performance against age-matched norms. In addition, quantitative estimates of cognitive function permit more accurate assessments of change after therapy. The neuropsychologist should be asked to establish the patient's areas of strength as well as weakness. This will be of help in counseling the family as well as in planning therapy. However, neuropsychological testing should never be considered a substitute for a careful clinical examination.

Neuropsychological testing cannot completely differentiate psychological from "organic" factors in test performance.

A speech and language evaluation may be useful for many patients. An occupational therapy and vocational therapy assessment is useful not just for purposes of planning therapy but also for observing patients in situations that simulate real-life challenges.

CT or MRI scans may also be useful, not only to exclude potential late neurologic sequelae of head injury but to assess the degree of hydrocephalus ex-vacuo and cerebral contusion that may be present. I attempt to correlate the degree of damage seen on imaging studies with estimates of injury from the history and clinical examination. Electroencephalography (EEG) is generally not useful except to exclude epileptiform activity. Quantitative EEG and evoked potentials have not yet proven their clinical utility, in my opinion.

SUGGESTED READING

Alexander MP. Neuropsychiatric correlates of persistent postconcussive syndrome. J Head Trauma Rehabil 1992; 7:60–69.

Alexander MP. Some neurobehavioral aspects of closed head injury. In: Mueller J, ed. Neurology and psychiatry: A meeting of minds. Basel: S Karger, 1989:175.

Alexander MP. The role of neurobehavioral syndromes on the rehabilitation and outcome of closed head injury. In: Levin HS, Grafman J, Eisenberg HM, eds. Neurobehavioural recovery from head injury. New York: Oxford University Press, 1987:191.

Bachman DL. The diagnosis and management of common neurologic sequelae of closed head injury. J Head Trauma Rehabil 1992; 7:50–59.

Levin HS, Benton AL, Grossman RG. Neurobehavioral consequences of closed head injury. New York: Oxford University Press, 1982.

Levin HS, Handel SF, Goldman AM, et al. Magnetic resonance imaging after 'diffuse' nonmissle head injury. Arch Neurol 1985; 42:963–968.

Teasdale G, Jennett B. Assessment of coma and impaired consciousness: A practical scale. Lancet 1974; ii:81–84.

Wilson JTL, Wiedmann KD, Hadley DM, et al. Early and late magnetic resonance imaging and neuropsychological outcome after head injury. J Neurol Neurosurg Psychiatry 1988; 51:391–396.

Wood RL. Brain injury rehabilitation: A neurobehavioural approach. Rockville, Md: Aspen, 1987.

SYMPTOMATIC HYDROCEPHALUS IN THE ELDERLY

NEILL R. GRAFF-RADFORD, M.B.B.Ch., M.R.C.P. (UK)
JOHN C. GODERSKY, M.D.

Patients with possible symptomatic hydrocephalus, also termed normal pressure hydrocephalus or NPH, are often encountered in clinical practice and comprise up to 6 percent of patients in some dementia studies. To the neurologist the commonly asked question is, "Which patients with the clinical triad of dementia, gait abnormality, and incontinence of urine, together with the radiologic finding of hydrocephalus, should be recommended for shunt surgery?" The basis of this question is that only half the individuals with this constellation of findings improve with surgery. Moreover, shunt surgery has about a 30 percent long-term complication rate. An important corollary question is, "Why do half the patients with the clinical triad and hydrocephalus fail to

improve with surgery?" One of the answers to this latter question is that each of the clinical findings associated with symptomatic hydrocephalus is common in the elderly and may have multiple causes. Severe dementia may occur in up to 5 percent of people over 65 years and a milder form may be present in many more. Incontinence occurs in 15 percent of women and 10 percent of men over 70 years. Gait abnormality is also common in the elderly and has been shown to have multiple causes. The cerebral ventricles increase in size with age, and ventriculomegaly is a common accompaniment of Alzheimer's disease. Since none of its cardinal findings is specific to symptomatic hydrocephalus, it is not surprising that a patient can exhibit the typical clinical triad plus computed tomography (CT) hydrocephalus, and yet not respond to surgery. How can the neurologist best make the decision regarding recommendation for surgery? This is the question addressed in this chapter.

ASSESSING PATIENTS FOR SHUNT SURGERY

History

Several important questions should be asked when taking a history from these patients and their families.

How long has the patient been demented? If this exceeds 2 years it is less likely that the patient will respond to surgery. Note that the question is not how long the patient has had gait abnormality but how long the patient has been demented. Please refer to Table 1

This chapter is based upon another chapter, Graff-Radford NR, Godersky JC. A clinical approach to symptomatic hydrocephalus in the elderly. In: Morris JC, ed. Handbook of dementing illness. New York: Marcel Dekker, 1993 (in press); with permission.

Table 1 Variables Predicting Surgical Outcome in Symptomatic Hydrocephalus

Variable	No. of Patients	Odds Ratio	p Value*	95% Confidence Interval for Odds Ratio†	Correct Classification	
					Unimproved	Improved
Age	30	1.031	0.59	0.919–1.157		
Education	30	0.906	0.41	0.716–1.146		
Sex	30	4.615	0.215‡	0.423–233.0		
Gait abnormality (yrs)	30	1.133	0.51	0.789–1.626		
Incontinence (yrs)	30	1.441	0.402	0.614–3.408		
Dementia (yrs)	30	9.002	<0.001	1.542–52.56	5/7	21/23
Order of onset (gait versus dementia)	30	0	0.009‡	0–0.425	3/7	23/23
% time B-waves present	28	0.969	0.04	0.937–1.001	2/6	22/22
% time pressure > 15 mm Hg	28	0.968	0.055	0.930–1.006	0/6	22/22
% time pressure > 20 mm Hg	28	0.979	0.23	0.940–1.020		
Visual naming test	25	0.941	0.093	0.875–1.013	2/7	17/18
Visual naming, pass/fail	25	8.750	0.058‡	0.887–113.3	5/7	14/18
Cerebral blood flow (anterior/ posterior ratio slice 4)	30	1.120	<0.001	1.026–1.224	5/7	22/23
CSF conductance	23	0.254	0.956	0–infinity		
CSF conductance, 0.08 as cutoff value	23	1.071	1.00‡	0.065–67.354		

From Graff-Radford NR, Godersky JC. Variables predicting surgical outcome in symptomatic hydrocephalus in the elderly. Neurology 1989; 39:1601–1602; with permission.
*p value based on likelihood ratio test.
†Based on Wald test (which is slightly different from likelihood ratio test) and on Fisher's exact test when this test was used.
‡p value based on Fisher's exact test.

to see how reliable this information was in our series in predicting surgical outcome.

Which started first, gait abnormality or dementia? If the gait abnormality began before or at the same time as dementia, then there is a better chance for successful surgery. If dementia started before gait abnormality, shunting is less likely to help (see Table 1).

Is there a history of alcohol abuse? Alcohol abuse is a poor prognostic indicator.

Is there a secondary cause of hydrocephalus? Examples include subarachnoid hemorrhage, meningitis, previous brain surgery, and head injury. If any of these are present, the chances of improvement with surgery are better.

Examination

On examination, the following issues should be addressed.

Measure the head circumference. If greater than 59 cm in males or 57.5 cm in females (>98th percentile for head circumference) the patient may have congenital hydrocephalus that has become symptomatic in later life.

Exclude diseases that may mimic symptomatic hydrocephalus such as Parkinson's disease, cervical spondylosis with spinal cord compression, progressive supranuclear palsy, multisystem degenerative disorder, phenothiazine use, Alzheimer's disease with extrapyramidal features, and multiple subcortical infarctions. This is sometimes easier said than done, but keeping this differential diagnosis in mind during the history and examination is helpful.

Neuropsychological Evaluation

Look for evidence of aphasia. If there is evidence of aphasia, such as anomia, this is a poor prognostic indicator for surgical success (see Table 1).

Cerebrospinal Fluid Drainage Procedures

If the patient's gait improves after a large quantity of cerebrospinal fluid (CSF) is removed by lumbar puncture (30 to 50 ml, and this can be repeated daily), the patient would be a good candidate for shunt surgery.

A modification of this technique is continuous CSF drainage via a catheter placed in the lumbar CSF space and connected to a drainage bag. The height of the bag is adjusted to allow drainage of 5 to 10 ml per hour and yet avoid CSF hypotensive symptoms of headache and nausea. This is a closed system and allows an average of 150 ml drainage per day. The closed system helps prevent infection, and the thin tube prevents rapid CSF drainage, reducing the risk of subdural hemorrhage. There are other methods of doing this. Hanley et al use a larger (16 gauge) catheter through which CSF pressure can also be monitored. They pay attention to the level of the drainage bag, aiming to drain 240 ml per day. To minimize infection the drainage system is kept in for only 2 to 5 days. If symptoms of headache and nausea develop, one should be concerned that too much CSF is being drained.

There are shortcomings to these diagnostic tests. We have seen patients who eventually responded to shunt surgery but who showed no obvious improvement for the first postsurgical week. The drainage test often gives a false-negative result in these patients. On the other hand, when the drainage is performed, the patient may appear improved for the duration of the test (the placebo effect) but not maintain the response, leading to a false-positive result. In addition, meningitis and subdural hematoma are possible complications of the continuous CSF drainage procedures.

Computed Tomography and Magnetic Resonance Imaging

Some factors should be addressed when looking at the CT or magnetic resonance imaging (MRI).

Hydrocephalus must be present. The modified Evans ratio (maximum width of the frontal horns to measure of the inner table at the same place) should be greater than 0.31.

Is cortical atrophy prominent? Extensive cortical atrophy reduces but does not eliminate the chance of improvement with surgery.

The pattern of atrophy may be useful diagnostically. Does it involve the medial temporal lobes as is seen in Alzheimer's disease? Although data on this point are lacking, it may be that prominent medial temporal cortical atrophy lessens the chances for surgical improvement because these patients may have Alzheimer's disease.

Is there evidence of congenital hydrocephalus? For example, is there aqueductal stenosis or an Arnold-Chiari malformation?

Newer MRI techniques such as Cine-MRI involving the analysis of a CSF flow void in the aqueduct of Sylvius may be helpful in predicting who will respond to a shunt. Bradley and colleagues have recently shown that this finding on MRI correlates with a good or excellent long-term response to surgery. They recommend that if the patient fulfills the clinical picture for symptomatic hydrocephalus and has a flow void on MRI, the patient should be considered for surgery.

Regional Cerebral Blood Flow

It has been reported that regional cerebral blood flow (rCBF) is decreased in the frontal areas in hydrocephalus and in the parietotemporal areas in Alzheimer's disease. On the presumption that many of the nonimproved group have Alzheimer's disease, which we have confirmed in two who came to autopsy, we tried to differentiate those who will respond to shunt surgery from those who will not based on the pattern of preoperative rCBF. To do this, we calculated the ratio of frontal over posterior rCBF, expecting a lower frontal-posterior ratio in true symptomatic hydrocephalus and a higher ratio in pseudosymptomatic hydrocephalus patients who have Alzheimer's disease. In fact, this has been a good method of predicting surgical outcome: the ratio predicted 5:7 unimproved and 22:23 improved patients in our series (see Table 1).

Cisternography

Our experience with cisternography is limited, but the literature suggests that there are numerous cases with a positive test (radioisotope seen within the ventricles 48 to 72 hours after being injected in the lumbar area) who do not improve with surgery and patients with equivocal or negative tests who do improve. Further, the test itself may be difficult to interpret. Black et al, in a review of their experience with this test, found the following: of 11 patients who had a positive test, nine improved and two did not. Of six patients who had mixed results, three improved and three did not. Of six who had negative results, four improved and two did not. They suggest a positive test is helpful but an equivocal or negative test is not. A recent study by Vanneste et al reported that "cisternography did not improve the diagnostic accuracy of combined clinical and computerized tomography in patients with presumed normal-pressure hydrocephalus." We do not use cisternography.

CEREBROSPINAL FLUID PRESSURE MONITORING

There have been reports of a significant relationship between measures of intracranial CSF pressure monitoring and surgical outcome for symptomatic hydrocephalus. In Borgesen and Gjerris's study and in our study, the greater the percentage of time B waves were present, the greater the chance of a good outcome. Also, in our series, the longer the pressure was more than 15 mm Hg the better the chance of successful surgery (see Table 1). This implies that increased pressure may be pathogenic in symptomatic hydrocephalus.

These data raise the issue of what is meant by *normal pressure hydrocephalus.* Does it mean normal pressure at one spinal tap, or does it imply that pressure remains normal all the time? We do not know what 24 hour CSF pressure recordings in normal people would show. It follows that we do not know if the pressure is abnormal in those who respond to surgery compared to those who don't. For this reason, at present, we prefer the term *symptomatic hydrocephalus* over *normal pressure hydrocephalus.*

Infusion Tests

Borgesen and Gjerris described the CSF conductance test, in which CSF absorption is measured at different CSF pressures. They reported in their series a greater than 90 percent accuracy in predicting short-term prognosis following shunt surgery and about an 85 percent accuracy in predicting long-term prognosis. The concept is that the greater the pressure needed to obtain a fixed amount of absorption, the better the chances of that patient improving with shunt surgery. Borgenson and Gjerris reported that a conductance of less than 0.08 predicted a favorable outcome. In our study, we found no significant correlation between CSF conductance and improvement (see Table 1). However, we chose our patients based on the conductance result, so this was not an independent variable. In addition, most of our patients had idiopathic hydrocephalus, whereas many of Borgenson and Gjerris's patients had secondary hydrocephalus. The conductance test, which relates to CSF absorption, may be a better predictor of outcome in secondary hydrocephalus, in which an absorption defect may be causative.

ASSESSING PATIENT IMPROVEMENT

Traditionally, patient improvement has been assessed on a 5-point rating scale. This may be problematic because levels on the scale overlap and the measurement is subjective. We have tried to develop more objective measures and use the following:

Serial Videotaping of Gait

Preoperatively and 2 and 6 months postoperatively, we videotape the patient's neurologic examination, including walking. Scales have been developed and published to measure the patient's gait performance both qualitatively and quantitatively.

Katz Index of Activities of Daily Living

The Katz Index rates the patient on six items: bathing, dressing, toileting, transferring, continence, and feeding. The worst score for each item is 3 and the best is 1. Thus the worst obtainable score is 18 and the best is 6. There is a written description for each score in each item. We regard a change of 2 or more in this index as significant. This allows measurement of small but funtionally important changes. An example of a 2-point improvement on this index might be as follows: a change from "occasional urinary accidents" to "controls urination and bowel movements completely by self" (1-point improvement) plus a change from "moves in and out of bed or chair with assistance" to "moves in and out of bed as well as chair without assistance" (1-point improvement).

Neuropsychological Testing

Our patients receive a battery of neuropsychological tests pre- and 2 and 6 months postoperatively. These tests sample orientation, intelligence, verbal and visual memory, language, visuospatial functioning, and executive control. We judge the patient neuropsychologically improved when there has been a significant increase in the test scores in two or more neuropsychological areas evaluated, provided there is no decline in another area. Only about 50 percent of those responding overall to shunt surgery improve cognitively by the above criteria.

RECOMMENDING PATIENTS FOR SHUNT SURGERY

Bearing the above information in mind we recommend the following. Take a careful history from the patient and the family. Try to establish time of onset of dementia and gait abnormality by asking questions such as, "How did the patient walk last Christmas or on their last birthday?" Noting the differential diagnoses mentioned above, ask appropriate questions to find other causes of the constellation of findings. Has the patient had cervical spondylosis or a previous neck injury? Has the patient been a heavy drinker? Is there another cause for urinary difficulty such as prostatism or the birth of multiple children? What medications does the patient take? Are there symptoms of autonomic dysfunction such as postural hypotension? Is there a secondary cause for hydrocephalus such as a head injury, meningitis, or subarachnoid hemorrhage? Has the patient had a large head since childhood? Does the patient have symptoms of Parkinson's disease involving the hands, such as micrographia or tremor?

On examination, measure the head size, measure the postural blood pressure, look for signs of Parkinson's disease involving the arms (making parkinsonism more likely), look for vertical gaze paresis (unusual in symptomatic hydrocephalus in the elderly), look for upper motor neuron signs in the legs and or lower motor neuron signs in the arms (making one suspicious of cervical spondylosis). Do formal psychometric testing looking for evidence of aphasia, especially anomia. Obtain a head CT and/or MRI. Analyze it, keeping in mind the points mentioned earlier in the section on CT and MRI. If necessary, order a cervical MRI. Make a videotape of the patient walking about 20 yards, turning, and walking back.

At this point you may be able to make your decision about surgery. If you are still uncertain, perform daily serial lumbar punctures for 3 to 5 days, videotaping the patient before and after. If the patient improves, surgery is likely to help, but if there is no improvement, a benefit from surgery cannot be ruled out. Continue to follow and reassess the patient as needed. Before recommending surgery, be sure to point out that complications occur in about 30 percent of patients undergoing shunt surgery. Also tell the patient and family that even if the patient improves, it is likely that the patient won't return to normal. In those that respond favorably, gait and incontinence usually improve, but cognition improves in only 50 percent. These are important improvements and may prevent a patient from being placed in a nursing home, but the patient and family should have realistic expectations. If at this stage you are still unsure of what to do, you can defer the decision and let the patient return in 3 months, repeating the videotape at that time. Longitudinal information documenting that the problem is stable or progressive may factor into your decision. Alternative diagnostic tests such as cerebral blood flow, CSF pressure monitoring, infusion studies, and continuous CSF drainage studies are not universally available, but can be used as adjunctive information in the centers that use these tests.

SUGGESTED READING

Black PMcL. Idiopathic normal pressure hydrocephalus. Neurosurg 1980; 52:371–377.

Borgesen SE, Gjerris F. The predictive value of conductance to outflow of CSF in NPH. Brain 1982; 105:65–86.

Bradley WG, Whittemore AR, Kortman KE, et al. Marked cerebrospinal fluid void: Indicator of successful shunt in patients with suspected normal-pressure hydrocephalus. Radiology 1991; 178:459–466.

Fisher CM. The clinical picture in occult hydrocephalus. Clin Neurosurg 1977; 24:270–315.

Graff-Radford NR, Godersky JC. Normal pressure hydrocephalus: Onset of gait abnormality before dementia predicts a good surgical outcome. Arch Neurol 1986; 43:940–942.

Graff-Radford NR, Godersky JC. Symptomatic congenital hydrocephalus in the elderly simulating normal pressure hydrocephalus. Neurology 1989; 39:1596-1600.

Graff-Radford NR, Godersky JC, Jones MP. Variables predicting outcome in symptomatic hydrocephalus in the elderly. Neurology 1989; 39:1601–1604.

Graff-Radford NR, Rezai K, Godersky JC, et al. Regional cerebral blood flow in normal pressure hydrocephalus. J Neurol Neurosurg Psychiatry 1987; 50:1589–1596.

Haan J, Thormeer RTWM. Predictive value of temporary external lumbar drainage in normal pressure hydrocephalus. Neurosurgery 1988; 22:388–391.

Hanley DF, Borel CO, Herdman S. Normal-pressure hydrocephalus. In: Johnson RT, ed. Current therapy in neurological disease 3. Philadelphia: BC Decker, 1990:305.

Peterson RC, Mokri B, Laws ER. Surgical treatment of idiopathic hydrocephalus in elderly patients. Neurology 1985; 35:307–311.

Vanneste J, Augustijn P, Davies GAG, et al. Normal-pressure hydrocephalus. Arch Neurol 1992; 49:366–370.

Wikkelsö C, Anderson H, Blomstrand C, et al. Normal pressure hydrocephalus: Predictive value of the cerebrospinal fluid tap-test. Acta Neurol Scand 1986; 73:566–573.

POSTCONCUSSIVE HEADACHE

R. NORMAN HARDEN, M.D.

Although the clinical diagnosis of postconcussive headache (PCHA) is easily made, trauma can cause a variety of headache syndromes. Proper management requires a specific diagnosis and specific therapy. The personal cost to the patient and the financial cost to society are significant. An aggressive and methodical approach to these patients is required for a successful outcome.

Between 5 and 10 percent of the general population seek medical care for headache and 40 percent of North Americans suffer severe headache during their lives. Approximately 8 percent of ongoing headaches are estimated to be postconcussive. Between 75,000 and 3 million U.S. citizens are head injured each year, representing over $2 billion in yearly losses. Between 12 and 80 percent of patients have headache after trauma. Headache lasts longer than 2 months in approximately 40 to 60 percent of patients hospitalized for head trauma. Over 90 percent of these patients report head pain within 24 hours, and up to 100 percent of those over 50 years of age experience head pain after injury. Approximately 60,000 people are disabled each year from postconcussive headache.

Headache is the most frequent symptom of the postconcussive syndrome. The syndrome usually includes depression, insomnia, and some degree of cognitive impairment. It may include anxiety states and a wide array of neurologic signs or symptoms. There appears to be an inverse relationship between the severity of the injury and headache. The incidence of headache increases with the frequency of litigation, and settlement may contribute to the ultimate recovery of these patients. The development of PCHA is unrelated to sex, occupation, IQ, the duration of loss of consciousness, or presence of amnesia, electroencephalogram (EEG) abnormalities, fracture, or blood in cerebrospinal fluid. Patients with lacerations or a prior history of headache show an increased incidence of PCHA.

PCHA can be of almost any headache type. In this chapter I first discuss general principles of headache diagnosis and then the various specific diagnoses often seen in victims of head trauma. The Headache Classification Committee of the International Headache Society (IHS) has generated the most uniformly accepted criteria for headache diagnosis. The IHS has designated a general category of "headache associated with head trauma," which is divided into acute post-traumatic headache, if the headache lasts less than 8 weeks after the trauma, and chronic post-traumatic headache, if it persists more than 8 weeks. In addition to this general diagnosis, a more specific headache diagnosis is suggested by the IHS because more specific diagnoses will lead to specific therapies.

GENERAL DIAGNOSTIC PRINCIPLES

Patient History

In addition to a general history, important points to be elicited in the evaluation of PCHA include the circumstances of the injury, with particular attention to the forces involved. Whether the injury was work-related may be relevant. The location, duration, and radiation of the pain are important, as are aggravating and alleviating factors. It is important to explore the temporal patterns of, and limitations caused by, the headache. Inquire whether the headache is associated with nausea, photophobia, phonophobia, or sensory alterations. Any history of disease of the sinuses, teeth, ear, nose, or throat is relevant. The integrity of the senses must be assessed. Questions as to the existence of numbness, weakness, spasm, fasciculation, incontinence, loss of consciousness, epilepsy, or dizziness are relevant. I find it very useful to ask for the patient's self-diagnosis because this provides insight into the cause of the PCHA. We know that PCHA patients are more likely to have a history of headache of some type, and characterization of this could be useful. Ask for the effect of stress, fatigue, and posture on the headache. Ask about the patient's sleep pattern (particularly in reference to insomnia) and history of changes in personality, degenerative joint disease, or spondylosis.

A list of past and current medications will be helpful in guiding therapy. Use of and response to alcohol, tobacco, caffeine, and street drugs are all relevant. In women, the use of birth control pills and the effect of menses on the headache must be known. Previous head and neck injury should be recorded along with surgeries, psychiatric interventions, and allergies. Family medical history should pursue a history of headache. Social history should include whether or not the patient is currently working, as well as the history of work satisfaction and marital status. The number of children, their ages, and the patient's educational level and military participation can provide insight. One needs to know the source of income and the litigation status. Questions to elicit psychological state must be asked.

Patient Examination

In addition to a general physical examination including vital signs, special attention should be paid to the head, its shape and the presence of any lesions. Careful examination of nose, ears, teeth, throat, sinuses, and temporomandibular joints (TMJ) is also required. TMJ auscultation, palpation, and checking for trigger points and maximum opening girth of the mouth are essential points of the TMJ examination. The carotids should be examined for bruits and tenderness. Examination of the thyroid for nodes and lesions is necessary. A careful neurologic exam is obviously indicated, with special attention to the cranial nerves. Anosmia is considerably more common in those head injury patients who develop PCHA. In addition to visual acuity and perimetry, the fundi should be examined carefully. Cervical range of motion should be assessed for flexion, extension, side-to-side movement, and rotation. The curvature of the spine should be noted with attention to any deviations from normal. Kernig's and Lhermitte's signs should be checked. The presence of trigger points, spastic muscles, and percussion tenderness should be noted, especially in the neck.

Tests

A variety of tests may be indicated, especially imaging of the head such as magnetic resonance imaging (MRI) or computed tomography (CT) scanning. Cervical spine films should include flexion, extension, and oblique views. The patient's presentation may indicate EEG, sleep studies, and audiology. A variety of psychological tests including the Minnesota Multiphasic Personality Inventory (MMPI), state-trait anxiety inventory, and a depression scale (Beck, Zung, or Hamilton) should be part of the general workup. Other tests that may be indicated are VER, BAER, electromyogram, bone scan, myelogram, and thermography. Laboratory tests should include a complete blood count with differential and a SMA-7. Westergren sedimentation rate, thyroid functions, Folate, B_{12}, and serum protein electrophoresis should be considered.

SPECIFIC HEADACHE SYNDROMES

Migraine (Vascular) Headache

When it was noted that histamine could exacerbate or precipitate a PCHA, it was suggested that PCHA was primarily vascular. Since the principal pain-mediating structures in the head are the large vessels, particularly the veins and venous sinuses, this was a reasonable theory. Angiography performed at the time of head injury has occasionally shown arterial spasm associated with the injured part of the brain. A biphasic cerebrovascular response is seen in experimental trauma. At first an increase in the rate of fill and flow in the brain is seen, and then, approximately an hour later, spasm with decreased cerebral blood flow occurs. These experiments suggest that cerebral autoregulation may be lost after trauma. Decreased cerebral oxidative metabolism has sometimes been seen after head trauma. The impairment of blood flow may be serious, leading to rapid post-traumatic atrophy. Diffuse ischemic parenchymatous damage and areas of demyelination have been noted, even after apparently mild head injury. Changes are also noted in vascular compliance, which may predispose to orthostatic changes and orthostatic triggers for PCHA.

The IHS criteria for migraine require an idiopathic headache disorder manifesting as attacks lasting 4 to 72 hours. Headache may occur with or without aura or neurologic prodrome. The typical characteristics of the headache are unilateral location, pulsating quality, pain of moderate or severe intensity, aggravation by routine physical activity, and the associated symptoms of nausea, photophobia, and phonophobia. Two symptoms referable to the basilar circulation would meet the criteria for basilar migraine. Other, less common migraine types can also be defined, such as ophthalmoplegic or retinal migraine.

Cluster Headache

Cluster headache is frequently seen after head trauma. Post-traumatic migraine and post-traumatic cluster headaches account for at least one-third of the PCHA that we see. Of 100 patients with cluster headache, 41 had a history of head trauma, 20 of whom had lost consciousness. The mean latency between trauma and headache occurrence was 9 years.

The IHS criteria for cluster headache requires attacks of severe pain that is unilateral and periorbital.

The attacks usually last between 15 and 180 minutes and can occur from once every other day up to 8 times a day. They are often associated with conjunctival injection, lacrimation, nasal congestion, rhinorrhea, forehead and facial sweating, myosis, ptosis, and eyelid edema. The attacks occur in series lasting for weeks or months, the so-called cluster periods. The attacks are separated by periods of remission that can last for months to years. Approximately 10 percent of patients have chronic symptomatology.

Extracranial Lacerations and Meningeal Scar

The meninges and scalp skin are pain-sensitive. Headache may be due to damage to these structures, probably a deafferentation type of pain phenomenon. These patients show a local throbbing and tenderness in the area of the laceration. They may also show numbness at the site of injury, with diffuse burning pain in the general area.

Cervicogenic Headache

Animal experiments have shown that a 25 mile per hour vehicle collision is sufficient to cause shear in cerebral tissue and strain or rupture of cervical ligaments. Head rotation has been shown to be a significant factor in producing those injuries. Even whiplash without a direct blow can cause contusion. The whiplash type of postconcussive headache is probably a significant and underdiagnosed contributor to post-traumatic headaches. There are no specific IHS criteria for cervicogenic headache, but the most appropriate category is "headache associated with disorder of the cranium or neck." If there is clinical or laboratory evidence of a disorder in the cranium, or if there is pain localized to the neck and occipital region that may radiate elsewhere, this category can be used. The two subcategories, cranial bone disorders and neck disorders, may occur independently or simultaneously. They are usually associated with limitations in range of movement and changes in neck muscle contour, texture, or tone, as well as abnormal tenderness, trigger points, and taut bands of neck muscles.

Muscular Headache

Soft tissue injuries in the trapezius and strap muscles, either primary or secondary to spasm caused by cervicogenic injury, can contribute to headache. This pain problem is called the myofascial pain syndrome, and such pain in the neck is often referred to the head.

Sympathetic Denervation

This type of head pain is seen primarily following blows to the carotid sheath. The head pain is often associated with sympathetic changes and probably reflects damage to the cervical sympathetic system. It may take on the characteristics of a facial reflex sympathetic dystrophy.

Cranial Neuralgia

The trigeminal nerves and other cranial sensory nerves are subject to deafferentation pain after injury. We often see post-traumatic trigeminal neuralgia, which is characterized by brief "electrical" shooting pains. A trigger area can usually be identified. Pain after sinus surgery and dental procedures is also fairly common. The IHS criteria merely require pain in the distribution of a nerve or plexus that has either a persistent or a neuropathic (ticlike) quality. In these syndromes, even criteria-based diagnosis is vague.

Traumatic Temporomandibular Joint Syndrome

Patients with this syndrome experience malocclusion, decreased opening width, tenderness, and clicking. This is a frequent and underdiagnosed cause of post-traumatic head pain.

The IHS criteria place TMJ dysfunction in the category of headaches associated with "facial structure disorders." Required for diagnosis are positive X ray or bone scan findings and pain of mild to moderate intensity located at the TMJ or referred from there. The criteria also require at least two of the following: pain of the jaw precipitated by movement or clenching, decreased range of movement, auscultated noise during joint movements, tenderness of the joint capsule.

Psychosomatic Headache

The DSM IIIR defines psychosomatic pain as pain existing without evidence of organic damage. This is probably not a useful category in reference to post-traumatic headaches and should only be utilized after careful attempts at excluding other diagnoses.

DIFFERENTIAL DIAGNOSIS

One must rule out the obvious entities of subarachnoid hemorrhage, subdural hematoma, meningitis (especially with a laceration), and facial or orbital injury. Traumatic TMJ and dental injury are often overlooked, as stated above.

PROGNOSIS AND NATURAL HISTORY

After 1 year, 30 percent of patients with PCHA still have headache, and after 3 years, 15 percent remain symptomatic. With penetrating wounds, as many as 60 percent may have headache symptoms even after 15 years. Those older than age 45 are more likely to experience prolonged symptoms. The duration of disability is more closely related to other symptoms of the post-traumatic syndrome, such as depression or cognitive impairment. Continued disability is associated with such factors as middle age, single marital status, lower socioeconomic group, industrial accidents, unskilled occupations, and previous behavioral abnormalities. The use of a consistent, methodical, and multimodal approach to the diagnosis of PCHA increases the chance of arriving at a specific headache classification and thereby designing an effective treatment regimen.

SUGGESTED READING

Dalessio DJ. Wolff's headache and other head pain. 5th ed. New York: Oxford University Press, 1987.

Goldstein J. Post traumatic headache and the post concussion syndrome. Med Clin North Am 1991; 641–652.

Lance JW. Mechanism and management of headache. 4th ed. Boston: Butterworth Scientific, 1982.

Raskin NH. Headache. 2nd ed. New York: Churchill Livingstone, 1988.

IDIOPATHIC INTRACRANIAL HYPERTENSION (PSEUDOTUMOR CEREBRI)

JAMES J. CORBETT, M.D.

Idiopathic intracranial hypertension (IIH), also known as pseudotumor cerebri or benign intracranial hypertension, is a syndrome of increased intracranial pressure, headache, and papilledema that occurs most commonly in obese women. Men are also affected but less frequently (8:1 ratio). Children are affected with equal sex incidence, but it is much less common in children than in adults. To qualify for the diagnosis there should be no focal neurologic signs other than abducens nerve palsy; normal computed tomography (CT) or magnetic resonance imaging (MRI) findings; cerebrospinal fluid (CSF) pressure greater than 200 mm H_2O; and normal CSF constituents (see Table 1).

SYMPTOMATIC INTRACRANIAL HYPERTENSION

This diagnosis includes all other identifiable conditions that are known to cause elevated CSF pressure in which no focal neurologic deficits occur. Conditions that alter CSF protein or cellular content, such as spinal cord tumors, Guillain-Barré syndrome, and infections, as well as various toxins and medications have been associated with intracranial hypertension (Table 2). For many of these conditions a clear, rigorous cause and effect relationship has never been established. Despite the appearance of cause and effect, correction of organ failure or removal of reputed toxins and medications has not been systematically studied to see whether CSF pressure returns to normal after treatment. The most commonly implicated medications are excess vitamin A, tetracyclines, lithium, and nalidixic acid. The most intriguing organ failure associations are uremia and hypoparathyroidism.

CONFIRMING THE DIAGNOSIS

Lumbar Puncture

Before a patient is labeled with IIH, a lumbar puncture (LP) must be performed to confirm normal CSF constituents and pressures of greater than 200 mm H_2O. If the patient is massively obese, LP under fluoroscopy or a cervical puncture should be used. An extra long, 6 inch anesthesia needle should be used if the lumbar spine is obscured by fat. CSF pressure should be measured with the legs extended and the neck in a neutral position. *Obesity alone does not elevate CSF pressure.* If CSF pressure is less than 200 mm H_2O, repeat the LP in a couple of days to see if the pressure is elevated. If more than two normal pressures are recorded and it is urgent to establish the diagnosis, 24 to 48 hours of continuous CSF pressure recording should be made using either a subarachnoid bolt or an intraventricular cannula. In patients with IIH, this test will show episodic severe elevation of intracranial pressure. Under no circumstances should a patient be given the label of IIH without strict adherence to the modified Dandy Criteria.

Imaging Studies

In the days before CT, angiography and pneumoencephalography were the basic tools used to identify

Table 1 Modified Dandy Criteria for the Diagnosis of Idiopathic Intracranial Hypertension

---

Signs and symptoms of increased intracranial pressure

Absence of localizing findings on neurologic examination

Absence of deformity, displacement, and obstruction of the ventricular system and otherwise normal neurodiagnostic studies except for increased cerebrospinal fluid pressure

Awake and alert patient

No other cause of increased intracranial pressure present

Modified from Wall M. Idiopathic intracranial hypertension. Neurol Clin 1991; 9:74; with permission.

Table 2 Differential Diagnosis of Idiopathic
Intracranial Hypertension*

Highly Likely
  Decreased flow through arachnoid granulations
    Scarring from previous inflammation, such as meningitis or
      sequel to subarachnoid hemorrhage
  Obstruction to venous drainage
    Venous sinus thromboses
      Hypercoagulable states
      Contiguous infection, such as middle ear or mastoidotitic
        hydrocephalus
    Bilateral radical neck dissection
    Superior vena cava syndrome
    Increased right heart pressure
  Endocrine disorders
    Addison's disease
    Hypoparathyroidism
    Obesity
    Steroid withdrawal
  Nutritional disorders
    Hypervitaminosis A (vitamin, liver, or isoretinoin intake)
    Hyperalimentation in deprivation dwarfism
  Arteriovenous malformations

Probable Causes
  Anabolic steroids (may cause venous sinus thrombosis)
  Chlordecone (kepone)
  Ketoprofen or indomethacin in Bartter's syndrome
  Systemic lupus erythematosus
  Thyroid replacement therapy in hypothyroid children
  Uremia

Possible Causes
  Amiodarone
  Diphenylhydantoin
  Iron deficiency anemia
  Lithium carbonate
  Nalidixic acid
  Sarcoidosis
  Sulfa antibiotics

Causes Frequently Cited That Are Unproven
  Corticosteroid intake
  Hyperthyroidism
  Hypovitaminosis A
  Menarche
  Menstrual irregularities
  Multivitamin intake
  Oral contraceptive use
  Pregnancy
  Tetracycline use

---

*To be included in any category, the patient had to fulfill the modified
Dandy Criteria.
  From Wall M. Idiopathic intracranial hypertension. Neurol Clin 1991;
9:74; with permission.

patients with IIH. Angiography—digital venous subtraction or intra-arterial angiography aiming to visualize the venous structures—is still the standard way to identify patients suspected of having a major venous sinus occlusion.

CT scans with and without contrast can identify abnormalities suggesting secondary causes of intracranial hypertension, such as large ventricles, intracranial masses, and ventricular shift. Tumors are rarely missed. Most CT scanners are also limited to patients who weigh less than 300 pounds. This is an occasional

obstacle, as with MRI, when the patient is massively obese.

MRI is the ideal imaging modality for IIH except for the size and weight limitations of the machines. About a third of patients are claustrophobic enough that the symptom restricts the use of MRI.

Laboratory Studies

Except for serologic tests for syphilis, serum calcium levels and studies for systemic lupus erythematosus, it is fruitless to perform extensive endocrinologic studies unless there is clinical evidence of some endocrine disease. Occasional patients have amenorrhea and galactorrhea related to their empty sella, a common consequence of IIH.

Studies of CSF have not been helpful in the basic understanding of IIH. About 25 percent of patients have CSF protein less than 20 mg per deciliter. Any more than 5 mononuclear cells should prompt investigation for occult tumor, chronic infection, or inflammation such as sarcoidosis. Single brief CSF pressure measurements are not a reliable guide to the status of the patient's CSF pressure or response to medication. Papilledema frequently improves despite the persistence of high CSF pressure measured during ordinary LP.

Visual evoked potentials (VEP) are of no help to determine the severity of visual loss until visual loss is very extensive. VEP test central vision optimally. Peripheral visual loss, the earliest and commonest defect, remains undetected until very late in the course.

Ophthalmologic Studies

Ophthalmologic studies are the cornerstone of proper diagnosis of IIH. Once the CT or MRI and LP confirm the diagnosis, it is time to investigate the degree to which the papilledema has affected vision.

Most patients with IIH first see a neurologist because of headache, whereas patients with visual complaints (double vision, "blurry" vision, or transient episodes of visual blackout) usually arrive first in the ophthalmologist's office. A small percentage of IIH patients are symptom-free and are accidentally found to have papilledema during an ophthalmoscopic examination for some unrelated problem.

The major complication for the patient with IIH is permanent visual loss. Thus a neurologist must also consult an ophthalmologist to help manage the visual aspects of the patient's problem. In truth it is the ophthalmologist whose visual field studies hold the key to the long-term medical and surgical management of these patients.

FOLLOW-UP

Visual acuity, visual fields using standard kinetic, static, or high-pass quantitative ring perimetry, ophthalmoscopy with fundus photographs, and intraocular

Table 3 Approach to Diagnostic Follow-Up of the Patient with Idiopathic Intracranial Hypertension

How to Follow the Patient with IIH
Visual acuity – Snellen
Contrast sensitivity – Vistech or Pelli-Robson
Visual fields – Goldmann, Humphrey 30-2, Ophthimus
Color vision tests – AO 14 plate test or Ishihara test
Intraocular pressure measurement
Fundus photographs

How Not to Follow the Patient with IIH
Repeated lumbar puncture
Visual evoked potentials
Measurement of the blind spot
Visual acuity alone without other tests of optic nerve function

pressure measurement should be performed on a regular basis. Unless, as a neurologist, you are able to perform these studies, the patient must be followed at timely intervals (1 to 3 months) by an ophthalmologist. The do's and don'ts of optimal follow-up are outlined in Table 3. Visual failure is silent. It is not necessarily accompanied by severe headache, and exactly like glaucoma, visual field loss proceeds from the periphery to the center. Visual acuity (central vision) is the last part of the visual field to be affected. Visual acuity is one of the few ophthalmologic studies a neurologist performs. Visual acuity measurement provides very little warning of impending visual loss until it is too late.

Repeated LP, both for therapy and "to see how the pressure is doing," is the diagnostic mainstay of the neurologist. Unfortunately, CSF pressure varies widely from day to day as well as throughout the day. Thus CSF pressure measurements provide no useful information regarding the success of therapy. A repeat LP does not need to be performed unless the patient requests it for headache relief. CSF pressures provide no guideline for surgical intervention.

HOW OFTEN SHOULD THE PATIENT BE FOLLOWED?

If the patient has visual field loss at the first visit, it is prudent to see the patient in follow-up within 2 to 4 weeks. All patients should be cautioned that they should return earlier if their vision is worsening. If visual loss is rapid, medical management should be abandoned and surgical treatment undertaken.

If the visual field is stable, patients can be seen in follow-up at monthly intervals until one is relatively certain that visual loss is not progressing. At that point follow-up can be extended to 3 or 6 month intervals.

Fundus photographs are important in the same way that chest X rays are useful in following a patient with tuberculosis. Photographs provide objective evidence of change or lack of change in appearance and they provide documentary evidence of the evolution of swelling.

SUGGESTED READING

Corbett JJ. Diagnosis and management of idiopathic intracranial hypertension (pseudotumor cerebri). Focal Points 1989; 7:1–12.

Corbett JJ, Nerad JA, Tse DT, Anderson RL. Results of optic nerve sheath fenestration for pseudotumor cerebri. Arch Ophthalmol 1988; 106:1391–1397.

Corbett JJ, Savino PJ, Thompson HS, et al. Visual loss in pseudotumor cerebri: Follow-up of 57 patients from five to 41 years and a profile of 14 patients with permanent severe visual loss. Arch Neurol 1982; 39:461–474.

Corbett JJ, Thompson HS. The rational management of idiopathic intracranial hypertension. Arch Neurol 1989; 46:1049–1051.

Digre KB, Corbett JJ. Pseudotumor cerebri in men. Arch Neurol 1988; 45:866–872.

Ireland B, Corbett JJ, Wallace RB. The search for causes of idiopathic intracranial hypertension. Arch Neurol 1990; 47:315–320.

Kosmorsky G. Idiopathic intracranial hypertension (pseudotumor cerebri). Ophthalmol Clin North Am 1991; 4:557–574.

Wall M. Idiopathic intracranial hypertension. Neurol Clin 1991; 9:73–94.

Wall M, George D. Visual loss in pseudotumor cerebri: Incidence and defects related to visual field strategy. Arch Neurol 1987; 44: 170–175.

FACIAL PAIN

J. KEITH CAMPBELL, M.D., F.R.C.P (Ed)

In considering facial pain, I generally include pain in the forehead even though this is more often considered as head pain. For this discussion, therefore, facial pain is defined as pain in the anterior half of the head. This avoids the artificial and clinically inappropriate exclusion of pain in the distribution of the first or ophthalmic division of the trigeminal nerve, a structure that is intimately involved in the transmission and pathogenesis of many types of facial pain.

Pain in the face, while most often perceived via the trigeminal nerve, may be carried by sensory fibers in the facial nerve, autonomic nerves, and the glossopharyngeal and vagus nerves. In many instances it is not possible to determine the neural pathways involved, while in others the pain may be central in origin or due to deafferentation of the facial structures.

A detailed classification of facial pain was recently developed by the International Headache Society (see Suggested Reading), and while it is useful for reminding us of many of the types and causes of facial pain, it is not practical for everyday use in a clinical setting. I prefer a general grouping of facial pain into two major categories: those pains due to a lesion or lesions that can be identified on examination or by special investigations, and those pains where no structural abnormality can be identified. The latter category refers to pains of poorly understood pathogenesis such as migraine, cluster headache, referred pains, and "atypical facial pain."

Table 1 is a bare bones, eclectic listing of facial pains

Table 1 Facial Pain

A. With Demonstrable Causes

Nasopharynx, Nose, Sinuses	*Eye and Orbit*	*Dental*
Infection	Glaucoma	Teeth
Tumor	Inflammation	Cracked
Bony abnormalities	Tumor	Caries
Wegener's granuloma	Pseudotumor	Abscess
	Refractive error (rare except in children)	Temporomandibular joint arthritis
	Tolosa-Hunt syndrome	Trauma
		Myofascial pain
		Temporomandibular dysfunction
Skull and Cervical Spine	*Intracranial Lesions*	*Cranial Nerve Lesions*
Primary and secondary tumors	Tumors	Herpes zoster
Fibrous dysplasia	Benign	Geniculate herpes
Osteomyelitis	Malignant	Compressive lesions
Degenerative joint and cervical disk disease	Primary	Trauma
Neck-tongue syndrome	Secondary	Surgical interruption
	Infection	Deafferentation pain
	Abscess	Granulomatous
	Subdural empyema	Sarcoid
	Gradenigo's syndrome	Chronic meningitis
	Paratrigeminal syndrome	Lyme disease
		Connective tissue disease
Vascular Causes	*Referred Pain*	
Dissection of carotid artery	Angina	
Intracranial	Carcinoma lung	
Aneurysm	Cervical spine	
AVM		

B. With No Demonstrable Cause

Neuralgias	*Migraine Type*	*Cluster and CPH*
Trigeminal	Facial migraine	Lower and upper patterns of Ekbom
Glossopharyngeal	Vascular facial pain	Raeder's syndrome
Nervus intermedius	Carotidynia	"Obsolete" neuralgias
		Ciliary
		Sphenopalatine
		Petrosal
Undiagnosed Facial Pain		
Atypical facial pain		
Atypical odontalgia		

AVM = arteriovenous malformation; CPH = chronic paroxysmal hemicrania.

with and without demonstrable (by clinically available tests) causes. It is far from complete but is intended to provide a useful list of conditions to be considered in the differential diagnosis of facial pain.

CLINICAL APPROACH TO THE DIAGNOSIS OF FACIAL PAIN

The following discussion makes the assumption that pain is the primary complaint and that there is no complaint of greater neurologic significance, such as diplopia, facial or tongue weakness, or indeed any focal neurologic deficit. The presence of such a deficit or complaint would clearly take precedence in the differential diagnosis and in the schema of testing.

As with all neurologic conditions, evaluation begins with the careful acquisition of a history, followed by a complete physical examination, followed by those specialty evaluations such as the ophthalmic, ear, nose, and throat, and dental examinations that are indicated by the history and examination, and, finally, by the appropriate laboratory and imaging studies.

Obtaining the History

After confirming the demographic information, I ask how long the pain has been present, whether it is one-sided or bilateral, and whether it is continuous or intermittent. I ask the patient to indicate the site of the pain and request that it be mapped out, with one finger if possible. It is then determined whether the pain has any trigger mechanisms. Having obtained a general idea of the location and temporal profile of the pain, I then ask patients to go back in their mind to when the pain began and to relate the story to me. Most patients will speak for only a few minutes before pausing for guidance on how to continue to provide key diagnostic information. The details in this initial "bolus" are usually sufficient to proceed to the next stage in which I ask if the pain wakens them from a sound sleep or whether it is present on awakening at their normal getting-up time; and if so, whether it would feel better to remain in bed or whether getting up and having breakfast or a cup of coffee modifies the pain. If the pain is not present on awakening, I ask them when it usually first appears during the day. I then ask them to relate their "average day," including those factors that influence the pain, both worsening and relieving it. I determine if the pain is still present at bedtime, whether it keeps them awake, and if the pain is accompanied by other symptoms. I ask whether they or their relatives note any changes in their facial appearance during the attacks and whether the pain is worsening, remaining steady, or improving over time. When appropriate, this line of questioning can be extended to determine the behavior of the discomfort over days, weeks, and months.

The line of questioning then becomes more specific and is determined to a large extent by the information obtained in the preliminary assessment described above. Some of the specific questions relate to trigger factors the patient may have noted, such as touching the face, brushing the teeth, shaving, chewing, swallowing, heat, cold, the consumption of alcohol, neck movements, and brushing the hair. The effects of coughing, straining, sneezing, and the head low position are determined. I ask the patient and the relatives to describe the subject's behavior during an episode of pain. Are they restless, withdrawn, or quiet? Can they describe the associated autonomic symptoms, if any, such as tearing, redness, or pallor of the face, drooping of the eyelids, and changes in the pupil size? This latter is rarely reported appropriately. Most commonly, a large pupil is reported even though it may be contralateral to the pain, when the smaller pupil is the pathologic one.

I inquire if the subject has a prior warning of the pain before it develops, whether the pain is influenced by the menstrual cycle, the use of medications including oral contraceptive agents and hormones, and whether treatments already prescribed have influenced the pain. I ask if the patient has had the same pain earlier in life and if they have other facial or head pains.

The history also includes a review of the subject's other health problems, medications being used for unrelated conditions, and what investigations have already been done. The family history is obtained, and finally I ask the patient if they have a theory as to the cause of the pain.

By engaging the patient in the process of following the trail of clues to the diagnosis and by showing a genuine interest in trying to understand the temporal profile, the aggravating and relieving factors, the location and type of pain, and its effects on the subject's life, it is often quite easy to reach a diagnosis, or at least a short differential diagnosis, prior to the examination.

Physical Examination

I perform an examination that is initially directed to the head and neck and then takes in the remainder of the neurologic, neurovascular, and general examination. I palpate the head, examine the teeth and mouth, palpate the temporomandibular joints while the patient opens and closes the mouth, examine cervical spine mobility, check the ears, and, when appropriate, don a glove and feel the floor of the mouth and the muscles of mastication bimanually. The teeth are inspected for signs of bruxism, uneven wear, and the general state of the dentition or fit of the dentures. Dentures "worn" in the pocket or left on the bedside table may be a clue to the cause of the pain!

The head and neck examination includes testing all the cranial nerves and the special senses, with the exception of taste, as it is rarely of diagnostic significance.

Formulation of the Diagnosis and Special Examinations

At this stage, I have frequently formulated a diagnosis or at least a short list of conditions likely to be responsible for the pain.

The cause of many facial pains is so obvious that the necessary specialty examinations or investigations needed to confirm the diagnosis or exclude alternative conditions are clear. For example, localized dental pain on chewing, on exposure of the teeth to a thermal stimulus, or pain in the region of the temporomandibular joint on chewing or talking leads me to request an oral surgery and dental consultation. Pain and tenderness in the cheek or over the frontal sinuses, or a history of epistaxis, purulent nasal discharge, nasal blockage, unilateral hearing loss, or ear pain naturally prompts a referral to an ear, nose, and throat (ENT) colleague. Deep central facial pain, especially in an older patient and especially if there is any abnormality of cranial nerve function, also mandates an ENT examination to exclude a nasopharyngeal lesion (carcinoma or granuloma) or a sinus neoplasm.

Pain around an eye, a history of diplopia, a change in visual acuity, or any abnormality on examination of the eyes prompts a consultation with an ophthalmologist.

I look upon these specialty examinations as an extension of the neurologic examination. If the specialist in any of the fields mentioned requires specific imaging or other tests, I follow their advice. If the specialized examination has revealed the cause to be outside my sphere of expertise, the patient is passed to the appropriate colleague for definitive management.

Concurrent with the specialty examinations, key imaging and other studies are obtained (Table 2). Computed tomography (CT) and magnetic resonance imaging (MRI) of the head are studies that have revolutionized the diagnosis of head and face pain. Even a negative result is of great value. The specific procedure requested is largely determined by the differential diagnosis. CT of the sinuses, skull base, facial bones, and of the intracranial contents may be sufficient for diagnosis, especially if performed with and without contrast enhancement. MRI examination is superior for the posterior fossa, the facial soft tissues, and for demonstrating the trigeminal nerves intracranially. Cervical spine films with flexion, extension, and oblique views may be helpful to determine the cause of face pain referred from the high cervical spine.

Conventional angiography is occasionally needed if a vascular abnormality such as a dissecting aneurysm of the carotid artery or an intracranial aneurysm or vascular malformation is suspected. The need for this type of invasive procedure is relatively rare and has recently become even less common with the advent of MRI angiography, even though this technique is not yet as definitive.

Other tests may be needed, including electromyography of cranial innervated muscles, electrical elicitation of the blink reflex, and visual and auditory evoked responses. Radionuclide scanning may be helpful to detect a tumor or infection of the cranial and facial bones. The evaluation is completed by a chest roentgenogram or chest CT scan if referred pain from a lung cancer is suspected.

Table 2 Investigations for Facial Pain

Imaging Studies
  MRI of head and paranasal sinuses with enhancement
  CT of head and paranasal sinuses with enhancement
  Dental films
  TMJ studies—CT, MRI
  Radioisotope bone scan
  MRI angiography
  Cerebral angiography
  Cervical spine films and MRI of cervical spine (rarely)
  Chest radiography

Blood Tests
  Sedimentation rate
  Antinuclear antibody titer
  Full blood count
  Chemistry profile
  Lyme serology
  Antineutrophil cytoplasmic antibodies

MRI = magnetic resonance imaging; CT = computed tomography; TMJ = temporomandibular joint.

In addition to health-related screening blood tests, including a sedimentation rate, specific testing may be needed: the Lyme serology, antinuclear antibody test in those subjects in whom a connective tissue disease may be present, and the antineutrophil cytoplasmic antibody test for patients suspected of having Wegener's granuloma. Finally, a temporal artery biopsy may be required for confirmation of temporal (giant cell) arteritis. If this is performed, a long segment (4 or 5 cm) of artery should be removed unilaterally. If histologically negative on that side, the opposite vessel should also be removed.

Specific Pain Syndromes

Trigeminal neuralgia (tic douloureux) is most commonly seen in middle-aged or older subjects. It is more common in women but can occur in subjects of almost any age and in both sexes. The pain is unilateral in most instances and must be confined to the distribution of one or more divisions of the fifth cranial nerve. When there is a history of bilateral attacks, the possibility of multiple sclerosis comes to mind.

Tic douloureux is characterized by paroxysmal pain of great intensity but short duration. It is generally described as a bolt of lightning, an electric shock, or a lancinating pain. It can occur as an isolated, unprovoked jabbing pain or as a series of such pains. A majority of subjects quickly identify the triggering factors already mentioned and go to extreme lengths to avoid precipitating the pain by one of the tactile triggers. The pain rarely occurs at night or awakens the subject. It is most commonly felt in the second and third divisions of the nerve but may be confined to one such division. It is least common in the ophthalmic division in isolation but more commonly affects this branch in conjunction with pain below the eye. The trigger area is usually in the same distribution as that affected by the lancinating pain. The pain rarely affects the tongue even when the mandibular division of the nerve is involved. Exacerbations and remissions are common.

In older subjects, the paroxysms of pain may be so frequent that the subject will describe the pain as lasting minutes to hours, but if questioned closely, they usually agree that this "envelope" of pain is made up of multiple paroxysms. When the pain has been occurring for days, there is a residual soreness or aching in the face between the paroxysms.

Occasionally I see a patient in such extreme pain that they cannot give the history, for each attempt to speak provokes a further volley of painful jabs. Until recently, I gave such patients carbamazepine or phenytoin by mouth and postponed completion of the history until they were more comfortable. A recently described technique of anesthetizing the ipsilateral conjunctival sac with several drops of the local ophthalmic anesthetic proparacaine (0.5 percent) has proven most effective in several patients and surprisingly gives a period of freedom from pain lasting from hours to days.

After the pain of trigeminal neuralgia is "fired" several times, there is sometimes a refractory phase lasting a variable time during which the history can be completed or the subject can quickly finish a meal before the pain is once more triggered.

The examination for idiopathic trigeminal neuralgia is normal. Specifically, there is no involvement of the motor division of the nerve and no sensory loss. Unilateral lack of dental hygiene and a reluctance to shave or apply makeup may be noted.

Although the cause of the condition is often vascular compression of the sensory root of the nerve between the gasserian ganglion and the pons, examination by CT, MRI, or angiography is not helpful, because the vessel responsible is usually a displaced, but otherwise normal, superior cerebellar vessel and the imaging techniques are not yet sufficiently detailed to confirm the relationship of the vessel to the main sensory root of the nerve. I always advise a CT scan or preferably an MRI scan to exclude a larger lesion such as a meningioma or neuroma compressing or arising from the nerve.

Glossopharyngeal neuralgia is much less common than tic douloureux but occurs in the same age group. The pain is also less sharp and probably less severe than fifth nerve neuralgia. It is felt in the throat, the base of the tongue, and tonsillar fossa. It is almost invariably triggered by swallowing and not by chewing. Like tic, it may go into remission.

Temporary relief from the pain after the application of a topical anesthetic to the tonsillar fossa and adjacent portions of the pharynx is almost diagnostic. An MRI scan with enhancement is the investigation of choice because it is the most appropriate way of excluding a structural lesion, other than a loop of a posterior fossa vessel, compressing the nerve.

Nervus intermedius neuralgia is an extremely rare cranial neuralgia. I have seen only three examples in 30 years. The pain is felt deep in the ear and is like the two neuralgias already described. It occurs spontaneously or is triggered by talking, chewing, swallowing, or touching the pinna. It may develop spontaneously or occur in the symptomatic form, a far more common variety, when it is associated with a herpetic eruption in the ear and ipsilateral soft palate—the syndrome of geniculate herpes or Ramsay Hunt syndrome. Identification of the herpetic lesion during the acute stage makes the diagnosis clear, and further investigations are not required.

Vascular face pain is a term used advisedly, which may not be scientifically correct. By this I mean pain in the face that is related to migraine, vasomotor rhinitis, and a bewildering range of poorly understood facial pains that are throbbing and made worse by exposure to heat, ingestion of alcohol, and other vasodilators. Tenderness of the ipsilateral carotid artery may be noted, and if the pain is episodic, may lead to the diagnosis of carotidynia. Investigations are almost invariably unhelpful, and the diagnosis depends upon the history of other migrainous features, the response to vasoactive drugs, and failure to determine any other cause for the pain.

A more dramatic and important vascular lesion that can present with unilateral facial or more commonly retro-orbital pain is that which accompanies a dissection of the ipsilateral carotid artery. The presence of a Horner's syndrome on the side of the pain is an important clue to this disorder. Angiography or an MRI angiogram may be necessary.

Finally, a brief word about that most troublesome disorder, atypical facial pain or atypical odontalgia. It is, in my experience, a term that is too readily applied to any pain in the face of unknown cause. Professor Neil Raskin, an authority on head and face pain, makes the important point that it should be called *facial pain of unknown cause.* I agree with this, because it is not safe to dismiss it as an idiopathic facial pain and to blame it on stress or depression until a thorough evaluation has been carried out and time has elapsed to see if the cause becomes apparent. Despite this exhortation to keep an open mind, if *typical* atypical facial pain exists, it is generally described as a deep, boring, poorly localized facial pain that may be felt unilaterally, usually in the maxillary region, but often becomes bilateral. There are no trigger mechanisms, and the features of the pain do not conform to those specific facial pain syndromes described above. The condition is most commonly diagnosed in women of middle age or older, many of whom are depressed, but there is no certainty that depression is the cause. It may well be the effect of the unresolved pain. Treatment is difficult.

Our dental and oral surgery colleagues see a similar facial pain to which they apply the term *atypical odontalgia.* It is one of the forms of facial pain that is not understood, although some authorities believe that microabscess cavities in the maxilla or lower jaw are responsible. This has not been my experience or that of my dental and oral surgery colleagues.

Facial pain due to migraine, the so-called lower half headache, the pain of cluster headache, and the pain of chronic paroxysmal hemicrania should be identifiable on the basis of the history of the attacks and the associated autonomic features. Nevertheless, imaging studies should be obtained because there are reports of each of these pains occurring as a result of some structural lesion, even though in the vast majority of cases no such abnormality can be demonstrated.

Facial pain due to herpes zoster of the fifth nerve is easily diagnosed once the rash is present but may initially be a cause for confusion. Once the dermatologic manifestations have subsided, some subjects, especially the elderly, develop postherpetic neuralgia, a condition that is extremely difficult to treat but one that is easily diagnosed if the history of the skin eruption is obtained or if the postherpetic scarring is observed.

COMMENTS

In summary, when dealing with facial pain obtain a full history, perform a thorough examination, do not hesitate to ask your colleagues for help to do those parts of the evaluation you are not trained to do, obtain the appropriate imaging and other tests, keep an open mind when the diagnosis is not apparent, and be prepared to use the test of time: the cause may become clear.

SUGGESTED READING

Bongers KM, Willigers HMM, Koehler PJ. Referred facial pain from lung carcinoma. Neurology 1992; 42:1841–1842.

Campbell JK. Facial pain due to migraine and cluster headache. Semin Neurol 1988; 8:255–347.

Campbell JK, Caselli RJ. Headache and other craniofacial pain. In: Bradley WG, Daroff RB, Fenichel GM, Marsden CD, eds. Neurology in clinical practice. Boston: Butterworth-Heinemann, 1989.

Headache Classification Committee of the International Headache Society. Classification and diagnostic criteria for headache disorders, cranial neuralgias, and facial pain. Cephalalgia 1988; 8(suppl 7):9–96.

Rovit RL, Murali R, Jannetta PJ. Trigeminal neuralgia. Baltimore: Williams & Wilkins, 1990.

Solomon S, Lipton RB. Facial pain. In: Mathew NT, ed. Neurologic clinics. Philadelphia: WB Saunders 1990: 8:913.

NECK AND LOW BACK PAIN

RICHARD L. STRUB, M.D.

Pain in the low back and neck is a very common symptom, most often merely a nuisance or minor inconvenience. The pain itself, however, can be disabling or can represent the initial symptom of a serious spinal or systemic disease.

The majority of patients seen in the office or emergency room with neck or low back pain have symptoms either as a result of an injury or from chronic degeneration of the supporting tissues of the spine (intervertebral disks, muscles, ligaments, and facet joints). Pain may be the only symptom, or it may occur in association with other neurologic symptoms and signs, the latter situation being far more important. The pain from disks and facets is not always midline or directly paraspinous. For example, in the lumbar area it is often referred to the medial or lateral hip region and at times can radiate to the anterior thigh. The neurologic involvement in the lumbar spine usually involves the lumbosacral nerve roots, but rare disease in the upper lumbar spine (L1 or L2) can cause damage to the conus medullaris. In the cervical spine both the cervical nerve roots and the spinal cord can be involved.

The other major group of back pain patients usually has a more serious underlying cause for back pain: infection in the vertebrae, epidural space, subarachnoid space, or disks; metastatic cancer; multiple myeloma; vertebral collapse; arthritis (ankylosing spondylitis); or diseases of abdomen, pelvis, or thorax that refer pain to the spine. Pain from these conditions tends to be constant, progressive, and not relieved by positional change, unlike mechanical strain or degenerative diseases where pain is intermittent and relieved by postural change, especially after lying down.

The clinical history and examination, both physical and radiologic, that are necessary to diagnose the myriad conditions presenting with back pain are outlined and discussed here. Because the general clinical approach and cause of pain are quite similar in the cervical and lumbar areas, both are discussed together. It is suggested that the reader review the anatomy of the spine in conjunction with the clinical information in this chapter.

The differential diagnosis of spinal disease is included in the history and examination sections as well as in tabular form in the last section. In this way the relevance of each historical fact, symptom, and sign can be fully appreciated during the data-gathering process.

HISTORY

There are three aspects of the history of neck or back pain that establish a framework for the diagnosis. The first is the history of antecedent trauma. Many patients experience their initial, and subsequent, episodes of pain as a result of trauma. The type of trauma varies, from the all too common flexion/extension injuries associated with motor vehicle accidents, to trauma associated with lifting, rising too quickly, turning rapidly, straining such as when coughing, or bending over with legs straight. If a definite history of trauma is present and the symptoms commenced suddenly or shortly thereafter, the clinician can be reasonably certain that the trauma is the cause of the pain and can concentrate the clinical approach on the neurologic examination. In unusual cases, the pathophysiology of post-traumatic back pain may be complex; for example, where the trauma has caused collapse of a vertebra that is osteoporotic or involved with metastatic disease. This possibility must be considered in the elderly patient or those with known primary cancer.

The second important bit of historical information is the time course of the symptoms and their relation to body position and movement. Sudden pain is usually seen with trauma but can arise spontaneously from such rare causes as the rupture of an arteriovenous malformation of the spinal cord, or an extramedullary cord tumor that causes a block of spinal fluid flow. Pain that is chronic and intermittent over many months or, more commonly, years is almost always secondary to degenerative or chronic musculotendinous disease, with or without disk involvement. If the patient is over 40 years old, it is likely that the pain and neurologic problems arise at least in part from degenerative disk disease and facet arthropathy. In patients whose pain emanates primarily from injury or degeneration in the spine's support tissues, there is usually a history of pain fluctuating with movement and change in position. Pain is usually lessened by lying on the side but not the stomach, worsened by sitting, getting up, or twisting, and often relieved somewhat by walking. With an acutely herniated disk the patient will usually report that coughing and sneezing reproduce the pain quite dramatically.

The most worrisome time course for neck and back pain is slowly progressive and unrelenting. This suggests a serious pathologic process such as tumor or infection as the cause. In such cases the pain is constant but may be exacerbated by a rapid change in position. Constant pain can also be referred from an intra-abdominal, pelvic, or thoracic lesion, so history-taking in the patient with constant pain must be expanded to include the possibilities of systemic infection, cancer, multiple myeloma (in males over 40), ulcer, inflammatory bowel disease, pelvic disease including pregnancy, and urinary tract problems. Pain may also be accompanied by other neurologic symptoms in these conditions, when neural tissue is affected by the primary pathologic process.

There are two special situations in which position-related pain can be diagnostic. When pain is only present while lying in bed, it may be due to an extramedullary tumor that blocks venous or spinal fluid flow. When lumbar pain is present primarily when standing or walking, the symptom suggests spinal instability with subluxation.

A third situation in which symptoms vary with activity is lumbar stenosis. In this condition there is extensive degenerative disease in the lumbar spine such that the neural foramina are all narrowed. As the patient walks, the lumbar nerve roots rub against the spurs and degenerated calcified disk margins, producing progressive paresthesias and weakness.

The third and by far the most important aspect of the history of spinal pain is the assessment of neurologic involvement. In the neck one must be concerned with both spinal cord and cervical root involvement. Root symptoms (Table 1) include focal atrophy and weakness, localized paresthesias, and radiating pain. Some patients report that the radicular symptoms can be provoked by tilting the head to the side of the lesion, strong evidence that a nerve root is pinched by extruded disk material or spurs. Spinal cord symptoms include gait problems from

Table 1 Neurologic Signs and Symptoms with Irritation or Damage to Specific Nerve Root

Root	Disk	Pain	Sensory Changes	Motor Signs	Reflex Changes
C5	C4–5	Lateral neck, shoulder, and upper arm	Over deltoid	Deltoid and external rotators of arm	None or partial decrease in biceps
C6	C5–6	Arm to thumb	Thumb (palmar surface) and index finger	Biceps and brachioradialis (weak arm flexion); finger and wrist extension	Biceps
C7	C6–7	Lateral arm to middle finger	Middle finger	Triceps (arm extension); finger and wrist flexors	Triceps
C8	C7–T1	Lateral arm to little finger	Little finger	Intrinsic hand muscles	None
L4	L3–4	Anterior thigh	Anteromedial thigh and knee	Quadriceps	Patellar (knee jerk)
L5	L4–5	Lateral thigh, anterior leg, dorsum of foot, and great toe	Anterior (dorsum) foot, particularly web between great and 2nd toe	Weak dorsiflexion of great toe	None
S1	L5–S1	Posterior thigh and leg, leg to heel, lateral foot, and 4th and 5th toes	Lateral foot and 4th and 5th toes	Weak plantar flexion of foot	Achilles (ankle jerk)

bilateral leg spasticity, sensory symptoms in trunk and legs, clumsy hand coordination, or a *change* in bowel, bladder, and sexual function, primarily in males. It is not sufficient to ask if the patient is constipated. The history of a recent *change* is the critical fact when spinal cord involvement is suspected. With spinal cord lesions, the sensory symptoms can fluctuate considerably. At times the sensory symptoms can ascend and descend in several hours' time. In other cases a distinct sensory level is observed by the patient. For example, the patient may notice a change in the ability to feel hot water below a given level when in the bathtub. The spinal cord lesions that must be considered in back pain patients are (1) spinal stenosis with cord impingement from degenerative disk and articulatory facet hypertrophy and (2) extramedullary lesions, primarily tumor. Intramedullary lesions such as primary spinal cord tumors cause spinal cord symptoms but *rarely* cause neck pain.

In lumbar disease, bowel and bladder function can sometimes be affected. This can occur either from a high lumbar lesion that affects the conus medullaris or from lesions involving the cauda equina.

Progressive, severe pain that is both in the low back and radiates into one or both legs suggests involvement of multiple spinal roots. This is seen in spinal stenosis, carcinomatous meningitis, arachnoiditis, carcinomatous invasion of the pelvis and lumbosacral plexus (in this case usually unilateral), and lumbosacral plexitis (again usually unilateral). Constant neck, shoulder, and upper arm pain is also seen in inflammation (brachial plexitis) and tumor invasion of the brachial plexus.

It must not be forgotten that neck pain can also be a sign of infectious meningitis. This possibility must always be considered in patients who are immunosuppressed either from acquired immunodeficiency syndrome or from specific immunosuppressive medications, including prednisone.

EXAMINATION

A systematic examination (Table 2) starts with an inspection of the spine. First note muscle spasm and curvature. Muscle spasm due to underlying tissue injury or inflammation produces a scoliosis toward the side of the pathology. With bilateral mechanical injury there is loss of the normal lumbar or cervical lordosis. Loss of the gluteal fold unilaterally indicates an S1 nerve root lesion, usually secondary to root damage from a herniated

Table 2 Examination Outline

1. Inspection and palpation
2. Range of motion
3. Gait
4. Strength
5. Reflexes
6. Sensory examination
7. Straight-leg raising and hip examination
8. Abdominal, pelvic, and rectal examinations, if indicated

nuclear pulposis. A sharply angulated flexion of the lumbar or thoracic spine (gibbus deformity) indicates an anterior collapse of one or more vertebrae from trauma, osteoporosis, or metastatic or inflammatory disease. Mid-line dimples or hair patches should also be noted. These signal the possible presence of a spinal dysraphism. The muscles should also be inspected for atrophy and fasciculations. Diffuse fasciculation suggests motor neuron disease (amyotrophic lateral sclerosis), a condition that can present with pain in the paraspinous muscles. Focal fasciculations may be present in a denervated muscle, as is seen in radiculopathy from acute or chronic disk disease.

Palpation of the spine is also very useful. Palpation of paraspinous muscles will verify the impression of spasm. If a patient has an infection of the vertebra, disk (diskitis—usually postoperative or post–lumbar puncture), or epidural space (epidural abscess), the vertebrae are often exquisitely sensitive. Metastatic disease of the spine also produces tenderness. Palpate the spinous processes carefully and do not percuss with the reflex hammer unless hand palpation is negative. In suspected S1 nerve root damage, palpation of the sciatic notch may verify the sensitivity of the sciatic nerve at that level.

The second step in the examination is the assessment of range of motion of both neck and lumbar region. Pain and a rotational impairment are usually more pronounced toward the side of the pathology.

Thirdly, watch the patient walk. In spinal cord lesions the patient's gait may be spastic and stiff-legged, with a tendency to circumduction and scissoring. The patient with pain tends to move the spine little when walking, and pain often limits full gait evaluation. Patients with an L5 or S1 radiculopathy tend to walk on their toes on the side of the lesion to avoid stretching the root (Neri's sign). Having the patient walk first on the toes, then the heels is very important. Toe-walking requires maximum calf strength and assesses S1 nerve root integrity. Trying to assess gastrocnemius strength by having the patient push against the examiner's hand is far less likely to pick up subtle weakness than toe-walking. Heel-walking with feet dorsiflexed tests anterior tibial muscle (L4 and L5) strength and is an excellent way to identify both subtle and significant weakness. In patients with spinal stenosis there is often bilateral, at times asymmetric, L5 and S1 radiculopathy such that the patient can neither toe- nor heel-walk. After gait testing and with the patient still standing, test individual muscles of the upper extremity for signs of focal weakness. Focal weakness indicates focal denervation, which in turn usually points to radiculopathy (see Table 1).

With the patient seated, test the strength of the proximal leg muscles. Distal muscles are more easily tested with toe- and heel-walking. In the sitting position, test the muscle stretch reflexes (deep tendon reflexes). If there is root impingement from (1) an acutely herniated disk (nucleus pulposis), (2) an extramedullary tumor, or (3) a degenerative disk with facet spurring, the reflex at that level will be reduced or absent (see Table 1). In a degenerative process (cervical spondylosis or lumbar stenosis), multiple roots may be involved and more than one reflex affected. In cervical spondylosis or an acute cervical disk lesion (Fig. 1), the cervical radiculopathy may be associated with spinal cord findings, such as Babinski's signs and hyperreflexia in the lower extremities with ankle clonus.

With the patient still seated, test the sensory system. The goal of the sensory examination is to localize any neurologic impairment (Table 3).

The final aspect of the neurologic examination is the straight-leg raising test. With the patient supine, raise the leg straight up by the heel. If the patient has an acutely herniated disk with entrapment of the S1 nerve root, significant radiating pain can be elicited at angles of as little as 25 degrees. On occasion, pain will be elicited in the leg opposite to the one being raised. This is strongly suggestive of an acutely ruptured disk. The straight-leg raising test (Lasègue's sign) is more likely to be abnormal and diagnostic in younger patients (less than 40 years).

Table 3 Sensory Examination

1. Establish a sensory level with a pin—this identifies the level of spinal cord involvement. If a level is established, see if there is an asymmetry. A decrease in sensation on one side suggests an asymmetric spinal cord lesion (Brown-Séquard).

2. Search for isolated dermatomal sensory loss—this indicates a nerve root lesion secondary to isolated disk or multiple level degenerative disease.

3. Proprioceptive testing in hands—abnormalities suggest a posteriorly placed lesion such as a foramen magnum meningioma.

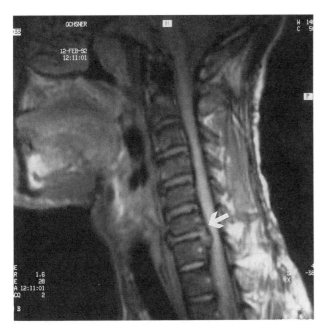

Figure 1 Sagittal cervical magnetic resonance imaging scan of herniated disk (*arrow*).

With the patient supine, hip pathology can also be evaluated by having the patient flex the leg (this removes the stretch from the sciatic nerve), then externally rotate the hip. This maneuver will not be painful with root disease but can be in primary hip disease (Patrick's sign).

In patients with constant pain who have not had trauma, additional physical examinations are necessary. If the pain, for example, is in the low back and buttocks, a rectal and pelvic examination is needed to rule out tumor or abscess. With flank, thigh, and mid-lumbar pain, the lower abdomen as well as the rectum should be examined.

LABORATORY EVALUATION

The basic studies used to evaluate spine disease are the electromyogram (EMG) to verify nerve root disease;

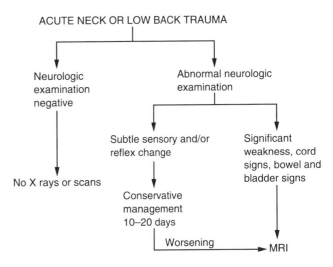

Figure 2 Imaging algorithm for the patient with acute neck or low back trauma. MRI = magnetic resonance imaging.

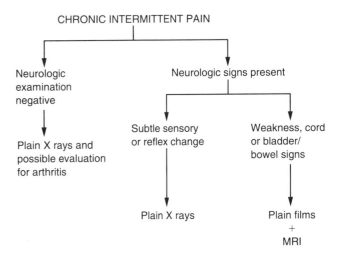

Figure 3 Imaging algorithm for the patient with chronic intermittent back or neck pain.

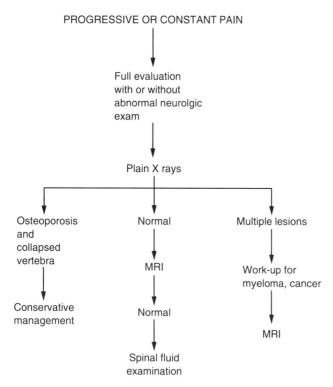

PROGRESSIVE OR CONSTANT PAIN

Full evaluation
with or without
abnormal neurolgic
exam

Plain X rays

Osteoporosis and collapsed vertebra → Conservative management

Normal → MRI → Normal → Spinal fluid examination

Multiple lesions → Work-up for myeloma, cancer → MRI

Figure 4 Imaging algorithm for the patient with progressive or constant back or neck pain. MRI = magnetic resonance imaging.

plain X rays to evaluate for congenital abnormalities and bone density, disk degeneration, spur formation, metastatic or infectious disease, and spinal instability; magnetic resonance imaging (MRI) for spinal cord tumor, disk (see Fig. 1), abscess, syrinx, and other soft tissue changes; and myelography with computed tomography (CT) in cases where disease is strongly suspected and MRI inconclusive. Cerebrospinal fluid analysis should be performed if carcinomatous or infectious meningitis is suspected. See Figures 2, 3, and 4 for a basic approach to diagnosis. Plain films of the neck and lumbar region should include anterior-posterior, lateral, and oblique views.

BASIC SYNDROMES

The following sections outline the typical clinical and laboratory presentation of the major neck and back syndromes frequently encountered by neurologists.

Simple musculotendinous neck or back pain:

1. Acute onset
2. Muscle spasm and stiffness
3. Pain with sitting and movement but relief lying down, particularly on one side
4. Negative neurologic exam
5. No imaging studies necessary

Acute disk rupture:

1. History of trauma or minor twist or bend of spine
2. Radiating pain
3. Muscle spasm and stiffness
4. Focal neurologic symptoms and signs
5. Positive straight-leg raising
6. Evaluate with X ray and MRI

Chronic degenerative spine disease:
   A. Cervical spondylosis with or without myelopathy
      1. Pain with neck rotation
      2. Root signs and symptoms—may be bilateral or multiple
      3. Possible spinal cord findings
      4. Plain X ray in all patients; MRI and EMG if the neurologic examination is abnormal or neurologic symptoms are present
   B. Lumbar spinal stenosis
      1. Low back pain
      2. Paresthesias and weakness when walking (lumbar claudication)
      3. Multiple lumbosacral root signs
      4. X ray, EMG, and MRI
   C. Spine instability
      1. Pain upon standing and walking
      2. May or may not have abnormal neurologic findings
      3. Plain X rays *very* important
         (a) Supine cross-table lateral. This shows spinal alignment in the relaxed position.
         (b) Standing (weight-bearing) flexion and extension lateral views. This demonstrates motion (subluxation), which can stretch soft tissues and compromise nerve roots.
      4. MRI or CT with or without myelography may be necessary to fully assess the degree of degenerative change and neural compromise.
   D. Chronic progressive pain
      1. History may suggest systemic disease (e.g., cancer of breast, lung, prostate, kidney, thyroid, or stomach, or multiple myeloma; rheumatoid arthritis; immunosuppression; sepsis; tuberculosis).
      2. General physical includes abdominal, rectal, and pelvic examination.
      3. Vertebrae may be tender.
      4. Neurologic examination may show spinal cord involvement.
      5. Medical tests may include sedimentation rate, immunoelectrophoresis, and rheumatoid factor, depending upon the case.
      6. Plain spine films.
      7. MRI, CT, radioisotope bone scan.
      8. Other consultations and evaluation that may be indicated in the individual patient.
   E. Miscellaneous causes of back pain
      1. Facet syndrome—localized unilateral paraspinous pain
      2. Pyriformis muscle syndrome—pain with abduction of hip

3. Abdominal or thoracic aortic aneurysm
4. Aortic dissection
5. Aortic occlusion
6. Spondylolisthesis
7. Post-polio syndrome

SUGGESTED READING

Adams RD, Victor M. Pain in the back, neck and extremities. In: Principles of neurology. 4th ed. New York: McGraw-Hill, 1989:155.

Cervical Spine Research Society. The cervical spine. Philadelphia: JB Lippincott, 1989.
Finneson BE. Low back pain. 2nd ed. Philadelphia: JB Lippincott, 1981.
Macnab I, McCulloh JA. Backache. 2nd ed. Baltimore: Williams & Wilkins, 1989.

SPORTS INJURIES

BARRY D. JORDAN, M.D.

Until recently, sports neurology has been an unrecognized clinical subspecialty among neurologists and sports medicine physicians. Neurologic injuries in sports are infrequent, but these injuries may be associated with significant morbidity and mortality that introduces a tremendous economic and emotional burden on the athlete's family and society. Accordingly, it is necessary for the non-neurologist involved with sports medicine to be knowledgeable about the diagnosis, management, and treatment of neurologic injuries and disorders that may be encountered in the recreational and competitive athlete. Furthermore, neurologists acquainted with the pathophysiology of nervous system injuries and disorders should become involved in exploring how sporting activities cause neurologic disease. This chapter highlights the more important and controversial clinical syndromes encountered in sports neurology.

ACUTE BRAIN INJURY

Acute brain injury can occur in almost any sport. However, there are certain sports, in particular contact and collision sports, that have an increased risk of brain injury (Table 1). Cerebral concussion represents the most common type of acute brain injury in sports. Diffuse axonal injury and focal intracranial hematomas are rare but represent a major percentage of catastrophic injuries in sports and are associated with significant morbidity and mortality.

The major concern with acute brain injury in sports is the proper evaluation of the concussed athlete and subsequent determination of when it is appropriate to return to competition. This concern is typically encountered in boxing, football, ice hockey, and the martial arts. In addition to the Glasgow Coma Scale, there are two

Table 1 High-Risk Sports for Head Injury

Boxing	Auto racing
Football	Equestrian sports
Ice hockey	Motorcycle racing
Martial arts	Sports diving
Rugby	Bicycling
Wrestling	Snow skiing
Soccer	

Table 2 Cantu Grading System for Concussion in Sports

Grade	Criteria for Return to Play
1. *Mild:* No loss of consciousness; post-traumatic amnesia less than 30 minutes	May return to play if asymptomatic for 1 week.
2. *Moderate:* Loss of consciousness less than 5 minutes in duration or post-traumatic amnesia lasting longer than 30 minutes but less than 24 hours in duration	May return to play if asymptomatic for 1 week.
3. *Severe:* Loss of consciousness for more than 5 minutes or post-traumatic amnesia for more than 24 hours	Should not be allowed to play for at least one month. May then return to play if asymptomatic for 1 week.

frequently utilized evaluation or grading scales of acute head injury in sports (Tables 2 and 3). An athlete with transient loss of consciousness for 1 minute would be a moderate injury on the Cantu scale (see Table 2) and a severe injury on the scale of the Colorado Medical Society (CMS) (see Table 3). An athlete experiencing post-traumatic amnesia for 8 hours, without loss of consciousness, would be considered a moderate injury on both scales.

Careful scrutiny of these scales reveals obvious discrepancies in the classification of head injury. The CMS grading system is more appropriate in grading the milder forms of head trauma (without loss of consciousness), whereas the Cantu scale is more appropriate in grading more severe head trauma (with loss of consciousness). A more comprehensive scale should encom-

Table 3 Colorado Medical Society (CMS) Grading System for Concussion in Sports

Grade	Criteria for Return to Play
1. *Mild:* Confusion without amnesia; no loss of consciousness	May return to play if asymptomatic at rest and exertion after at least 20 minutes observation.
2. *Moderate:* Confusion with amnesia; no loss of consciousness	May return to play if asymptomatic for 1 week.
3. *Severe:* Loss of consciousness	Should not be allowed to play for at least 1 month. May then return to play if asymptomatic for 2 weeks.

Table 4 Proposed Grading System for Concussion in Sports

Grade	Criteria for Return to Play
1. *Mild:* Confusion without amnesia; no loss of consciousness	May return to play if asymptomatic at rest and exertion after at least 20 minutes of observation.
2. *Mild-Moderate:* Confusion with amnesia lasting less than 24 hours; no loss of consciousness	May return to play if asymptomatic for 1 week.
3. *Moderate-Severe:* Loss of consciousness with an altered level of consciousness not exceeding 2–3 minutes; post-traumatic amnesia lasting more than 24 hours	Should not be allowed to play for at least 1 month. May then return to play if asymptomatic for 1 week.
4. *Severe:* Loss of consciousness with an altered level of consciousness exceeding 2–3 minutes	Should not be allowed to play for at least 1 month. May then return to play if asymptomatic for 2 weeks.

pass the best qualities of both scales. This scale should distinguish a concussion without amnesia from a concussion with confusion and amnesia, as in the CMS grading scale. All athletes with loss of consciousness should not be included together. There are athletes who experience transient episodes of altered consciousness and who then respond quickly within a few minutes. On the other hand, there are individuals with transient loss of consciousness who do not return to a normal level of consciousness within a short period of time (2 to 3 minutes). The latter group should be transported to the hospital for evaluation, whereas the former may be observed at the place of competition, provided they are neurologically asymptomatic and exhibit a normal neurologic examination.

In view of the limitations of the Cantu and CMS grading systems, a new grading system is proposed that categorizes head injuries in sports into four grades: mild, mild-moderate, moderate-severe, and severe (Table 4).

Despite the potential disparities in the grading of head injuries, there are certain universal principles in the management of head trauma. First, any athlete in a contact or collision sport who experiences a concussion should be removed from competition and should not return to play until he or she is asymptomatic. The determination of return to play obviously depends on the severity of the head injury. An athlete with loss of consciousness or amnesia should not return to play that day. Any athlete who does not recover from a concussion within a few minutes should be sent for neurologic evaluation.

Returning a symptomatic athlete to competition may predispose the athlete to the second impact syndrome. This syndrome has been described primarily among football players. These individuals typically experience symptoms consistent with the postconcussion syndrome (headache, decreased concentration, impaired memory, and dizziness) and are allowed to return to play. While symptomatic, these individuals may encounter a second, relatively mild head injury, but they experience an exaggerated neurologic response, resulting in coma and possibly death. The mechanism of this injury is thought to be secondary to loss of vasomotor autoregulation, resulting in hyperemia and brain swelling.

CHRONIC BRAIN INJURY

Chronic brain injury (CBI) in sports represents the long-term cumulative effect of multiple concussive and subconcussive blows to the head. This condition has been described, mostly among retired boxers, as the "punch-drunk syndrome," "dementia pugilistica," or chronic traumatic encephalopathy. However, a milder form has been described among soccer players who "head" the soccer ball with a high frequency. Theoretically this clinical syndrome can also be anticipated in American football.

Approximately 20 percent of retired professional boxers exhibit CBI. They tend to be less skilled boxers who have poor defensive skills and are notorious for their ability to take a punch. However, more highly skilled scientific boxers can also develop this syndrome with long exposure to boxing. Documented risk factors for CBI in boxing include later retirement (over 28 years of age), increased duration of career (more than 10 years), and a greater number of bouts (more than 150 fights). Boxers afflicted with the advanced form of CBI may experience personality changes or impaired intellectual function, ranging from slow mentation or forgetfulness to severe dementia. Motor disturbances may include cerebellar dysfunction, extrapyramidal disorder of the Parkinson type, slurred speech, and ataxia. Pathologically, these boxers exhibit varying combinations of brain atrophy, cavum septum pellucidum, degeneration of the substantia nigra, and Purkinje cell reduction in the cerebellum. Pathologically, CBI associated with boxing also resembles Alzheimer's disease by the presence of neurofibrillary tangles, beta-amyloid protein deposition in diffuse plaques, ubiquiten immunoreactivity in neurofibrillary tangles, and reduced choline acetyltransferase activity in the nucleus basilis of Meynert.

Milder or subclinical CBI may be encountered in active amateur and professional boxers. Clinically these boxers may exhibit mild difficulties with memory, concentration, and attention identifiable by neuropsychological testing. However, applying standardized neuropsychological test norms to the boxing population is plagued with socioeconomic and educational bias. Neuroimaging techniques such as computed tomography (CT) or magnetic resonance imaging (MRI) may demonstrate brain atrophy or progressive changes indicative of the cumulative effect of head trauma.

Soccer players have been observed to exhibit abnormalities on CT, electroencephalography (EEG), and neuropsychological testing similar to those encountered among boxers. On CT scanning, approximately one-third of retired soccer players demonstrated brain atrophy. It has been postulated that repetitive "heading" of the soccer ball may be responsible for this finding. Also of note, cavum septum pellucidi were noted in 6 percent of retired soccer players. It has also been demonstrated that soccer players display a higher frequency of EEG disturbances than the normal population, and that 80 percent of soccer players experience mild to severe neuropsychological impairment involving attention, concentration, memory, and judgment.

Although infrequently reported in the clinical literature, CBI probably occurs in American football. The retirement of Al Toon, a wide receiver on the New York Jets of the National Football League, during the 1992 season, is indicative of this problem. According to news reports, he retired from professional football after sustaining his ninth cerebral concussion. Apparently, each successive concussion was associated with longer periods of postconcussive symptoms. The prevalence and magnitude of CBI among football players remains to be determined.

CERVICAL SPINE INJURIES

A variety of cervical spine injuries can be encountered in sports (Table 5). Certain sports, such as diving, football, trampoline, and equestrian sports, entail the potential risk of cervical spine injury. Diving injuries are usually associated with the participants diving head first into shallow water. Cervical spine injuries associated with the trampoline and horseback riding are usually associated with falls. In football, fractures of the cervical spine may occur secondary to axial loading on a flexed cervical spine. Flexion of the cervical spine reduces the cervical lordosis and results in a straightening of the cervical spine, which predisposes it to the effects of axial loading. Football players with loss of the cervical lordosis and narrowing of the cervical spinal canal may be at increased risk of catastrophic cervical spine injuries.

The evaluation and management of the athlete who

Table 5 Cervical Spine Injuries in Sports

Stable cervical sprain
Muscle strain
Nerve root/brachial plexus injury
Intervertebral disk injury
Vertebral subluxation without fracture
Fracture and dislocation
Spinal cord neurapraxia

experiences transient neurologic symptoms attributable to the cervical spinal cord, cervical nerve roots, or brachial plexus require careful consideration. It is essential that the team physician involved with football be able to distinguish the usually benign "stingers" or "burners" (stretch injuries to the brachial plexus or cervical nerve roots) from the more ominous transient neurapraxia of the cervical spinal cord. The characteristic clinical presentation of neurapraxia of the cervical spinal cord is transient paresthesias of all four extremities, with or without transient quadriparesis. Typically these symptoms last approximately 10 to 15 minutes and resolve completely. Incomplete resolution of symptoms by 24 to 48 hours suggests more serious injury to the cervical spine. Any football player who experiences this transient neurapraxia of the cervical spinal cord should be removed from play and treated as a cervical spine fracture until plain radiographs fail to demonstrate a fracture or cervical instability. Once it has been established that the athlete has a stable cervical spine, without fracture, an MRI scan of the cervical spine should be obtained. This imaging technique will identify those athletes with structural lesions, such as disk herniation or osteophyte formation, that significantly encroach upon and narrow the cervical spinal canal, causing a developmental spinal stenosis.

Controversy exists as to whether athletes with a normal MRI or mild spinal stenosis with a normal neurologic examination should be allowed to return to play after an episode of transient quadriparesis. Obviously the decision is difficult, and each case should be interpreted individually. Although it is not clear whether transient quadriparesis predisposes to catastrophic cervical spine injury, it is probably justifiable to exercise caution and prohibit continued participation in football, especially in those athletes who have experienced multiple injuries.

SUGGESTED READING

Cantu RC. Guidelines for return to contact sports after a cerebral concussion. Physician & Sportsmed 1986; 14(10):75–83.

Jordan BD. Medical aspects of boxing. Boca Raton, Fl: CRC Press, 1993.

Jordan BD, Jahre C, Hauser WA, et al. CT of 338 active professional boxers. Radiology 1992; 185:509–512.

Jordan BD, Jahre C, Hauser WA, et al. Serial computed tomography in professional boxers. J Neuroimag 1992; 2:181–185.

Jordan BD, Tsairis P, Warren RF. Sports neurology. Rockville, Md: Aspen Publishers, 1989.

Jordan BD, Warren RF, Tsairis P, et al. How to evaluate transient quadriparesis. Physician & Sportsmed 1992; 20(2):83–90.

Kelly JP, Nichols JS, Filley CM, et al. Concussion in sports: Guidelines for prevention of catastrophic outcome. JAMA 1991; 266: 2867–2869.

Saunders RL, Harbough RE. The second impact in catastrophic contact sports head trauma. JAMA 1984; 252:538–539.

Sortland O, Tysvaer AT. Brain damage in former association football players: An evaluation by cerebral computed tomography. Neuroradiology 1989; 31:44–48.

Torg JS. Athletic injuries to the head, neck, and face. St Louis: Mosby, 1991.

MYOFASCIAL PAIN SYNDROME

ROBERT D. GERWIN, M.D.

Myofascial pain is pain of muscle origin. Described and characterized by Dr. Janet G. Travell over the past 50 years, the syndrome of myofascial pain is both a common cause of pain in its own right and a complication of a variety of other medical and dental problems. The determination that pain is of myofascial origin is made primarily by physical examination. Corroborative laboratory studies are available, but for most clinicians the hands-on examination remains the most practical, indeed the essential, diagnostic tool. At the heart of the myofascial pain syndrome (MPS) is the myofascial trigger point (MTrP), an exquisitely tender region of a discrete, taut band of muscle that is responsible for the symptoms of MPS.

Current research indicates that the trigger point is associated with the muscle spindle. A characteristic pattern of referred pain, initiated by stimulation of the MTrP but experienced at a distant site, exists for each muscle. Range of motion at joints moved by affected muscles is limited by the taut bands with trigger points (TrPs). Weakness without muscle atrophy occurs, and altered limb temperature and piloerection are among the sympathetic disturbances seen in association with the TrP. These features of the MTrP provide the basis for diagnosis of MPS by physical examination (Table 1).

MPS can be an acute condition, usually restricted to a regional or local group of muscles. It is frequently a chronic condition, however, of greater than 6 months duration, and may persist for years if not effectively treated. Perpetuating factors lead to the persistence of MTrPs and include mechanical stressors, such as skeletal structural variations and postural imbalances, and systemic medical disorders, such as nutritional and hormonal inadequacy states. Identification of perpetuating factors is part of the evaluation of MPS and requires a thorough history, physical examination, and appropriate laboratory tests.

HISTORY

The history focuses on the chief complaint: A description of the location of the pain, its duration, and its inception is obtained. The distribution of pain provides clues about referred pain patterns that can be explored during the physical examination. A diagram of the distribution of pain, burning or uncomfortable sensations, and numbness prepared by the patient is very useful in understanding the extent of the pain problem. Marking the physical findings of structural asymmetries, MTrPs, and sensory changes on another body diagram provides a companion picture that, when coupled with the patient's drawing, graphically illustrates the extent and distribution of MTrPs and the structural factors that may be contributory.

Home and work activities that aggravate the pain are evaluated. Occupational stresses on body mechanics affecting posture are examined by a work history and by use of photographs of the subject in the workplace. Symptoms of cold intolerance, sleep disturbance, headache, chronic fatigue, bowel dysfunction, frequent infections, or postexercise cramps can indicate underlying medical disorders. Concurrent medical problems such as sciatica, multiple sclerosis, residual effects of polio, gout, and stroke can cause MPS and lead to persistent MTrPs. The dietary history includes the extent and source of animal protein in the diet, the amount of caffeine and alcohol consumed, and the use of nutritional supplements in order to identify inadequacy states and assess nutritional needs. A smoking history is obtained since smoking increases the requirement for vitamin C. A history of drug intake includes drugs previously taken for pain, with their dosage when known, birth control pills, and recreational or illicit drugs. The effect pain has on the patient, the family, and work is assessed through a social history. This information provides the background for modifying pathologic or inappropriate coping strategies that may have developed in response to the pain.

Table 1 Diagnostic Steps in the Evaluation of Myofascial Pain Syndrome (MPS)

Evaluate for body asymmetry.
Assess range of motion.
Identify taut bands by palpation.
Identify trigger area of exquisite tenderness within taut band.
Produce local twitch response by palpation of the trigger point.
Map referred pain zones.
Assess for perpetuating factors in chronic MPS, and for coexistent conditions in both acute and chronic MPS.

PHYSICAL EXAMINATION AND LABORATORY STUDIES

The diagnosis of the MTrP is made first and foremost by manual physical examination. The diagnostic process starts when the patient is first seen walking into the examination room or sitting in a chair. Asymmetry of shoulder height may reflect a structural or functional scoliosis or a leg-length or pelvic height inequality that perpetuates MTrPs in the low back, neck, and shoulder regions. Short upper arms in relation to torso height frequently lead to a slouched sitting posture, or to leaning to one side to reach the armrest, aggravating low back or quadratus lumborum TrPs. The foot is examined for a longer second than first metatarsal bone, a variation in foot structure that produces pronation of the foot and internal rotation of the lower limb at the hip, resulting in TrPs in the peroneus longus, vastus medialis, and gluteus medius and minimis, and pain in the ankle, knee, leg, and buttocks. Rounded shoulders, forward head position, and excessive or flattened cervical or lumbar lordotic curvatures result in increased activity of antigravity muscles and can perpetuate MTrPs.

Range of motion is assessed to identify those muscles that cannot be stretched or elongated fully because of taut muscle bands. The head and neck are tested in active and passive movement in extension, flexion, lateral bending, and rotation, noting asymmetrical movements that could reflect limitations imposed by the taut band. Movement at the waist is studied in extension for the abdominal obliques, the rectus abdominis, and iliopsoas muscles, and in lateral bending and flexion for the quadratus lumborum, abdominal obliques, and erector spinae muscles. Internal and external rotation of the thigh at the hip evaluates the piriformis and the other short external rotators, the semitendinosus, semimembranosus, tensor fascia lata, and the anterior fibers of the gluteus minimis and medius. Range of motion of the shoulder joint is evaluated for external rotation by wrapping the arm behind the head and touching the opposite corner of the mouth with the fingertips. This maneuver evaluates the ability of the subscapularis muscle to lengthen. Attempting to touch the opposite scapular spine behind the back tests the ability of the infraspinatus and teres minor muscles to lengthen. Muscles that have restricted range of motion are thoroughly examined for MTrPs. Application of intermittent cold and stretch after testing range of motion is both therapeutic and diagnostic, relieving some of the discomfort caused by stretching and confirming the impression that restricted movement is caused by muscle and not joint dysfunction.

Identification of the MTrP requires knowledge of muscle surface anatomy and of muscle action. The MTrP itself is examined using gentle palpation to identify taut bands and tender points. While palpating for TrPs, the physician asks the patient if any tender or painful spot that is encountered reproduces pain that is commonly felt and if palpation of the tender point produces pain or an odd sensation that is felt elsewhere; that is, if stimulation of the tender TrP refers pain to a distant site. Involuntary withdrawal, or the "jump sign," indicates that a tender trigger area has been encountered.

The subject is made comfortable with the limbs supported. The muscle to be examined is placed in mid-position where possible, neither fully lengthened nor shortened. Palpation is performed either flat or by pincer grasp. If the muscle lies against bone, as does the infraspinatus muscle or the gluteal muscles, it may be palpated by moving the fingers across the muscle, perpendicular to the direction of the fibers, feeling for the taut band. Once the taut band is felt, it is searched for the tender trigger area. Snapping the taut band results in a local twitch response (LTR) that is confined just to the taut band and does not involve the entire muscle. An active TrP that is either spontaneously painful or that is painful on palpation usually reproduces the patient's pain problem and usually produces a characteristic pattern of pain referral, more often than not distal to the TrP. The patterns of pain referral for a particular muscle are generally reproducible day to day for each patient and are reproducible from patient to patient. It is helpful to map these patterns on a body diagram as part of the patient's record. Cervical vertigo, or loss of equilibrium caused by chronic MTrPs in the upper cervical segments or the sternocleidomastoid muscle, is evaluated by having the patient walk with the eyes closed, by tandem walking, and by the Romberg test.

The usual laboratory tests are of little diagnostic value in the identification of MPS. The hemogram, blood and urine chemistries, radiologic and magnetic resonance imaging studies, and the usual electrodiagnostic studies of nerve conduction and electromyography do not identify the TrP or the cause of myofascial pain. They are invaluable, however, in assessing associated conditions that coexist with or perpetuate MPS. A recent finding that the MTrP has a low-amplitude persistent discharge (100 to 1,000 μv) resembling an end-plate muscle fiber discharge has diagnostic implications, although it is not suitable as a routine diagnostic test. Thermography demonstrates an area of increased heat emission in the vicinity of the MTrP. Coupled with dolorimetry, which shows an area of increased sensitivity to pressure, thermography is an objective laboratory test that helps to confirm the presence of a MTrP.

Finally, a comprehensive physical examination, including tendon reflexes and sensory examination, provides necessary information about causative or concurrent medical conditions that can either initiate, aggravate, or perpetuate myofascial pain.

DIFFERENTIAL DIAGNOSIS

The differential diagnosis of MPS includes consideration of those neuromuscular conditions that resemble MPS, particularly those that produce referred or radiating pain. Hence, cervical and lumbar radiculopathies and nerve entrapment syndromes are looked for routinely. They are usually diagnosable through a combination of historical data highly suggestive of radiculopathy, such as increased pain with coughing or numbness in a limb, and such physical signs of nerve dysfunction as weakness, muscle atrophy, absent tendon reflexes, or sensory loss. Identification of MTrPs in an individual with the "failed low back syndrome" of persistent pain after lumbar laminectomy or fusion is of great importance because the postoperative pain can be of myofascial origin and not due to recurrent radiculopathy. Inflammatory disorders of muscle show a much more generalized proximal weakness and diffuse tenderness than is seen in MPS, often a skin rash and an elevated serum creatine phosphokinase. Lyme disease can cause fatigue and muscle soreness but is more apt to show specific signs of peripheral neuropathy. An elevated Lyme antibody titer aids in the diagnosis. The examiner must be mindful that MPS may coexist with any of these conditions, compounding the difficulty in diagnosis.

Fibromyalgia (FM) can be difficult to distinguish from MPS when multiple muscles in different regions of the body are affected in MPS. Both conditions can be chronic. The sleep disorders that occur in the two conditions are qualitatively different, however. Nonrestorative sleep with intrusion of alpha activity in delta sleep, though not confined to FM, is nonetheless more characteristic of FM than of MPS. Sleep disturbance in MPS is more likely to be the result of pain. When pain is controlled, sleep tends to be restorative in MPS. Chronic fatigue is very common in FM but is not necessarily seen in MPS. Symptoms such as irritable bowel syndrome, Raynaud's phenomenon, dysmenorrhea, headaches, and stiffness are associated with FM but not with MPS. The chief difference, however, is in the diffuse involvement of muscle in FM, contrasted with the focal involvement of muscle in MPS. The entire muscle is likely to be tender in FM, whereas myofascial TrPs are very discrete within the muscle. The American College of Rheumatology 1990 criteria specify 18 points that should be examined in patients suspected of having FM to ensure that the elicited tenderness is diffuse, not localized. MPS TrPs, on the other hand, are discrete, and muscle involvement is focal within any single muscle. The muscles affected in MPS can be either a few muscles within a functional muscle unit or many muscles within a region of several functionally related muscle groups. While MPS can be multifocal, affecting different areas of the body, it remains within distinct functional muscle groups. Persons with fibromyalgia can also have MTrPs superimposed on the underlying FM, thereby compounding the difficulty in separating the two conditions. However, if one keeps in mind that the MTrP is a response of muscle to injury or stress and not a systemic illness like FM, it is not difficult to understand that TrPs may be present in persons with FM.

In conclusion, MPS is characterized by discrete areas of exquisite tenderness in taut bands in specific muscles. The exquisitely tender areas refer pain to distant sites either spontaneously or when stimulated, a central feature of MPS. Palpation can also elicit a LTR. The taut bands restrict movement and can cause weakness. These physical findings are identifiable by manual examination and serve as the basis for the diagnosis of MPS.

SUGGESTED READING

Gerwin RD. The clinical assessment of myofascial pain. In: Turk DC, Melzack R, eds. Handbook of pain assessment. New York: Guilford Press, 1992: 61.

Simons DG. A myofascial pain syndrome due to trigger points. In: Goodgold J, ed. Rehabilitation medicine. St. Louis: Mosby–Year Book, 1988: 686.

Simons DG. Single muscle myofascial pain syndromes. In: Tollison CD, ed. Handbook of chronic pain management. Baltimore: Williams & Wilkins, 1989: 490.

Travell JG, Simons DG. Myofascial pain and dysfunction: The trigger point manual. Vols 1 & 2. Baltimore: Williams & Wilkins, 1983, 1992.

CAUSALGIA AND REFLEX SYMPATHETIC DYSTROPHY

ROBERT J. SCHWARTZMAN, M.D.

Reflex sympathetic dystrophy (RSD) is a syndrome that is primarily caused by peripheral tissue injury. It is characterized by severe pain, edema, autonomic dysfunction, and a particular movement disorder. In its later stages, autoimmune dysfunction, trophic changes, and severe disability supervene. The entire process evolves through three major stages. Early in its course, RSD is sympathetically maintained but with time becomes sympathetically independent. The process spreads in a characteristic pattern to involve formerly uninjured tissue. Specific injuries are more likely than others to incite the process. Thermography, triple phase bone scanning, plain film, and magnetic resonance imaging findings may support the diagnosis. In its early stages, relief by sympathetic blockade in addition to characteristic clinical findings confirms the diagnosis. Sympathetic blockade is ineffective when the illness is sympathetically independent. Patients can be cured in its early stage, but with time this becomes much more difficult. If the process is sympathetically independent, cure is rarely achieved. Patients remain in a sensitized state for a varying period of time once they have had RSD. If reinjured during this period, they are more liable to get RSD in the recently injured area.

RSD is caused by peripheral nerve, plexus, and soft tissue injury in the vast majority of cases. In those instances where central nervous system injury is noted, the central injury may cause a further peripheral nerve or plexus injury that incites the process. In soft tissue and ligament injury, the "C" fiber, A-delta, and deep muscle pain afferents are most likely responsible for initiating the process. There are no reports of RSD following sunburn or blistering skin lesions. It has been suggested that injury to those nerves that have the greatest number of sympathetic fibers is most likely to cause RSD. These include the median, sciatic, and peroneal nerves as well as the brachial plexus. If the process follows a partial peripheral nerve injury, it is usually termed *causalgia*. The process does not follow a complete nerve transection. About 50 percent of all cases follow ligamentous and soft tissue injury. Flexion-extension or neuropractic brachial plexus injuries are a very common cause of upper extremity RSD. A Colles' fracture with median nerve damage and poor carpal tunnel surgery are also common initiating factors for upper extremity RSD. About 50 percent of all patients with RSD were casted and immobilized after their initial injury. In the lower extremity, trimalleolar (plantar nerves) and fibular fracture (peroneal nerve) are frequently associated with partial neuropractic nerve injury and RSD. Unusual but not uncommon causes of RSD are thrombophlebitis, ergotrate and phenobarbital use, radiculopathy from surgery or disk disease, tumor, syrinx, stroke, and spinal cord injury.

CLINICAL PICTURE

RSD evolves insidiously through consistent stages. Stage I disease (acute) follows injury within hours to days. A few patients suffer almost instant continuous pain, while others may note the characteristic pain several days to as long as a few weeks from the time of injury. In general, the pain starts within a matter of hours after injury. In those patients with delayed pain, other manifestations of the illness, such as edema, autonomic instability, or movement abnormalities, may precede the pain.

The pain is frequently more severe than expected for the type or degree of injury. It is burning, diffuse, deep, and usually distal in the extremity even if the inciting injury is proximal. It extends beyond a nerve or dermatomal distribution and is exacerbated by movement, emotional upset, and dependent posture. It is frequently more severe on the dorsal than on the ventral aspect of the affected extremity. Characteristically, many patients suffer hyperalgesia (lowered pain threshold and enhanced perception of a painful stimulus), allodynia (pain from innocuous mechanical or thermal stimuli),

and hyperpathia (severe pain from a stimulus that reaches maximum intensity too rapidly and decays slowly).

Spontaneous exacerbations of pain are common, and the pain frequently spreads in a mirror distribution to the opposite extremity or contiguously over the ipsilateral side of the body. Although the pain is characteristically burning in nature, some patients describe it as crushing or lancinating at some point in their illness. Most patients shield the affected part from all stimuli, and some attain a measure of relief by packing it in ice or wrapping it tightly in cloth. The affected extremity is rarely moved spontaneously.

In stage I disease, the pain is sympathetically maintained in that it can be relieved by adrenergic blockade. However, there is a significant group of patients that have hyperthermic, hyperemic extremities that are not relieved by sympathetic blockade even in this early stage. In general, stage I disease (acute) lasts approximately 6 months and is associated with edema, temperature change, increased hair and nail growth, and difficulty with movement of the affected part.

Stage II disease (dystrophic) in general lasts from 6 months to 2 years and is characterized by an increase and spread of the pain that is now invariably associated with sleep disruption, anxiety, and severe depression. The edema is now indurated and brawny and the skin is hyperhidrotic and cool. Most patients demonstrate dusky cyanosis and clear livedo reticularis of the skin. X-ray of affected bones reveals the characteristic cystic and subchondral erosion of early Sudeck's atrophy. Hair loss is prominent in areas that earlier had shown exuberant dark thickened growth, and the nails become ridged, dull, and brittle.

In stage III disease, the pain spreads proximally and at times covers almost all of the body surface. There are some patients who never experience spread of their pain from the initially injured area. Hyperalgesia, allodynia, and hyperpathia dominate the clinical picture. The pain no longer responds to adrenergic blockade in any form and is now sympathetically independent. The movement disorder of RSD usually becomes a prominent part of the symptom complex in late stage III patients. It consists of difficulty in initiating movements, weakness, spasms, tremor, increased reflexes, and dystonia. In lower extremity involvement, the foot is plantar flexed and inverted while the upper extremity is held in flexion at the elbow and wrist. If the hand is involved, the fourth and fifth fingers are flexed tightly into the palm. The movement disorder is present to some degree in all patients. It is frequently ascribed to pain or hysteria. The dystonic postures persist during sleep. The skin is thin, atrophic, reddened, and shiny. There is loss of subcutaneous tissue and muscle. The fascia is thickened and contractures are prominent. Radiographs demonstrate diffuse demineralization and marked ankylosis of the small bones of the hands and feet. Approximately 40 to 50 percent of patients at this stage of illness have a positive triple phase bone scan.

There are two prominent variants of RSD, and

several clinical aspects of the syndrome that are easily identified but frequently cause a great deal of confusion. The first variant, the ABC syndrome (angry backfiring "C" nociceptors), is a manifestation of probable neuropeptide release (substance P and calcitonin gene-related peptide) from their terminal storage vesicles in "C" nociceptors. The neuropeptides produce vasodilation of the vasculature in the affected part with consequent hyperemia and hyperthermia. The patient suffers the burning pain of RSD from the orthodromic "C" fiber stimulation. The Triple Cold syndrome manifests itself as a cold extremity that when tested is hypoesthetic to cold stimuli, which the patient describes as burning and painful. It is postulated that there is concomitant damage of sympathetic fibers (with hypersensitivity of remaining alpha$_1$ adrenergic receptors on the vasculature and consequent vasoconstriction), cold A-delta fibers, and activation of "C" fibers. There may be loss of A-delta temperature modulation of "C" fiber afferents at the dorsal horn level.

Clinical aspects of RSD that give rise to diagnostic problems are the following: (1) the disease frequently spreads with time; (2) if both lower extremities are involved, the patients have difficulty urinating and are constipated; (3) if the upper extremities are involved, particularly from a brachial plexus injury, patients complain of blurred vision in the ipsilateral eye; (4) the process may be dissociated (patients may have pain in the affected extremity as well as autonomic dysfunction and movement abnormalities in nonpainful extremities); (5) the illness depresses all patients, but there is no evidence that these patients have more psychiatric illness than the general population; and (6) RSD in one part of the body apparently sensitizes some patients to the development of the process in a newly injured area. This may occur within hours.

The clinical signs and symptoms of each stage of RSD overlap and evolve insidiously. A clear breakpoint in the illness occurs when those patients formerly sympathetically maintained (as regards pain) become sympathetically independent (no longer respond to sympathetic blocks). At this point, cure is extremely difficult.

DIAGNOSIS

The diagnosis of RSD is primarily clinical. However, it may be supported by a response to sympathetic blockade, thermography, triple phase bone scanning, and laser Doppler fluxmetry. The major pitfalls in interpretation of sympathetic blockade are the placebo response (in up to 30 percent of patients) and the interpretation of what constitutes a positive response. Many patients feel that a block has failed if the pain relief is only transient (less than 3 hours). If the pain is significantly relieved for any length of time, it is sympathetically maintained, and that is strong evidence for RSD. A series of blocks (at least three) with adequate temperature rise (at least 3°) of the affected part is necessary to be certain that the pain block was effective. Several groups employ the intravenous phentolamine test, which blocks adrenergic receptors systemically, as their screening test for sympathetically maintained pain. The advantage of this technique is its ease of delivery and placebo control, because the patient does not know whether saline or drug has been administered through the intravenous catheter. Those who respond to intravenous phentolamine will not require sympathetic blocks. A few patients will respond to prolonged epidural block for 3 to 5 days when they have failed direct paravertebral sympathetic blocks. It must always be remembered that in stage II and III disease RSD may no longer be sympathetically maintained but have progressed to sympathetically independent pain.

Very small fibers, 1 micron in size, cannot be studied by standard electromyogram techniques. Unfortunately, "C" fibers and sympathetic fibers are in this size range and must be evaluated by functional methods in RSD patients. Thermography is an excellent tool for this type of evaluation and demonstrates temperature change not in a single dermatomal (usually two or more) or strictly nerve distribution in RSD patients. It may also demonstrate temperature change in the uninvolved extremity because the process frequently spreads to the contralateral side.

Dynamic vascular scanning utilizing ^{99m}Tc human serum albumin (HSA) has been used to stage and monitor therapy in patients with RSD. It demonstrates abnormal pooling of isotope in the involved area approximately 50 percent of the time.

Skeletal radiographs demonstrate subchondral and periarticular bone resorption in a majority of patients with late stage disease.

RSD may be the human counterpart of neurogenic inflammation. Recent studies suggest that painful stimuli initiate a cascade of chemical events in the central pain projecting neurons of the spinal cord that changes their response to further incoming signals. Exciting new pharmacologic strategies are being developed to block this excitotoxic barrage and desensitize the spinal cord.

SUGGESTED READING

Beacham WS, Perl ER. Characteristics of a spinal sympathetic reflex. J Physiol (Lond) 1964; 173:431–448.

Bennett GJ. Development and plasticity in the superficial dorsal horn. In: Cervero G, Bennett GJ, Headley PM, eds. Processing of sensory information in the superficial dorsal horn of the spinal cord. New York: Plenum Publishing, 1989.

Bennett GJ. The role of sympathetic nervous system in painful peripheral neuropathy. Pain 1991; 45:221–223.

Blumberg H. Development and treatment of the pain syndrome of reflex sympathetic dystrophy: Clinical picture, experimental investigation, and neuropathophysiological consideration. Der Schmerz 1988; 125–143.

Blumberg H, Griesser HJ, Hornyak ME. Mechanisms and role of peripheral blood flow dysregulation in pain sensation and edema in reflex sympathetic dystrophy. In: Stanton-Hicks M, Janig W, Boas RA, eds. Reflex sympathetic dystrophy: Current management of pain. Germany: Kluwer, 1990: 81.

Brain SD, Williams TJ. Inflammatory edema induced by synergism between calcitonin gene-related peptide (CGRP) and mediators of increased vascular permeability. Br J Pharmacol 1985; 86:855–860.

Dougherty PM, Willis WD. Enhancement of spinothalamic neuron responses to chemical and mechanical stimuli following combined micro-iontophoretic application of N-methyl-D-aspartic acid and substance P. Pain 1991; 47:85–93.

Dubner R. Pain and hyperalgesia following tissue injury: New mechanisms and treatments. Pain 1991; 44:213–214.

Dubner R, Ruda MA. Activity-dependent neuronal plasticity following tissue injury and inflammation. Trends Neurosci 1992; 15:3.

Levine JD, Dardick SJ, Basbaum AI, Scipio E. Reflex neurogenic inflammation. I. Contribution of the peripheral nervous system to spatially remote inflammatory responses that follow injury. J Neurosci 1985; 3:1380.

Schwartzman RJ. Reflex sympathetic dystrophy. In: Frankel HL, ed. Handbook of clinical neurology: Spinal cord trauma. New York: Elsevier, 1992: 61.

Schwartzman RJ, Kerrigan J. The movement disorder of reflex sympathetic dystrophy. Neurology 1990; 40:57–61.

Schwartzman RJ, McLellan TL. Reflex sympathetic dystrophy: A review. Arch Neurol 1987; 44:555–561.

INTRACRANIAL HYPOTENSION

SUSAN C. PANNULLO, M.D.

When a patient suffers from postural headaches following a lumbar puncture, the diagnosis of a low pressure headache, or intracranial hypotension, is generally clear. Postural headaches may follow a variety of procedures, including diagnostic lumbar punctures, myelography, and spinal anesthesia. Thirty percent of diagnostic lumbar punctures in one series were complicated by subsequent headache. These headaches are attributed to a dural tear producing a cerebrospinal fluid (CSF) leak with consequent lowering of the intracranial pressure.

A similar syndrome of headache and a variety of associated symptoms may occur after minor trauma to the head or buttocks, after coughing, or without an obvious precipitating cause. In this setting, the diagnosis of intracranial hypotension may be unclear, provoking an extensive search for the cause of the patient's symptoms. Diagnostic tests may in fact be confusing to the clinician, and may exacerbate the patient's headache.

The purpose of this chapter is to help the clinician make a diagnosis of intracranial hypotension and to understand the laboratory and radiographic findings that may accompany low CSF pressure. Early recognition of the syndrome of intracranial hypotension prevents unnecessary workup and allows appropriate management of this generally benign, self-limited condition.

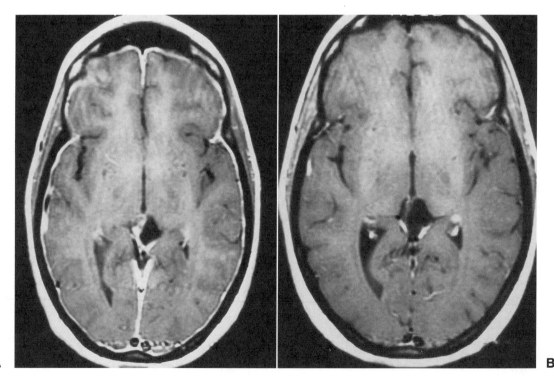

A   B

Figure 1 *A,* Meningeal enhancement in a patient with intracranial hypotension. *B,* Resolution of enhancement following symptomatic improvement.

CLINICAL SIGNS AND SYMPTOMS

The headache of intracranial hypotension is elicited or exacerbated by upright position and is improved or absent when the patient is recumbent. Patients describe the headache as primarily frontal, occipital, or both. Nausea and vomiting are common and may be precipi-

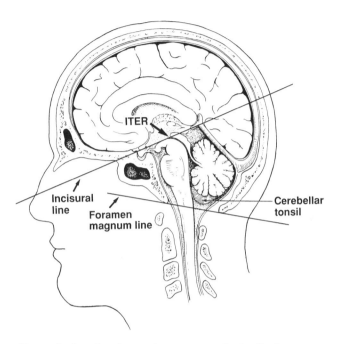

Figure 2 Landmarks used to measure brain displacement. (From Reich JB, Sierra J, Camp W, et al. Magnetic resonance imaging measurements and clinical changes accompanying transtentorial and foramen magnum brain herniation. Ann Neurol 1993; 33:159–170; with permission.)

tated by sitting or standing. Vertigo, diplopia, tinnitus, neck stiffness, and photophobia may accompany the headache and may raise concern about a more serious process when the postural nature of the headache is unrecognized. Impaired taste and numbness inside the mouth are also reported.

Simple bedside examination may suggest the presence of intracranial hypotension. The patient with low CSF pressure will generally be lying flat because symptoms are reduced in this position. Ask the patient to sit upright, with legs dangling over the edge of the bed. The patient with intracranial hypotension will complain of onset or worsening of headache, may appear suddenly pale and ill, and often vomits. A unilateral or bilateral sixth nerve palsy may also be elicited or enhanced with the patient in upright position.

Valsalva's maneuver may exacerbate headache and associated signs and symptoms in the patient even when supine, possibly by enhancing an abnormal gradient between intracranial vasculature pressure and CSF pressure. Orthostatic changes in blood pressure and pulse may occur if the patient has become dehydrated from vomiting and anorexia but are not believed to be part of the underlying process. The remainder of the neurologic examination should be normal in a patient with uncomplicated intracranial hypotension. Careful funduscopic exam should be performed to exclude papilledema, which is not observed with low CSF pressure.

CEREBROSPINAL FLUID

With the signs and symptoms described above, a diagnosis of intracranial hypotension may be made and further evaluation is generally unnecessary. However,

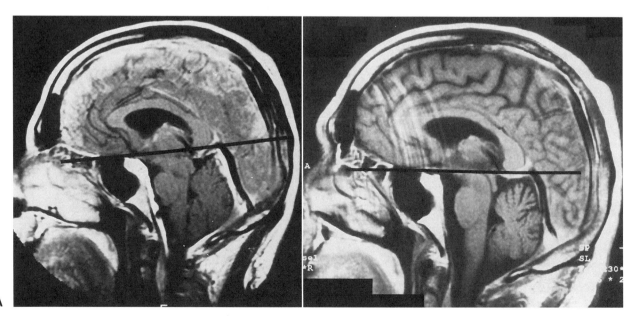

Figure 3 *A,* Downward displacement of the iter. *B,* Return of the iter to normal position.

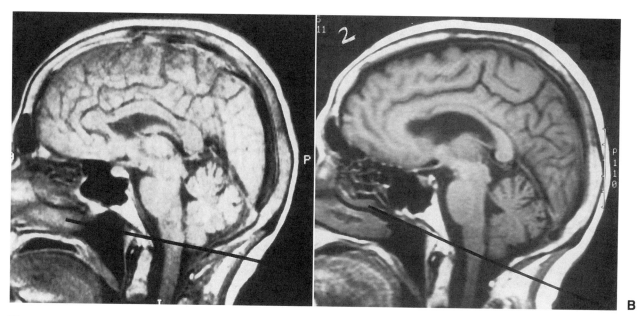

Figure 4 *A,* Downward displacement of the cerebellar tonsils below the foramen magnum. *B,* Resolution of tonsillar herniation.

when there is no clear cause for a dural tear, the diagnosis may be less clear. In this case, lumbar puncture may be useful in confirming the presence of low CSF pressure.

The CSF pressure will generally be less than 70 mm H_2O. In some patients, CSF is obtainable only with the patient in an upright position. The CSF pressure may even be negative relative to atmospheric pressure, causing a sucking sound when the dura is punctured. Valsalva's maneuver or *gentle* aspiration with a syringe may help produce a CSF sample, although sometimes fluid cannot be obtained.

Abnormalities of CSF chemistries and cell counts may prompt concern about an infectious or malignant disease process in patients with intracranial hypotension. CSF pleocytosis, red blood cells, and elevation of CSF protein are frequently found in patients with low CSF pressure. These abnormalities may be due to tearing of meningeal blood vessels by a sagging brain or to compensatory vasodilatation with diapedesis of cells and protein into the subarachnoid space. In most cases, one set of negative cultures and one negative cytology should rule out the presence of meningeal infection or cancer. Repeated lumbar (or cisternal) punctures are not warranted in most patients, and in fact may worsen or prolong symptoms.

DIAGNOSTIC IMAGING

When the diagnosis of intracranial hypotension remains unclear, the neurologic workup may include computed tomography (CT) or magnetic resonance imaging (MRI). CT is of little value in this situation because it is less sensitive than MRI in examination of

the meninges and posterior fossa. Gadolinium-enhanced MRI may help support the clinical diagnosis of intracranial hypotension, although when the syndrome is unrecognized an MRI may produce diagnostic confusion. MRI findings of meningeal enhancement, subdural effusions, and downward displacement of the brain have been described recently in patients with intracranial hypotension. MRI may also be normal.

The meningeal enhancement pattern (Figure 1) may be difficult to distinguish from that seen in meningeal cancer or infection. The enhancement tends to surround both supra- and infratentorial compartments, although it generally does not involve the brain stem or depths of cortical sulci. A contiguous, linear pattern is usually seen. Subdural effusions may occur but do not generally produce mass effect. The venticles should not be enlarged. Meningeal enhancement and subdural effusions are believed to be due to the same tearing or leaking of meningeal vessels that produces the CSF abnormalities found in this syndrome.

Measurements of the position of the brain within the cranial vault, utilizing the opening of the sylvian aqueduct (the iter) and the cerebellar tonsils as reference points on midline sagittal images (Figure 2), may reveal significant downward displacement (Figures 3 and 4), believed to be due to downward sagging of an unsupported brain. Without appropriate clinical history, the tonsillar herniation may be misinterpreted as a Chiari malformation.

As the clinical syndrome of intracranial hypotension resolves, the MRI abnormalities improve. The meningeal enchancement clears, the effusions diminish, and the brain rises back to its normal position within the cranium. The abnormal MRI findings may persist to some degree several months after the patient's symptoms have resolved. However, some decrease in meningeal enhancement usually accompanies symptomatic improvement. Thus, serial MRI scans, at onset of symptoms and at 2 weeks to 1 month following symptom improvement, may be used to confirm the clinical diagnosis of intracranial hypotension and to document improvement over time or after intervention.

Radionuclide cisternography has been recommended in the past to demonstrate, and in some cases localize, a CSF leak. This technique may occasionally be helpful in targeting a region for an epidural blood patch but is probably unnecessary in the usual diagnostic workup for intracranial hypotension.

COMMENTS

Intracranial hypotension is a clinical syndrome that may occur with or without an obvious precipitating cause such as lumbar puncture or trauma. The clinical diagnosis hinges upon recognition of the postural nature of the patient's headache. The diagnosis may be confirmed by the finding of low CSF pressure on recumbent lumbar puncture. The presence of CSF pleocytosis, red blood cells, and elevated protein are not inconsistent with a diagnosis of intracranial hypotension and should not confound the diagnosis. Patients with intracranial hypotension may have abnormal findings on MRI scans, including enhancement of the meninges with gadolinium, subdural effusions, and downward displacement of the brain. The clinical syndrome and MRI abnormalities generally resolve on their own. Extensive workup is generally not helpful and may be misleading. Patients should be treated symptomatically, although when the headache is protracted, epidural blood patch may be necessary to hasten recovery.

Acknowledgement. The author wishes to thank Jerome B. Posner, M.D., for his assistance in the preparation of this chapter.

SUGGESTED READING

Bell WE, Joynt RJ, Sahs AL. Low spinal fluid pressure syndromes. Neurology 1961; 10:512–521.

Gaukroger PB, Brownridge P. Epidural blood patch in the treatment of spontaneous low CSF pressure headache. Pain 1987; 29:119–122.

Pannullo SC, Reich J, Krol G, et al. MRI changes in intracranial hypotension. Neurology (in press).

Rando TA, Fishman RA. Spontaneous intracranial hypotension: Report of two cases and review of the literature. Neurology 1992; 42:481–487.

Reich JB, Sierra J, Camp W, et al. Magnetic resonance imaging measurements and clinical changes accompanying transtentorial and foramen magnum brain herniation. Ann Neurol 1993; 33: 159–170.

Spielman FJ. Post-lumbar puncture headache. Headache 1982; 22: 280–283.

DIZZINESS

DAVID A. DRACHMAN, M.D.

For many physicians, the prospect of evaluating a new patient with the complaint of "dizziness" is among the most dismaying in all of medicine. Not only do they have little idea of the many problems *other* than inner ear disease that may produce versions of this complaint, but for most physicians, even the structure of the vestibular labyrinth is at best a dim recollection. The purpose of this chapter is to provide a logical guide to the medical understanding of dizziness, and a method for sorting out the diagnoses of patients with this complaint.

To begin, it is important to recognize that dizziness is a *complaint,* not a disease. More than 60 different conditions may result in this complaint, either as the initial symptom or as an important and often disabling aspect of some other underlying disease process. The vestibular labyrinth, central and peripheral nervous systems, emotional state, eyes, heart, peripheral vascular system, respiratory system, kidneys, hematologic status, and joints of the spine and lower extremities may all contribute to symptoms referred to as "dizziness." Despite the apparent variety and complexity of underlying problems, most of the diseases causing dizziness fall into a few categories, within which the individual diseases are easily sorted out.

DIZZINESS AND VERTIGO

While *vertigo* etymologically means "a turning sensation" (from the Latin vertere), dizziness is actually a much more inclusive term for a broad variety of unfamiliar—and generally unpleasant—sensations. Since the sensations *are* unfamiliar, most people, including physicians, have difficulty describing with precision what they are experiencing when dizzy. Many people think dizziness *should be* a rotational phenomenon and so initially say they feel as if they are spinning, whether they experience a rotational sensation or not. Others use terms like *light-headed* to describe their problem. After listening to many thousands of such complaints, we have found that they can be categorized into four types:

- Type 1—True vertigo, with a definite *rotational* component

- Type 2—A syncopal-like sensation, as if the patient is *about to faint*
- Type 3—Dysequilibrium: a disorder of *balance and gait, without* an abnormal head sensation, sometimes called "dizziness in the feet"
- Type 4—Lightheadedness: an *abnormal head sensation* other than types 1-3

Spinning, faintness, loss of balance, and lightheadedness may seem to be quite different sensations, and at first we wondered why patients with these sensations would all say they were "dizzy." Eventually we recognized that the common denominator among the wide variety of conditions that present as dizziness was *spatial disorientation,* or a feeling of *uncertainty of position or motion in space.*

While this common aspect does not identify specific diagnostic entitities producing dizziness, it does provide the key to comprehension of the underlying physiologic mechanisms. Adequate and accurate sensation and perception of the environment, integration of the sensory information into a comprehensive picture, and appropriate motor response are necessary to assure orientation over time. When one or more components of this process are disordered, dizziness often results.

PATIENT EVALUATION

History

History-taking is always a three-stage process. While generic questions (How long have you had it? What makes it better, worse?) apply equally well to many problems, complaint-specific questions provide useful information to sort out the underlying causes. Finally, disease-specific questions are necessary to identify the specific diagnosis. In order to ask complaint- and disease-specific questions, however, the physician must know what to look for. Although clinical settings differ, the five most common categories of dizziness (comprising more than 85 percent of all dizziness) are listed in Table 1.

Four *complaint-specific* questions can narrow the possibilities:

Table 1 Five Common Causes of Dizziness

Cause	% of Patients
Vestibular disorders	38
Hyperventilation syndromes*	23
Multisensory disorders	13
Psychiatric disorders	9
Cerebrovascular disease	5

*More than half have associated anxiety attacks.

1. What type of dizziness does the patient have? Type 1, true rotational vertigo, occurs almost exclusively with vestibular disorders—either peripheral or central. A patient who experiences an unequivocal turning sensation and no other symptoms of dizziness has a disorder involving this system. Type 2, a syncopal-like sensation, strongly suggests a decrease of blood flow to the brain. Cardiovascular problems such as arrhythmias or orthostatic hypotension—not cerebrovascular problems—are the most common cause of this complaint. Type 3, dysequilibrium without a head sensation, raises the possibility of cerebellar ataxia, Bruns (frontal lobe) apraxia of gait, a dorsal column or peripheral nerve sensory impairment, or impaired motor control, such as parkinsonism. Type 4, lightheadedness other than types 1 to 3, is a less specific complaint. It suggests a fractional or poorly described version of the previously mentioned problems, psychiatric-hyperventilation syndrome, or multisensory dizziness due to impairment in several sensory modalities.

2. How old is the patient? The patient's age is important in identifying likely causes of dizziness and excluding others. Vestibular disorders can occur at any age, but panic states, hyperventilation, and multiple sclerosis are more common in young adults, while parkinsonism, multisensory dizziness, and strokes are rare except in the elderly.

3. What is the relation of symptoms to position or motion? Orthostatic hypotension occurs only in the upright position and benign positional vertigo only on rapid positional change, for example. Multisensory dizziness occurs when the patient is walking and turning and is absent when still or seated. On the other hand, the vertiginous episodes of Ménière's disease occur without regard to position or motion, as may cardiac arrhythmias.

4. What is the course of the dizziness? Episodic vertigo beginning abruptly on change of position and lasting under a minute virtually defines benign positional vertigo. Dizziness due to cardiac arrhythmias is always of sudden onset and offset. Variable lightheadedness of gradual onset lasting hours or more is more common in psychiatric problems or as the late residual of peripheral vestibulopathy.

Disease-specific questions—for example, the association of hearing loss and tinnitus with Ménière's disease—are discussed below with the individual entities. It is always useful for the neurologist to run through a review of the neurologic system to consider the possibility that some neurologic disorder not obviously suggested by the symptoms, or whose association with dizziness is unfamiliar, might be either causing or contributing to the patient's dizziness.

Neurologic Examination

The purpose of the neurologic examination in the dizzy patient is to identify a number of specific neurologic patterns that may occur in patients with dizziness (Table 2). For example, in the elderly patient with vertigo, the question invariably arises as to whether the vertigo is due to a stroke. Since infarction exclusively in the territory of the vestibular branch of the internal auditory artery is very rare, the neurologist's task is to determine whether the vertigo is due to a brain stem lesion involving nearby structures in addition to the vestibular nuclei. Neighborhood signs include facial weakness or numbness, dysarthria, cerebellar signs, Horner's syndrome, or long tract signs. The absence of all of these findings is a strong indication of peripheral, rather than central, vestibular disease in an elderly patient with vertigo. Similarly, vertigo in the young adult raises the possibility of multiple sclerosis, to be ruled out by neurologic evaluation. Negative, as well as positive, findings thus provide valuable information that helps to establish the diagnosis. While meticulous examination of nervous system function is the hallmark of the neurologist, it is important to keep in mind the limited (albeit important) number of neurologic entities that are relevant to the complaint of dizziness, as indicated in Table 2.

Neuro-otologic Testing

Since disorders of the inner ear are an important cause of dizziness, tests of both hearing and vestibular function form part of every dizziness evaluation. Identification of two-digit whispered numerals from a distance of 6 feet to either side of the patient, with the opposite ear blocked, is a sensitive screen for hearing loss. The familiar Weber and Rinne tests are useful in distinguishing bone- from air-conduction disorders. In the Hennebert test the examiner pumps air into the external ear canal, using a closed otoscope with a rubber bulb attached to its side-port. Vertigo may be produced in patients with a fistula of the round or oval window of the labyrinth. The Quix test is performed by having the patient stand with arms extended and index fingers pointed at the examiner's fingers, similarly extended.

The patient's aim will drift to one side or the other if there is a vestibular imbalance.

Dizziness Simulation Battery

In many instances, the dizziness simulation battery has provided the crucial information necessary to identify the cause of dizziness. This is a series of eight maneuvers (Table 3) designed to help both the patient and the examiner to identify accurately the type and cause of symptoms. Some of the maneuvers produce dizziness in all patients, while others induce it only in those with an underlying disorder. As each maneuver is done, the patient is asked whether the test-evoked dizziness is similar in *character*, but not necessarily in *severity*, to his or her own dizziness. Identification of a provoked sensation of dizziness is often more reliable than a verbal description, especially if a single maneuver exclusively reproduces the patient's own symptoms.

Laboratory Tests (Table 4)

The extent of the laboratory tests performed in a patient with dizziness varies with the patient's medical background, the suspicions of the examining physician, and the acuteness or chronicity of the symptoms. In an otherwise healthy young patient who abruptly develops symptoms and physical signs of benign positional vertigo,

Table 2 Neurologic Patterns in Patients with Dizziness

Brain stem lesion (such as stroke)
Cerebellopontine angle syndrome
Multiple sclerosis
Cerebellar ataxia
Benign positional vertigo
Multisensory dizziness
Bruns' (frontal lobe) apraxia of gait
Parkinsonism
Astasia-abasia
Migraine syndrome
Shy-Drager syndrome (orthostatic hypotension,
   multiple system disorder)
Agoraphobia

Table 3 Dizziness Simulation Battery

Maneuver	Cause of Symptoms
1. Orthostatic blood pressure testing	
2. Carotid sinus sensitivity	
3. Potentiated Valsalva maneuver	Cardiovascular
4. Head-turn (airplane follow)	
5. Walk-turn	Multisensory
6. Nylen-Barany	
7. Barany rotation	Vestibular
8. Hyperventilation (30 sec)	Hyperventilation—
9. Patient's own maneuvers	Psychiatric

Table 4 Laboratory Tests for Dizziness

1. Routine hematology, SMA-12, electrolytes
2. ECG, Holter monitor*
3. MMPI, psychometric evaluation*
4. SPEP, thyroid functions
5. Electronystagmography, audiometry
6. MRI scan*
7. EEG,* 24 hour EEG monitor*
8. BAER*
9. 5 hour GTT*
10. Tilt-table,* cardiac electrophysiologic studies*

*Optional, as indicated by other findings
MMPI = Minnesota Multiphasic Personality Inventory, SPEP = serum protein electrophoresis, MRI = magnetic resonance imaging, EEG = electroencephalogram, BAER = brain stem auditory evoked responses, GTT = glucose tolerance test.

which resolve in a few days, the workup can well be limited to the electronystagmogram, with audiometric studies if hearing is compromised. When dizziness lasts more than a few days, however, it is both efficient and economical to obtain the complete battery of relevant tests, not only to identify specific causes of dizziness, but to rule out other possibilities. We have found, for example, that obtaining the Minnesota Multiphasic Personality Inventory (MMPI) at the outset in every patient with dizziness is a valuable strategy. It takes no examiner time and gives a generally reliable insight into a range of relevant psychiatric problems. This strategy is especially useful because it is much more comfortable to tell patients that this is part of our routine battery for dizziness than to have them return 2 weeks later, when all other tests have proven negative, and suggest a referral to a psychiatrist! As a rule, we have found that while the positive yield for some tests, such as thyroid functions, may not be high for dizziness, the assurance that a patient is *not* hypothyroid is a useful negative in arriving at a secure diagnosis.

Electronystagmography (ENG) (Table 5) is of value in identifying unilateral or bilateral peripheral vestibular deficits (labyrinth, eighth nerve) and distinguishing them from central vestibular disease. Recording of the amplitude, speed, and duration of ocular movements is first made during a series of maneuvers in which ocular tracking and head positioning are evaluated. Caloric testing is carried out with the patient positioned so that the horizontal semicircular canals are vertical (head elevated 30 degrees), and each ear is irrigated with cool and warm water or air to produce a flow of endolymph by convection, mimicking the flow produced by head rotation. Modern ENG systems provide readouts of the speed of the slow phase of the nystagmus, and the amplitude, and compute any side-to-side differences or failure to respond. Other abnormalities beyond the scope of this chapter may indicate a disorder of central vestibular pathways.

Audiometric studies are helpful in assessing the auditory pathways, especially in Ménière's disease and cerebellopontine angle tumors. Routine pure-tone audiometry indicates whether a hearing loss is present and may distinguish common causes (aging, otosclerosis, acoustic trauma) from cochlear and nerve disorders. Site of lesion studies, such as speech discrimination, alternate binaural loudness balance (ABLB), threshold tone decay, Békésy, and acoustic reflex tests may improve

Table 5 Electronystagmographic Patterns

Normal*
Unilateral labyrinthine (canal) paresis*
Positional nystagmus and vertigo*
Spontaneous nystagmus—unidirectional
Bilaterally unresponsive labyrinths
Central disorders: poor ocular fixation suppression, perverted nystagmus
Ocular motility disorders

*Most common findings

accuracy of diagnosis. Brain stem auditory evoked response (BAER) studies are especially valuable in screening for acoustic neuromas and can distinguish brain stem from peripheral cochlear or eighth nerve disorders.

Imaging studies, including computed tomography or magnetic resonance imaging (MRI) scans, are not part of the routine evaluation of most complaints of dizziness, including episodic vertigo, although they have an important place in more complex neurologic problems. Serious diagnostic evaluation of acoustic neuromas (which almost never present with episodes of true vertigo and are well screened with BAER), strokes, cerebellar or brain stem tumors, or other disorders with intracranial neurologic findings requires imaging studies, based on the neurologic evaluation.

ARRIVING AT A DIAGNOSIS: DISEASES PRODUCING DIZZINESS

Some diseases producing dizziness have an easily recognized, stereotypical pattern, while others require detailed analysis of all the data. To complicate matters, about 10 to 15 percent of patients have more than one cause of dizziness. In any case, arriving at the diagnosis is much easier if one has in mind the broad range of disorders that can cause dizziness (Table 6), and especially the five groups of conditions that make up more than 85 percent of diagnoses (see Table 1)—vestibular disorders, hyperventilation syndromes, multisensory disorders, psychiatric conditions, and brain stem strokes.

Vertigo and Vestibular Disorders

The first diagnostic decision to be made is whether the patient has true rotational vertigo. As noted, many patients refer to any complaint of dizziness as "spinning" or "turning," but true vertigo can be characterized by descriptions of being "on a merry-go-round" (subjective visual movement of the environment) and the association with nausea or vomiting. Most important, however, is the identification of vertigo induced by Barany rotation and by no other dizziness simulation maneuver as *like the patient's own complaint.*

If the patient has true vertigo, the physician must then decide whether it is peripheral or central in origin. In most cases, the absence of a history or physical findings of central nervous system involvement indicates peripheral vestibular disease. Neighborhood neurologic symptoms or signs such as facial weakness or numbness, dysarthria, weakness, or long-tract signs suggest central vestibular disease.

Among the peripheral vestibular disorders, Ménière's disease is identified by the concurrence of fluctuating hearing loss and tinnitus with a characteristic low-frequency loss on audiometry. Benign positional vertigo is diagnosed in patients whose vertigo is *exclusively* precipitated by change of position—often con-

Table 6 Important Clinical Disorders Producing Dizziness

Peripheral vestibular disorders
  With vertigo:
    Benign positional vertigo
    Acute peripheral vestibulopathy
    Acute and recurrent peripheral vestibulopathy
    Ménière's disease
  Without vertigo:
    Bilateral vestibular paresis (drug-induced)

Hyperventilation syndromes
  With underlying psychiatric disorder
  Without underlying psychiatric disorder

Multiple sensory deficits
  Three or more: peripheral neuropathy, visual impairment,
    vestibular hypoactivity-imbalance, cervical spondylosis, hearing
    loss
Psychogenic Disorders
  Depression
  Anxiety, hyperventilation
  Agoraphobia-panic state
  Astasia-abasia
Cerebrovascular Disorders
  Brain stem cerebrovascular accident with neighborhood signs
  Isolated ischemia of vestibular system (central and/or
    peripheral) — *rare*
Cardiovascular Disorders
  Orthostatic hypotension
  Cardiac arrhythmias
Other
  Parkinsonism, progressive supranuclear palsy
  Multiple sclerosis
  Hypothyroidism
  Cerebellar degeneration
  Acoustic neuroma, cerebellar tumor
  Subdural hematoma
  Normal pressure hydrocephalus
  Hypoglycemia

firmed on ENG. Acute peripheral vestibulopathy and the recurrent form lack the auditory problems of Ménière's and have vertigo both with and without change of head position. Bilateral loss of labyrinthine function, such as due to aminoglycoside antibiotics, may begin with vertigo but results in unsteadiness and difficulty seeing objects clearly when the patient is in motion, due to loss of the vestibulo-ocular reflex.

Viral infections are often suspected of causing vestibular syndromes, but only herpes zoster has been proven to be a causative agent, generally associated with the rash of shingles.

The most difficult diagnosis of vestibular disorders is that of the patient who has largely recovered from a mild peripheral vestibulopathy and now has mild unsteadiness and imbalance when walking in the dark, in the absence of vertigo. A good history of preceding vertigo can be illuminating in these cases. Decreased or asymmetrical vestibular function is found on ENG.

The most common central vestibular disorders are brain stem ischemia or stroke and multiple sclerosis. Since stroke is largely a disease of the elderly, and multiple sclerosis of the young, suspicion of these two conditions rarely occurs in the same individual. Brain

stem stroke that results in vertigo is due to ischemia in a branch of the basilar-vertebral system, most commonly the AICA, which supplies the vestibular nuclei and the peripheral labyrinth via the internal auditory artery. Even in elderly patients with risk factors for stroke, however, vertigo in the absence of other brain stem symptoms or signs does not justify the diagnosis of stroke. Multiple sclerosis may occasionally present with vertigo in young patients but far more commonly occurs in the setting of other previous neurologic symptoms, such as optic neuritis.

Cerebellopontine angle tumors are often considered in patients with vertigo, but rarely if ever produce a syndrome of episodic vertigo of abrupt onset, and virtually never in the absence of other findings. More commonly, these tumors produce gradual unsteadiness, hearing loss, and facial weakness with cerebellar and long-tract signs.

Other central conditions causing vertigo include the rare vertiginous migraine, which is diagnosed by its temporal association with other migraine features. More often, patients may have both migraine and a vestibular disorder, both of which are common. Epileptic seizures exceedingly rarely present exclusively with dizziness (so-called tornado epilepsy), although a feeling of dizziness is fairly commonly experienced as part of complex partial seizures.

Faintness (Syncopal and Seizure Disorders)

Syncope is invariably a cardiovascular disorder, due to inadequate flow of blood to the brain as a whole. In presyncope, the patient feels lightheaded, as if about to faint, without actually losing consciousness. Most people recognize this symptom as one commonly experienced on suddenly standing up after lying down, with dimming of vision and perhaps distortion of sounds momentarily. The conditions in which this symptom presents as dizziness include cardiac arrhythmias; orthostatic hypotension; cough, micturition, or vasovagal syncope; and hypersensitivity of the carotid sinus.

In addition to the typical description of symptoms, the dizziness simulation maneuver of a potentiated Valsalva maneuver will reproduce a syncopal-like sensation for many people. Orthostasis produces dizziness only in those with abnormal hypotension, however. Careful stimulation of one carotid sinus at a time produces faintness in those with hypersensitivity. Questions regarding the relation of symptoms to position, subjective palpitations, head-turning, micturition, and cough are helpful. Useful tests include the Holter monitor, and in some cases tilt-table studies or electrophysiologic stimulation cardiac evaluation.

Dysequilibrium (Impaired Balance)

This cause of dizziness is largely seen in the elderly and includes Bruns' apraxia of gait and normal pressure hydrocephalus (NPH), parkinsonism (and progressive supranuclear palsy), astasia-abasia, and cerebellar disorders. In patients with diffuse or frontal lobe disease, such as multiple strokes, a variably unsteady gait may be seen, together with an apraxic inability to hop on one foot. The findings in NPH are often similar. In both conditions, mental changes, incontinence, and extrapyramidal features may also be present. After a careful neurologic examination, neuroimaging procedures such as MRI are most useful here. Parkinsonism should be suspected early in any elderly person with a deteriorating gait. The clinical findings are well described elsewhere. Astasia-abasia is uncommon and refers to impaired balance and gait on a psychiatric basis. This may be seen in young and old patients alike. The inconsistency of gait disturbance and objective neurologic findings, together with an abnormal conversion pattern on the MMPI, are diagnostically useful. Among the most confusing gait disorders may be the early manifestations of a noninherited cerebellar degeneration, such as that seen in alcoholism, the Dejerine-Thomas form of olivopontocerebellar degeneration, or carcinomatous cerebellar degeneration. Once suspected, however, the clinical picture, often supplemented by neuroimaging findings of cerebellar atrophy, together with the features that are well described elsewhere, are diagnostic.

Lightheadedness

Poorly described lightheadedness accounts for more than half of the complaints of dizziness and includes the broadest range of disorders. This complaint includes two groups of problems: first, patients with either fractional forms of vertigo, syncope, or dysequilibrium or poorly described symptoms, and second, those with multisensory dizziness, hyperventilation, and psychiatric disorders.

For those patients who in reality have one of the other complaints of dizziness, the dizziness simulation battery is often extremely useful in clarifying the nature of their problem by permitting them to *recognize* a symptom, rather than having to describe it de novo. Since dizziness is a subjective symptom, we inevitably place considerable reliance on the nature of the description by the patient.

Multisensory dizziness occurs most frequently in elderly patients when more than two sensory channels of orienting information are impaired or distorted. Elderly diabetic patients with peripheral neuropathy, cataracts, cervical spondylosis, and impaired hearing or vestibular function are typical of this group. The inadequacy of sensory perceptions when they are walking, particularly in a confusing environment such as a shopping center, leads to the complaint of dizziness. The neurologic examination often best defines many of the underlying sensory deficits that contribute to the patient's disorientation. The ENG, audiometric evaluation, and imaging of the cervical spine add to the diagnosis. Such patients often walk much better if given the examiner's finger to touch while walking. This additional sensory channel may stabilize their gait, and response to this maneuver provides further diagnostic information.

Hyperventilation syndrome is a common cause of dizziness in younger patients. In the majority, but not all, it has a psychiatric basis. A history of perioral and digital paresthesias and difficulty breathing are helpful but seldom present. The clinical observation that the patient sighs repeatedly during an interview is often missed but is strongly suggestive. The identical reproduction of all symptoms by 30 seconds of hyperventilation, and no other maneuver in the dizziness simulation battery, is virtually diagnostic. If symptoms are aborted by the rebreathing of air into a plastic bag, this confirms the diagnosis.

Psychiatric disorders contribute both to the hyperventilation syndrome and astasia-abasia, but they are often the sole cause of complaints of dizziness. The most important psychiatric disorders causing dizziness are agoraphobia-panic state, anxiety, and depression. Patients with agoraphobia avoid open spaces, crowds, elevators, parties, or other situations where, if suddenly overcome, they would have difficulty extricating themselves. Unable or unwilling to describe these feelings, many patients use the term *dizziness* instead. Conversely, it is worth knowing that patients with unpredictable episodic vertigo may develop secondary agoraphobia, with the realistic fear of losing orientation and control in these circumstances. In each of these conditions, appropriate questions should be asked regarding the symptoms of anxiety, loss of energy and interests, together with sleep and sexual disorders or avoidance of the circumstances described above. The MMPI routinely obtained in dizzy patients often provides valuable confirmatory evidence for the diagnosis, and the absence of other objective findings is a necessary corollary.

Multiple Diagnoses

About one patient in eight will have dizziness with more than one cause. This often confuses the physician, since we expect to arrive at a single answer, using the principle of Ockham's razor. Recognition that overdetermination rather than underdetermination of the cause is a common situation should remind the physician of the need to be comprehensive in the evaluation of the dizzy patient.

COMMENTS

The complaint of dizziness opens the door to a broad range of diagnostic possibilities. Once the nature of the complaint has been narrowed down to one of the four dizziness types, by history and by use of the dizziness simulation battery, the identification of the specific cause becomes much simpler. The physician knows that the condition is vestibular, cardiovascular, multisensory, a disorder of balance and gait, or psychogenic in the large majority of cases. It is important to use a systematic approach, however, especially in older patients or those with more than one cause for the dizziness. A comprehensive evaluation is the most reliable way of arriving at a secure diagnosis.

SUGGESTED READING

Baloh RW. Dizziness in older people. J Am Geriatr Soc 1992; 40:713–721.

Baloh RW, Honrubia V. Clinical neurophysiology of the vestibular system. ed 2. Philadelphia: FA Davis 1990.

Caplan LR. Transient vertigo, drop spells and cerebrovascular disease. In: Barber H, Sharpe J, eds. Chicago: Year Book Medical Publishers, 1988:239.

Drachman DA, Hart CW. An approach to the dizzy patient. Neurology 1972; 22:323–334.

Zee DS. The management of patients with vestibular disorders. In: Barber H, Sharpe J, eds. Vestibular disorders. Chicago: Year Book Medical Publishers, 1988:254.

CONGENITAL AND DEVELOPMENTAL DISORDERS

INHERITED NEURODEGENERATIVE AND NEUROGENETIC DISEASES

WILLIAM G. JOHNSON, M.D.

Genetic neurologic disorders range from rare to common, from disorders of infancy to disorders of the aged, and from disorders occurring in many members of large families to sporadic cases.

In the aggregate, neurogenetic disorders are relatively common and occur commonly in differential diagnoses. Once the diagnosis is known, it is an easy matter to find sources of information concerning specific diseases. However, the usual problem confronting clinicians is the patient presenting in the office with a complaint and an unknown diagnosis. The following is an approach to the diagnosis of inherited neurodegenerative disorders.

At the time of the initial visit, it is usually not clear whether the patient has a genetic neurologic disease or a nongenetic disorder. Our evaluation for patients is divided into four steps: (1) history and examination, (2) family history and genetic evaluation, (3) comparison with genetics source material, and (4) laboratory evaluation.

HISTORY AND EXAMINATION

The clinical history, physical examination, and neurologic examination are the most important steps in the evaluation of the patient with suspected genetic neurologic disease. The usual natural history of these disorders is insidious onset and slow progression. Disorders that are present at birth and static thereafter are not usually genetic. Likewise, disorders with sudden onset and a static course are not usually genetic. There are exceptions to these conventions, however. Some forms of alpha-mannosidosis have the appearance of a static encephalopathy. Congenital myopathies appear static yet are usually genetic. Spina bifida cystica, a genetic disorder with multifactorial inheritance, is present at birth. Homocystinuria, Fabry's disease, and MELAS, a mitochondrial disorder, may present with stroke.

In children, development and acquisition of milestones are usually occurring at the typical time of onset of neurodegenerative processes. Therefore, the initial finding may be a slowing of acquisition of developmental milestones, followed by a plateau when milestones are neither gained nor lost, followed by the progressive loss of milestones. Diagnosis is more difficult in this situation and may require a high index of suspicion.

In addition to the natural history, the clinical history can give information about what other systems are involved. Auditory or visual disturbances are important. The finding of cataract or retinal vascular abnormality may suggest galactosemia or Von Hippel-Lindau's disease. Deafness complicating a neurologic disorder could have many causes, including neurofibromatosis or mucopolysaccharidosis. Seizures occur in many neurodegenerative diseases such as Lafora's body disease, Sanfilippo's disease, the gangliosidoses, and some leukodystrophies. Outside the nervous system, specific system involvement may be an important clue to diagnosis.

The physical examination is important because any associated physical finding may make the diagnosis easier. The finding of a sacral dimple suggests a form of spinal dysraphism. The finding of pigmented or depigmented skin lesions may suggest neurofibromatosis, tuberous sclerosis, or other neurocutaneous disorders. The finding of dysostosis multiplex suggests mucopolysaccharidosis. Anosmia may suggest a range of disorders from Kallmann's syndrome to Alzheimer's or Parkinson's disease. Examination of the face is particularly important because many genetic disorders, especially in children, have characteristic facies.

The neurologic examination is important because it determines which systems are affected. For example, dementia plus chorea suggests Huntington's disease. Dementia plus dystonia plus pyramidal tract involvement suggests Hallervorden-Spatz disease. Cerebellar plus pyramidal involvement suggests a spinocerebellar degeneration. Dementia plus demyelinating motor neuropathy suggests a leukodystrophy, such as metachromatic leukodystrophy.

The natural history, the pattern of involvement in

the nervous system, and the findings outside the nervous system create the framework from which a diagnosis can be established.

FAMILY HISTORY AND GENETIC EVALUATION

A careful family history is the next step in diagnosis of inherited neurodegenerative diseases. A detailed family history may require only a few minutes if it is entirely negative or if little information is available. On the other hand, it may require over an hour. For this reason, family histories are often taken by genetic counselors. It is particularly important to determine accurately the clinical picture of any affected relatives, even if they do not have exactly the same disorder as the patient. An affected family member may be a genetic compound and have a somewhat different disorder caused by different alleles at the same gene locus. Clinicians often forget to question the patient or parent about parental consanguinity or the geographic and ethnic origin of grandparents. The finding of parental consanguinity suggests a recessive disorder. The finding of a maternal and a paternal grandparent with the same ethnic or geographic origin, both perhaps coming from the same small town in another country, supports the possibility of a recessive disorder. Certain recessive disorders have a high frequency among members of a specific ethnic group, such as Tay-Sachs disease in individuals of Ashkenazi Jewish background or aspartylglycosaminuria in individuals of Finnish background.

Autosomal Dominant Inheritance

Inheritance of an autosomal dominant disorder is vertical (that is, through successive generations) from parent to child to grandchild. Males and females are affected with equal frequency and with equal severity. There is no increased frequency of parental consanguinity as there is with autosomal recessive inheritance. Children of an affected parent have a 50 percent risk of receiving the harmful gene and therefore a 50 percent risk of being affected. Half sibs through the affected parent have the same risk of being affected as full sibs, in sharp contrast to the situation with autosomal recessive diseases, where the risk to half sibs is very small. Male-to-male transmission occurs in autosomal dominant inheritance and should always be looked for. Male-to-male transmission cannot occur in X-linked dominant pedigrees and may not occur in small autosomal dominant pedigrees simply by chance.

Dominant Lethal Traits

This group of dominant disorders is mentioned separately because its inheritance pattern is different. Dominant lethal disorders are those in which an affected individual does not reproduce. The disorder is not necessarily lethal to the patient, and because the patients do not reproduce, the disease cannot be transmitted from parent to child. Therefore, nearly all cases are sporadic and result from new mutation of a parental germ cell. When one searches the literature and finds that all published cases of a disorder are sporadic, it is not reasonable to conclude therefore that the disorder is nongenetic. The happy practical result of this situation, however, is that the recurrence risk for the next pregnancy is nearly zero for parents who have had a child affected with a dominant lethal disorder.

Penetrance and Expressivity

These features are especially characteristic of dominant rather than recessive inheritance. *Penetrance* is the fraction of individuals with an abnormal allele who actually have the abnormal phenotype. In individuals who are known to carry the abnormal gene but who have the normal phenotype, the abnormal gene is said to be *nonpenetrant.* Obviously, whether or not an individual is affected can be defined or determined in different ways. Different ways of determining the abnormal phenotype will give different numerical values for penetrance.

Expressivity is the degree of clinical involvement in an individual with the abnormal gene. It is especially characteristic of dominant disorders that two individuals carrying the same abnormal gene, perhaps sibs in the same family, may vary greatly in the severity of their disease. Nonpenetrance is an extreme form of variable expressivity.

Autosomal Recessive Inheritance

Inheritance of a disorder transmitted in autosomal recessive fashion is horizontal rather than vertical. Affected individuals are usually seen only in a single sibship where the parents are unaffected but are both heterozygotes for the harmful gene. Collateral sibships are occasionally affected. Of course, disorders occurring in a sibship are not necessarily genetic; infectious disorders may cluster in a sibship. Males and females are affected with equal frequency and with equal severity.

Autosomal recessive disorders have an increased incidence of parental consanguinity, unlike dominant disorders. In general, the rarer the disorder, the greater the fraction of families with parental consanguinity. A corollary to this is that rare recessive disorders are most likely to be found in inbred genetic isolates. Recessive disorders also frequently show striking ethnic predilections, a fact that is helpful in diagnosis. Another corollary is that heterozygotes for some autosomal recessive disorders have increased frequency in specific ethnic groups, which has made possible carrier testing for such disorders as Tay-Sachs disease, thalassemia, and sickle cell disease.

X-Linked Inheritance

X-Linked Dominant Inheritance

X-linked dominant pedigrees show vertical transmission and look like autosomal dominant pedigrees except that in X-linked dominant pedigrees (1) male-to-male transmission does not occur, (2) all daughters of an affected male are affected, (3) females are more frequently affected than males, (4) females are less severely affected than males, and (5) occasional female heterozygotes show nonpenetrance, probably as a chance result of preponderant Lyon inactivation of the X-chromosome carrying the abnormal gene.

Since X-linked dominant pedigrees look so much like autosomal dominant pedigrees, X-linked dominant inheritance can easily be overlooked unless every apparently autosomal dominant pedigree is carefully examined for the features just mentioned.

X-Linked Recessive Inheritance

X-linked recessive inheritance somewhat resembles autosomal recessive inheritance, especially if only a single sibship is considered. However, in larger pedigrees the appearance is different from either autosomal dominant recessive or autosomal dominant inheritance. Transmission is diagonal rather than vertical or horizontal: affected males are connected on the pedigree through unaffected females. Only males are affected, but no male-to-male transmission occurs. Occasional female heterozygotes may be affected, probably as a chance result of preponderant Lyon inactivation of the X-chromosome carrying the normal gene.

Metabolic Interference

Metabolic interference is a postulated mechanism in which two alleles at a locus or two alleles of genes at different loci cause a harmful effect only when they are present together in the same individual. In some instances, these pedigrees are strikingly unusual. Examples include (1) a disorder limited to females, apparently dominant or recessive, especially a disorder passed to affected females through unaffected males; (2) a disorder occurring in all members of a large sibship with normal parents; (3) a disorder occurring in all members of a large sibship with one parent similarly affected; (4) an apparently dominant disorder with females more severely affected than males; or (5) an apparently X-linked dominant disorder in which males are not more severely affected.

A number of pedigrees have been reported that are explained by the metabolic interference hypothesis but are not easily explained by any other known pattern.

Multifactorial-Threshold and Polygenic Disorders

These disorders occur more commonly in the population than the Mendelian disorders. The pattern of inheritance is quite different from the Mendelian patterns just discussed. However, in practice it is difficult to distinguish between autosomal dominant inheritance with greatly reduced penetrance, disorders exhibiting genetic heterogeneity, and multifactorial-threshold inheritance. The disorders that best fit this model, such as neural tube defects, cleft lip, cleft palate, diabetes, and some form of epilepsy and mental retardation, are not

good examples of neurodegenerative disorders. Some neurodegenerative disorders that do fit the multifactorial-threshold model, such as Parkinson's disease, are probably better described as autosomal dominant with reduced penetrance.

The Sporadic Case

The commonest presentation for genetic disorders in small human families is probably the sporadic case. If the clinician waited for a second case in a family before suspecting a genetic disorder, most genetic disorders would escape diagnosis. The following is a partial list of diagnostic possibilities for the sporadic case:
- Autosomal dominant (reduced penetrance)
- Autosomal dominant (new mutation)
- Autosomal recessive
- X-linked recessive (male only)
- X-linked dominant (female or male)
- Multifactorial-threshold disorder of polygenic inheritance
- Nonpaternity
- Adopted child
- Nongenetic (phenocopy)

COMPARISON WITH GENETICS SOURCE MATERIAL

Genetics source material is indispensable in the diagnosis of neurogenetic disorders, even for the experienced clinician, because there are so many different disorders. It is therefore helpful to use books, databases, telephone consultation with an experienced geneticist, or all of these in approaching the diagnosis of many cases.

Some useful reference books for neurogenetic diagnosis are listed in the Suggested Reading. Of these, the most useful is McKusick's catalog. I keep it by my telephone for reference during telephone consultations. The book is organized by specific disorders, each with a 6-digit "McKusick number." Autosomal dominant disorders begin with 1, autosomal recessive disorders begin with 2, and X-linked disorders begin with 3. Over 5,000 gene loci are listed, most representing Mendelian disorders. The most useful feature of the book for diagnosis is an index of signs, symptoms, and disease features at the end. For example, retinitis pigmentosa, deafness, mental retardation, and hypogonadism lead one directly to entry 268020, where a description of the disorder with reference to the literature is found. Other useful features include lists of disorders and gene loci associated with each of the chromosomes. The same information, more recently updated, is also available on an on-line database, OMIM (On-line Mendelian Inheritance in Man).

An extensive list of diagnostic features of specific genetic metabolic diseases, such as age of onset, dementia, myoclonus, corneal opacity, unusual facies, and skull abnormalities, is found in Rudolph's textbook *Pediatrics*. Useful, well-indexed, and well-illustrated compendia of many genetic, chromosomal, and congenital disorders are found in Smith's *Recognizable Patterns of Human Malformation* and Bergsma's *Birth Defects Compendium*. Finally, *Atlas of the Face* by Gorlin and Goodman, as well as Smith and Bergsma, are useful picture books with which to compare the facies of a patient in the office with the facies characteristic of a wide variety of genetic disorders.

LABORATORY EVALUATION

The laboratory evaluation for suspected neurogenetic disorders can be quite extensive. Usually it is best to proceed from diagnoses suggested by the clinical examination and genetic evaluation. The usual laboratory evaluation consists of three parts:

1. Biochemical or molecular study of blood, urine, or cultured skin fibroblasts
2. Electrophysiologic and roentgenographic studies
3. Light and electron microscopic study of biopsy material

Many genetic metabolic disorders can be readily diagnosed by means of relatively noninvasive studies (Group 1). Three kinds of specimens are useful: blood, urine, and cultured skin fibroblasts. It is important to check the requirements of the laboratory performing the assays *before* any specimens are taken.

Biochemical and Molecular Studies

Serum, plasma, leukocytes, and cultured skin fibroblasts are good sources of enzymes for many specific and nonspecific biochemical studies. Urine is a good source of metabolites such as mucopolysaccharides, oligosaccharides, aminoacids, and organic acids for biochemical studies. Blood leukocytes and skin fibroblasts are good sources of DNA for DNA-based diagnostic testing. Immortal cell lines can be prepared from leukocytes using EB virus and from cultured fibroblasts using SV40 virus.

Skin punch biopsy for fibroblast culture is readily carried out as an office procedure by the medical geneticist or the dermatologist in consultation. Immediately after biopsy, the piece of skin should be placed into a sterile solution for culture. If a skin punch biopsy for electron microscopy is required, this can be taken at the same time.

DNA-based diagnosis is highly useful for disorders for which mutations in the disease gene are known or for which DNA markers tightly linked to the disease gene are known. For example, in Huntington's disease, fragile X syndrome, X-linked spinobulbar muscular atrophy, myotonic dystrophy, and one type of dominant cerebellar ataxia, the expanded trinucleotide repeats associated with disease are usually readily detectable even in single individuals without testing the entire kindred. In other disorders, such as tuberous sclerosis, where only linked

markers are yet available, it is necessary to test the entire kindred in order to determine the risk that a specific individual carries the disease gene. Even then, the results usually carry a significant margin for error, especially when the disease can be caused by more than one gene locus.

For enzyme deficiency disorders, DNA-based diagnostic testing of patients and carriers is not likely to replace enzyme-based testing in the near future, except in some specific instances. If only a few mutations account for all or nearly all cases of a specific enzyme deficiency encountered, then DNA-based diagnosis will gradually move from the role of a confirmatory test or a subtyping test to the primary testing modality for that disease. However, if many mutations are commonly encountered among patients with a specific enzyme deficiency, enzyme-based diagnosis will remain the primary testing modality.

Electrophysiologic and Roentgenographic Studies

These studies are nonspecific but often very helpful. Decreased nerve conduction velocities indicating demyelinating neuropathy are useful in the leukodystrophies and a number of hereditary motor and sensory neuropathies. Electromyography provides a useful indication of muscle disease or denervation from neuropathy or anterior horn cell diseases. The electroretinogram is abolished in patients with the neuronal ceroid lipofuscinoses and other patients with pigmentary retinal disorders. Visual evoked responses are helpful to document optic atrophy. Roentgenographic changes are helpful in the diagnosis of the mucopolysaccharidoses, GM1-gangliosidosis, and other disorders.

Biopsies

Biopsies are a valuable additional modality for diagnosis of degenerative neurologic diseases, even though brain biopsies are rarely performed nowadays. Much of the information obtainable by brain biopsy is now obtainable by various peripheral biopsies, which are much more simply performed and at far lower risk. For some disorders, such as the ceroid lipofuscinoses, brain biopsy remains the definitive diagnostic test. In other situations, such as atypical GM2-gangliosidosis, it remains a useful confirmatory test. In other cases, cultured fibroblasts are required for metabolic testing as in Niemann-Pick disease type C.

Rectal biopsy remains useful as both a screening and confirmatory test because it is the simplest and safest source of nerve cell bodies for electron microscopic study. Careful positioning and embedding of the specimen are essential since submucosal ganglion cells are sparse.

Sural nerve biopsy remains useful for electron microscopic study of myelin. Biopsy may be performed at the ankle with skin biopsy or at the calf with skin and muscle biopsy.

Skin biopsy is useful since so many structures such

as sweat glands, hair follicles, blood vessels, and some myelinated nerve fibers can be seen. The procedure is the simplest diagnostic test for Lafora's disease (a form of recessive progressive myoclonus epilepsy), which has characteristic inclusions only in sweat gland duct cells of the skin. The neuronal ceroid lipofuscinoses have curvilinear bodies or fingerprint bodies in multiple cell types in skin.

Bone marrow aspirate can be examined by both light and electron microscopy. This is a useful screening procedure because many lysosomal diseases have foam cells or otherwise distinctive abnormal storage cells in the marrow. Likewise, on peripheral smear, many lysosomal diseases produce vacuoles or abnormal granules in lymphocytes or monocytes, making this a simple and useful, though nonspecific and nondefinitive, screening test.

Conjunctival biopsy is also a useful nonspecific source of tissue for screening ultrastructural studies. Like skin, it contains many different structures and is especially rich in myelinated nerve fibers.

Muscle biopsy is often examined in neuromuscular disorders, but it has also become important in the search for ragged red fibers, which often indicate the presence of a mitochondrial disorder.

Finally, in patients with abnormalities noted at birth, the placenta should not be overlooked as a source of tissue for ultrastructural, biochemical, or molecular study.

UNDIAGNOSED PATIENTS

Although the combination of clinical acumen, genetic evaluation, and intensive laboratory study will result in successful diagnosis for many patients, many cases will remain undiagnosed. Since neurogenetics is a growing and rapidly evolving field, it is important to follow undiagnosed patients at regular but not necessarily frequent intervals. This follow-up, often over years, will be rewarded with successful diagnosis in many of these cases, some of them with new, previously undescribed disorders.

SUGGESTED READING

Bergsma D. Birth defects compendium. 2nd ed. New York: Alan R. Liss, 1979.

Johnson WG, Rapin I. Progressive genetic metabolic diseases. In: Rudolph AM, ed. Pediatrics. 19th ed. Norwalk, CT: Appleton & Lange, 1991:1849.

Jones KL. Smith's recognizable patterns of human malformation: Genetic, embryological, and clinical aspects. 3rd ed. Philadelphia: WB Saunders, 1982.

McKusick VA. Mendelian inheritance in man: Catalogs of autosomal dominant, autosomal recessive, and X-linked phenotypes. (2 vols.) 10th ed. Baltimore: Johns Hopkins University Press, 1992.

Vogel F, Motulsky AG. Human genetics: Problems and approaches. 2nd ed. New York: Springer-Verlag, 1986.

ARNOLD-CHIARI MALFORMATION

NEVILLE W. KNUCKEY, M.D.

Arnold-Chiari malformations are congenital anomalies involving the brain stem and the cerebellum and are associated frequently with hydrosyringomyelia. This chapter considers the Arnold-Chiari malformations as two syndromes based on pathologic anomalies and clinical presentation. The first syndrome presents in childhood and consists of two different pathologic abnormalities: the Arnold-Chiari type 2, characterized by displacement of the brain stem and cerebellum into the upper cervical canal, and the Arnold-Chiari type 3, characterized by displacement of the cerebellum into a high cervical meningocele. Hydrosyringomyelia is estimated to occur in 50 to 80 percent of childhood cases. The second syndrome presents in adulthood and is pathologically characterized as the Arnold-Chiari type 1 by displacement of the cerebellar tonsils into the upper cervical canal with variable displacement of the medulla. Hydrosyringomyelia is variable and estimated to occur in 20 to 75 percent of Arnold-Chiari type 1 cases.

CLINICAL PRESENTATION

Childhood Syndrome

Children have different clinical symptoms depending on their age at presentation. Infant presentation occurs in the first few months of life, usually associated with a myelomeningocele and hydrocephalus repaired at birth. The typical presentation includes stridor, poor feeding, nasal regurgitation, and periods of apnea. Neurologic examination is likely to reveal inspiratory wheeze, depressed gag reflex, vocal cord abductor paralysis, retrocollis, and generalized hypertonia.

A late presentation of the childhood syndrome typically involves a child who is 2 to 5 years old. The child often has a more insidious onset of truncal or limb ataxia. Neurologic examination reveals horizontal and rotatory nystagmus, twelfth nerve palsy, spastic quadriplegia, and truncal ataxia. Spinal examination is essential in order to ascertain the presence of scoliosis.

Adult Syndrome

Adult patients with an Arnold-Chiari malformation usually present with a constellation of symptoms and signs. Most patients have a dominant mode of presentation, however. One is the posterior fossa presentation, which involves compression at the foramen magnum resulting in (1) paroxysmal intracranial hypertension, (2) cerebellar dysfunction, or (3) the foramen magnum compression syndrome. The other dominant presentation involves obstruction of the spinal fluid circulation resulting in hydrocephalus or hydrosyringomyelia. The mean age of presenting adults is 40 years with a slight female predominance. The average duration of symptoms is 3.5 years.

Posterior Fossa Presentation

The posterior fossa presentation results from crowding of the foramen magnum by the cerebellar tonsils with compression of the brain stem and the cerebellum. The first manifestation of this presentation is paroxysmal intracranial hypertension. Patients typically have occipital-cervical headache precipitated by bending forward or coughing. The headache may be associated with vomiting, blurred vision, or dizziness. Neurologic examination is usually normal. Paroxysmal headaches are the principal presenting symptom in 21 percent of patients, but headaches are reported in over 40 to 65 percent of patients.

The second manifestation involves compression of the brain stem resulting in cerebellar dysfunction, with complaints of gait and truncal/limb ataxia. Neurologic examination reveals nystagmus, dysarthria, and limb ataxia. Cerebellar symptoms are the principal presentation in approximately 10 percent of patients, but 30 to 45 percent of patients reveal cerebellar symptoms and signs upon detailed neurologic examination.

The third and most common manifestation is the foramen magnum compression syndrome, which is the presenting symptomatic complex in 38 percent of patients. These patients present with a constellation of headaches, nystagmus, ataxia, dysphagia, and motor weakness. Neurologic examination is variable, with a combination of bulbar, cerebellar, corticospinal, spinothalamic, and dorsal column signs. In these patients a predominantly affected neurologic structure cannot be clinically isolated.

Presentation with Obstruction of the Spinal Fluid Circulation

Hydrosyringomyelia is common in patients with the Arnold-Chiari malformation, resulting from obstruction of the cerebrospinal fluid (CSF) pathways at the foramen magnum. The hydrosyringomyelia syndrome is the principal presenting syndrome in 20 percent of patients, and 60 to 75 percent of patients with the Arnold-Chiari malformation have symptoms or signs of hydrosyringomyelia. The usual symptoms include sensory disturbances such as limb pain or sensory dysesthesias. In 90 percent of patients, neurologic examination reveals sensory changes, most commonly dissociated sensory loss in a cape distribution. Motor weakness is found in over 80 percent of patients, but its distribution is variable. The motor weakness is most commonly associated with upper limb wasting and weakness, but lower limb spasticity is also common. When the hydrosyringomyelic cavity is predominately in the cauda equina, patients may present with lower motor neuron signs and sensory disturbance in the legs. General spinal examination is essential because a scoliosis is found in 30 percent of patients.

Obstruction of the CSF pathways may result in syringobulbia or hydrocephalus. Syringobulbia is the presenting symptom in only 3 percent of cases. However, cranial nerve involvement is found in 25 percent of patients with a hydrosyringomyelic cavity. The ninth to twelfth cranial nerves are most frequently involved. Hydrocephalus is uncommon and is present in only 10 percent of patients.

NEURORADIOLOGIC STUDIES

Neuroradiologic investigations are critical to diagnosis of the Arnold-Chiari malformations (Fig. 1). Sagittal and axial magnetic resonance imaging (MRI) is the investigation of choice. MRI replaces myelography and angiography except in unusual circumstances. MRI with gadolinium is essential to exclude other lesions at the foramen magnum, such as intraosseous tumors (Fig. 2) and abscess. The initial investigations must include cranial and cervical MRI. If the cervical MRI demonstrates cervical hydrosyringomyelia, a thoracic and lumbar MRI scan is indicated. The MRI in an adult patient with an Arnold-Chiari type 1 will demonstrate displacement of the cerebellar tonsil, which has a peglike configuration, below the foramen magnum and decreased CSF around the lower brain stem. Patients with symptomatic Arnold-Chiari malformation always have tonsillar herniation 3 mm below the foramen magnum. Tonsillar displacement of less than 2 mm is not considered significant. Adult patients with a symptomatic Arnold-Chiari malformation and hydrosyringomyelia have an increased incidence of brain stem abnormalities visualized on MRI. These brain stem anomalies are generally not visualized in patients without hydrosyringomyelia. The anomalies include greater tonsillar herniation, low pontomesencephalic junction, and "kinking" of the brain stem.

Careful inspection of the bony architecture of the foramen magnum is required in order to exclude basilar invagination with displacement of the odontoid peg into the foramen magnum. If the bony outline is poorly visualized on MRI, computed tomography visualization of the region is essential. Defining basilar invagination is critical because, when present, surgical posterior fossa decompression is associated with an increased incidence of postoperative complications.

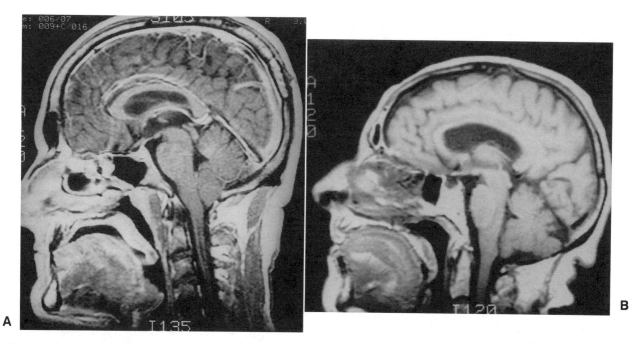

Figure 1 *A,* Cranial magnetic resonance imaging (MRI) showing displacement of the cerebellar tonsils through the foramen magnum with compression of the brain stem. *B,* The normal position of the cerebellar tonsillar above the foramen magnum.

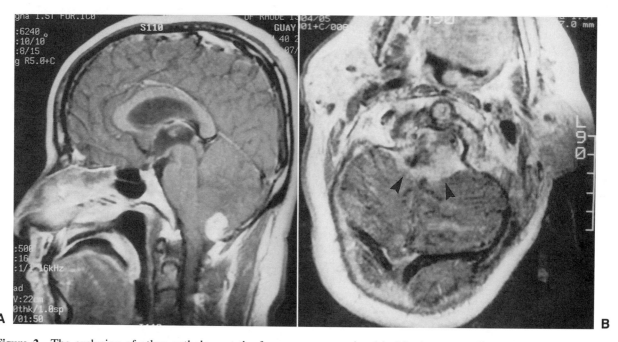

Figure 2 The exclusion of other pathology at the foramen magnum is critical in the correct diagnosis of a patient with Arnold-Chiari malformation. Gadolinium cranial MRI scans show patients with tonsillar hemangioblastoma *(A)* and foramen magnum meningioma *(arrowheads) (B).*

MRI characteristics in children with the Arnold-Chiari type 2 malformation demonstrate beaked colliculi, elongated aqueduct, dilated supracerebellar CSF space, medullary and tonsillar herniation through the foramen magnum, and kinking of the cervicomedullary junction (Fig. 3). The type 2 Arnold-Chiari malformation is frequently associated with anomalies such as agenesis of the corpus callosum and enlargement of the massa intermedia.

High-quality spinal MRI is essential in the diagnosis of hydrosyringomyelia and to help formulate the appropriate operative management. Hydrosyringomyelia is best visualized on T1-weighted axial and sagittal MRI (Fig. 4). The hydrosyringomyelic cavity is demonstrated

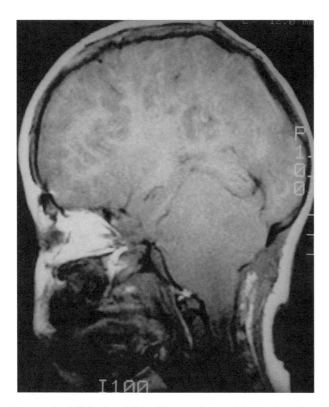

Figure 3 MRI of a child with type 2 Arnold-Chiari malformation shows displacement of the cerebellum and medulla through the foramen magnum.

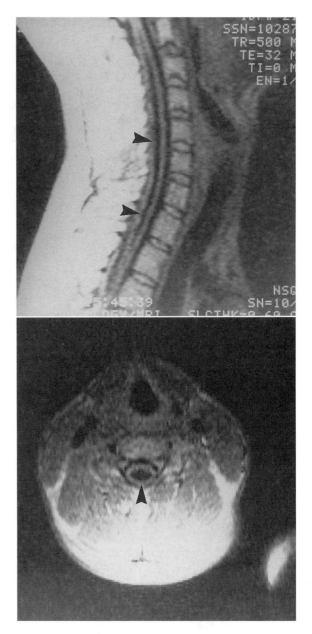

Figure 4 Sagittal and axial MRI scans show cervical hydrosyringomyelia that extends from C1 to the upper thoracic cord.

as a low-intensity area within the spinal cord. The hydrosyringomyelic cavity is frequently eccentrically located toward the posterior horns between the posterior and lateral columns of the spinal cord. While the extent of the hydrosyringomyelic cavity is variable, MRI has demonstrated that it rarely communicates with the fourth ventricle.

Syringobulbia is characterized by thin, irregular, slitlike clefts or cavities within the brain stem. The brain stem cavities are usually continuous with the hydrosyringomyelic cavity, but there is usually no obvious communication with the fourth ventricle. The cavity extends an average of 8 mm above the foramen magnum. Spinal MRI with gadolinium is critical in order to exclude other lesions such as spinal cord tumors.

PITFALLS IN DIAGNOSIS

The principal pitfall in diagnosis of the Arnold-Chiari malformation is a failure to consider and exclude tumors, infection, hemorrhage, and aneurysms that present with foramen magnum symptoms and signs. These lesions are excluded by high-quality MRI with gadolinium. More difficult is the exclusion of multiple sclerosis. Evaluating the patient who has idiopathic dizziness also poses problems. The correct diagnosis of an Arnold-Chiari malformation depends on displacement of the cerebellar tonsils through the foramen magnum by more than 2 mm.

SUGGESTED READING

Barkovich AJ, Wippold FJ, Sherman JL, Citrin CM. Significance of cerebellar tonsillar position on the MR. Am J Neuroradiol 1986; 7:795–799.

Bell WO, Charney EB, Bruce DA, et al. Symptomatic Arnold-Chiari malformation: Review of experience with 22 cases. J Neurosurg 1987; 66:812–816.

Dyste GN, Menezes AH, VanGuilder JC. Symptomatic Chiari malformations: An analysis of presentation, management, and long-term outcome. J Neurosurg 1989; 71:159–168.
Pillay PK, Award IA, Little JR, Hahn JF. Symptomatic Chiari malformation in adults: A new classification based on magnetic resonance imaging with clinical and prognostic significance. Neurosurgery 1991; 28:639–645.
Saez RJ, Onofrio BM, Yanagihara T. Experience with Arnold-Chiari malformation, 1960 to 1970. J Neurosurg 1976; 45:416–422.

AQUEDUCTAL STENOSIS

MARK LUCIANO, M.D., Ph.D.
PETER McL. BLACK, M.D., Ph.D.

The cerebral aqueduct is the cerebrospinal fluid (CSF) passage between the third and fourth ventricles. It is approximately 1.5 cm in length and an average of 0.8 mm^2 in cross-sectional area in the adult and 0.5 mm^2 in the child. Although its diameter is quite variable, it is usually more than large enough to conduct CSF from the third to the fourth ventricle. When it is sufficiently narrowed or occluded, however, an obstructive pattern of hydrocephalus develops in which the lateral and third ventricles dilate while the fourth ventricle remains relatively normal. Complete obstruction may sometimes lead to a "blow-out" of the ventricular walls of the third ventricle, which can restore CSF circulation. However, untreated complete stenosis can also result in death because of progressive hydrocephalus.

Noncommunicating, or "triventricular," hydrocephalus, with CSF building up behind an aqueductal stenosis, is often contrasted with generalized ventriculomegaly resulting from a "communicating hydrocephalus," where there is decreased CSF absorption around the base of the brain or convexities. In practice, however, communicating and noncommunicating hydrocephalus may not be so easily separated, because anatomic changes resulting from a communicating hydrocephalus may eventually cause aqueductal stenosis. This changes communicating hydrocephalus into noncommunicating hydrocephalus. The two types of hydrocephalus may also coexist in varying degrees. This has practical implications for both diagnosis and treatment.

Aqueductal stenosis may be classified as congenital or acquired. Congenital aqueductal stenosis is a narrowing or forking of the aqueduct, either alone or in association with Arnold-Chiari malformation, Dandy Walker syndrome, X-linked hydrocephalus, or other disorders. With improved magnetic resonance imaging (MRI) techniques, some cases believed to be idiopathic congenital aqueductal stenosis are now known to result from small, previously undetected periaqueductal tumors such as low-grade astrocytomas (Fig. 1). This is especially true in patients with onset of symptoms in early

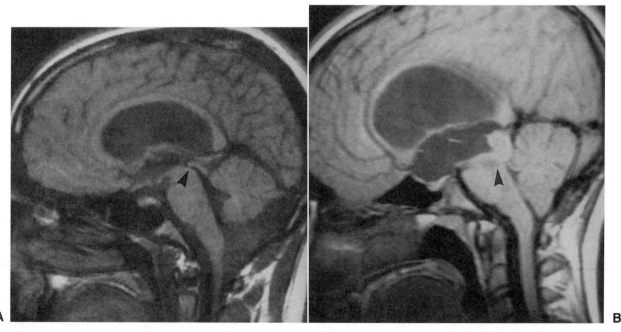

Figure 1 T1 weighted sagittal MRI scans of patients presenting in the second decade with headache and papilledema. *A*, Partial proximal stenosis. *B*, A tectal tumor with high-grade stenosis and dramatic enlargement of the third ventricle.

adulthood. Some instances of aqueductal stenosis may also arise from a postinflammatory gliotic membrane.

Acquired aqueductal stenosis may result from bacterial infections (ventriculitis), congenital toxoplasmosis, viral illnesses such as mumps, or, less frequently, intraventricular hemorrhage. It may also occur secondary to mechanical obstruction by a brain stem or pineal region tumor or from a vascular malformation such as a vein of Galen aneurysm.

DIAGNOSIS

Clinical Presentation

Patients with aqueductal stenosis may present in infancy, childhood, or adulthood. Congenital forms appear most often in the first 3 months of life, with a second peak of occurrence at 3 years. Late onset "congenital" aqueductal stenosis develops in childhood or young adulthood with gradual obstruction of the aqueduct. Adult forms usually present in early adulthood with subtle symptomatology. Overall, aqueductal stenosis presents later than communicating hydrocephalus in the pediatric age group. There is no male versus female predominance.

The presenting symptoms are those of increased intracranial pressure. Headache, lethargy, and nausea are common initial symptoms. Paralysis of downward gaze and abducens palsies are also seen. These may rapidly progress to coma because this form of hydrocephalus is less well tolerated than communicating forms, perhaps because of the steep intracranial pressure gradient or the more rapid rate of onset.

Because the third ventricle may be severely affected in aqueductal stenosis, symptoms related to hypothalamic dysfunction can also occur. Presenting endocrine symptoms such as amenorrhea, obesity, diabetes insipidus, precocious puberty, acromegaly, and dwarfism have been reported. Rarely, visual acuity can also be affected through pressure on the optic chiasm by enlargement of the third ventricle.

Clinical Tests

The diagnosis of aqueductal stenosis can be readily made with contemporary imaging techniques. Computed tomography (CT) scan shows large lateral and third ventricles with a normal or only slightly enlarged fourth ventricle. MRI with gadolinium is useful for the detection of small periaqueductal masses. When available, MR flow imaging may demonstrate increased turbulence in the aqueduct or total cessation of flow. Volumetric imaging reveals considerably larger lateral and third ventricles than fourth.

A lumbar puncture is not needed and is not advisable because of the risk of downward herniation. A ventriculostomy reveals elevated lateral ventricular pressures but is not usually performed for diagnostic purposes. It may, rarely, be needed for emergent decompression.

Further Evaluation

Determination of the cause of aqueductal stenosis is important in determining appropriate treatment and follow-up. Underlying causes may require specific treatment. For example, a recent ventriculitis or intraventricular hemorrhage may explain the onset of obstructive hydrocephalus, and a period of time for the treatment of infection or hemorrhage may be required before definitive shunting. In some cases, MRI may suggest a vascular malformation requiring arteriogram and subsequent treatment such as radiosurgery or endovascular embolization.

It is important to rule out a tectal neoplasm as the cause of aqueductal stenosis. This is especially true in any patient with late onset aqueductal stenosis (child or young adult) without other apparent cause. Gadolinium-enhanced MRI has effectively demonstrated these tumors and is useful in following these patients. Biopsy may ultimately be required, but this carries significant risk. A rule we have found helpful is to biopsy a lesion that appears extrinsic and larger than 1 cm. Smaller lesions may be followed with MRI studies every 6 months to 1 year. If they do not increase in size, treatment of the hydrocephalus may be all that is required. If the tumors expand or become more symptomatic by disordering eye movements, they may be biopsied or debulked. Most often these masses are low-grade astrocytomas or gliomas. Depending on the age of the child and the biopsy result, radiation treatment, including radiosurgery, stereotactic radiotherapy, or chemotherapy may be indicated.

CSF DIVERSION

Although the primary treatment for hydrocephalus is CSF diversion via shunt placement, not all ventriculomegaly needs to be shunted. Some patients present with large ventricles consistent with aqueductal stenosis but without any obvious symptoms or signs of increased pressure. Large ventricles and thinned cortex are not always the result of acute pressure compression but may be due to previous insult and not reversible by CSF diversion. Misguided CSF diversion in these asymptomatic patients can result in ventricular collapse, resulting in subdural hematomas and symptomatic central nervous system compression. To avoid inappropriate shunting in questionably symptomatic patients with large ventricles, we obtain a better idea of the intracranial pressure through continuous monitoring with a fiber-optic subdural bolt. If there are no pressure waves, observation without shunting is the best approach.

OUTCOME

With effective shunting, patients with aqueductal stenosis can do very well. More than half of the patients will be independent and able to work, with perhaps some cognitive neurologic deficit. Giuffre et al reported that

35 percent of nontumor cases shunted in infancy did well, and 24 percent had residual deficits. Cagnoni et al found that 61 percent of patients were working at follow-up. Endocrine problems often resolve after shunting. Generally, patients diagnosed when they are older than 1 to 2 years have a better outcome. The prognosis also depends on the severity of presenting hydrocephalus and its response to shunting. It has been suggested that a frontal cortical mantle width less than 3 cm after shunt placement predicts a significant residual neurologic deficit. Prompt recognition and treatment of aqueductal stenosis is essential to a potentially good outcome.

Acknowledgment. Pat Barnes provided the MRI scans shown here.

SUGGESTED READING

Cagnoni G, Guizzardi G, Giardina F, Mennonna P. Follow up and surgical considerations on a series of patients operated on for non tumoral aqueductal stenosis. J Neurosurg Sci 1986; 30:77–79.
Giuffre R, Palma L, Fontana M. Infantile nontumoral aqueductal stenosis. J Neurosurg Sci 1986; 30:41–46.
Hanigan WC, Morgan A, Shaaban A, Bradle P. Surgical treatment and long-term neurodevelopmental outcome for infants with idiopathic aqueductal stenosis. Childs Nerv Syst 1991; 7:386–390.
Jellinger G. Non tumoral aqueductal stenosis. J Neurosurg Sci 1986; 30:1–16.
Rotilio A, d'Avella D, de Blasi F, et al. Disendocrine manifestations during non tumoral aqueductal stenosis. J Neurosurg Sci 1986; 30:7–76.
Steinbock P, Boyd MC. periaqueductal tumor as a cause of late-onset aqueductal stenosis. Childs Nerv Syst 1987; 3:170–174.

CEREBROVASCULAR DISEASE IN THE NEWBORN

JOELLE MAST, M.D., Ph.D.

Cerebrovascular disease in the neonate, as in older patients, can be divided into ischemic and hemorrhagic injuries. The cause of cerebrovascular disease in the neonate differs from that in older patients because of hazards unique to intrauterine development, labor and delivery, and especially to entering the world prematurely. Because of the immaturity of the nervous system, clinical presentation also differs. The expression of cortical damage is incomplete. For example, spasticity may not become apparent for weeks. Focal injuries do not necessarily result in lateralized signs, and lateralized signs may not reflect a focal injury. Thus, localization based on the physical examination alone is difficult, if not impossible. Consequently, there is increased reliance on ancillary tests. As in older patients, history provides major diagnostic clues. In the case of the neonate, maternal history, details of labor and delivery, and gestational age are necessary components of the history. This chapter will discuss the types of ischemic and hemorrhagic injuries found in the neonatal population, with emphasis on clinical diagnosis.

ISCHEMIA

In both premature and full-term infants, the most common cause of nonhemorrhagic cerebrovascular disease is a diffuse injury such as hypoxic-ischemic injury in the perinatal period. This frequently results in diffuse brain damage. However, it is also the leading cause of focal stroke in newborns. Other causes of neonatal stroke are embolic or thrombotic events. Because of its importance, diffuse hypoxic/ischemic injury will be discussed separately from other causes of cerebrovascular disease.

Hypoxic-Ischemic Injury

Cause

Hypoxic-ischemic injury accounts for 20 percent of all perinatal deaths. Most cases occur either prenatally or during labor and are secondary to placental insufficiency. Associated factors include maternal hypertension, vascular disease, drug use (such as cocaine), maternal hypotension or hypoxia, infection, or physical causes such as umbilical cord compression or placental abruption.

Clinical Findings

The typical history is that of an infant with poor Apgar scores who requires resuscitation, ventilation, and pressor support at birth. It is important to keep in mind that infants who have not been asphyxiated may have low Apgar scores. By themselves, Apgars do not reveal anything about the nature of injury, its duration, or (except in the extreme) its severity. With very low Apgars that are carried out for 10 minutes or more, such as 0, 1, and 2, the prognosis is poor. High Apgars, such as 9 and 10, are a reliable sign that an infant has not suffered significant hypoxic-ischemic insult in the perinatal period.

Clinically, there is a dynamic progression in the examination of an infant who has suffered significant hypoxia-ischemia (Table 1). The exam at 0 to 12 hours reveals depressed nervous function. Seizures, taking the form of posturing and tonic seizures in pre-term and clonic seizures in full-term infants, may occur at 6 to 12 hours. Organ system failure is often apparent. At 12 to 24 hours, the neonate frequently shows increased alertness. Jitteriness and autonomic hyperactivity are common. Lethargy during this time period is a poor prognostic sign. Seizures are common and difficult to control. It is important to differentiate seizures from jitteriness. The latter will be altered by passive restraint or by extension or flexion at a joint, whereas seizure activity will be unaffected. Deterioration occurs at 24 to 72 hours coincident with maximal cerebral edema. Seizures, if present, may be difficult to control. Involvement of other organ systems typically improves, while continued involvement of other systems, such as the presence of oliguria beyond 36 hours, is a poor prognostic sign.

Diagnostic Tests

The neonate, especially the premature infant, has a very limited exam. Infants less than 28 weeks gestational age may lack pupillary responses as well as primitive reflexes such as the Moro or palmar grasp. Even the term infant functions at a predominantly brain stem level. Because of this, ancillary tests play a key role in neonatal neurology. The electroencephalogram (EEG) is a measure of cerebral activity. In a *term* infant, EEG changes parallel the time course of cerebral swelling and also the degree of encephalopathy. Early on, or with mild asphyxia, voltage reduction and slowing are common. At 24 hours, or with moderate asphyxia, a burst suppression pattern is frequently seen. At the height of edema, or with severe asphyxia, there may be marked attenuation of background or electrocerebral silence. Long-term, the EEG may reflect ongoing cerebral dysfunction or epileptiform activity. With focal injury, the EEG may show focal slowing or voltage reduction over the affected area. Focal epileptiform activity may also be seen.

Prognostically, background is more important than epileptiform activity. Infants with a history of hypoxia whose EEG has a normal background, except for the presence of rhythmic delta frontally or multifocal sharp waves, usually suffer no sequelae. The EEG of the *premature* infant is less sensitive to hypoxia. In fact, an abnormal EEG in a premature infant with a history of recent hypoxia suggests that other injuries such as intraventricular hemorrhage are present.

Radiologic studies identify the extent and nature of cerebral injury, distinguishing hemorrhage from infarction. Acute hypoperfusion affecting the parasaggital area or the deep gray or periventricular white matter may show increased echos on head ultrasonography (HUS). With swelling, slitlike ventricles are apparent on HUS and the entire brain may take on a bright appearance. Real-time HUS may demonstrate changes in arterial pulsations in blood vessels within the lesion. After 2 weeks, encephalomalacia secondary to infarction and tissue destruction should be evident.

Computed tomography (CT) is preferred to evaluate the brain parenchyma because HUS may miss focal areas of infarction. Immediately after the insult, CT may be normal. However, at 2 to 4 days, abnormalities such as loss of gray-white junction, areas of patchy hypodensity in the white matter, diffuse hypodensity of the hemispheres with sparing of the cerebellum, and, occasionally, high density in the central gray matter may be apparent. With severe hypoxic injury, hyperdensity outlining the gyri may be seen. This reflects cortical necrosis. Cortical volume loss will usually be evident by 10 to 14 days. Particular neuropathologic patterns and their long-term clinical correlates are listed in Table 2.

Magnetic resonance imaging (MRI) is superior to both HUS and CT in evaluating parenchymal lesions in term infants. However, in most medical centers MRI is difficult to perform on an emergency basis. CT is also preferred because of the ease of monitoring unstable patients in the scanner. In term infants, MRI reveals the same stages of infarction seen in older patients. Imaging may have important legal implications in terms of estimating a lesion's age. An MRI or CT performed early may show that the insult occurred in utero and was the *cause,* rather than the *result,* of low Apgars. Intravascular enhancement is seen in the first 2 days after injury. Meningeal enhancement may also be apparent by day 2 or 3. Parenchymal enhancement occurs last, on day 5 to 7. This is due to a damaged blood-brain barrier and assumes two patterns: cortical or subcortical gyriform enhancement, and wedge-shaped transcortical enhancement.

CT and MRI are not as sensitive for parenchymal lesions in infants less than 35 weeks gestational age because of poor myelination. However, serial MRI studies are very useful in evaluating the development of myelination and gyration in infants born prematurely.

Evoked potential tests are less useful. Normal sensory evoked potentials and brain stem auditory evoked potentials are correlated with good outcome.

Table 1 Hypoxic-Ischemic Encephalopathy: Clinical Findings (All Need Not Be Present)

0–12 hours	12–24 hours	24–72 hours
Lethargy	Hypervigilance	Stupor
Irregular respirations	Irregular respirations	Irregular respirations or apnea
Reactive pupils	Reactive, dilated pupils	Sluggish or nonreactive pupils
Ophthalmoplegia	Ophthalmoplegia	Ophthalmoplegia
Extensor posturing	Extensor posturing	Extensor posturing
Seizures (6–12 h)	Seizures	Seizures
Major organ involvement	Organ involvement	Improvement of other organs
DTRs present	DTRs present	DTRs depressed-absent

DTRs = deep tendon reflexes.

Table 2 Neuropathologic Patterns Seen After Hypoxia-Ischemia

Pattern	Age	Location	Clinical Outcome
Parasaggital infarction	Term	Parasaggital cortex (posterior > anterior)	Spastic quadriparesis (proximal > distal), possible developmental delay, learning disability
Selective neuronal necrosis	Term	Hippocampus, Purkinje cells in cortical layers III, V, VI	Spastic or hypotonic quadriparesis, developmental delay, bulbar or pseudobulbar palsy
	Preterm	Inferior olives, pons, subiculum	Same as term
Status marmoratus	Term	Thalamus, basal ganglia	Choreoathetosis, developmental delay
Periventricular leukomalacia	Preterm	Periventricular white matter	Spastic diplegia, developmental delay
Focal ischemic necrosis	Term	Variable	Spastic mono-, hemi-, di-, or quadriparesis, developmental delay
	Preterm	Variable	Same as term

Adapted from Volpe JJ. Intraventricular hemorrhage in the premature infant—current concepts: Part II Ann Neurol 1989; 25:106–116; with permission.

Abnormal studies that improve with time are also encouraging.

Prognosis

Neonates are relatively resistant to hypoxic damage. The majority (60 to 80 percent) are neurologically normal, but 10 to 20 percent die, and 10 to 20 percent have permanent sequelae. The presence of hypoxic-ischemic encephalopathy (HIE) is somewhat predictive. If infants show no neurologic symptoms after birth, it is very unlikely they will have any long-term neurologic sequelae. Even with mild encephalopathy, sequelae are very uncommon. With moderate HIE, approximately 20 to 25 percent will have some morbidity such as spasticity, seizure disorder, or developmental delay. Severely affected infants with diffuse, bilateral cerebral injury, if they live, will have microcephaly, spastic quadriparesis, and severe developmental delay. Duration of neurologic abnormalities is also predictive. If neurologic signs persist past 2 weeks, the prognosis is worse. Other factors associated with poor outcome are listed in Table 3. Despite the presence of seizures in the Table, the majority of infants with seizures following a hypoxic-ischemic episode are normal at age 7 years. In general, serial EEG studies documenting improvement and normal development of background activity suggest a good prognosis regardless of the age of the infant.

HUS will frequently show areas of parenchymal echodensity. If these are persistent and bilateral, they are associated with neurologic sequelae. Parenchymal echodensities shaped like flares and disappearing by 10 days are not associated with any morbidity. Bilateral diffuse injuries on CT or MRI are associated with poor outcome. It is difficult to predict the nature of sequelae with unilateral focal lesions.

Focal Infarction: Thrombotic and Embolic Injury

Cause

With the increased survival in neonatal intensive care units and improved radiologic capabilities, more

Table 3 Poor Prognostic Factors Following a Hypoxic-Ischemic Event

Apgars less than or equal to 6 at 5 minutes
Need for ventilatory support beyond 5 minutes
Seizures in the first 6 hours of life
Seizures lasting more than 30 minutes
Seizures persisting beyond 72 hours despite treatment
Tonic or myoclonic seizures

cases of cerebral vascular disease secondary to thrombus or embolus are being reported. Embolic and thrombotic causes of stroke are listed in Table 4. Infants born to mothers with lupus or with anticardiolipin antibody may have infarction secondary to hyperviscosity. Arterial infarction has been associated with deficiencies of proteins S and C and of antithrombin III.

Clinical Findings

Examination in an infant with a focal cerebral injury is usually nonspecific. There may be increased lethargy, hypotonia, poor feeding, or decreased suck and root. Rarely, a mild hemiparesis may be evident on close examination. Focal seizures, although nonspecific, are a valuable warning sign. In the term infant, focal clonic jerking is the most common seizure type. However, subtle seizures such as eye deviation are reported. These are frequently accompanied by other manifestations of seizures such as focal tonic seizures. History provides clues to the diagnosis, as does physical examination. For example, limb ischemia at birth is correlated with cerebral thrombosis.

Diagnostic Tests

The majority of infants with focal infarcts do not have focal seizures. However, even fewer have focal clinical signs, making EEG an important diagnostic tool. *In term infants, repetitive lateralized motor seizures should raise the suspicion of focal injury.* This is especially true if there is normal background activity and focal electro-

Table 4 Causes of Stroke in Neonates

Embolic	Thombotic
Placental tissue	Trauma to vessels
Congenital heart disease	Polycythemia
Twin-to-twin transfusion	Hyperviscosity
Vessel thrombus	Tumor/infection
	Coagulation anomalies

graphic abnormalities on the corresponding side. These take the form of voltage attenuation and focal slowing. Increased sharp waves may be seen overlying the affected areas.

HUS may be normal or show nonspecific, diffuse increased echogenicity. Real-time echo may reveal decreased flow through a major vessel. CT is sensitive 24 hours after injury. If no lesion is seen on an early CT and the patient has focal seizures, the CT should be repeated or an MRI performed. MRI provides the most information about age of the lesion and subsequent development.

Prognosis

Prognostically, focal lesions in the neonate result in less morbidity than similar lesions in older patients. The motor strip is vulnerable, but lesions in regions such as the frontal lobe may not be clinically evident. This is presumably due to the plasticity of the developing brain.

HEMORRHAGE

The epidemiology of intracranial hemorrhage has changed in recent years. Hemorrhage due to peri- or intraventricular hemorrhage (PIVH) has increased because more premature infants are surviving. Hemorrhage due to trauma has decreased because obstetric practice has improved.

Periventricular Hemorrhage

Cause

PIVH is most common in premature infants weighing less than 1,500 grams. Bleeding occurs in the subependymal tissue of the germinal matrix overlying the head of the caudate. The pathogenesis of PIVH is related to the anatomy of the area and to changes in intravascular inflow and outflow that occur in the premature infant. The germinal matrix is a highly vascularized capillary bed fed by the anterior and middle cerebral arteries, penetrating branches of the meningeal arteries, and the anterior choroidal branch of the internal carotid artery. The vessels in the germinal matrix lack a muscular coat and are prone to rupture with increases in arterial or venous pressure. Venous drainage flows anteriorly to the head of the caudate, where it joins the internal vein and then turns posteriorly

to join the vein of Galen. The site of most intraventricular hemorrhages in premature infants is adjacent to this turning point. It should be noted that in infants less than 28 weeks gestational age, the mass of the germinal matrix is located posteriorly, and consequently most hemorrhages in this age group occur over the body of the caudate. In term infants, most intraventricular hemorrhages occur within the choroid plexus.

Intraventricular hemorrhage is classified according to severity. There are multiple grading systems. Grade I hemorrhage is confined to the subependymal region. Grades II and III represent more severe degrees of intraventricular hemorrhage, with dilatation of the ventricles in III. Grade IV, if used, refers to hemorrhage into the parenchyma as well as intraventricular hemorrhage.

Parenchymal hemorrhage in the setting of PIVH is most common in premature infants less than 34 weeks gestational age (20 to 25 percent in major centers). The younger the infant, the greater the incidence of PIVH. In infants less than 700 grams, 60 percent have major intraventricular bleeds. Between 26 and 34 weeks, the germinal matrix undergoes a dramatic involution, virtually disappearing by 36 weeks. The parenchymal hemorrhage usually represents hemorrhagic infarction, bleeding into an area that has suffered a prior hypoxic-ischemic insult. This typically occurs at the angle where the medullary veins converge to join the terminal vein.

PIVH is associated with fluctuating cerebral blood flow (CBF). Autoregulation of CBF is tenuous and is easily lost with hypercarbia and hypoxemia. Hypotension accompanying asphyxia leads to decreased CBF. Treatment of hypotension with volume re-expansion increases CBF and may predispose to hemorrhage within damaged areas. Increases in CBF are also associated with labor, increased PCO_2, ligation of patent ductus arteriosus, pneumothorax, seizures, ECMO, and noxious procedures such as tracheal suctioning and abdominal examination. Increased venous pressure accompanies labor and is exacerbated by asphyxia and respiratory distress. In addition, large fluctuations in CBF occur on a second-to-second basis in infants with respiratory distress. Most of the time, these occur in intubated, nonparalysed infants who are breathing against the ventilator. Evidence suggests that paralysis may decrease the incidence of PIVH in these infants.

Clinical Findings

The majority of PIVH occurs within the first 72 hours of life. In the very premature (less than 700 grams), the time frame is broader—the first 18 hours to 14 days of life. Clinical presentation falls into three categories. The *catastrophic syndrome* presents as a sudden deterioration in status with hypotension, bulging fontanel, respiratory disturbances or apnea, stupor, sluggish or absent pupils, absent oculocephalic reflexes, decerebrate posturing, seizures, and flaccidity. A drop in hematocrit often accompanies this. Prognosis is very poor. The *saltatory syndrome* presents as a decrease in level of consciousness, activity, and muscle tone. Deterioration may take place over a period of hours to days in a stepwise progression. Eye movement abnormalities and respiratory disturbances may be present. *Silent bleeds* may account for 25 to 50 percent of PIVH in neonatal intensive care units. These are usually diagnosed on routine HUS.

Intraventricular hemorrhage in the term infant has a broad range of onset, from the first few days to weeks of life. Infants typically become irritable and jittery. They may develop seizures. Intraventricular hemorrhage of any cause can lead to obstruction of CSF outflow, resulting in obstructive hydrocephalus and also to an obliterative arachnoiditis resulting in communicating hydrocephalus. This can present as full fontanel, enlarging head circumference, or apnea.

Diagnostic Tests

Laboratory diagnosis of PIVH is typically made by HUS. These studies should be performed in the first 3 days of life and repeated at 2 weeks in infants at risk. This enables early detection of bleeds and ensures that later bleeds will also be picked up. Correction of any coagulopathy is essential. All high-risk infants should have daily head circumferences. In addition, serial HUS studies are necessary because a significant amount of ventricular enlargement can occur in the absence of any change in head circumference. HUS is noninvasive and ideal for following ventricular size. CT or MRI should be performed if there is a suggestion of parenchymal involvement or in any infant with focal findings on exam, focal seizures, or a focal EEG.

Prognosis

Prognosis is related to the grade of PIVH. The presence and extent of intraparenchymal hemorrhage is predictive of short-term outcome. Long-term prediction is less certain. If parenchymal damage is bilateral and extensive, the infant will suffer major neurologic sequelae. With focal small bleeds, sequelae are variable. Morbidity with PIVH is also related to hydrocephalus and intraparenchymal damage secondary to ischemia.

Hemorrhage Other Than PIVH

Cause

Trauma, aneurysms, arteriovenous malformations (AVMs), hypertension, tumor, and bleeding disorders also cause parenchymal hemorrhage in neonates. Subdural hemorrhage, now relatively rare, is seen after traumatic birth. It is more common in term infants than in neonates. Risk factors are rapid labor, cephalopelvic disproportion, and breech or face-brow presentation. In addition, subdural hemorrhage is associated with extreme molding, either vertical or fronto-occipital. Therefore, any abnormal clinical sign in the setting of extreme molding should alert the clinician to the possibility of subdural hemorrhage.

Subarachnoid hemorrhage (SAH), unrelated to intraventricular hemorrhage, and spontaneous parenchymal hemorrhage are more common in premature than full-term infants. Both are associated with birth trauma and also with hypoxia. Intraparenchymal hemorrhage in the neonate is most often cerebellar. One reason for this is the compliant skull of the infant. Pressure during delivery, resuscitation, or care-taking results in forward motion of the squamous bone causing a tentorial tear and sometimes a cerebellar laceration. Another reason is that the cerebellum has a capillary bed in the folia, subpial, and external granule layers that is similar to the germinal matrix. This is vulnerable to trauma and the changes in CBF that accompany hypoxia.

Hypertension is also associated with cerebral hemorrhage. It should be noted that infants with coarctation of the aorta have been reported with cerebral hemorrhages due to hypertension that is relatively mild. Aneurysms are also associated with coarctation and may be the source of bleeding. The location of aneurysms is the same as in older patients.

AVMs that present as hemorrhage in the neonatal period typically involve the vein of Galen. Infants with vein of Galen AVMs usually have high-output cardiac failure. There may be obstructive hydrocephalus. Infarction, either bland or hemorrhagic, can occur secondary to a "steal" phenomenon.

Tumors presenting in the neonatal period and associated with hemorrhage are: teratomas, gliomas, and medulloblastomas. In the neonatal period, as opposed to childhood, the majority of tumors are supratentorial.

Coagulation disorders include disseminated intravascular coagulation, thrombocytopenia of any cause (maternal, drug-induced, infection), and deficiencies of coagulation factors (hemophilia, liver disease, vitamin K deficiency, maternal drug use). Anticonvulsants associated with hematologic abnormalities include Dilantin, primidone, methsuximide, and phenobarbital. Vitamin K should be given 24 hours prior to delivery if a mother is taking any of these drugs.

Clinical Findings

Clinical presentation of other types of hemorrhage depends upon location. With subdural hemorrhages involving tentorial tears, there is posterior fossa compression. Some patients may rapidly develop stupor, skew deviation of the eyes, abnormal pupillary reflexes, irregular respirations, and other signs of brain stem compression. Others present less dramatically with irritability or lethargy and the slow development of a bulging fontanel from outflow obstruction, or a seventh nerve palsy. Subdurals over the convexity may be asymptomatic, or the patient may be hyperalert. With expansion of the bleed, focal signs such as a hemiparesis or pupillary asymmetry will develop.

Infants with SAH are usually asymptomatic except for seizures and irritability. Rarely, the bleed is large enough to result in decreased hematocrit and hypovolemia. SAH can be complicated by hydrocephalus secondary to arachnoiditis.

The presentation of parenchymal hemorrhage will depend on the location of the bleed. Cerebellar hemorrhage, the most common site in the neonate, is characterized by flaccidity, tonic posturing, and brain stem signs such as respiratory irregularities, skew deviation, and facial palsy.

Diagnostic Tests

Lumbar puncture (LP) is indicated in any infant with a deterioration in status of unclear cause. [Although rare, herniation does occur in neonates. Therefore, an infant with focal or brain stem signs should not have an LP until CT or MRI is performed.] As in adults, a CSF profile of elevated protein, hypoglycorrachia, and increased red blood cells is expected with SAH or intraventricular hemorrhage. The hypoglycorrachia takes a few days to develop in the neonate and lasts for weeks. It is probably secondary to decreased glucose transport into the CSF. HUS is not the test of choice prior to CT, because it may miss hemorrhages that occur in the posterior fossa or over the convexities. MRI is the most sensitive tool for evaluating the parenchyma. However, difficulty monitoring vital signs may preclude its use in an unstable patient. EEG frequently reflects focality with voltage attenuation, slowing, or epileptiform activity over the damaged area.

Prognosis

Once again, prognosis depends upon the amount of parenchymal damage.

COMMENTS

Cerebrovascular disease in the neonate is usually due to a perinatal event rather than an ongoing disease process. A careful history will usually suggest the cause of the disorder. The result is usually a static motor deficit, fitting the definition of cerebral palsy. Depending on the extent of injury, some degree of developmental delay may result. Since neonates have an immature central nervous system, the full extent of neurologic damage can only be appreciated over time. Because of limitations in the examination of a neonate, ancillary tests are usually necessary for confirmation of diagnosis and for prognosis. However, the key to prognosis is change. The physical exam should be consistently developing with time. Corresponding changes should be present on EEG and MRI. Thus, serial studies from different modalities are very useful. Lack of change suggests underlying damage and calls for further evaluation to delineate any special needs the child may have.

SUGGESTED READING

Allan WC, Riviello JJ. Perinatal cerebrovascular disease in the neonate: Parenchymal ischemic lesions in term and preterm infants. Pediatr Clin North Am 1992; 39:621–650.

Clancy R, Malin S, Laraque D, et al. Focal motor seizures heralding stroke in full-term neonates. Am J Dis Child 1985; 139:601–606.

Hill A, Martin DJ, Daneman A, Fitz CR. Focal ischemic cerebral injury in the newborn: Diagnosis by ultrasound and correlation with computed tomographic scan. Pediatrics 1983; 71:790–793.

Mannino FL, Trauner DA. Stroke in neonates. J Pediatr 1983; 102:605–610.

Mantovani JF, Gerber GJ. "Idiopathic" neonatal cerebral infarction. Am J Dis Child 1984; 138:359–362.

McArdle CB, Richardson CJ, Hayden CK, et al. Abnormalities of the neonatal brain: MR imaging. AJNR Am J Neuroradiol 1987; 163:395–403.

Ment LR, Duncan CC, Ehrenkranz RA. Perinatal cerebral infarction. Ann Neurol 1984; 16:559–568.

Sarnat HB, Sarnat MS. Neonatal encephalopathy following fetal distress: A clinical and electroencephalographic study. Arch Neurol 1976; 33:696–705.

Volpe JJ. Intraventricular hemorrhage in the premature infant—current concepts: Parts I and II. Ann Neurol 1989; 25:3–11, 109–116.

PHAKOMATOSES

ALLAN E. RUBENSTEIN, M.D.

The term *phakomatosis* was coined by Van der Hoeve from the Greek "Phakos," which has a number of meanings, including birthmark. The term refers to disorders in which abnormal growth potential exists primarily in ectodermally derived tissue. For phakomatoses that have skin lesions, *neurocutaneous syndrome* is a more descriptive term. The phakomatoses additionally include genetically determined familial cancer syndromes involving neural tissues, such as von Hippel-Lindau disease. This chapter focuses on the most common of the phakomatoses: neurofibromatosis 1 and 2, tuberous sclerosis, von Hippel-Lindau disease, and Sturge-Weber syndrome.

NEUROFIBROMATOSIS

The disorder, originally described by Von Recklinghausen in 1882, is now termed neurofibromatosis type 1

(NF-1). NF-2 refers to a separate genetic disorder characterized by bilateral vestibular schwannomas, meningiomas, and spinal cord neurofibromas, previously known as central NF. NF-1 is frequently mentioned as the "Elephant Man's" disease, though substantial evidence has been available for at least 5 years to demonstrate that the so-called Elephant Man did not have NF but probably had Proteus syndrome.

NF-1 is by far the most common of the neurocutaneous syndromes, with an incidence of 30 to 40 per 100,000 live births. There is no known racial, geographic, or ethnic predilection. NF-1 is an autosomal dominant disorder with a sporadic mutation rate of approximately 50 percent, which is probably due to the large size of the NF-1 gene. There is substantial variability of expression. Nonpenetrance is almost unheard of.

In 1987, a National Institutes of Health consensus conference developed inclusive clinical criteria for the diagnosis of NF-1 (Table 1). No single sign of NF-1 is pathognomonic. Individuals who meet only one of the criteria should be considered NF-1 suspects and followed as such. Café-au-lait spots may be present at birth or develop up to approximately age 7 (Fig. 1). Examination of the skin with an ultraviolet (Wood's) lamp is useful in identifying subtle pigmentation in light-skinned individuals. Numerous conditions may be associated with café-au-lait spots (Table 2), though typically less than six are present in these disorders. Many normal individuals have one to three café-au-lait spots. A recent study of 41 children with six or more café-au-lait spots showed that signs of NF-1 eventually developed in 24 (59 percent).

Axillary or groin freckling is relatively specific to NF-1 (Fig. 2). It can be present at birth but typically develops later in childhood. In children with multiple café-au-lait spots, axillary or groin freckles are the most common feature to appear to confirm the diagnosis of NF-1. Occasionally diffuse freckling of the entire torso appears in NF-1.

Dermal neurofibromas typically appear in late childhood or adolescence. They usually present as small lumps under the surface of the skin, often with a pinkish or purplish color. When they become larger, they may be pedunculated, which is often the case in adults (Fig. 3).

Plexiform neurofibromas are large, isolated lesions, which often grow along peripheral nerves or nerve roots. Plexiform neurofibromas are often congenital and may be quite disfiguring due to associated regional hypertrophy and overlying pigmentation (Fig. 4). Isolated dermal and spinal root neurofibromas may be seen in the absence of the NF-1 gene. Plexiform neurofibromas are more specific.

When dermal neurofibromas appear in association with other signs of NF-1, it is usually not necessary to obtain pathologic confirmation of the diagnosis. Xan-

Table 2 Conditions Associated with Mutiple Café-au-Lait Spots

Neurofibromatosis type 2
Polyostotic fibrous dysplasia
Tuberous sclerosis
Multiple mucosal neuroma syndrome
Bloom's syndrome
Ataxia telangiectasia
Fanconi's anemia
Multiple lentigines syndrome
Russell-Silver syndrome
Bannayan-Riley-Ruvalcaba syndrome
Manffucci's syndrome
Jaffe-Campanacci syndrome

Table 1 Diagnosis of Neurofibromatosis Type 1*

1. Six or more café-au-lait macules over 5 mm in greatest diameter in prepubertal individuals and over 15 mm in greatest diameter in postpubertal individuals
2. Freckling in the axillary or inguinal regions
3. Two or more neurofibromas of any type or one plexiform neurofibroma
4. Two or more Lisch nodules (iris hamartomas)
5. Optic glioma
6. A distinctive osseous lesion such as sphenoid dysplasia or thinning of long bone cortex with or without pseudoarthrosis
7. A first-degree relative (parent, sibling, or offspring) with NF-1 by the above criteria

*The diagnostic criteria are met in an individual if two or more of the features listed are present.

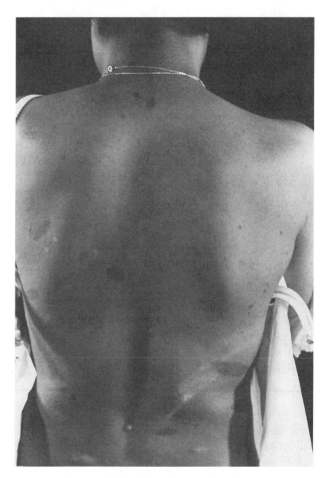

Figure 1 Café-au-lait spots.

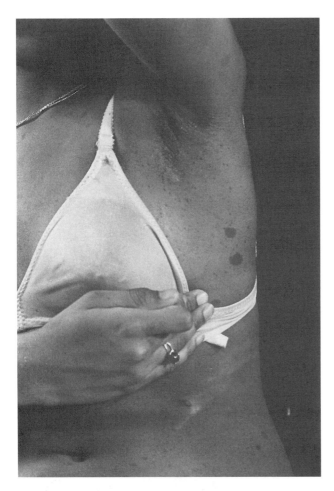

Figure 2 Axillary freckling.

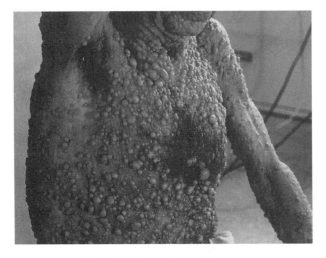

Figure 3 Dermal neurofibromas.

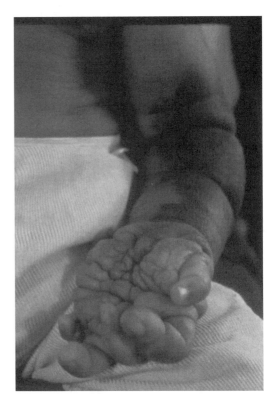

Figure 4 Plexiform neurofibroma with overlying pigmentation and associated soft tissue hypertrophy.

thogranulomas appear with increased frequency in children with NF-1, though they are rare. They are waxy, yellowish, small lumps on the skin, which usually develop in the first 5 years. Xanthogranulomas have been reported to occur in association with xantheleukemia in

NF-1, though in my 6 cases they were benign and disappeared after 1 to 2 years. I occasionally see adults referred with the diagnosis of NF-1 on the basis of multiple lumps on the skin who actually have multiple lipomas. It is usually not difficult to distinguish large, subcutaneous lipomas from neurofibromas, particularly in the absence of other signs of NF-1.

Lisch nodules are melanocytic hamartomas of the iris, which typically appear in late childhood or adolescence (Fig. 5). They are named after a German ophthalmologist who described them in 1937. Examination of the iris through an otoscope head is a useful way to search for the nodules, though a slit-lamp is necessary to distinguish the nodules, which have depth to them, from common iris freckles, which do not. A recent study of iris nodules claimed that their frequency in adults with NF-1 is 100 percent. In my experience the frequency is closer to 90 percent. A slit-lamp examination becomes important when the diagnosis is in doubt; that is, when only one of the other diagnostic criteria is present in an older child or adult.

The incidence of optic gliomas in NF-1 varies in different series from 3 to 15 percent. Optic gliomas typically develop in the first 5 years of life and may be chiasmatic or involve one or both optic nerves. They are frequently asymptomatic and nonprogressive and therefore often cannot be diagnosed clinically. A magnetic resonance imaging (MRI) scan is preferable to computed tomography (CT) because MRI can more easily

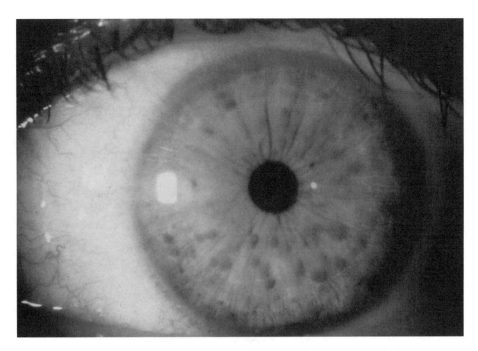

Figure 5 Multiple Lisch nodules.

distinguish dural ectasia of the optic canal, a phenomenon seen in NF-1, from true optic nerve thickening. We do not routinely perform MRI scans for diagnostic purposes on children with NF-1.

A variety of skeletal lesions are seen in NF-1, of which scoliosis is by far the most common. Sphenoid wing dysplasia, which occurs rarely in NF-1, is specific enough to be included as a diagnostic criterion. It is typically unilateral and involves the greater wing. It is frequently associated with pulsating exophthalmos and congenital plexiform neurofibroma of the orbit. Congenital thinning of long bones, often with pathologic fracture and pseudoarthrosis, is also rare in NF-1 but useful as a diagnostic criterion. This typically presents as thinning and anterolateral bowing of the tibia, though it can also involve other long bones, including the radius and ulna.

A first-degree relative with NF-1 is a very important criterion because it obviates the need for one of the two clinical signs of the disorder required to confirm the diagnosis. Because the signs of NF-1 can be subtle in an adult with mild involvement, both parents of a child suspected of having NF-1 should be examined.

A variety of other clinical findings, while not among the diagnostic criteria, are seen frequently enough in NF-1 to suggest the diagnosis in an NF-1 suspect. These include macrocephaly in the absence of hydrocephalus; short stature; and learning disability. In addition, two imaging findings are useful in diagnosis. Posterior vertebral scalloping due to dural ectasia may occur in up to 20 percent of cases of NF-1 (Fig. 6). Abnormal signals on MRI scan have been described in up to 60 percent of children with NF-1 (Fig. 7). They typically appear on T2-weighted images, do not enhance with gadolinium, have no obvious mass effect, and are not seen on CT

scan. They are presumed to be clinically insignificant. Because the percentage of adult NF-1 cases with unidentified bright objects appears to be substantially less, they may disappear with age. There are no adequate pathologic studies of such lesions.

The identification of the NF-1 gene on chromosome 17 has allowed the use of gene linkage for diagnosis in families in which confirmed cases are available for testing in two different generations. While this technology is important for prenatal diagnosis, it is expensive and requires the availability and cooperation of multiple family members. As a result, gene linkage has not been widely utilized for presymptomatic diagnosis. Linkage studies have confirmed that the Watson syndrome (familial café-au-lait spots, pulmonary stenosis, and mental retardation) is localized to the NF-1 gene. The cloning of the NF-1 gene should eventually lead to a direct gene test for NF-1. Progress in finding detectable mutations of the NF-1 gene has been slow, however. Recently, several individuals with NF-1, mild retardation, and dysmorphic facies have been shown to share a common large deletion of the NF-1 gene. Direct gene testing should eventually determine whether or not segmental NF, in which signs of NF-1 are restricted to a single region of the body, represents variability of the NF-1 gene, a somatic mutation, or another phenomenon.

NF-2 is a rare autosomal dominant disorder with a high sporadic mutation rate. Penetrance is assumed to be 100 percent. Unlike NF-1, expression is not variable, and practically everyone with the NF-2 gene eventually develops bilateral vestibular schwannomas.

The diagnosis of NF-2 is usually made when an imaging study confirms the presence of bilateral vestibular schwannomas (Table 3). A contrast-enhanced MRI

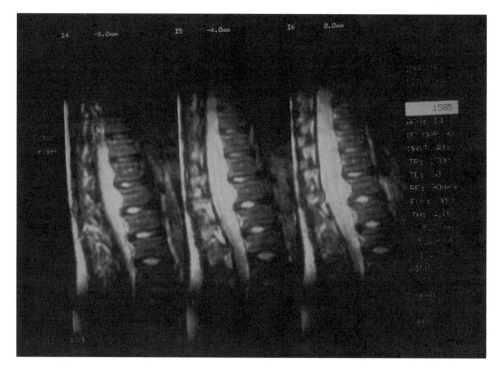

Figure 6 MRI of spine demonstrating vertebral scalloping due to dermal ectasia.

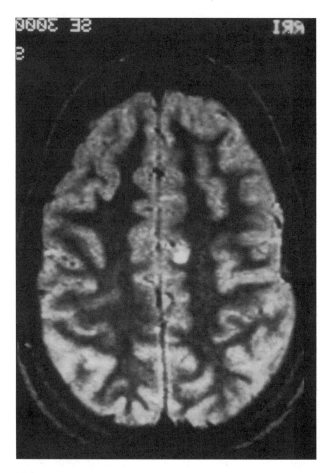

Figure 7 MRI of brain demonstrating unidentified bright object (UBO) on T2-weighted image.

Table 3 Diagnosis of Neurofibromatosis Type 2

Bilateral masses of the eighth cranial nerve seen with appropriate imaging techniques (computed tomography or magnetic resonance imaging) or
A first-degree relative with NF-1 and either:
  Unilateral mass of the eighth cranial nerve
  or
  Two of the following:
    Neurofibroma
    Meningioma
    Glioma
    Schwannoma
    Juvenile posterior subcapsular lenticular opacity

scan is the imaging procedure of choice. The usual presentation of vestibular schwannomas is tinnitus, hearing loss, or both, with speech discrimination being affected early and prominently. The age of onset ranges from childhood to the late 60s, but most symptoms develop in the second decade of life. Many NF-2 patients have two to three café-au-lait spots. It is unusual for there to be more than six. A few raised plaques representing schwannomas may be present on the skin. It is claimed that such lesions can be distinguished clinically from dermal neurofibromas. In my experience the distinction may require a biopsy. Multiple meningiomas of the brain, multiple spinal cord neurofibromas, multiple schwannomas of cranial or peripheral nerves, and occasional brain or spinal cord gliomas may develop in NF-2. A single neural tumor in an individual who has a first-degree relative with NF-2 confirms the diagnosis. Posterior subcapsular cataracts occur in 50 percent of NF-2 cases. They are considered a diagnostic criterion when they are seen in juveniles. Lisch nodules are not seen in NF-2. It has been suggested that NF-2 has two clinical forms with differing prognoses: a mild form in which only bilateral vestibular schwannomas appear, and a severe form in which these lesions develop along with multiple other brain and spinal cord tumors. Gene linkage testing for NF-2 has recently become available. The recent cloning of the NF-2 gene on chromosome 22 raises hopes that a direct gene test will be developed. The diagnosis of a unilateral vestibular schwannoma in an individual under the age of 20 should raise the suspicion of NF-2. The multiple meningioma syndrome, while extremely rare, may be familial and may be confused with NF-2, particularly if bilateral cerebellopontine angle masses are present. While NF-1 and NF-2 have some overlapping signs, vestibular schwannomas are rare in NF-1 and ubiquitous in NF-2.

TUBEROUS SCLEROSIS

The tuberous sclerosis complex (TSC) was originally described by Bournevelle in 1880. Vogt described the triad of facial angiofibromas, mental retardation, and seizures in 1908, which for many years was considered the classical presentation of TSC. Modern imaging techniques have demonstrated that the disorder is truly a complex of numerous lesions involving a number of organs (Table 4). Affected individuals need not have any of Vogt's triad of symptoms.

TSC is an autosomal dominant disorder with what appears to be a very high sporadic mutation rate. Penetrance is considered to be almost 100 percent. There are numerous phenotypes to TSC, which reflects variability of expression and possibly genetic heterogeneity. Linkage studies suggest a locus on chromosome 9 in some kindreds and chromosome 11 in other kindreds, none of whom have distinctive phenotypes.

The diagnostic criteria for TSC are listed in Table 5. The primary features of TSC are each pathognomonic, and documentation of a single one confirms the diagnosis. While the diagnosis of TSC may be raised as early as the third trimester, when fetal echocardiography can detect cardiac rhabdomyomas, the usual presentation to a neurologist is an infant or young child who has infantile spasms. Mental retardation is directly related to the age of onset of seizures, with the severest retardation occurring when seizures develop before the age of 2 years. A careful search for hypomelanotic macules with a Wood's lamp is important; 90 percent of cases of TSC have more than four. A variety of connective tissue hamartomas are seen in TSC. A fibrous plaque found on

Table 4 Tuberous Sclerosis Complex: Major Findings

Findings	(%)
Cutaneous	
Hypopigmented macules	90
Facial angiofibromas	50
Forehead plaque	25
Shagreen patch	20–40
Ungual fibromas	15–50
Neurologic	
Seizures	85
Mental retardation	50–60
Giant cell astrocytomas	5–10
Cranial Imaging Findings	
Subependymal nodules	90
Cortical lesions (either calcified or low density)	50
Renal	
Angiomyolipomas	60
Cysts	20
Cardiac	
Rhabdomyomas	50–60
Skeletal	
Sclerotic patches	60
Pseudocysts	60
Periosteal new bone	60
Others	
Poliosis	20
Gum fibromas	10
Dental pits	70
Pulmonary	
Honeycomb lung	Rare

Table 5 Diagnostic Criteria for Tuberous Sclerosis Complex (TSC)

Primary Features
 Facial angiofibromas*
 Multiple ungual fibromas*
 Cortical ungual fibromas*
 Cortical tuber (histologic confirmation)
 Subependymal nodule or giant cell astrocytoma (histologic confirmation)
 Multiple calcified subependymal nodules protruding into the ventricle (radiographic confirmation)
 Multiple retinal astrocytomas*
Secondary Features
 Affected first-degree relative
 Cardiac rhabdomyoma (histologic or radiographic confirmation)
 Other retinal hamartoma or achromic patch*
 Cerebral tubers (radiographic confirmation)
 Noncalcified subependymal nodules (radiographic confirmation)
 Shagreen patch*
 Forehead plaque*
 Pulmonary lymphangiomyomatosis (histologic confirmation)
 Renal angiomyolipoma (radiographic or histologic confirmation)
 Renal cysts typical of TSC (histologic confirmation)
Tertiary Features
 Hypomelanotic macules*
 "Confetti" skin lesions*
 Renal cysts (radiographic confirmation)
 Randomly distributed enamel pits in deciduous or permanent teeth or both
 Hamartomatous rectal polyps (histologic confirmation)
 Pulmonary lymphangiomyomatosis (radiographic confirmation)
 Cerebral white matter "migration tracts" or heterotopias (radiographic confirmation)
 Gingival fibromas*
 Angiomyolipoma: nonrenal (histologic confirmation)
 Infantile spasms
Definite TSC: One primary feature or two secondary features or one secondary plus two tertiary features
Probable TSC: One secondary plus one tertiary feature, or three tertiary features
Suspect TSC: One secondary feature or two tertiary features

*Histologic confirmation is not required if the lesion is clinically obvious.
 Developed by a National Tuberous Sclerosis Association Professional Advisory Board committee.

the forehead and occasionally on the eyelid, cheek, or scalp is often present at birth. Facial angiofibromas usually do not develop until after the age of 3. They may appear up to puberty. Shagreen patches and ungual fibromas typically appear in the second decade. An MRI or CT scan of the brain is a necessity in the evaluation for TSC. While the calcification nearly always seen in subependymal nodules is better visualized with CT, MRI can detect these lesions and is more sensitive than CT in the detection and delineation of cortical tubers. A careful opthalmologic examination is additionally necessary to search for retinal hamartomas, which are usually asymptomatic. Renal and cardiac ultrasound and a skeletal survey are not usually necessary to make a diagnosis but are indicated to define the extent of involvement after a diagnosis has been made.

VON HIPPEL-LINDAU DISEASE

Von Hippel described familial retinal angioma in 1911. Lindau described familial angiomas in association with cerebellar hemangioblastoma in 1926. Von Hippel-Lindau disease (VHL) is an autosomal dominant disorder that is quite rare. Like NF-1 and TSC, there is substantial variability of expression, and penetrance is assumed to be almost complete. Sporadic mutations are much less common than in those disorders, however. As a result, most diagnoses are made in individuals at risk for the disorder. The gene for VHL has been localized to chromosome 3, and markers flanking the gene have been defined, though gene linkage diagnosis is not yet clinically available.

Table 6 lists the major manifestations of VHL. Table 7 lists diagnostic criteria for VHL. The majority of patients with VHL have retinal and central nervous system (CNS) hemangioblastomas. At least one large kindred has been described in which the commonest lesion was pheochromocytoma, and CNS hemangioblastomas were uncommon. This kindred mapped to the VHL locus, suggesting that, as in NF-1, there may be multiple alleles at the same locus with distinct phenotypes.

The retinal hemangioblastoma, or angioma, is typically the earliest sign of the disorder. These lesions usually appear late in the second decade of life but have been seen in younger children. An adequate screen for retinal angiomas requires a sophisticated ophthalmologic evaluation. Large angiomas appear as red-orange masses with a pair of dilated vessels running between the lesion and the disk, which represent a dilated feeding artery and draining vein. Large lesions may cause retinal detachment or macular edema. Small lesions are asymptomatic and may be on the periphery. They are best searched for with indirect ophthalmoscopy. If this is negative, a fluorescein angiogram should be performed, which may detect leakage from small lesions.

CNS hemangioblastomas may involve the cerebellum, medulla, or spinal cord and rarely affect other areas

Table 6 Von Hippel-Lindau Disease: Major Findings

Organ	Lesion	Patients Affected (%)
Eye	Hemangioblastoma; retina, optic disc	24–73
Central nervous system	Hemangioblastoma; cerebellum, medulla oblongata, cord	22–66
Kidney	Cysts, cancer, hemangiomas, adenomas	56–83
Pancreas	Cysts, cancer, hemangioblastoma, hemangiomas	9–72
Adrenal	Pheochromocytoma, adenomas, cysts, cortical hyperplasia	7–17
Epididymis	Cysts, hemangiomas, adenomas	7–27
Liver	Cysts, adenomas, hemangiomas	17

Table 7 Diagnostic Criteria for Von Hippel-Lindau Disease

CNS and retinal hemangioblastoma
or
CNS or retinal hemangioblastoma plus one of the following:
  Renal, pancreatic, hepatic, or epididymal cysts
  Pheochromocytoma
  Renal cancer
or
First-degree relative plus:
  CNS or retinal hemangioblastoma
  Renal, pancreatic, or epididymal cysts
  Pheochromocytoma
  Renal cancer

CNS = central nervous system.

of the brain. Cerebellar hemangioblastomas often cause the first symptom in VHL patients and are the most common cause of morbidity and mortality. The signs and symptoms of cerebellar hemangioblastomas are similar to those of other cerebellar tumors, with headache and vomiting, gait disorder, vertigo, and diplopia the common symptoms. An adequate evaluation for VHL requires an MRI or CT scan of the brain.

Additional tests required to evaluate an individual who has either a retinal or CNS lesion include renal ultrasound, CT scan of the abdomen, and urinary pheochromocytoma screen. When there is an affected first-degree relative, confirmation of additional lesions other than retinal or CNS lesions is not necessary for diagnosis but should be performed to complete the evaluation.

STURGE-WEBER SYNDROME

In 1879 Sturge described a child with a congenital nevus of the face and partial seizures and correctly suggested that a similar nevus over the cortex might be the cause of the seizures.

Weber reported a case in 1922 and described the

linear calcifications of the cerebral cortex, which are uniformly present in adults with Sturge-Weber syndrome (SWS). SWS is considered a congenital malformation. Practically all cases are sporadic. There have been a few reports of familial cases. The classical signs of the syndrome are a congenital venous angioma of the face, ipsilateral venous angioma of the leptomeninges, and choroidal angioma (Table 8). In order to make the diagnosis, clinical or imaging evidence of cerebral angiomatosis should be present.

The usual presentation of a suspect is an infant with a facial venous angioma, the port wine stain. This is typically present at birth and occurs in approximately 87 percent of cases of SWS. The nevus is usually in the distribution of the trigeminal nerve on one side of the face, though occasional cases are bilateral, and other areas of the body may be affected. The infant in most cases will have partial motor seizures, which occur in at least 75 percent of cases and have their onset in early infancy. An electroencephalogram (EEG) should be performed and is invariably abnormal, though there are no EEG abnormalities unique to SWS. A CT scan should demonstrate cortical calcifications in infancy, though typical "railroad track" calcification is usually not dense enough to be noted on skull radiograph until the age of 1 year. Older children additionally demonstrate cortical atrophy. Cerebral arteriography will demonstrate a variety of abnormalities indicative of extensive leptomeningeal angiomatosis, though this is usually not necessary to make a diagnosis.

Choroidal angiomas occur in about 40 percent of SWS cases and should be carefully searched for in an infant with any of the other signs of SWS. In most cases

Table 8 Diagnostic Criteria for Sturge-Weber Syndrome

Leptomeningeal angiomatosis with or without either of the following:
   Facial angioma
   Choroidal angioma

the choroidal angioma is ipsilateral to the facial nevus and is associated with glaucoma or buphthalmos, though a choroidal angioma may be present in their absence.

SUGGESTED READING

Glenn GM, Daniel LN, Choyke P. Von Hippel-Lindau (VHL) disease: Distinct phenotypes suggest more than one mutant allele at the VHL locus. Hum Genet 1991; 87:207–210.
Gomez MR. Neurocutaneous syndromes. Boston: Butterworth, 1987.
Johnson WG, Gomez MR. Tuberous sclerosis and allied disorders. Ann NY Acad Sci 1991; 615:1–389.
Korf BR. Diagnostic outcome in children with multiple café-au-lait spots. Pediatrics 1992; 90:924–927.
Moore AT, Maher ER, Rosen P, et al. Ophthalmological screening for Von Hippel-Lindau disease. Eye 1991; 5:723–728.
Northrup H, Wheless JW, Bertin TK, et al. Variability of expression in tuberous sclerosis. J Med Genet 1993; 30:41–43.
Rubenstein AE, Korf BR. Neurofibromatosis: A Handbook for patients, families and health care workers. New York: Thieme, 1986.
Seizenger BR, Rouleau GA, Ozelius LJ, et al. Von Hippel-Lindau disease maps to the region of chromosome 3 associated with renal call carcinoma. Nature 1988; 332:269–269.
Stumpf DA, Alksene JF, Annegers JF, et al. Neurofibromatosis. Arch Neurol 1988; 45:575–578.
Truhan AP, Filipek PA. Magnetic resonance imaging: Its role in the neuroradiologic evaluation of neurofibromatosis, tuberous sclerosis, and Sturge-Weber syndrome. Arch Dermatol 1993; 129:219–226.

DEVELOPMENTAL DYSLEXIA

RUTH NASS, M.D.

Developmental dyslexia is a common problem, affecting 5 to 15 percent of school-age children. Like other learning disabilities and developmental disorders, it is about two to three times more common in boys than in girls.

Developmental dyslexia is in essence an unexpected difficulty in learning to read. It often occurs with another learning disability, such as difficulty with attention or math, but sometimes occurs in its pure form. The diagnosis of dyslexia is based on both exclusionary and inclusionary criteria:

1. Strictly speaking, the dyslexic child should have no major neurologic abnormalities, meaning no cerebral palsy. However, children with cerebral palsy whose reading skills are below that expected for their intellectual abilities do meet educational criteria for the diagnosis of dyslexia. Many dyslexic children have soft signs on neurologic examination (see below).
2. The major sensory functions must be normal. The child should not be blind or deaf. However, children who are blind or deaf may be dyslexic, if they have reading difficulties out of proportion to their other academic and intellectual abilities. Because of the lack of language input, deaf children often have more trouble learning to read than blind children.
3. The strict diagnostic criteria do not allow for major psychiatric problems, such as psychosis or depression. However, problems with self-esteem are often a reactive secondary issue in the learning disabled child.
4. Normal intelligence using either a verbal or nonverbal measure is required. Note that chil-

dren with dyslexia often have language problems. Hence verbal IQ may not accurately reflect overall intellectual abilities.

5. The dyslexic child must have been in a social-educational environment conducive to learning to read; several studies of inner city school children have demonstrated that enrichment programs help some nonreaders become readers.

The most commonly used diagnostic criterion for dyslexia is that the child must read one and one-half to two grades below actual or expected grade level. However, consideration must be given to the fact that different types of reading tests yield different reading levels. A child with true dyslexia may have trouble on the Gray Oral Reading Test, which is timed and requires comprehension of what is read, but may not have trouble on the Wide Range Achievement Test, a single word reading test that only requires phonetic decoding. Hence a variety of reading measures must be used to make the diagnosis. Intelligence is an important factor in determining what grade level of reading is expected. Otherwise we would underestimate the incidence in the child with high IQ, who should be reading above grade level, and overestimate the incidence in the child with low-normal IQ, who may actually not be able to read at grade level despite having no special reading problems. Regression equations correlating reading score, age, and IQ in the social and educational milieu of the individual child have been developed to deal with these issues. Low achievement in reading needs to be differentiated from real reading disability. Defining reading discrepancy (disability) as more than 1.5 standard deviations between IQ and reading cluster scores, and defining low reading achievement as scoring in the lowest 25th percentile on the reading cluster tests, investigators found that 78 percent of those with reading disability were also low reading achievers. However, only 40 percent of the low reading achievers met criteria for reading disability. Compared to those with both low achievement in reading and reading disability, those who were only low reading achievers had lower IQ scores and lower overall reading scores.

Since we do not expect children to read until first grade, a strict definition makes a diagnosis of dyslexia impossible before the third grade. A history of language delay is often predictive of dyslexia, however. Definitions should not pre-empt consideration of early intervention in the at-risk child. In addition, a 2 year discrepancy reflects a greater disability for the older than for the younger child. Finally, the age of the person affects our ability to make the diagnosis. Diagnosing residual dyslexia in the adolescent or adult often requires looking at spelling skills as well as reading skills in a wide range of situations. Attitudes toward reading (e.g., pleasure reader or not) are often useful clues to a residual disability in the older person.

Dyslexia is often an inherited disorder. Family history is positive in 50 to 80 percent of children. In Denckla's cohort of 52 pure dyslexics, 40 had a positive family history. The high concordance in monozygotic twins is consistent with a genetic basis for the disorder. Siblings and offspring are also frequently affected. Several recent large family studies document autosomal dominant transmission, although there is still considerable debate over single gene versus polygenetic transmission. Galaburda and Geschwind suggest that symptom constellations of allergies, autoimmune diseases, migraines, sinistrality, and learning disabilities occurring in a single dyslexic individual or among family members are also common.

PSYCHOMETRIC WORK-UP

The reading process is complex and requires many cognitive skills. Deficits in any one area can result in overall reading problems. Four major neuropsychological syndromes have been documented in dyslexics: (1) language disorder syndrome, (2) articulatory graphomotor disorder syndrome, (3) sequencing disorder syndrome, and (4) visuoperceptual disorder syndrome. Although visuoperceptual problems used to be thought the most common cause for dyslexia, they have turned out to be the least common. The language disorder syndrome is the most common.

The *language disorder syndrome* (occurring in 30 to 70 percent of the dyslexic population) is defined by anomia and impaired comprehension of language, impaired repetition, or impaired speech sound discrimination. Rapid automatized naming tasks, which pick up slow naming, and line drawing tests of object naming, which pick up dysphasic errors, are particularly sensitive measures. Children with this dyslexia subtype tend to have lower verbal IQ (VIQ) than performance IQ (PIQ). Among children with a language disorder syndrome, there is often a history of language delay.

In the *articulatory graphomotor disorder syndrome* (15 to 50 percent), sound blending is impaired, buccal lingual difficulties and disarticulation are present, and graphomotor skills are weak. Here, PIQ equals VIQ, motor milestones are often delayed, and the neurologic examination is more often abnormal.

In the *sequencing disorder syndrome* (10 to 15 percent), defective short-term visual and verbal memory, difficulty with rote series, and difficulty with syntax are noted. Here, again PIQ equals VIQ.

Finally, in the *visuoperceptual disorder syndrome* (5 to 15 percent), visual reasoning, reproduction of geometric designs, and some math skills, such as working in columns, are impaired. VIQ tends to be higher than PIQ.

The classic finding of letter reversals is particularly common in the latter two syndromes. Note, however, that letter reversals are also seen as part of the process of normal reading acquisition. Reversals of *b* and *d* in writing can be normal through age 7 years. Table 1 lists some of the tests psychologists use to assess cognitive and academic skills in children with learning disabilities.

In addition to these underlying neuropsychological syndromes, dyslexia can be analyzed by type of reading processing impairment. There appear to be at least two ways to read a word: phonetically (letter by letter) or

Table 1 Basic Neuropsychological Battery
to Assess Dyslexia

Naming tasks: Boston Naming Test, Oldfield Naming, Rapid
  Automatized Naming
Language comprehension: Token Test, stories, relational sentences
Repetition tasks: words, Spreen Benton sentences
Auditory discrimination tasks: Goldman Fristoe
Sound blending tasks
Articulation tasks
Segmentation tasks
Visuo-motor tasks: Bender Gestalt, Rey Complex Figure, Draw-A-
  Person, Beery Visuo-Motor Integration
Sequencing tasks: rote series (days, months)
Memory: Digit Span, Benton Visual Retention Test
Visuo-perceptual tasks: Ravens Matrices, Motor Free Test
Reading tests: silent, oral with and without comprehension, Gray
  Oral Reading Test (WRAT-R), Gates-MacGinitie
Spelling tests: WRAT-R
Math tests: WRAT-R, Key Math

From Nass R. Rapid assessment of the mental status exam of the child.
Emerg Med Clin North Am 1987; 739–750; with permission.

Table 2 Soft Signs in Learning Disabled Children

Arms extended: drop or spread
Head rotation: arms drop or spread
Hop, one-foot stand
Finger and foot tapping
Choreiform movements
Associated and mirror movements
Finger nose, finger pursuit, tandem
Diadochokinesis
Copy finger movements
Double simultaneous stimulation
Finger agnosia
Head: extraocular muscles-movements
Strabismus or cannot converge
Hold lateral gaze
Grimace, raise brow
Tongue waggle
Speed of speech

From Touwen BCL, Prechtl HFR. The neurological examination of the
child with minor central nervous system anomalies. London: Spastic International, 1970; with permission.

visually (by sight as a whole). Some children have trouble with the visual route to reading and are called *surface* or *dyseidetic* dyslexics. They cannot read irregular words, which are not spelled the way they sound. Other children have trouble with the phonetic route to reading and are called *deep* or *dysphonetic* dyslexics. They cannot sound out unfamiliar words and cannot read phonetically regular nonwords. Dyslexia may represent a failure to pass through any one of the stages of normal reading acquisition. Remediation often trades on the child's strength.

NEUROLOGIC EXAMINATION

The neurologic examination of the child with dyslexia is similar to that of children with all types of learning disabilities. There are an excess of soft neurologic signs. A number that are reliably found are listed in Table 2. *Developmental soft signs* are findings that would be normal if the child were younger, such as mirror movements or overflow. In Denckla's series of pure dyslexics, 38 of 52 had such signs. *Classic pastel soft signs* are traditional neurologic signs found in a mild form, such as minimally asymmetric deep tendon reflexes. In Denckla's series, 11 of 52 had pastel signs. Both right and left hemisyndromes were demonstrated, although the side did not clearly correlate with the neuropsychological profile. Only three of 52 children had no soft signs. Most investigators report a marked decline in number of soft signs after puberty. Notably, motor coordination difficulties do not necessarily affect athletic prowess.

LABORATORY EVALUATION

Routine computed tomography or magnetic resonance imaging (MRI) is not generally indicated in the standard evaluation of dyslexia, unless there are addi-

tional neurologic symptoms like seizures or headache, or unless the examination reveals focality. Rumsey and colleagues found on MRI no specific, consistent, focal abnormalities among a group of severe dyslexics. Since girls are less often affected, the threshold for imaging them should be lower. Other possible red flags include left-hander with negative family history of learning disabilities or left-handers with negative family history of left-handedness (possible pathologic left-handers), very specific disability, large VIQ-PIQ split, or decline in IQ. Brain tumors and arteriovenous malformations rarely manifest only as dyslexia.

With respect to the electrophysiologic assessment of dyslexia, routine electroencephalogram (EEG) is generally not helpful. EEG abnormalities are common in the normal child, and minor nonspecific abnormalities are common in the learning disabled population. Finding these abnormalities does not aid diagnosis or treatment. In addition, EEG findings once considered abnormal have, at other times, been considered normal. For example, 14 and six positive spike pattern, once considered a marker of epilepsy, appears to be a common age-dependent EEG finding. Lombroso and co-workers determined this by obtaining EEGs on high school students at a top prep school. Duffy et al, using the BEAM technique, compared dyslexic boys to controls during active tasks like reading, writing, and listening. Differences in electrical activity were seen in the left hemisphere, particularly in Broca's and Wernicke's areas and in the supplementary motor area bilaterally. The left hemisphere differences are consistent with dyslexia as a left hemisphere-language disorder. The supplementary motor areas may be involved in the subvocalization process that accompanies reading and thus be differentially involved in normal and dyslexic readers.

With respect to outcome, adults with a history of dyslexia take less pleasure in reading than spouses or friends. Like other learning disabilities, there is often lower school attainment, academic and social success.

Hartzell and Compton report no difference in level of job satisfaction, although job choices differ. Not surprisingly, positive factors include high IQ and socioeconomic status. Since dyslexia is neurologically based, reading difficulties never completely disappear, although compensation may be excellent.

SUGGESTED READING

Denckla MB. Dyslexia. In: Blaw M, Rapin I, Kinsbourne M, et al, eds. Topics in child neurology. New York: Spectrum Press, 1977 243–262.

Duffy FH, Denckla MB, Bartels PH, Sandini G. Dyslexia: Regional differences in brain electrical activity by topographic mapping. Ann Neurol 1980; 7:412–420.

Funnucci J, Whitehouse C, Issacs S, Childs B. Derivation and validation of a quantitative definition of specific reading disability in adults. Dev Med Child Neurol 1984; 26:143–153.

Galaburda A, Geschwind N. Cerebral lateralization. Cambridge, MA: MIT Press, 1987.

Hartzell H, Compton C. Learning disability: 10 year follow-up. Pediatrics 1984; 74:1058–1064.

Lombroso C. Ctenoids in healthy youths: Controlled study of 14 and 6 spike and wave. Neurology 1966; 16:300–305.

Mattis S, French JH, Rapin I. Dyslexia in children and young adults: Three independent neuro-psychological syndromes. Dev Med Child Neurol 1975; 17:150–163.

Nass R. Rapid assessment of the mental status exam of the child. Emerg Med Clin North Am 1987; :739–750.

Penington BF, Gilges JW, Pauls D, et al. Evidence for major gene transmission of developmental dyslexia. JAMA 1992; 266:1527.

Rudel R. Learning disability: Diagnosis by exclusion and discrepancy. J Am Acad Child Psychiatry 1980; 19:547–578.

Rudel R. The definition of dyslexia. In: Duffy F, Geschwind N, eds. Dyslexia. Boston: Little, Brown, 1987.

Rumsey J. MRI in developmental dyslexia. Arch Neurol 1986; 43:1043–1044.

Touwen H, Prechtl H. The neurological exam of the child with minor nervous system dysfunction. Philadelphia: JB Lippincott, 1970.

Yule W, Rutter M. Reading and intelligence. In: Knights R, Bakker J, eds. Neuropsychology of language disorders: Theoretical approaches. Baltimore: University Park Press, 1976.

MENTAL RETARDATION

HART PETERSON, M.D.

Mental retardation can be defined as a fixed lag in the development of normal cognitive function. It is differentiated from dementia, which is generally progressive and occurs in a previously normal individual. Mental retardation arises early in life from abnormalities in the prenatal, perinatal, or postnatal period. Almost any irreversible childhood encephalopathy can result in mental retardation, but the precise cause is rarely important in its diagnosis or management.

The diagnosis of mental retardation in young children is generally suggested by documenting delayed developmental milestones. Differentiating delayed motor development, as seen in cerebral palsy or infantile spinal muscular atrophy, from delayed mental development is particularly difficult in patients under a year of age. The rate of development of speech in the second year is a key milestone, since it is relatively independent of motor skills. In older children, developmental lags may be more apparent, and the degree of handicap may be roughly quantitated. A very crude estimate of mental age may be made by comparing age of development of key landmarks to the norm. For example, a child who first walks at age 2 and says numerous single words at age 2 ½ is functioning at approximately 50 percent of age expectation. A child of 4 who is just starting to talk and walk is functioning at 25 percent of age expectation, or a 1 year mental age.

Formal psychometrics can be carried out at any age.

Under age 6 these are unreliable predictors of later intelligence except when markedly abnormal. I generally recommend postponing formal testing until it is required to make clinical decisions, such as deciding whether a child should go into regular or special education kindergarten.

Classifying the child by severity of mental retardation can be done by IQ score or by functional ability. The functional classification is clinically more useful. Children with IQs of 55 to 70 are considered educable or mildly retarded. They are children one hopes to teach reading, writing, and computational skills so that they can live independently in the community. Children with IQs of 25 to 55 are considered trainable or moderately retarded and are not candidates for complete independence. They may be able to master self-care and simple vocational skills and be able to communicate. Children with IQs less than 25 are considered severely or profoundly retarded and require a high degree of care. Their communication skills are generally absent or rudimentary, and they are dependent in most activities of daily living.

GOALS OF DIAGNOSIS

It is extremely important to understand the goals of diagnosis. With certain exceptions, mental retardation will be apparent from history-taking. An elaborate neurologic workup is required in only a minority of cases.

Medical treatment is a laudable goal but is infrequently applicable. Examples that come to mind are shunting of hydrocephalus and surgically correcting multiple premature craniosynostoses. Metabolic diseases such as phenylketonuria or hypothyroidism are important to detect in the young because they can be treated. Modern gene therapy may soon add to the list of metabolic diseases amenable to treatment.

Prognosis is of extreme importance to parents. Many parents feel that a mentally retarded child will never develop at all and cannot learn. This is usually untrue and needs to be explained. A precise diagnosis occasionally permits a prediction of shortened life expectancy, as might be the case in trisomy 13 or anencephaly. The same prediction can be made for a profoundly retarded, nonambulatory, non–self-feeding child regardless of cause. Certain progressive diseases are traditionally listed as causes of mental retardation. An example is mucopolysaccharidosis type I (Hurler's disease). Individuals with this condition rarely reach their twentieth birthday.

Genetics are usually far from the parents' minds when the initial determination of mental retardation is made, but genetic and chromosomal causes of mental retardation are common. If a specific syndrome that produces mental retardation is diagnosed and its genetics are understood, this information can be provided to the parents to assist them in planning future pregnancies. In a growing number of metabolic diseases, such as Tay-Sachs disease, carrier detection can be carried out and amniocentesis offered in at-risk pregnancies. I strongly recommend Tay-Sachs carrier testing be carried out in husband and wife who are of Ashkenazic Jewish background.

Chromosome testing is desirable when the mental retardation syndrome includes multiple congenital anomalies. This is important not only for the parents, but possibly for siblings, since carriers of a balanced translocation are at greatly increased risk for similar problems when they reach reproductive age.

Identification of the fragile X chromosome syndrome cannot be made in a routine karyotype. It must be specifically sought. This disease can also be diagnosed by DNA analysis. Individuals with this syndrome are generally male, mildly retarded, and may have features of autism. The clinical phenotype of long face, large ears, and large testicles is not usually apparent in childhood. Asymptomatic sisters of such boys are at increased risk of carrying this chromosome and transmitting it to their children. I recommend a fragile X search when there are autistic features or where more than one male in the family is retarded without explanation. It is not yet clear whether girls with learning disabilities should be tested for the fragile X chromosome.

Medical needs can be anticipated when specific causes of mental retardation are recognized. For example, individuals with neurofibromatosis are at increased risk for scoliosis, optic nerve tumors, and hypertension. Individuals with tuberous sclerosis occasionally develop hydrocephalus due to growth of benign giant cell astrocytomas adjacent to the foramen of Monro. Individuals with Down's syndrome are at increased risk of subluxation of C1 cervical vertebra on C2 due to minor trauma in adolescence or later.

A *realistic plan* is the goal of your workup. The bulk of management of the retarded individual is through educational and psychological support. Mentally retarded individuals have all the medical needs of their normal counterparts and frequently more. It is important to remember that mentally retarded individuals do not surrender their intrinsic rights as citizens.

DIFFERENTIAL DIAGNOSIS

A number of conditions need to be differentiated from mental retardation, either because they require an alternative approach to management or because they may coexist with mental retardation.

Cerebral palsy syndromes are generally difficult to differentiate from mental retardation in patients under 1 year of age. About 50 percent of children with cerebral palsy show some degree of mental retardation. This is especially true of microcephalic children with spastic quadriplegia, a syndrome common after neonatal hypoxic ischemic encephalopathy. About 50 percent of children with choreoathetoid cerebral palsy have mental retardation. Individuals with spastic hemiplegia and spastic diplegia are much less likely to be mentally retarded.

Progressive diseases are misdiagnosed as mental retardation with some frequency. Fortunately, these are relatively uncommon. The identification of a progressive neurodegenerative disease requires documentation of deterioration of neurologic status on examination or by history. Many of these diseases are fatal, and most are inherited in an identifiable fashion. Children with the acquired immunodeficiency syndrome may have static or progressive mental retardation, but a progressive systemic disease. Girls with Rett syndrome appear to deteriorate beginning at about age 1, but then seem to stabilize at a low functioning level of mental function. Children with mental retardation *do not deteriorate,* although they may appear to do so when intensive support systems are withdrawn.

Pervasive developmental disorder (PDD) and other severe disorders of language must be identified. Mental retardation is common in PDD (autism), but PDD is a disorder of relatedness and socialization.

Deafness is important in the differential diagnosis of a child with delayed speech. Mere hearing of sounds does not establish that hearing is normal. Children with high-tone hearing loss have trouble hearing the sounds of consonants and understanding language, although they may be well aware of noise in their environment. All children with delayed language not otherwise explained should have their hearing tested. Modern neurophysiologic methods permit hearing testing in the young and uncooperative patient.

Attention deficit hyperactive disorder (ADHD) is easily confused with mental retardation. Both groups of children have school problems, and mentally retarded children may be impulsive, distractable, and hyperactive. This is an area where the psychologist has the best tools. Children with ADHD symptoms frequently respond well to stimulants such as methylphenidate, dextroamphetamine, or pemoline.

Epilepsy is not to be confused with mental retardation, but since both conditions are reflections of altered brain function they are commonly seen in the same individual. Management of epilepsy is not altered in the retarded except that administration of anticonvulsant medication commonly requires supervision. The principle of optimum seizure control with minimal sedation is the same. Phenobarbital, which has been displaced in popularity by the emergence of newer anticonvulsants, can aggravate hyperactivity in the mentally retarded.

Psychosocial factors are of enormous importance because they may be susceptible to social intervention. We know that a child's intelligence is best correlated with the mother's intelligence and education level. We know that children from single parent families and especially homeless children have a disproportionate incidence of school failure.

WORKUP

History

It is useful to divide the history into prenatal, perinatal, and postnatal periods. Prenatal factors of special interest include exposure of the mother to toxins, alcohol, drugs, infection, or radiation. A history of maternal infection, abnormal weight gain, abnormal bleeding, or toxemia is potentially important. Perinatal factors include prematurity, low birth weight, hypoglycemia, abnormal labor and delivery, low Apgar scores, and postnatal evidence of hypoxic-ischemic encephalopathy. A low 1 minute Apgar score indicates only a need for resuscitation, whereas a low 5 minute Apgar score begins to identify a small percentage of children who will exhibit neurologic defects later on. The longer the Apgar is depressed, the greater the probability that the child will ultimately show neurologic problems. Hypoxic-ischemic encephalopathy is a well-defined and readily apparent clinical syndrome in the postnatal period. Moderate or more severe degrees of mental retardation are rarely, if ever, due to hypoxic-ischemic encephalopathy in the absence of associated cerebral palsy. Other postnatal factors should also be assessed. Head trauma and infection of the central nervous system are the most important. Lead encephalopathy is an uncommon cause of mental retardation. Asymptomatic elevated blood lead levels, which are believed by some to be associated with mild reductions in IQ, do not explain significant mental retardation.

A detailed family history is essential. It is not sufficient to ask if there is a family history of neurologic disease, since many families do not understand the term. Specific neurologic disorders such as epilepsy, cerebral palsy, and blindness should be asked about. Always ask about consanguinity, especially in families from the Middle East where marriage between relatives such as cousins is encouraged by social custom. Consanguinity greatly increases the incidence of recessively inherited diseases.

Physical Examination

Important clues to mental retardation may emerge from the physical examination. Head circumference should be appropriate to age. Microcephaly, regardless of body size, predicts mental retardation and other possible neurologic defects. Macrocephaly may be familial and is not uncommon in large children. Hydrocephalus represents one of the most treatable causes of mental retardation in children.

A careful examination of the skin is of great value. More than six café au lait spots is associated with neurofibromatosis. A facial vascular nevus suggests Sturge-Weber syndrome. Not all individuals with these nevi have the pial angioma that causes the syndrome. A simian crease is a congenital malformation commonly seen in Down's syndrome. The adenoma sebaceum or fibroadenomata of the face, periungual fibromata, and shagreen patches of tuberous sclerosis are not usually seen in infancy, but depigmented nevi or ash leaf spots can sometimes be made out on careful examination of the skin. An ultraviolet or Wood's lamp is helpful in finding these spots in fair skinned children. Depigmented spots are most often a nonspecific finding so that their presence should be interpreted with caution.

A careful eye exam is frequently useful. Chorioretinitis suggests prenatal infection, especially toxoplasmosis. Retinal colobomata is a congenital abnormality suggesting an insult during pregnancy. The retinal gliomas of tuberous sclerosis strongly resemble retinoblastomas. Optic hypoplasia suggests an insult during pregnancy, and optic atrophy suggests a disorder affecting white matter. A cherry red spot, actually a surround of pallor making the macula seem red, suggests ganglioside storage.

A clustering of congenital malformations suggests a prenatal cause. Some common ones include hypertelorism, epicanthal folds, low set or malformed ears, a high arched palate, and clinodactyly.

Physicians seeing retarded children should have access to some simple office psychological tests to help decide who should be referred for formal testing. For young children, the Denver Developmental Screening Test is easily administered and scored. The Peabody Picture Vocabulary Test is also easily administered and scored and gives a quick estimate of intelligence in English-speaking children from age 4 on. For those willing to spend an initial few hours learning to score it, the Goodenough Draw a Person Test provides a remarkably accurate and quick estimate of intelligence in children aged 4 to 10. This test has the considerable virtue that it almost never overestimates the intelligence.

Laboratory Studies

Most mentally retarded children do not require an elaborate laboratory investigation. As previously noted, treatable causes should be excluded wherever possible. Very young children with microcephaly should have TORCH (toxoplasmosis, rubella, cytomegalovirus, and herpes) antibody titers and, where possible, syphilis and human immunodeficiency virus testing. I routinely screen for urine and blood aminoacids and organic acids and hypothyroidism in young mentally retarded children.

A good rule of thumb is: Don't do a test unless you can anticipate how a normal or abnormal result will help you understand and manage the case. Magnetic resonance imaging and computed tomography (CT) are good examples to consider. Diagnosis of hydrocephalus will clearly lead to therapy. Radiologic documentation of the degree of asphyxia or the presence of a neuronal migration defect is helpful in prognostication. However, brain imaging of most mentally retarded children is neither indicated nor helpful. Skull x rays have no place in the evaluation of mental retardation. If a skull x ray is needed, a CT scan should be substituted since it reveals vastly greater information at only slightly greater cost and radiation exposure. Chromosome testing has been previously discussed. Electroencephalograms are commonly abnormal in the mentally retarded but, except where seizures are suspect, are of little value. Evoked potentials can demonstrate the anatomic integrity of the optic and auditory pathways and the spinal cord, but contribute little in evaluating a retarded child. PET scanning and electrical brain mapping are research tools that have no place in the routine evaluation of mental retardation.

SUGGESTED READING

Eyman PK, Grossman HJ, Chaney RH, Call TL. The life expectancy of profoundly handicapped people with mental retardation. N Engl J Med 1990; 323:584–589.

Freeman JM, Nelson KB. Intrapartum asphyxia and cerebral palsy. Pediatrics 1987; 82:240–249.

Gomez MR, ed. Neurocutaneous diseases: A practical approach. Boston: Butterworths, 1987.

Paneth N, Stark RI. Cerebral palsy and mental retardation in relation to indicators of perinatal asphyxia. Am J Obstet Gynecol 1983; 147:960–966.

PSYCHIATRIC DISORDERS

SOMATIZATION DISORDER

RICHARD J. GOLDBERG, M.D.

Somatization may be defined as the manifestation of psychological distress in the form of physical symptoms. Somatizing patients can be extremely frustrating to physicians, and their symptoms can lead to repeated unnecessary medical testing that drives up health care costs. In itself, somatization is not a diagnostic entity, since the process appears as a component of many disorders. This chapter reviews the formal diagnosis of somatization disorder and presents a clinically useful classification and differential diagnosis.

RESEARCH AND CLINICAL DEFINITIONS

The phenomenon of somatization encompasses a wide variety of terms and related disorders. Because of research on the validity and reliability of somatization disorder, much of the current literature has focused on that disorder. *Somatization disorder* is defined in DSM-IIIR based on observable symptoms that have some stability and predictive value. DSM-IIIR requires the presence of 13 out of a possible 35 symptoms (Table 1).

While describing an important subset of patients, the definition of somatization disorder is too narrow to be useful for practicing physicians. When the full criteria for somatization disorder are applied, many of the cases seen in clinical practice are excluded. Somatization disorder has a prevalence of about 0.03 to 0.7 percent. Such patients are usually female and show a pattern of symptom presentation beginning before age 30. However, somatizing patients are a major component of medical practice. It has been concluded that between 25 and 75 percent of patients seeing a primary care physician present primarily with somatic complaints as a manifestation of psychosocial distress. Less rigorous criteria have been proposed, and their predictive value is being explored.

A useful classification for the clinician dichotomizes somatizing patients into the following categories, determined by the temporal duration of the symptoms.

1. Acute somatized symptom(s): These consist of physical manifestations of current psychosocial distress generally lasting weeks to months. In general, these patients have a high level of premorbid function.
2. Chronic somatized symptom(s): These symptoms represent more chronic forms of somatization, including those that do not meet the full criteria for the disorder as defined in DSM-IIIR, and are generally present for months to years.

There are distinct management strategies for each of these categories.

PSYCHIATRIC DIFFERENTIAL DIAGNOSIS

Not all somatizing patients have an identifiable psychiatric disorder, but many do. Therefore, clinicians should always search for some underlying psychiatric disorder, most notably affective or anxiety disorders, before settling on somatization as a diagnosis.

Depression

Depression is the most common psychiatric disorder underlying somatization. Therefore, for any somatizing patient, the clinician should inquire about the potential presence of the full symptom complex of depression. A somatized physical complaint can be the "leading edge" of underlying depression. The physician should inquire about sleep and appetite disturbance, depressed mood, fatigue, loss of concentration, anhedonia, and suicidal ideation. When present with somatized symptoms, depression should be treated first, and it is likely that the somatized symptoms will disappear.

At times, patients may be depressed with the only presenting symptom being a somatized symptom. For example, there are many patients, especially but not exclusively elderly, who complain of a single serious medical symptom, such as abdominal or rectal pain. Some of these patients will vehemently deny other symptoms of depression, resent the implication that they

300

Table 1 Diagnostic Criteria for Somatization Disorder*

A. A history of many physical complaints or a belief that one is sickly, beginning before the age of 30 and persisting for several years.

B. At least 13 symptoms from the list below. To count a symptom as significant, the following criteria must be met:

   1. No organic pathology or pathophysiologic mechanism (e.g., a physical disorder or the effects of injury, medication, drugs, or alcohol) to account for the symptom or, when there is related organic pathology, the complaint or resulting social or occupational impairment is grossly in excess of what would be expected from the physical findings
   2. Has not occurred only during a panic attack
   3. Has caused the person to take medicine (other than over-the-counter pain medication), see a doctor, or alter life-style

Symptom List

Gastrointestinal symptoms:
   1. **Vomiting (other than during pregnancy)**†
   2. Abdominal pain (other than when menstruating)
   3. Nausea (other than motion sickness)
   4. Bloating (gassy)
   5. Diarrhea
   6. Intolerance of (gets sick from) several different foods

Pain symptoms:
   7. **Pain in extremities**
   8. Back pain
   9. Joint pain
   10. Pain during urination
   11. Other pain (excluding headaches)

Cardiopulmonary symptoms:
   12. **Shortness of breath when not exerting oneself**
   13. Palpitations
   14. Chest pain
   15. Dizziness

Conversion or pseudoneurologic symptoms:
   16. **Amnesia**
   17. **Difficulty swallowing**
   18. Loss of voice
   19. Deafness
   20. Double vision
   21. Blurred vision
   22. Blindness
   23. Fainting or loss of consciousness
   24. Seizure or convulsion
   25. Trouble walking
   26. Paralysis or muscle weakness
   27. Urinary retention or difficulty urinating

Sexual symptoms for the major part of the person's life after opportunities for sexual activity:
   28. **Burning sensation in sexual organs or rectum (other than during intercourse)**
   29. Sexual indifference
   30. Pain during intercourse
   31. Impotence

Female reproductive symptoms judged by the person to occur more frequently or severely than in most women:
   32. **Painful menstruation**
   33. Irregular menstrual periods
   34. Excessive menstrual bleeding
   35. Vomiting throughout pregnancy

*American Psychiatric Association: Diagnostic and Statistical Manual of Mental Disorders 3rd ed. revised (DSM-III-R). American Psychiatric Association, 1987.
†The seven items in boldface may be used to screen for the disorder. The presence of two or more of these items suggests a high likelihood of the disorder.

may be depressed, and show offense at the suggestion that the physical symptom may be "all in their head." Some of these patients may acknowledge a few symptoms of depression but rationalize them by such statements as, "Of course I can't sleep. That pain keeps me up. Would you feel like eating if you were worried about this pain all the time?" It is not uncommon for such patients to pass through the hands of multiple specialists, with repeated invasive tests. At some point a clinician should abandon the "rule out" mentality and opt for an empirical treatment trial for depression. It has been the experience of many medical-psychiatry units that such patients often respond to aggressive treatment for depression, including electroconvulsive therapy. Such patients always generate controversy among providers, who divide into groups and debate the diagnosis. One way to rationalize the approach to treat depression is that everything else has been tried.

Anxiety Disorders

Anxiety disorders are also extremely common as the underlying cause of physically unexplained symptoms in the general population, with a prevalence of about 5 to 10 percent overall. In patients presenting with repeated physical symptoms and no apparent medical explanation, the following anxiety disorders should be considered.

Panic disorder, which has a prevalence of about 2 percent, presents with episodic physical symptoms that may be primarily cardiac, pulmonary, or neurologic. Among the neurologic symptoms, episodic dizziness or vertigo accounts for about 20 percent of panic presentations, headache for about 10 percent, and syncope for another 10 percent. As with depression, there are times when the anxiety component of the panic attacks seems minimal and the patient emphasizes the physical symptom.

Generalized anxiety disorder (GAD) may be the most common anxiety disorder other than simple phobias. Patients with GAD tend to worry excessively over a number of things, including physical symptoms, and are often extremely vigilant for physical perturbations, which they present to their physician. Patients with this pattern of behavior often have a long (if not life-long) pattern of such generalized anxiety. They often have a reputation among family and friends for being anxious.

Patients with *obsessive compulsive disorder (OCD)* present with repeated behaviors (compulsions) or repeated thoughts (obsessions). It is possible that OCD may manifest as hypochondriasis, with repeated thoughts of being sick. The presence of some physical symptoms amplified by obsessive attention may also appear as somatization. In some cases, especially of monosymptomatic preoccupations, trials of anti-OCD drugs such as clomipramine or fluoxetine, with or without augmentation by buspirone, may be of benefit.

Schizophrenia and Psychotic Disorders

Occasionally a patient with an underlying psychotic disorder will present with some medically unexplainable symptom. Usually the symptoms of psychotic patients tend to have a bizarre aspect. Naturally the clinician should ascertain the patient's past psychiatric history to see if there has been a previous diagnosis of psychosis. When the physical symptom is part of a schizophrenic disorder, adequate treatment of the schizophrenic psychosis with neuroleptics will often resolve the physical symptom component. In fact, somatized symptoms may

be one of the early symptoms of relapse in some schizophrenics going off their medication.

There are cases in which a nonschizophrenic patient has such an intense somatic preoccupation that it is labeled delusional. The identification of a delusion is somewhat arbitrary and is a matter of clinical judgment. Such patients may be considered candidates for a trial of neuroleptics. However, when the somatized symptom is isolated and not part of a broader psychotic disorder, neuroleptics are rarely successful. Nevertheless, a short-term trial, when other psychiatric diagnoses have been considered, is often warranted.

Conversion Disorder

Patients with conversion disorder present with a single physical symptom that appears in the context of some emotional distress. The symptom serves as a psychological defense against some unconscious conflict. For example, one patient presented with inability to move her right arm after a mastectomy. The initial differential diagnosis involved damage to axillary nerve plexus, or spinal cord involvement associated with disease or anesthesia complications. However, careful neurologic examination revealed that the motor loss did not fit the pattern of any possible physical disorder. Under hypnotic induction, the patient described an urge to kill herself by stabbing herself with a knife. The motor "loss" served as protection against this unconscious impulse. Over a course of brief therapy, the patient was able to come to terms with her extreme emotional response to her cancer diagnosis, and her arm symptom resolved. Thus, conversion disorder is a specific form of somatization.

Malingering

Malingering is defined as the conscious pursuit of an identifiable secondary gain through a physical symptom. For example, patients may complain of continued pain (or some other symptom) in order to obtain medical disability or compensation through a lawsuit. Therefore, in any somatizing patient, it is important to inquire about any pending legal action or disability-compensation issue. Patients with factitious disorders are also fabricating physical symptoms. However, unlike malingerers, their goals may appear less clear-cut, and the process producing the symptoms may be less consciously planned. (Malingering is discussed in greater detail in the following chapter.)

Hypochondriasis

Hypochondriasis is often confused with somatization in terminology. Hypochondriasis is the false belief that one has a disease. When there is no actual symptom present, the diagnosis of somatization is not relevant. However, when there is a concurrent medical disorder, exaggerated hypochondriacal concerns may be difficult to distinguish from somatization. As with somatization, hypochondriasis may be acute or chronic. It may also be a manifestation of underlying depression and disappear when the depression is resolved.

MEDICAL EVALUATION ISSUES

One of the major problems in making the diagnosis of somatization is that the definition requires the absence of an underlying physical cause. To begin with, the presence of some physical disorder does not rule out somatization. Somatized symptom(s) can co-occur with biomedically based symptoms. At times it can be very difficult to rule out physical causes in a patient who presents convincingly. There are also some relatively obscure or complex disorders that present with chronic physical symptoms which may elude diagnosis, such as fibromyalgia, polymyalgia rheumatica, Lyme disease, chronic fatigue syndrome, and multiple sclerosis.

While diagnostic vigilance is warranted, clinicians can get into trouble using a "rule out" mentality with somatizing patients. Such patients can lead the clinician down a path of endless diagnostic testing, each test suggesting that some physical disease may be present if only enough tests are done to find it. Excessive diagnostic testing also creates potential physical morbidity. At some point, the clinician must recognize the likelihood of somatization and move into the management strategy appropriate for such patients. Within this strategy, diagnostic testing is not totally excluded. However, it is used sparingly.

Once patients are identified as possible somatizers, their physical symptoms cannot be totally ignored. When symptoms are ignored, patients become more anxious, more insistent, or simply go to see another physician. One challenge with the somatizing patient is to assemble all previous diagnostic testing. It is an unfortunate consequence of our medical system that patients can see numerous physicians without consolidation of their medical records. Repeating all the tests not only wastes money but perpetuates a pattern of maladaptive behavior for the patient. After getting to know the patient, the physician diagnosing somatization must have the courage to limit diagnostic testing and move from the focused physical into the management strategy described below.

MANAGEMENT IN THE THERAPEUTIC RELATIONSHIP

Since the driving force behind somatization is psychosocial distress, it is necessary to review potential areas of distress in such patients. Common sources of distress involve work, finances, relationships, domestic violence, abuse, sexuality, and family.

Guidelines for Managing Patients with Acute Somatized Symptoms

There are no controlled studies on the value of psychotherapy in patients with brief forms of somatiza-tion. Somatization in patients undergoing transient stress is often time limited, and the patient recovers spontaneously. Nevertheless, the treatment approach involves the following:

1. Identify the relevant psychosocial distresses.
2. Perform brief physical assessment to assure the patient that a medical problem is not being overlooked.
3. Link the psychosocial distress to the symptom through an educational approach.
4. Reassure the patient that there is no disease requiring medical treatment.
5. Involve the patient in some treatment that will help address the underlying psychosocial distress.

Guidelines for Managing Patients with Chronic Somatized Symptoms

1. Reassurance that nothing is wrong does not help.
2. The patient does not want a diagnosis or symptom relief but rather an ongoing relationship and understanding.
3. The patient wants the physician to acknowledge that he or she is sick. The patient should not be told that there is no real problem. Instead the physician should show a willingness to help identify the problems the patient is facing. The physician should acknowledge the patient's plight.
4. Little is gained by a premature educational explanation that the symptoms are based on psychosocial distress. Such an explanation is eventually important but must be gradually introduced in the context of an ongoing trusting relationship and not come across as rejection.
5. A positive organic diagnosis does not cure these patients. The emphasis should be on functional level rather than on symptoms. It is important to assess the patient's coping resources.
6. Regularly scheduled appointments are required so the patient does not have to manifest symptoms to seek help.
7. The physician should reinforce nonillness behaviors and communications.
8. Diagnostic tests should be limited. Some focused examination can be helpful, with more reliance on signs than symptoms.

The recommendations for treating the chronic somatizing patient may seem complex, but they are not too difficult to put into practice. It has been demonstrated that primary care physicians are able to reduce medical care costs by instituting such management practices when they feel some confidence in the diagnosis supplied by a psychiatric consultant.

The most important aspect of the management strategy is to establish a trusting relationship. Many physicians assume that what a patient wants to hear is good news: "There is nothing wrong with you!" It turns out that this is exactly the wrong message to give chronic somatizing patients. While no one has exactly identified the psychodynamic basis for chronic somatization, it seems clear that such patients are seeking some relationship as an aspect of their illness behavior. Telling such patients that nothing is wrong basically tells the patient they do not have to be seen again. Such patients will merely accentuate their somatizing in order to accomplish one of their prime goals—an ongoing relationship with the physician. Therefore, physicians should just accept the fact that what the patient wants is a relationship, not a diagnosis. This oversimplified formula can provide the basis of a useful management strategy. Give the patient a relationship by regular scheduled brief visits, regardless of the patent's symptom status. Do not force the patient into having to produce symptoms in order to be seen. To have a chance to succeed in this strategy, it is crucial for the physician to recognize the frustration and anger that may emerge when dealing with these patients.

WORKING WITH PSYCHIATRY

Patients with longer, more chronic forms of somatization are often reluctant to consider psychiatric referral or psychotherapies because of a resistance to considering a psychological model. Yet making a referral to psychiatry can be an important, if difficult, hurdle. To begin with, there is a group of somatizing patients who will be offended by the implication of a psychiatry referral and will never go. This residual group is one of the most frustrating to deal with. However, most patients will accept such a referral if it is made in a reasonable way, which includes a credible explanation. There needs to be some discussion with the patient that includes the following elements:

1. That the patient may be under some stress (everyone is).
2. That whether or not the stress is directly causing the symptoms in question, that stress can exaggerate symptoms and interfere with treatment and resolution.
3. That it will be important to look further into this dimension as part of an overall evaluation.

If there is suspicion of a psychiatric disorder such as depression, anxiety, or neuropsychiatric disorder, a referral to a psychiatrist is necessary. In cases that seem clearly related to some identifiable stress, the use of a nonmedical mental health professional for stress management or supportive therapy may be indicated.

SUGGESTED READING

Brown FW. Somatization disorder in progressive dementia. Psychosomatics 1991; 32:463–465.

Escobar JI, Rubio-Stipec M, Canino G, et al. Somatic Symptom Index (SSI): A new and abridged somatization construct. J Nerv Ment Dis 1989; 177:140–146.

Goldberg RJ, Novack DH, Gask L. The recognition and management of somatization: What is needed in primary care training. Psychosomatics. 1992; 33:55–61.

Kaplan C, Lipkin M Jr., Gordon GH. Somatization in primary care: Patients with unexplained and vexing medical complaints. J Gen Intern Med 1988; 3:177–190.

Katon W, Lin E, Von Korff M, et al. Somatization: A spectrum of severity. Am J Psychiatry 1991; 148:34–40.

Kellner R, Hypochondriasis and somatization. JAMA 1987; 258: 2718–2722.

Simon GE, Von Korff M. Somatization and psychiatric disorder in the NIMH epidemiologic catchment area study. Am J Psychiatry 1991; 148:1494–1500.

Smith GR. The epidemiology and treatment of depression when it coexists with somatoform disorders, somatization, or pain. Gen Hosp Psychiatry 1992; 14:265–272.

Smith RL. Somatization disorder: Defining its role in clinical medicine. J Gen Intern Med 1991; 6:168–175.

MALINGERING

THOMAS J. GUILMETTE, Ph.D., A.B.P.P.
DUANE S. BISHOP, M.D.

Malingering is defined as the intentional production or exaggeration of symptoms that outweigh the objective medical findings, for the purpose of obtaining an external incentive such as financial compensation or the avoidance of an aversive environment, such as prison. The presence of both an external incentive and the intentional production or exaggeration of symptoms is necessary to consider the diagnosis of malingering.

Other psychiatric disorders such as Münchausen's syndrome (the psychological need to assume the sick role), conversion disorders, depression, and personality disorders can affect symptom presentation, but the diagnosis of malingering cannot be made in these conditions, because the exaggeration of deficits may not be intentional or there may not be an obvious secondary gain.

Within neurology, the exaggeration of symptoms for secondary gain is evident in cases where there is a strong financial incentive to exhibit impairment, such as in personal injury, disability, or forensic cases. Also, individuals with injuries that are considered mild to moderate are more likely to exaggerate symptoms than individuals with more severe injuries, because deficits in the latter group would be apparent even to the casual observer. More specifically, injuries resulting from mild to moderate head trauma where symptoms are largely subjective, such as headache and cognitive disorders, as well as injuries resulting in pain syndromes provide the greatest opportunity for malingering. Unfortunately, there have been few attempts (in the neurologic literature) to develop empirical methods of assessing exaggeration of symptoms. There has been far greater research in neuropsychology and psychiatry to develop validated methods of detecting simulated cognitive dysfunction and mental disorders.

This chapter focuses on patient characteristics and behavior that may raise the practitioner's index of suspicion that malingering may be present. Apart from a few select signs, however, no single, well-validated measure demonstrates conclusively that a patient is exaggerating symptoms. Thus the practitioner is forced to utilize and integrate data from a number of sources to determine if a pattern of deception is present. We will focus on examples that may be most common in personal injury cases, particularly those involving mild to moderate head trauma, because these injuries can present diagnostic dilemmas and are most easily simulated.

We begin with some myths and misconceptions about malingering in general.

MYTHS ABOUT MALINGERING

Myth 1: Any patient who is involved in a personal injury case or has a lawyer must be malingering. A neurologist evaluating a patient who is involved in personal injury litigation should consider malingering as a differential diagnosis, although the base rates of malingering are generally unknown. Studies that have looked specifically at the resolution of symptoms following settlement of a court case or that have attempted to determine base rates for malingering have revealed estimates as low as 1 percent and as high as 50 percent.

Myth 2: Malingering is easy to detect through face-to-face clinical interviews. The detection of lying during face-to-face interviews is fraught with error even for the most seasoned clinician. Relying on "gut instincts" rather than on specific aspects of a patient's presentation is likely to cause both under- and overdetection of malingering.

Myth 3: Only individuals with psychopathic personalities are likely to simulate deficits. Although there may be a high proportion of individuals with antisocial personality disorders who undergo forensic evaluations, particularly in criminal cases or to avoid prison, there is no empirical evidence to support the notion that a disproportionate number of patients in personal injury cases are sociopathic. By the same token, the absence of a criminal past history should not be used as a criterion in deciding that the patient will not exaggerate deficits. Last, individuals with a history of criminal behavior or antisocial personality are no more adept at faking symptoms or malingering than the general population.

Myth 4: Patients with genuine organic illnesses will not exaggerate their symptoms. Genuine neurologic disorder and malingering are not mutually exclusive. Thus you may be confronted with an individual who is fabricating all symptoms, which theoretically should be easier to detect, as well as by an individual who is simply exaggerating his or her level of dysfunction or symptomatology. You cannot automatically assume that individuals with objective medical evidence of a neurologic disorder will not further exaggerate their impairment for secondary gain.

Myth 5: The absence of objective medical evidence should automatically result in the diagnosis of malingering. The absence of "hard" neurologic findings should not definitively result in the diagnosis of malingering, particularly in the absence of secondary gain on the part of the patient. In addition, certain types of neurologic conditions may, by definition, result in a normal neurologic examination. The most notable disorder in this group is mild head injury, where subjective complaints predominate in the absence of any quantifiable deficits on neurodiagnostic or clinical examinations. Although there is still some controversy concerning postconcussive or post–head-injury syndromes, there is enough scientific evidence to support permanent disability even in the absence of definitive neurologic signs.

HOW TO DETECT MALINGERING

With few exceptions, there is no well-validated test to identify simulation of neurologic disorders. The clinician must look for a convergence of evidence that includes history, patient characteristics, injury parameters, incentive, interview behavior, and physical examination to support a malingering diagnosis. The weight each practitioner gives the variables described below depends on the type of error that he or she feels most comfortable committing: labeling someone a malinger who is not, or saying someone is not a malinger who is. The diagnosis of malingering needs to be taken very seriously because it is a label that carries significant medical-legal and financial ramifications. As such, the diagnosis of malingering needs to be made judiciously.

Listed below are characteristics of a patient's history or presentation that should alert the clinician to possible exaggeration of symptomatology.

1. *Late onset of symptoms.* Symptoms that are first reported several months postinjury or following a meeting with an attorney should arouse the suspicion that, at the very least, there may be some psychological component to symptom presentation. Although the effects of some injuries may not be evident until a patient tries to return to his or her normal routine, it is unusual for individuals who have resumed their normal lifestyle and who are functioning relatively well to suddenly deteriorate because of an injury that occurred several months previously. Generally speaking, earlier onset of symptoms is usually associated with greater genuine disability.

2. *Resistance to evaluation or treatment.* Patients who find excuses for not following through on treatment recommendations or follow-up evaluation may be trying to avoid scrutiny from medical professionals or diagnostic testing. Simulators may also be reluctant to engage in treatment for fear that their symptoms will be expected to lessen or dissipate. It is important to inquire why the patient has not complied with suggestions, because there are numerous other reasons why patients do not comply with treatment.

3. *Resistance to signing release forms to obtain additional background information or reports from other medical professionals.* Although patients may have legitimate reasons for not wishing to disclose reports from medical professionals or other sources, such as legitimate personality clashes with former treatment providers or other embarrassing non–injury-related information, a reluctance to disclose information can suggest that a patient is trying to hide contrary or conflicting findings or that other practitioners may have suspected malingering or exaggeration of deficit. When patients are reluctant to sign releases of information or if they have a great number of questions as to why the information we are requesting is necessary to obtain, we attempt to reassure them of the importance of gathering all pertinent information while simultaneously inquiring, in a nonthreatening manner, about their resistance.

4. *Evidence of lying about history.* Patients may make small errors or slightly under- or overestimate certain aspects of their history and functioning. When a blatant lie is detected, however, it should call into question all information the patient has provided. Fabricated stories about what other physicians have said or gross inaccuracies about occupational, military, or educational history, for example, must lead to doubting the veracity of the patient's report on all aspects of his or her functioning.

5. *Inconsistencies with physical examination as reported by other medical professionals or with your own examination conducted earlier.* It is important to take detailed notes about the patient's comments regarding his or her functional impairment and the extent of motor and sensory loss, so that other practitioners can replicate your findings or so that you can re-evaluate the patient at a later date to determine the consistency of the patient's symptomatology. Especially to the unsophisticated deceiver, it can be difficult to replicate the same symptoms in a physical examination over a period of several months. This is particularly true of motor tasks that require range of motion, speed, and strength, all functions that can be objectively assessed. It is incumbent upon the practitioner,

therefore, to try to use the most objective method possible to quantify the extent of impairment so that the results can be replicated later by the same or other neurologists.

6. *Nondermatomal sensory loss and giveway weakness.* In the case of sensory loss, measurements can be taken to localize the extent and pattern of the deficit and conclude whether it is consistent with neuroanatomic dermatomes. The ability to judge giveway weakness, however, may vary from clinician to clinician and may thus be a less reliable and valid measure. Because techniques and interpretations vary, this measure does not lend itself to replication by other practitioners.

7. *The presence of Waddell signs.* These signs include nonanatomic and superficial tenderness, the simulation of movement that the patient previously reported caused pain, inconsistent pain response from the patient while being distracted, weakness or sensory loss that is inconsistent with anatomic origin, and overreaction. Three or more of these signs is suggestive of a nonorganic basis for the patient's complaints.

8. *Marked pain behavior in your office that is inconsistent with the patient's report of functioning in other environments.* An example is the patient who is unable to sit for longer than a few minutes in your office yet was able to drive a long distance to get there. A report of severe, unremitting pain but undisturbed sleep is another example of an inconsistency between patient description of symptoms and functional capabilities. The malingerer may be less likely to undergo painful laboratory tests for diagnostic reasons. A history of pain-related litigation cases requires a careful scrutiny of the patient's records and may reveal prior evidence of malingering.

9. *Frequent "I don't know" responses to simple or easy questions.* Suspicion should be raised when patients are unable to provide even rudimentary autobiographical information, such as their home address, date of birth, or names of siblings, or when they give bizarre or blatantly incorrect responses to orientation questions or questions of common knowledge, such as the name of the president of the United States. The clinician should encourage the patient to make a guess and, if that fails, provide multiple choices. Patients who will not guess at questions, even when given three choices from which to choose, should make the physician suspicious of their effort and motivation.

10. *Evidence of exaggeration of pathology or "faking bad" on psychological testing.* Malingering research has revealed that the Minnesota Multiphasic Personality Inventory (MMPI) is one of the most sensitive measures of malingering

detection available. Several indices on the MMPI, including the validity scales, the subtle/obvious items, the Dissimulation Scale (a scale that separates individuals attempting to fake neurosis from patients who actually have neurotic conditions), and the number of critical items endorsed all provide important information regarding a patient's tendency toward defensiveness or symptom exaggeration. Referral to a psychologist for evaluation with the MMPI may assist the practitioner in the diagnosis of malingering.

11. *Failure on forced-choice testing procedures.* Forced-choice or symptom validity test procedures have been gaining greater support within the field of neuropsychology as a way of detecting feigned memory impairment. These procedures can also be effective in the detection of feigned visual, hearing, and sensory loss. The underlying principle in these procedures is to provide a patient with two possible responses from which they are to choose over several trials. Because each stimulus is provided an equal number of times, even patients who are guessing randomly because they don't know the correct answer should show at least a chance level of performance, or 50 percent correct. A score indicating significantly less than chance performance would be indicative of malingering.

The following are two examples of this forced-choice procedure. For assessment of a memory disorder, the patient can be shown one of two stimuli, such as a black pen or a yellow pencil, or one of two five-digit numbers, and asked to remember which stimulus they were shown after a 5 second delay period. The patient can then be shown both stimuli together and asked which one they just saw. If each stimulus is presented an equal number of times but in random order over several trials (30 or more), then random guessing will result in a chance level of performance. Because recall of this information is so simple, the use of this strategy in memory assessment can reveal poor motivation to perform well when the error rate exceeds 10 to 20 percent. When the performance is less than chance, a very strong case can be made for suspecting the intentional exaggeration of deficits.

In assessing sensory loss, one of two single digit numbers can be written on a patient's fingertip or in the palm of their hand, again over several trials, with the patient asked to state which number was just written. A significantly less than chance performance (an error rate of greater than 60 percent) would strongly suggest malingering. There are several variations of these procedures. Empirical evidence exists regarding their sensitivity to faked memory dysfunction. Although the underlying principle remains the same, these types of symptom validity test procedures can be made to appear more difficult then they actually are, which may be necessary for more sophisticated patients. More refined

methods have been developed within neuropsychology. Neuropsychological consultation may be quite helpful in differentiating exaggerated from objective memory deficits.

COMMENTS

The detection of malingering does not lend itself to the application of cutoff scores and hard pathognomonic signs. Rather, it requires the integration of convergent pieces of data obtained from the patient's history, interview, physical examination, and other corroborating sources. Research in this domain is in its infancy. What has emerged to this point is that there is no standard malingering profile. Patients may exaggerate symptoms or deficits to varying degrees, in varying ways, to various practitioners. The myths and fallacies about malingering also cloud the ability of practitioners to detect simulation. When there is a likelihood of significant secondary gain, it is best for the practitioner to consider malingering as a differential diagnosis. Personal injury cases involving mild to moderate head injuries or pain syndromes are more likely to be associated with the emergence of symptom exaggeration. However, it is also important to recognize that postconcussive symptoms do occur in the absence of objective neurologic findings, and thus absence of "hard" findings does not automatically warrant a diagnosis of malingering.

We suggest that a team of practitioners be utilized to evaluate patients when malingering is in question. Each professional can evaluate the patient with his or her own specialized diagnostic skills, and the patient's symptoms can be discussed and reviewed in a collaborative format. These types of evaluation teams should include individuals who are familiar with research in malingering detection and whose clinical areas, such as neuropsychology and psychiatry, can be helpful in differentiating genuine from fabricated symptoms.

SUGGESTED READING

Binder LM. Malingering detected by forced choice testing of memory and tactile sensation: A case report. Arch Clin Neuropsychol 1992; 7:155–163.

Binder LM. Deception and malingering. In: Puente A, McCaffrey R, eds. Handbook of neuropsychological assessment: A biopsychosocial perspective. New York: Plenum Press, 1992.

Guilmette TJ, Hart KJ, Giuliano AJ. Malingering detection: The use of a forced-choice method in identifying organic versus simulated memory impairment. Clin Neuropsychol 1993;7:59-69.

Pankratz L. Symptom validity testing and symptom retraining: Procedures for the assessment and treatment of functional sensory deficits. J Consult Clin Psychol 1979; 47:409–410.

Pankratz L, Binder LM, Wilcox LM. Evaluation of an exaggerated somatosensory deficit with symptom validity testing. Arch Neurol 1987; 44:798.

Rogers R. Clinical assessment of malingering and deception. New York: Guilford Press, 1988.

Waddell G, McCulloch JA, Kummel E, Venner RM. Non-organic physical signs in low back pain. Spine 1980; 5:117–125.

DISORDERS OF CONSCIOUSNESS

COMA

KAREN FURIE, M.D.
EDWARD FELDMANN, M.D.

Coma, derived from the Greek word for "sleep," is a state simulating sleep in which the patient fails to respond to external stimuli and initiates no voluntary activities. Brain stem and spinal reflexes may be preserved. It is important to distinguish coma (unarousable unresponsiveness) from other degrees of impaired arousal and responsiveness such as stupor (arousable, unresponsive), and obtundation (arousable, reduced level of alertness). These disorders must be distinguished from akinetic mutism (alert unresponsiveness) and the "locked in" syndrome (normal level of consciousness, unable to move). A vegetative state describes a state of chronic unresponsiveness in which there are normal sleep-wake cycles.

Coma is the result of either a lesion in the brain stem affecting the ascending reticular activating system or dysfunction of both cerebral hemispheres. The lesion may be structural or metabolic. Structural and metabolic abnormalities that cause coma are listed in Table 1. The neurologic examination can be used to localize the site of the lesion. The examination should focus on the respiratory pattern, pupillary response, eye movements, and motor response.

INITIAL EVALUATION

The history of pre-existing medical conditions, medications, and recent illness or trauma is invaluable but often difficult to obtain at the time of presentation. A description of the onset of coma, whether sudden or gradual, may be helpful in diagnosis. The former suggests a vascular event or seizure and the latter a toxic or metabolic process, or slowly enlarging mass.

The general physical examination can provide helpful clues to the cause of coma. The patient should be carefully examined for evidence of head or cervical spine trauma. Neck stiffness should be noted in assessing for

Table 1 Structural and Metabolic Causes of Coma

Supratentorial lesions
  Massive infarction with edema
  Bithalamic infarcts
  Venous sinus thrombosis
  Subdural hemorrhage
  Epidural hemorrhage
  Epidural empyema
  Intraventricular hemorrhage
  Pituitary apoplexy
  Intracerebral hemorrhage
  Abscess
  Tumor
  Post-traumatic

Infratentorial lesions
  Brain stem infarction
  Cerebellar infarction
  Brain stem hemorrhage
  Cerebellar hemorrhage
  Herniation
  Central pontine myelinolysis
  Demyelination
  Tumor
  Abscess
  Granulomatous infection

Metabolic
  Ischemic-hypoxic
  Hypoglycemia
  Diabetic ketoacidosis
  Wernicke's encephalopathy
  Hepatic encephalopathy
  Uremic encephalopathy
  Pancreatic encephalopathy
  Hypothyroidism/hyperthyroidism
  Addison's disease/Cushing's disease
  Electrolyte abnormalities (sodium, calcium, magnesium, phosphorus)
  Intoxication
  Seizure
  Meningitis/encephalitis

Adapted from Plum F, Posner JB. The diagnosis of stupor and coma. 3rd ed. Philadelphia: FA Davis, 1980; with permission.

possible subarachnoid hemorrhage or meningitis. There may be physical findings indicative of cardiac, hepatic, or renal dysfunction. The extremities should be examined for peripheral emboli or evidence of intravenous drug abuse.

The pattern of respiration can be helpful in localizing the lesion in a comatose patient. Cheyne-Stokes respirations occur with bihemispheric or diencephalic dysfunction. Lesions of the rostral pons or midbrain may be associated with neurogenic hyperventilation. In patients with hyperventilation, metabolic acidosis and hypoxemia should be excluded because these are far more common than primary neurogenic hyperventilation. Pontine lesions may cause apneustic breathing, characterized by a prolonged inspiratory phase and inspiratory and expiratory pauses. Ataxic respirations are seen with disruption of medullary respiratory pathways. Other reflexes mediated by the medulla are yawning, vomiting, and hiccupping.

Abnormal motor responses include decortication (upper extremity adduction and flexion, lower extremities extended and internally rotated) and decerebration (upper and lower extremities extended and internally rotated). Decortication typically occurs with hemisphere lesions, while decerebration is seen with lesions of the midbrain. Extension of the arms and flexion of the legs is observed in pontine dysfunction. The extremities are typically flaccid with lesions of the medulla. Asymmetric responses or frank hemiplegia suggest the presence of a focal, structural lesion.

The pupillary light reactions may be affected early in uncal herniation, but they are preserved until late in the course of metabolic coma. Exceptions include cerebral anoxic-ischemic insults, which result in pupillary dilation. Opiate drugs cause miosis, but the pupillary light reflex is preserved. Glutethimide (Doriden) produces asymmetric midposition, unreactive pupils. Anticholinergic toxicity can produce large, poorly reactive pupils. Structural midbrain lesions cause midposition, 4 to 5 mm, unreactive pupils. Dorsal tectal and pretectal lesions may cause pupils to react to accommodation but not to light. Pontine pupils are bilaterally miotic, which, although difficult to detect, have an intact light reflex. A lateral medullary syndrome may cause a Horner's syndrome (ptosis, miosis, anhidrosis). Uncal herniation is heralded by an ipsilateral dilated, unreactive pupil.

Eye movement is mediated by both the frontal lobes and brain stem nuclei and is therefore commonly affected in comatose states. In supratentorial lesions, the eyes deviate toward the lesion and away from the side of hemiplegia. In hemispheric lesions, whether the eyes are midline or horizontally deviated, the oculocephalic reflex is preserved. Roving eye movements are a common finding. With lesions of the midbrain, the eyes remain in the midline, and they do not respond to the vertical Doll's maneuver. Downward deviation of the eyes may be seen with compression of the tectum. With pontine lesions, eye movements are almost always abnormal. Internuclear ophthalmoplegia from a lesion of the medial longitudinal fasciuolis may be seen, or there may be skew deviation. In contrast to horizontal gaze deviation seen in hemispheric lesions, horizontal gaze deviations in pontine lesions cannot be overcome by the Doll's maneuver or caloric stimulation. Eyes deviate away from the side of pontine lesion and toward the side

of hemiplegia. Ocular bobbing, a periodic downward deviation, may also be seen.

When the Doll's maneuver fails to elicit a clear response, ice water calorics should be performed to test the integrity of the oculovestibular system. The external canal must first be examined to ensure that there is no obstructing cerumen or perforation of the tympanic membrane. In a normally awake patient, with the head elevated 30 degrees from horizontal, irrigation with 5 to 10 cc of ice water will produce nystagmus, with the slow phase ipsilateral to the stimulation. The opposite response is obtained if warm water is used. Nystagmus has a slow component mediated by the brain stem, followed by a cortically driven rapid phase. Nystagmus should not be present in true unresponsiveness, regardless of the location of the lesion. In comatose patients with hemispheric lesions and an intact brain stem, there is tonic conjugate deviation toward the irrigated ear with no nystagmus. An asymmetric response, with deviation of only the eye ipsilateral to irrigation, points to a pontine lesion involving the medial longitudinal fasciculus. Patients with midbrain destruction will also have an asymmetric response due to third nerve damage.

The presence of corneal reflexes and Bell's phenomenon indicates the integrity of the third, fifth, and seventh cranial nerves. An asymmetry in the responses can be a helpful indicator of a focal brain stem lesion. Bilaterally absent corneal reflexes may be due to sedative drugs or hypothermia.

ACUTE MANAGEMENT

An algorithm for initial evaluation and management of the comatose patient is illustrated in Figure 1. This scheme uses the neurologic examination, whether focal or nonfocal, as a significant branching point in determining the cause of coma. There are exceptions to these guidelines. For example, metabolic aberrations such as hyponatremia and hypoglycemia may produce focal neurologic deficits. Alternatively, structural abnormalities such as bifrontal subdural hematomas may cause few focal neurologic signs.

The issue of whether every patient should have a computed tomography (CT) scan of the head prior to a lumbar puncture remains debatable. In general, with a nonfocal examination, a mass-producing lesion capable of causing herniation is unlikely. Any patient who fails to arouse after identified metabolic abnormalities have been corrected should have a CT scan of the head and, if appropriate, a lumbar puncture.

Note the recent addition of flumazenil to the list of emergency drugs administered diagnostically and therapeutically to patients with coma of unknown cause. Flumazenil, a benzodiazepine antagonist, has been used successfully to reverse coma of unknown cause. Adverse effects of this drug include nausea, vomiting, depression, agitation, anxiety, and shivering. Benzodiazepine withdrawal with seizures, although rare, can occur.

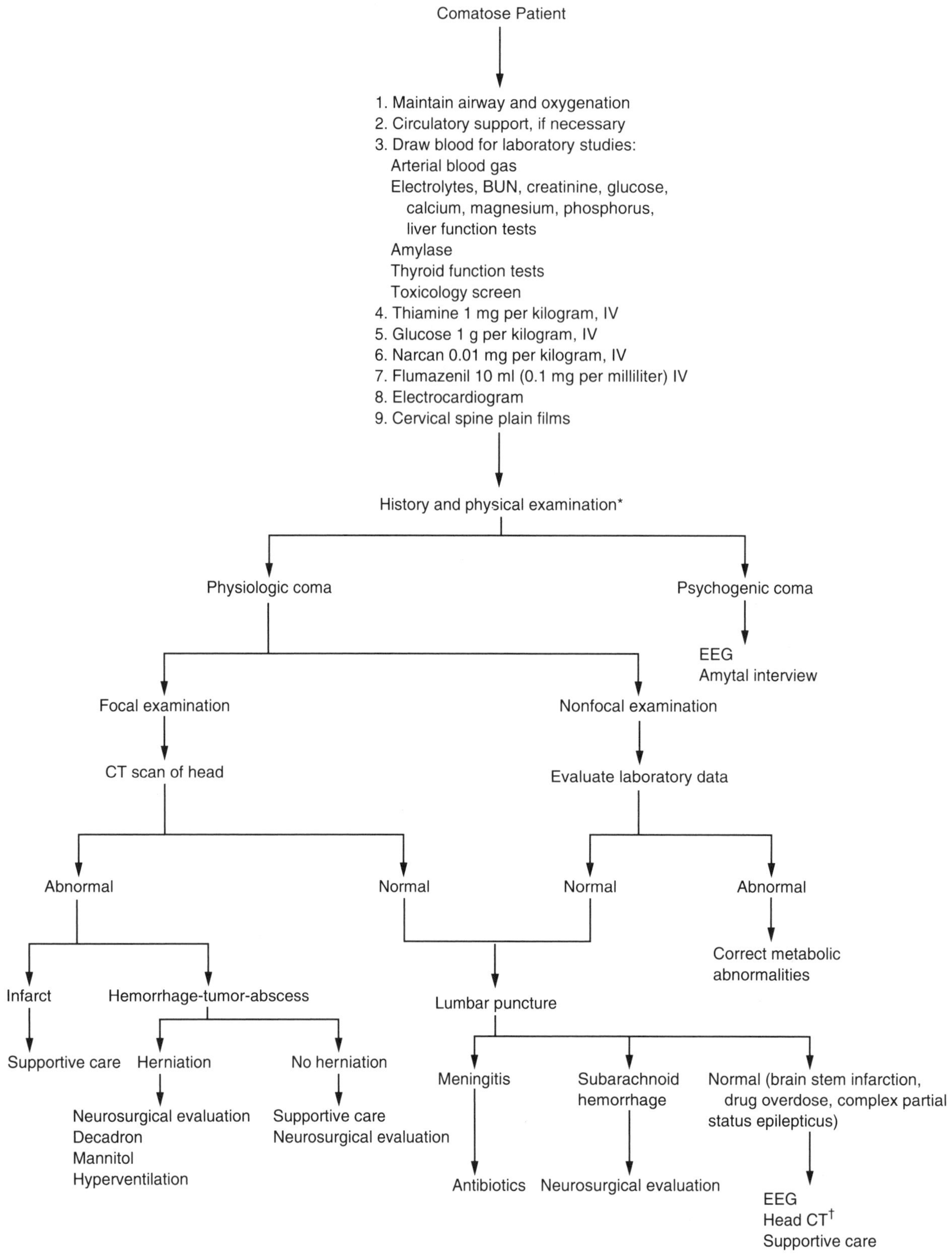

Comatose Patient

1. Maintain airway and oxygenation
2. Circulatory support, if necessary
3. Draw blood for laboratory studies:
   Arterial blood gas
   Electrolytes, BUN, creatinine, glucose,
      calcium, magnesium, phosphorus,
      liver function tests
   Amylase
   Thyroid function tests
   Toxicology screen
4. Thiamine 1 mg per kilogram, IV
5. Glucose 1 g per kilogram, IV
6. Narcan 0.01 mg per kilogram, IV
7. Flumazenil 10 ml (0.1 mg per milliliter) IV
8. Electrocardiogram
9. Cervical spine plain films

History and physical examination*

Physiologic coma → Psychogenic coma

Psychogenic coma → EEG / Amytal interview

Physiologic coma → Focal examination / Nonfocal examination

Focal examination → CT scan of head

Nonfocal examination → Evaluate laboratory data

CT scan of head → Abnormal / Normal

Evaluate laboratory data → Normal / Abnormal

Abnormal → Infarct / Hemorrhage-tumor-abscess

Abnormal (laboratory) → Correct metabolic abnormalities

Infarct → Supportive care

Hemorrhage-tumor-abscess → Herniation / No herniation

Herniation → Neurosurgical evaluation / Decadron / Mannitol / Hyperventilation

No herniation → Supportive care / Neurosurgical evaluation

Normal (CT and laboratory) → Lumbar puncture

Lumbar puncture → Meningitis / Subarachnoid hemorrhage / Normal (brain stem infarction, drug overdose, complex partial status epilepticus)

Meningitis → Antibiotics

Subarachnoid hemorrhage → Neurosurgical evaluation

Normal (brain stem infarction, drug overdose, complex partial status epilepticus) → EEG / Head CT† / Supportive care

Figure 1 Algorithm for acute coma management. * = Includes ice water calorics, when necessary. † = If head CT was negative on admission, patient may have brain stem infarction; repeat CT in 24 to 48 hours or obtain MRI. BUN = blood urea nitrogen; EEG = electroencephalogram; CT = computed tomography.

ANCILLARY TESTS

A noncontrast CT scan of the brain can reveal acute hemorrhages or mass lesions in the hemispheres. Unfortunately, the posterior fossa is often poorly visualized due to bony artifact. Magnetic resonance imaging (MRI) scanning provides more detail in those cases where posterior fossa pathology is suspected, and it has the advantage of magnetic resonance angiography (MRA) capability. MRI is rarely available on an emergency basis and cannot be used if the patient requires mechanical ventilation, except in specialized centers.

Electroencephalography (EEG) is frequently used as an adjunct to the neurologic examination. Supratentorial structural lesions such as infarct, hemorrhage, or tumor often show focal EEG slowing, although with involvement of the contralateral hemisphere, there may be diffuse slowing. Metabolic encephalopathies cause a slowing of the background rhythm and may show specific patterns such as the triphasic waves seen in hepatic and uremic encephalopathies. An alpha background rhythm has been reported in patients with hypoxic-ischemic encephalopathy, but this is extremely rare. A poor prognosis has been associated with patterns of burst suppression and periodic complexes. Patients in myoclonic status epilepticus, usually a consequence of ischemic-hypoxic injury, have an almost uniformly poor outcome. Infratentorial lesions also cause diffuse slowing.

Brain stem auditory evoked responses and long-latency auditory responses may be more sensitive than the oculocephalic reflex in detecting vestibular dysfunction. Bilaterally absent signals may be associated with a poor prognosis. Preliminary investigation has shown that somatosensory evoked potentials may also be useful, an absence or abnormal response correlating with poor outcome. Somatosensory evoked responses are superior to motor evoked responses (MEPs) in predicting outcome. Only the bilateral absence of MEPs could be associated with a poor prognosis. Evoked responses have been found to add to the clinical assessment in certain cases, particularly to confirm poor prognosis. The use of these evoked responses as ancillary tests remains inadequately studied at this time. There is little evidence to support their sole use to determine prognosis for quality of survival.

PSYCHOGENIC COMA

In psychogenic coma, the loss of consciousness is often incomplete, with the patient intermittently and surreptitiously waking up and performing purposeful movements. The causes of psychogenic coma include catatonic stupor, psychotic depression, conversion reaction, dissociative state, and malingering. Obtaining a history from family members and friends may help to distinguish these entities.

These patients may respond to deep pain. They should have normal vital signs and intact, symmetrical reflexes. It is not uncommon to note forceful contraction of the orbiculares oculi when trying to test pupillary and oculocephalic reflexes. The pupillary and corneal reflexes are present. However, the oculocephalic reflex may be absent in the conscious patient. Ice water calorics will be normal, with nystagmus, and this painful stimulus may elicit a violent arousal in some patients.

Ancillary tests that may confirm the diagnosis of psychogenic coma are an EEG and an Amytal (amobarbital) interview. The EEG will show an alpha background rhythm with no paroxysmal or lateralizing abnormalities. The Amytal interview, in which amobarbital is slowly infused intravenously, operates on the premise that true neurologic deficits will worsen with Amytal administration, whereas factitious symptoms will improve.

PROGNOSIS

The Glasgow coma scale (GCS) (Table 2) has been applied to victims of out-of-hospital cardiac arrest in order to predict outcome. Within 48 hours of resuscitation, a score of greater than 10 correlated with "successful" resuscitation (return to premorbid status, moderate or severe disability) and less than 5 with "failure" (death or vegetative state). The ability of the Glasgow coma scale to accurately predict a good outcome (positive predictive value) was 77 percent, whereas it could correctly identify a poor outcome (negative predictive value) in 97 percent of cases. When evaluated by cause of nontraumatic coma, patients with ischemic-hypoxic insults have the worst prognosis, followed by those with other types of metabolic coma. Drug-induced coma had the best prognosis for recovery.

In a study of 210 patients with hypoxic-ischemic coma (Levy et al, 1985), strong predictors of no recovery

Table 2 Glasgow Coma Scale

Response	Score
Verbal	
None	1
Incomprehensible	2
Inappropriate	3
Confused	4
Oriented	5
Eye opening	
None	1
To pain	2
To speech	3
Spontaneous	4
Motor	
None	1
Extensor posturing	2
Flexor posturing	3
Withdrawal	4
Localizes	5
Follows commands	6

included an absent pupillary reflex on initial exam, absent corneal reflexes at day 1, and decortication, decerebration, or absent appropriate localizing motor response at 3 days. Factors associated with a good outcome were verbal response at initial examination, and speech, spontaneous eye movements, and intact oculocephalic or oculovestibular reflexes present on subsequent examinations. The duration of coma was inversely related to the chance of a favorable prognosis.

A study of 500 patients with nontraumatic coma (Bates et al, 1977) established that 59 percent remained in a coma, and of these, two-thirds died in this state within 3 days. In another study (Sacco et al, 1990), 61 percent of patients with nontraumatic coma were dead or in a persistent vegetative state at 2 weeks. Levy et al found that almost 90 percent of their patients had a poor outcome: 57 percent of patients who remained in hypoxic-ischemic coma for more than 6 hours died, and

20 percent of these died the first day; 20 percent remained in a vegetative state; severe disability (10 percent) and moderate disability (3 percent) accounted for the remainder. Of the 10 percent who had a good outcome, the majority recovered within the first 3 days.

SUGGESTED READING

Bates D, Caronna JJ, Cartlidge NEF, et al. A prospective study of nontraumatic coma: Methods and results in 310 patients. Ann Neurol 1977; 2:211–220.
Levy DE, Bates D, Caronna JJ, et al. Prognosis in nontraumatic coma. Ann Intern Med 1981; 94:293–301.
Levy DE, Caronna JJ, Singer BH, et al. Predicting outcome from hypoxic-ischemic coma. JAMA 1985; 253:1420–1426.
Plum F, Posner JB. The diagnosis of stupor and coma. 3rd ed. Philadelphia: FA Davis, 1980.
Sacco RL, VanGool R, Mohr JP, Hauser WA. Nontraumatic coma: Glascow Coma score and coma etiology as predictors of 2-week outcome. Arch Neurol 1990; 47:118–1184.

BRAIN DEATH

JAMES L. BERNAT, M.D.

Brain death refers to human death as determined by tests showing permanent cessation of functioning of the critical neurons subserving the cerebral hemispheres, diencephalon, brain stem, and cerebellum. In those societies accepting the concept of brain death, when the tests are satisfied the patient is considered medically and legally dead irrespective of continued heartbeat, circulation, cellular metabolism, or other intact somatic physiologic functions. The majority of American states and European countries have drafted legislation enabling physicians to declare brain death.

Clinicians determining brain death should perfect and follow a systematic neurologic examination. Because the determination of brain death is literally a "life or death" decision, it is essential that clinicians perform and interpret the tests carefully and correctly. Following is my approach to the determination of brain death.

HISTORY

The diagnosis of brain death should be considered when a patient has been rendered deeply comatose and apneic by a profound, diffuse brain insult, such as a massive head injury or global hypoxic-ischemic neuronal damage from cardiopulmonary arrest, drowning, or suffocation. To maintain heartbeat, such a patient will have previously undergone endotracheal intubation and will currently be receiving positive pressure ventilation. Frequently the patient will have become hypotensive from maximal generalized vasodilatation and will have required vasopressor agents to maintain adequate arterial blood pressure. The patient's failure to recover evidence of brain functioning over time will have triggered the brain death evaluation.

The history should center on the cause of the brain insult to ascertain that it is an irreversible structural lesion and not a potentially reversible metabolic or toxic encephalopathy. Thus, the events leading up to the illness or injury, medications, possible drug ingestion, and past medical history should be sought.

EXAMINATION

The determination of brain death is a *clinical* neurologic assessment made at the bedside by an experienced clinician using an accepted test battery of neurologic examination techniques. I use the test battery published in 1981 by the Medical Consultants to the President's Commission for the Study of Ethical Problems in Medicine and Biomedical and Behavioral Research. These tests demonstrate *total* cessation of the clinical functions of the cerebral hemispheres and brain stem. The tests further demonstrate *irreversibility* when (1) the clinician knows that the brain dysfunction is caused by a structural lesion; (2) the profound brain dysfunction persists for an interval of time; and (3) potentially reversible causes of findings on the neurologic examination have been excluded (Table 1).

Table 1 Tests to Determine Brain Death

I. Proof of Cessation of Whole-Brain Functioning
   A. Coma, unresponsivity
   B. Apnea
   C. Brain stem areflexia
      1. Absent pupillary reflexes
      2. Absent corneal reflexes
      3. Absent oculovestibular reflexes
      4. Absent gag reflexes
      5. Absent cough reflexes

II. Proof of Permanence of Cessation of Whole-Brain Functioning
   A. Known pathologic cause sufficient to produce clinical state
   B. Exclusion of potentially reversible causes
      1. No central nervous system depressant drugs
      2. No neuromuscular blocking drugs
      3. No metabolic encephalopathies, including hypothermia, shock
   C. Two examinations separated by time interval

III. Confirmatory Tests
   A. Electrophysiologic
      1. Electroencephalography
      2. Brain stem auditory evoked responses
      3. Somatosensory evoked potentials
   B. Intracranial blood flow
      1. Contrast angiography
      2. Radionuclide angiography
      3. Xenon-enhanced computed tomography
      4. Transcranial Doppler ultrasonography

From Bernat JL. Brain death and withdrawal of life support in hopeless neurological diseases. In: Grotta JC, ed. Management of the acutely ill neurological patient. New York: Churchill Livingstone, 1993; with permission.

Coma and Unresponsivity

I first assess the patient's level of consciousness by asking the nurses about spontaneous movements, breathing, or any evidence of consciousness and by observing the patient's response to verbal and noxious stimuli. The brain-dead patient exhibits the most profound form of coma possible. The patient lies motionless when the ventilator is stopped, has no spontaneous movement, no posturing, and no response to noxious stimuli, bright lights, loud noises, or threats to the nasal airway. Reflexes integrated solely at a spinal cord level such as limb deep-tendon reflexes and triple-flexion Babinski's signs may be preserved despite brain death. Coma and unresponsivity show cessation of function of the cognitive, arousal, and motor centers of the brain.

I have seen the "Lazarus sign" occasionally during apnea testing. Here, the brain-dead patient may slowly elevate both arms and cross them over the chest touching the chin. This movement is believed to result from progressive ischemia of cervical spinal cord motor neurons producing spontaneous neuronal discharges that move the arms. The presence of this sign implies nothing about the state of *brain* neuronal functioning. Like the persistence of intact limb deep tendon reflexes, the Lazarus sign demonstrates only that the spinal cord has not been destroyed by the initial injury that produced brain death. Because of the possibility of provoking the

Lazarus sign and the confusion it might produce, I request that family members be absent when I perform brain death evaluations.

Absent Brain Stem Reflexes

I next test for absent brain stem reflexes. All reflexes subserved by the cranial nerves and integrated in the brain stem must be absent in brain death.

Pupillary light reflexes require cranial nerves II and III, the midbrain, and the sympathetic nervous system. I test them by shining a bright point light source at each pupil and observing for pupilloconstriction. Pupils in brain death are usually midposition in size (3 to 7 mm in diameter) as a result of sympathetic and parasympathetic denervation. They neither constrict to light nor dilate to dark. Pupillary light reflexes may be affected by medications given during resuscitation or previously ingested by the patient. Widely dilated pupils may result from atropine administration. Constricted pupils may result from opiate ingestion. The clinician should also consider that the pupils may have been unreactive prior to the brain insult.

Corneal reflexes require cranial nerves V and VII and the pons. I test them by stroking the cornea with the rolled tip of a cotton-tipped applicator and observe for a response. No direct or consensual blink response should be present in brain death.

Vestibulo-ocular reflexes require cranial nerves III, IV, VI, and VIII, the median longitudinal fasciculus, the pons, and the midbrain. I test them by observing horizontal eye movements in response to 50 ml of ice water injected into the external auditory canals (maximal ice water caloric test). First I inspect the canals otoscopically to assure that the ice water will have free access to the tympanic membranes. I modify a size 19 butterfly intravenous device by removing the needle and then attach it to a 50 ml syringe. I adjust the bed so the patient is supine with the head elevated to 30 degrees above the horizontal. I insert the open tip of the butterfly device into one external auditory canal until it is a few millimeters from the tympanic membrane. I then rapidly deliver the full ice water contents of the syringe into the canal. I ask an assistant to raise the patient's eyelids to observe for reflex eye movements. Then I perform the test on the other ear after a 5 minute interval. Brain-dead patients should have neither reflex horizontal eye movements nor any response whatsoever to this test.

Gag and cough reflexes require cranial nerves IX and X and are integrated in the medulla. I test them by observing for gagging or coughing when I stimulate the pharynx with a tongue depressor. I observe for coughing or "bucking" when the nurse or respiratory therapist irrigates and suctions the endotracheal tube.

Apnea

Apnea shows failure of the medullary breathing centers and is a critical brain death test. Older sets of brain death tests considered apnea simply as failure to breathe when the patient was disconnected from the ventilator for a few minutes. Such a definition is inadequate because the medullary breathing centers respond more to a hypercapneic than to a hypoxemic stimulus. The PA_{CO_2} must be permitted to exceed 60 mm Hg to permit maximal stimulation of the medullary breathing centers. Without such stimulation, the mere demonstration of temporary absence of breathing does not prove apnea.

I test apnea using the technique of apneic oxygenation. This procedure permits me to achieve a high PA_{CO_2} in the patient while protecting the PA_{O_2} from falling to dangerously low levels. I first determine that the patient's respiratory gas exchange is adequate to perform the apnea test safely. The apnea test is contraindicated if, because of cardiac or pulmonary disease, the patient's PA_{O_2} cannot be raised to at least 300 mm Hg. I ventilate the patient for 30 minutes with 100 percent oxygen ($FI_{O_2} = 1.0$). I choose ventilator settings to permit the PA_{CO_2} to normalize at approximately 40 mm Hg from the lower level at which comatose, intubated patients are usually maintained. If the patient has normal pulmonary function, the PA_{O_2} should reach at least 300 to 400 mm Hg. At this point I stop the ventilator and passively oxygenate the patient at 12 L per minute via a cannula through the endotracheal tube to the level of the carina, or using a T-piece. The patient's PA_{CO_2} rises during apnea at approximately 2.7 to 3.7 mm Hg per minute.

I calculate the duration of apnea to permit the PA_{CO_2} to reach 60 mm Hg. Beginning at $PA_{CO_2} = 40$ mm Hg, it takes approximately 6 or 7 minutes to achieve $PA_{CO_2} = 60$ mm Hg. The PA_{O_2} falls during this time but not to dangerously low levels because it began so high. It is unsafe to perform this test if very high PA_{O_2} levels are unattainable at the beginning of the test. I terminate the test prematurely if the patient becomes hypotensive or has ventricular ectopy during the test because these signs suggest critical hypoxemia. Ordinarily, the patient's pH falls and blood pressure rises during the apneic period.

I consider apnea to be present if I detect no respiratory excursion, sighing, hiccuping, or other evidence of spontaneous respiratory functions during maximal hypercapneic stimulation. Clinicians should take particular care to determine apnea properly because surveys of neurologists and neurosurgeons have shown that the majority of clinicians perform the test incorrectly.

Exclusions: Drugs, Hypothermia, and Shock

Brain death determination requires proof that a known structural lesion is sufficient to account for the patient's state and that reversible causes of global brain dysfunction have been excluded. If I do not know that the patient has a structural lesion and I cannot reasonably exclude the contribution of potentially reversible metabolic or toxic encephalopathies, I delay declaring brain death until I know with more certainty that the state is irreversible.

Toxic dosages of drugs depressing the central nervous system (CNS) are a common cause of coma in emergency room patients and can mimic all the clinical signs of brain death. For example, barbiturate coma can be sufficiently severe to produce coma, apnea, and brain stem areflexia as well as a flat electroencephalogram (EEG). Neuromuscular blocking drugs can induce a state of profound paralysis and produce apnea and brain stem areflexia.

I adopt one of several strategies if I cannot exclude the effects of CNS-depressing drugs. I order serum toxicologic screens. If these are positive for depressant agents, I continue to support the patient and wait for the depressant drugs to be metabolized, remembering that phenobarbital may persist in toxic concentrations for several days. Usually I order confirmatory tests of brain death to assess intracranial blood flow. When I am concerned about neuromuscular blocking drugs, if I can elicit limb deep tendon reflexes or if I can make a muscle contract by electrically stimulating its nerve, I can be sure that neuromuscular blocking agents are not present in degrees sufficient to interfere with brain death determination.

Severe hypothermia can also mimic brain death yet produce potentially reversible brain dysfunction. Brain death protocols require that the body core temperature exceed 90°F (32.2°C). When appropriate, I rewarm hypothermic patients according to standard protocols. When patients are severely hypotensive, I may attempt to achieve a systolic blood pressure greater than 90 mm Hg before I determine brain death.

Interval Between Examinations

Brain death usually cannot be determined on the basis of a single examination. At least two examinations should be performed, separated by a time interval. If global brain dysfunction is present on both examinations, I assume that it was present as well in the interval separating them. The recommended intervals between examinations vary as a function of the cause of brain death and the age of the patient.

I use the following examination intervals for patients over 1 year of age: 24 hours for patients with hypoxic-ischemic damage from cardiac arrest, 12 hours for patients with other known causes without confirmatory tests, and 6 hours for patients with known causes with positive confirmatory tests.

LABORATORY TESTS

Although brain death is primarily a clinical determination, in several instances I order laboratory tests to confirm the diagnosis. My most common reason for ordering confirmatory tests is that the clinical tests could not be performed safely or accurately. Patients with pulmonary edema, adult respiratory distress syndrome, pneumonia, or other causes of pulmonary failure may not be able to achieve PAo_2 levels high enough to safely perform the apnea test. Patients with perforated tympanic membranes cannot safely undergo the ice water caloric test for vestibulo-ocular reflexes. Patients with eye damage may not be able to have pupillary, corneal, or vestibulo-ocular reflexes assessed accurately.

Another reason I order confirmatory tests is to shorten the time interval between tests to expedite organ donation. Tests revealing absent intracranial blood flow can also confirm brain death even in the presence of toxic levels of depressant drugs. Finally, I find it desirable in some cases with medicolegal implications, such as homicide, to have "objective" documentation of the brain death determination in addition to my clinical report.

Confirmatory laboratory tests are of two types: those that measure neuronal electrical output and those that measure intracranial blood flow. Generally the electrophysiologic tests are more widely available, easier to perform at the patient's bedside, less invasive, and simpler to interpret. However, they are not as specific for confirming brain death as the tests of intracranial blood flow. To a great extent, the choice of which confirmatory test to use depends on which is most readily available.

When I use electrophysiologic confirmatory tests I choose both the EEG and the brain stem auditory evoked response (BAER). The EEG measures primarily hemispheric cortical activity, whereas the BAER assesses brain stem electrical conduction. The EEG alone is not a sufficient confirmatory test, because it may be isoelectric (flat) while the brain stem is undamaged. Further, the EEG is more susceptible to metabolic and toxic suppression than the BAER, so false-positive brain death confirmations with EEG alone will occur more often than with concomitant use of the BAER. Somatosensory evoked potentials show a characteristic pattern in brain death but, if used, should be ordered with EEG and BAER.

Tests of global intracranial blood flow (IBF) exploit the fact that there is a total cessation of circulation to the brain at some time in brain death. Several technologies have been developed to measure IBF. Early investigators showed that contrast angiography of the carotid and vertebral arteries disclosed absent intracranial blood flow. Later, less invasive portable isotope angiography with technetium-99 was used for the same purpose with a high degree of accuracy. More recently, xenon-enhanced computed tomography (CT) and single photon emission computed tomography with technetium-99 HM-PAD were shown to demonstrate absent regional intracranial blood flow. Most recently, transcranial Doppler (TCD) ultrasonography was shown to have characteristic findings of "reverberating blood flow" in brain death, revealing anterograde blood flow in systole and retrograde flow in diastole. With further development and availability, TCD will probably replace the other tests of IBF because of its ease, noninvasiveness, and accuracy.

BRAIN DEATH IN CHILDREN

For declaring brain death in children, I follow the guidelines of the Task Force for the Determination of Brain Death in Children. The guidelines provide that children older than 1 year be treated the same as adults. Children under 1 year of age must have a confirmatory EEG in addition to the clinical examination findings. Children aged 2 to 12 months require an examination interval of 24 hours regardless of pathogenesis. Children aged 7 days to 2 months require a 48 hour examination interval. Brain death cannot be declared in children under 7 days of age. Radionuclide angiography confirmatory tests can be performed and eliminate the need for the second examination and the EEG. The newer confirmatory tests (xenon-enhanced CT and TCD ultrasound) remain untested in this age group.

DIFFERENTIAL DIAGNOSIS

If the brain death physical assessment is performed properly, there will be no differential diagnosis. There has never been a substantiated report of a patient recovering after satisfying properly performed and interpreted brain death tests. The differential diagnosis becomes relevant only in the interpretation of specific tests. Unreactive pupils can be caused by atropine or other drugs or may be a pre-existing finding. Unresponsivity and apnea can be caused by metabolic or toxic encephalopathies or states of neuromuscular paralysis. Absent vestibular-ocular reflexes can result from previous ototoxic drug treatment. Isoelectric EEGs can be induced by toxic doses of CNS depressant drugs.

TIME OF DEATH

Death is declared at the time the patient fulfills the second set of brain death tests. Although this practice appears arbitrary, it is consistent with the timing of death declaration in other contexts. If organ transplantation is not being considered, I simply do not reattach the ventilator following the second apnea test. Asystole usually follows within 15 minutes of the conclusion of the apnea test.

ORGAN TRANSPLANTATION

Brain-dead patients should be considered potential candidates for multiorgan procurement, including heart, lungs, liver, kidneys, pancreas, intestines, and bone. When brain death declaration appears imminent following the first examination and the patient is a suitable organ donor, I ask the family to consider organ donation. If they are agreeable, I ask the organ transplantation nurse coordinator to speak with them. Should they consent to organ donation, the coordinator will ready the procurement team so that when the patient fulfills the second set of tests and is declared dead, the ventilator can be reattached and the patient moved expeditiously to the surgical suite for organ procurement.

No member of the organ procurement team should participate in the brain death determination, and no physician declaring brain death should participate in the organ procurement. Federal and some state laws now require physicians to ask families of brain-dead patients if they are interested in organ donation. Many families are very willing to proceed with organ donation.

OPPOSITION TO BRAIN DEATH

For religious reasons, some families indicate that they want the ventilator continued despite the declaration of brain death. When faced with this dilemma, I try to explain that their loved one is medically and legally dead and that nothing can possibly restore life. If the opposition on religious grounds remains intractable, I continue ventilator treatment and await the inevitable asystole in a few hours or days. Given the "zero" prognosis for recovery, however, I usually discontinue other aggressive therapies such as vasopressor drugs. I am firmer in my resolve to insist on brain death declaration if the opposition is solely on emotional grounds or may be a result of misunderstanding. The state of New Jersey recently enacted a statute prohibiting physicians from declaring brain death in patients when the physician is aware that the declaration would violate the patient's "personal religious beliefs."

LEGAL ASPECTS

As of August 1993, 45 states in the United States had enacted laws specifically recognizing brain death as a statutory definition of death, and most other states had recorded high court judicial precedents recognizing brain death as the standard of human death. Physicians in all jurisdictions can feel secure in declaring brain death when appropriate because it represents the standard of medical care in the United States.

Acknowledgment. Portions of this chapter are modified from Bernat JL. Brain death and withdrawal of life support in hopeless neurological diseases. In: Grotta JC, ed. Management of the acutely ill neurological patient. New York:Churchill Livingstone, 1993; with permission.

SUGGESTED READING

Belsh JM, Blatt R, Schiffman PR. Apnea testing in brain death. Arch Intern Med 1986; 146:2385–2388.

Bernat JL. Ethical issues in neurology. In: Joynt RJ, ed. Clinical neurology. Vol 1. Philadelphia:JB Lippincott, 1991:18.

Guidelines for the determination of death: Report of the Medical Consultants on the Diagnosis of Death to the President's Commission for the Study of Ethical Problems in Medicine and Biomedical and Behavioral Research. JAMA 1981; 246:2184–2186.

Kaufman HH, Lynn J. Brain death. Neurosurgery 1986; 19:850–856.

Pallis C. Brainstem death. In: Vinken PJ, Bruyn GW, eds. Handbook of clinical neurology. Vol 57. Amsterdam:Elsevier, 1990.

Petty GW, Mohr JP, Pedley TA, et al. The role of transcranial Doppler in confirming brain death: Sensitivity, specificity, and suggestions for performance and interpretation. Neurology 1990; 40:300–303.

President's Commission for the Study of Ethical Problems in Medicine and Biomedical and Behavioral Research. Defining death: Medical, legal, and ethical issues in the determination of death. Washington, DC:US Government Printing Office, 1981.

Reid RH, Gulenchyn KY, Ballinger JR. Clinical use of technetium-99m HM-PAO for determination of brain death. J Nucl Med 1989; 30:1621–1626.

Smith MC, Bleck TP. Techniques for determining brain death. J Crit Illness 1989; 4:67–73.

Task Force for the Determination of Brain Death in Children. Guidelines for the determination of brain death in children. Arch Neurol 1987; 44:587–588.

SLEEP DISORDERS

M. EILEEN McNAMARA, M.D.

To diagnose sleep disorders, a physician must assemble clues and use inductive reasoning because sleep disorders almost never present directly. By definition, the cardinal signs of sleep disorders occur when people are asleep, so patients are rarely aware of, or able to report accurately, what is happening. Rather, sleep disorders usually present with nonspecific complaints such as fatigue, depression, memory loss, confusion, or weakness. Moreover, many patients do not consider sleep problems as something to report to their neurologist the way they report changes in cognition or motor or sensory function, making accurate diagnosis even more difficult. Typically a patient is symptomatic for years and sees many physicians before an accurate diagnosis is made. This is all the more unfortunate because sleep disorders are common and a significant source of morbidity.

Careful history taking is crucial to diagnosis. The need for sleep varies in the general population, including both constitutionally short and long sleepers, but an individual's need for sleep is relatively fixed in adulthood until senescence. Variations from an individual's baseline need for sleep should raise clinical suspicion of a sleep disorder.

It is insufficient to ask a patient "How are you sleeping?" because the answer tends to be vague and unhelpful. Precise questions about sleep habits yield much more information (Table 1). Inquire both about how the patient slept when they felt well and how they sleep now. Determine whether the patient is sleeping more or less than their previous baseline. Common causes of disorders of excessive somnolence are listed in Table 2. Common causes of disorders of initiation or maintaining sleep, or decreased sleep, are listed in Table 3. Although there are exceptions, when patients report an increase in their need for sleep, a primary sleep disorder such as sleep apnea should be suspected. When patients report a decrease from their baseline need for sleep, a psychiatric disorder should be suspected.

When a patient reports altered sleep, first see if any medical or environmental factor can account for their symptoms. Review the patient's medications, and inquire about use of alcohol, caffeine, nicotine, cocaine, amphetamines, and other "recreational" drugs. A toxicology screen may be useful. Inquire about work and sleep habits and if the patient is on shift work or some other irregular schedule. Circadian sleep rhythms are easily disrupted, as anyone who has experienced jet lag

Table 1   Questions to Quantify Sleep

What time do you go to bed and turn off the light?
After you turn off the light, how long does it take you to fall asleep?
Do you wake up in the middle of the night? If so, how many times?
Are your awakenings brief or long? How long?
What time do you get up in the morning? Do you feel refreshed when you get up or are you still sleepy?
Do you nap in the day? How often? How long?

Table 2   Some Causes of Increased Sleep

Obstructive sleep apnea
Narcolepsy
Periodic leg movements of sleep
Drug use, medical or "recreational"
Toxin exposure
Idiopathic central nervous system hypersomnolence
Sleep deprivation
Delirium, stupor, and other medical conditions

Table 3   Some Causes of Decreased Sleep

Anxiety
Major depression
Sleep-wake circadian disruption from jet lag or shift work
Drug use or drug withdrawal
Restless legs

will know. Also inquire about how and where the patient usually sleeps. Is the environment noisy or hot? Does the patient sleep better at home or away from home? If no medical or environmental cause can be found to account for the patient's symptoms, primary sleep disorders should be considered.

INCREASED SLEEP

Obstructive Sleep Apnea

Obstructive sleep apnea (OSA) is one of the most common causes of hypersomnia. Patients with OSA report an increase in their total sleep time and often report daytime napping. Napping is not common among North American adults and should always be investigated. Patients usually do not complain of trouble falling asleep and usually do not complain of long nocturnal awakenings, although they may note multiple *brief* awakenings in their sleep. Apneas occur because of narrowing or collapse of the oropharynx during inspiration. The classic patient is an overweight, burly, middle-aged male, with a short thick neck. One report suggests that a neck size of 17 or greater should raise clinical suspicion of apnea. Multiple other structural problems may impede airflow as well, such as enlarged tonsils, a redundant soft palate, nasal obstruction, and retrognathia, so OSA also occurs in children, women, and thin people.

Ask if the patient snores. Snoring is a sign of partial airway obstruction, and the difference between snoring and an obstructive apnea is only one of degree. If the obstruction increases or ventilatory efforts decrease, apneas occur, the snoring stops, and the patient is suddenly quiet. The chest continues to move as the patient attempts to breathe, but the flow of air is halted. The patient usually awakens, probably with a protective snort or gasp. As the patient's sleep lightens, muscle tone and ventilatory effort improve and respiration begins again. The patient then falls asleep again, and the cycle begins anew. Patients usually do not remember their brief awakenings. Patients who report that they slept 10 hours may actually have had about 3 hours of sleep and 7 hours of near-suffocation events. A patient who complains of excessive sleepiness may actually be quite sleep deprived.

If a patient reports that their snoring is so loud their spouse has moved out of the bedroom, OSA should be strongly suspected. Many patients do not know that they snore, since they are asleep when it happens, and may deny that they snore even when they snore severely. Therefore, an interview with the bed partner, if available, can be invaluable. The report, "I thought he was dead and I shook him to wake him up," describing witnessed apneas, is virtually diagnostic.

Another common OSA symptom is morning headache, which may be due to the apneic events. Impotence is common in male apneics, although the mechanism is unclear. Hypertension is also commonly associated with OSA, but whether the hypertension is a cause, an effect, or just a temporal association also remains unknown. Another disturbing problem among these patients is a high number of motor vehicle accidents, probably due to drowsiness. Findley and colleagues reported that patients with severe apnea have four times more automobile crashes than do controls. Since this was a retrospective study that only counted survivors, the rate may be higher. It also appears likely that OSA may underlie some cases of sudden death during sleep, possibly from cardiac arrhythmia. The questions to ask of patients with suspected OSA are listed in Table 4.

If a patient is suspected of having OSA, the physical exam should include fundoscopy (because increased intracranial pressure may also cause somnolence), blood pressure, an examination of the thyroid (because hypothyroidism causes apnea and goiter can cause narrowing of the trachea), and a cardiac exam (because severe apnea with daytime hypoxemia and hypercapnia is associated with right heart failure). Neck size should be measured, and the head, neck, and chest should be examined for causes of potential airway obstruction. Screening laboratory work should include thyroid functions and thyroid-stimulating hormone to rule out hypothyroidism. Neurologic disorders associated with OSA include myotonic dystrophy, poliomyelitis, syringobulbia, acromegaly, spinal muscular atrophy, olivopontocerebellar degeneration, cluster headache, Cushing's disease, Klippel-Feil syndrome, multiple sclerosis, spinal cord injury, and stroke.

Studies have shown that the history and physical, although important, are not sufficiently sensitive or specific to confirm or exclude a diagnosis of OSA. If OSA is clinically suspected, the patient should be referred for polysomnography for definitive diagnosis.

Several electrodes are used in a sleep study, all of which are small and unobtrusive, thus permitting the most natural sleep possible. Electroencephalogram (EEG) and electromyogram (EMG) electrodes are used to stage sleep. The EEG of non-rapid eye movement (REM) sleep shows sleep spindles, K-complexes, and slow waves. The EEG of REM sleep looks more like wakefulness, with low-voltage fast activity. The flaccid hypotonia seen on EMG, however, distinguishes REM sleep from the awake state. The EMG is also useful to detect body movements such as the leg kicks of nocturnal myoclonus. Electrocardiogram (ECG) electrodes are applied to the chest. Apneas are commonly associated with cardiac ectopic beats or bursts of tachycardia.

Nasal and oral thermistors monitor airflow, while chest bands document respiratory effort. In OSA, the chest moves as the patient breathes, but no airflow registers from the mouth or nose. An oximeter, often a gentle clip on the finger or earlobe, documents changes in arterial oxygenation.

Up to 30 apneas lasting at least 10 seconds a night may be normal, but the OSA patient may have hundreds of events. Apneas last from 10 seconds to 2 minutes, during which time arterial oxygenation diminishes. Systemic blood pressure, heart rate, and intracranial

Table 4   Questions to Ask When Obstructive Sleep Apnea is Suspected

Are you sleeping more than usual? For how long?
(For men) What is your neck size?
Have your tonsils been taken out?
Do you have a deviated septum, sinus disease, postnasal drip?
Have you ever had a thyroid problem, hypertension, diabetes, impotence?
Do you snore? How loud? (Ask the bed partner, if available.)
Do you wake up with a headache?
Have you ever woken up gasping for air?
Have you gained weight?

pressure rise sharply. Cardiac arrhythmia may develop. The typical polysomnographic recording in OSA demonstrates a mix of obstructive and central apneas. Periodic leg movements are also commonly seen.

Narcolepsy

Another cause of hypersomnia is narcolepsy. While OSA usually begins in adulthood, narcolepsy often begins in adolescence, although accurate diagnosis may be delayed for years. Like apneics, narcoleptics describe "semi-irresistible" napping. In narcoleptics, naps are usually restorative, while apneics awake feeling unrefreshed. Both may dream during naps, but this report is more common in narcoleptics.

Even between naps, narcoleptics seldom feel fully alert. Half complain of memory problems, probably due to impaired attention. Some present with complaints of diplopia, probably due to drowsiness. The presentation of narcolepsy can be quite subtle, with patients mistakenly perceived as lazy or depressed. They often have problems in attention and concentration and with school or work failure.

Most narcoleptics report cataplexy as well, although the presentation can also be subtle. In full-blown cataplexy, there is loss of muscle tone with strong emotion, and the patient collapses. In subtle cases, which are the most common, the patient may report simply dropping things and feeling weak in the knees. Only a fraction of patients have the full "narcoleptic tetrad" of narcolepsy, cataplexy, hypnogogic hallucinations, and sleep paralysis. The absence of the full tetrad does not rule out the diagnosis.

The night-time sleep of narcoleptics can be normal, long, or short and disrupted, and particulars of the night-time sleep are not very helpful in making the diagnosis.

Narcolepsy is often a familial disorder, so it is helpful to inquire about the sleep habits of immediate family members. A history of napping in relatives should be regarded with suspicion (Table 5).

There is little in the physical examination that is specific for narcolepsy, although the examiner might try to induce strong emotion in the patient to see if a cataplectic event follows. It is probably wiser to try to make patients laugh than to make them angry. Also, care

Table 5 Questions to Ask if Narcolepsy is Suspected

Do you fall asleep during the day? When does this happen? How old were you when this started?
How do you feel when you laugh? Get mad? Do your muscles get weak?
Have you ever had unusual experiences just as you are falling asleep? (hypnogogic hallucinations)
Have you ever had unusual experiences just as you are waking up? (hypnopompic hallucinations or sleep paralysis)
Do you have any sleepy family members?

should be taken to prevent patients from falling and injuring themselves.

It can also be helpful to leave the patient in a quiet room to see if he or she will fall asleep. Narcoleptic naps are not "ictal," striking within seconds with abrupt transitions from wakefulness to sleep. Rather, they are "semi-irresistible" and occur under conditions of low stimulation. If the patient falls asleep, watch for rapid eye movements indicating early REM onset, or snoring indicating sleep apnea. Narcolepsy and sleep apnea can sometimes be diagnosed from the waiting room, as patients fall asleep waiting for their appointment. It is useful to have the front office staff alert you whenever a patient falls asleep, or snores, before their examination.

Narcolepsy is strongly associated with the human leukocyte antigen (HLA) DRw15, previously called DR2. It is positive in 91 to 100 percent of patients versus about 30 percent of the general population, and at times HLA typing can be helpful in excluding or confirming the diagnosis of narcolepsy. Blood work, however, does *not* replace the need for sleep studies. There are also rare reports of "symptomatic narcolepsy" from brain lesions, such as craniopharyngioma of the diencephalon, or lesions of the midbrain or pons. Cataplexy has been reported in a patient with a glioblastoma of the rostral brain stem and hypothalamus.

As mentioned, nocturnal sleep is quite variable in narcolepsy. Nocturnal polysomnography, while it can exclude other diagnoses such as sleep apnea, is not sufficient to make the diagnosis. The gold standard for the diagnosis of narcolepsy is the multiple sleep latency test (MSLT). The MSLT is performed the day after a night-time sleep study and consists of the polysomnograph recording of four or more scheduled naps at 2 hour intervals. Patients are allowed to attempt to sleep for about 20 minutes. If patients fall asleep in an average of less than 5 minutes, they are pathologically sleepy. Normals average 10 to 20 minutes. In addition, narcoleptics exhibit REM periods in two or more naps, with a REM latency of 15 minutes or less. Normal REM latency is usually greater than 60 minutes.

DECREASED SLEEP

Most sleep laboratories are reluctant to do polysomnograms on patients with insomnia because the yield of identifiable primary sleep disorders is low. Still, insom-

nia is a symptom of many identifiable illnesses, and it is better to identify and correct the underlying cause rather than just sedate the patient with hypnotics.

A common cause of insomnia is depression. Major affective disorder, or major depression, is associated with difficulty falling asleep, long nocturnal awakenings, and early morning awakenings. In my opinion, this triad of sleep complaints in the absence of daytime napping is virtually pathognomic for the illness. Primary sleep disorders may also cause nocturnal awakenings, but these are usually brief; and in other sleep disorders caused by medical factors, such as jet lag, there is usually catch-up daytime napping. Still, many patients when directly questioned will deny that they are depressed because of embarrassment or lack of understanding of their illness. Instead, they may note poor memory, lack of concentration, fatigue, anhedonia, decreased libido, loss of appetite, or irritability. While these symptoms are nonspecific, if they are associated with trouble falling asleep, long nocturnal awakening, and early morning awakening, depression should be strongly suspected.

It is not necessary to use a sedating antidepressant to treat depressed patients with insomnia. Sedating antidepressants such as Amitriptyline, Imipramine, and the other tricyclics have a high degree of anticholinergic side effects such as orthostatis, tachycardia, constipation, urinary retention, dry mouth, blurred vision, memory difficulties, and confusion. Moreover, patients usually complain of feeling drugged and "hung over." I much prefer to use a nonsedating antidepressant such as fluoxetine or sertraline, which have few side effects. When the depression is adequately treated, the sleep will normalize, and I use sleep patterns to gauge efficacy of treatment.

Restless legs is another interesting cause of trouble sleeping. Patients complain that as soon as they sit or lie down, they develop an unusual, uncomfortable feeling in their legs. If they stand up and bear weight upon their feet, their symptoms go away. This odd feeling is not a pain, cramp, or true dysesthesia but is very disagreeable. Since patients cannot lie down, they can't sleep until, presumably, fatigue overrides their other symptoms. Once asleep, however, the majority of patients then develop periodic leg movements (PLMs), which are semirhythmic stereotyped leg jerks that resemble the full Babinski's reflex, with dorsiflexion of the large toe and ankle, and knee and hip flexion. Movement occurs about every 20 to 40 seconds in clusters. The PLMs often disrupt sleep, and the patient complains of brief nocturnal awakenings and nonrestorative sleep. Patients with PLMs alone may complain of either trouble sleeping or hypersomnia. Restless legs and PLMs are usually idiopathic but have been associated with uremia, iron deficiency anemia, vascular insufficiency, and caffeine use. Most antidepressants, including tricyclics and fluoxetine, cause or aggravate PLMs. Restless legs is a clinical diagnosis based on the history. PLMs are diagnosed by characteristic findings on polysomnography of rhythmic anterior tibialis EMG artifact.

RECOMMENDATIONS

Clearly, discussing all the possible sleep disorders is outside the scope of this chapter. For the clinician, what is necessary is a high index of suspicion of the possibility of confounding sleep disorders whenever a patient presents with nonspecific or nonlocalizing complaints. The clinician should then review the patient's medications and medical history for possible problems and perform a thorough examination. If the history and physical suggest a possible sleep disorder, referral for polysomnography should be considered. The typical patient suffers from a sleep disorder for years and sees many physicians before an accurate diagnosis is made. Identifying a sleep disorder can result in a significant improvement in the patient's well-being and a gratifying experience for the clinician.

SUGGESTED READING

Aldrich MA. Narcolepsy. N Engl J Med 1990; 323:389–394.
Aldrich MS, Naylor MW. Narcolepsy associated with lesions of the diencephalon. Neurology 1989; 39:1505–1508.

Dement WC, Mitler MM, Roth T, et al. Guidelines for the multiple sleep latency test (MSLT): A standard measure of sleepiness. Sleep 1986; 9:519–524.
Ditta SD, George CFP, Singh SM. HLA-D-region genomic DNA restriction fragments in DRw15 (DR2) familial narcolepsy. Sleep 1992; 15:48–57.
Findley LJ, Fabrizio M, Thommi G, et al. Severity of sleep apnea and automobile crashes (letter). N Engl J Med 1989; 320:868–869.
Kales A, Cadieux RJ, Bixler ED, et al. Severe obstructive sleep apnea I: Onset, clinical course, and characteristics. J Chron Dis 1985; 38:419–425.
Montplaisir J, Godbout R, Boghen D, et al. Familial restless legs with periodic movements in sleep: Electrophysiologic, biochemical, and pharmacologic study. Neurology 1985; 35:130–134.
Montplaisir J, Lapierre O, Warnes H, et al. The treatment of the restless leg syndrome with or without periodic leg movements in sleep. Sleep 1992; 15:391–395.
Oates JA, Wood A. The diagnosis and management of insomnia. N Engl J Med 1990; 322:239–248.

ATTENTION DEFICIT HYPERACTIVITY DISORDER

RUTH NASS, M.D.

Attention deficit hyperactivity disorder (ADHD) is perhaps the most common of the learning disabilities (LDs), although it is not always considered a specific LD. Its prevalence in school-age children ranges from 1 to 20 percent, depending on the technique of ascertainment: parent versus child versus teacher assessment, particular questionnaire used, country of study (more common in the United States than in the United Kingdom), and age at ascertainment. ADHD can be diagnosed in the toddler and preschooler and can persist into adulthood. As with virtually all the other developmental disabilities, it is more common in males (four to eight times) than females. When affected, however, females are more severely affected. Females with ADHD tend to have lower IQs and more academic difficulties than males with ADHD.

Risk factors for ADHD identified by the National Collaborative Perinatal Project include family history of retardation, low socioeconomic status, smoking, anemia, breech birth, chorioamnionitis, low birth weight, and small head circumference. Suspect neurologic status in the perinatal period increased the risk of ADHD at age 7 years from 2 to 50 percent. In infancy, developmental delay and increased activity predicted ADHD at age 7 years. At age 4 years, visuo-motor, fine motor, and gross motor deficits, small head circumference, and refractive error predicted ADHD at age 7 years. Psychosocial risk factors for ADHD are also reported: the Kauai study showed an increased risk of 200 to 400 percent in the presence of such risk factors. In a Swedish case control study, unsatisfactory family life was the most important factor.

ADHD is often an inherited disorder. The disorder typically appears in males. However, females expressing ADHD appear to carry a greater gene load. Therefore, the risk to siblings of an ADHD proband is greater if the proband is a female or the maternal history is positive. Generally, the proband's father or maternal uncle have a history of similar problems in childhood. Children inheriting ADHD from their fathers tend to have more dysmorphic features (Table 1). As with other genetic disorders, there is a high concordance in monozygotic twins. There is an increased prevalence of alcoholism, hysteria, and sociopathy among parents, including biological parents where the proband is adopted. At least 10 percent of ADHD children probably carry the Tourette's syndrome gene, but do not evidence tics, although they may develop them when treated with stimulant medication such as methylphenidate.

HOW TO MAKE THE DIAGNOSIS

ADHD is defined as inappropriate inattention, impulsivity, distractibility, and hyperactivity for chrono-

Table 1 Physical Findings of Various Degrees in ADHD

Head:
  a. Electric hair: very fine hair that won't comb down; fine hair that is soon awry after combing
  b. Two or more whorls
  c. Abnormal head circumference

Eyes:
  a. Epicanthus: where upper and lower lids join the nose point of union; deeply covered; partly covered
  b. Hypertelorism: approximate distance between tear ducts: $>1\frac{1}{2}$ inches; $>1\frac{1}{4}$ but $<1\frac{1}{2}$ inches

Ears:
  a. Low seated: bottom of ears in line with mouth (or lower), area between mouth and nose
  b. Adherent lobes: lower edges of ears extend: upward and back toward crown of head; straight back toward rear of neck
  c. Malformed ears
  d. Asymmetric ears
  e. Soft and pliable ears

Mouth:
  a. High palate: roof of mouth definitely steepled; flat and narrow at the top
  b. Furrowed tongue (one with deep ridges)
  c. Smooth-rough spots on tongue

Hands:
  a. Fifth finger: markedly curved inward toward other fingers; slightly curved inward toward other fingers
  b. Single transverse palmar crease
  c. Index finger longer than middle finger

Feet:
  a. Third toe: definitely longer than second toe; appears equal in length to second toe
  b. Partial syndactylia of two middle toes
  c. Gap between first and second toe (approximately $\frac{1}{4}$ inch)

From Waldrop M, Pedersen F, Bell RQ. Minor physical anomalies and behavior in preschool children. Child Dev 1968; 39:391–400; © The Society for Research in Child Development, Inc.; with permission.

Table 2 Modified DSM-IIIR Criteria for Attention Deficit Hyperactivity Disorder

A. Disturbance compared with others of the same mental age of at least 6 months duration in eight of the following:
  1. Fidgets in seat
  2. Difficulty remaining seated
  3. Easily distracted
  4. Difficulty awaiting turn
  5. Blurts out answers
  6. Difficulty following through on instructions
  7. Difficulty sustaining attention
  8. Shifts tasks before completed
  9. Difficulty playing quietly
  10. Talks excessively
  11. Interrupts others
  12. Often does not seem to listen
  13. Loses things
  14. Reckless
B. Onset before 7 years
C. Does not meet criteria for pervasive developmental disorder

logical and mental age. A modified version of the DSM-IIIR criteria is given in Table 2. It is worth noting that the DSM-IIIR definition is a consensus, not a biologically validated definition. Further, behaviors subserved by the same neural system are listed as distinct in the DSM-IIIR definition, such as akathisia (often fidgets with hands or feet) and difficulty remaining seated. Also, behaviors subserved by different neural systems are lumped together. Consider "difficulty awaiting turn in game." Is the child aware of the rules of turn-taking (cognition)? Can he state the rules (language)? Can he analyze the situation and relate the rules to the specific situation (cognition)? Is he motivated to take turns (limbic-frontal)? Is he able to execute the plan (frontal)? Can he inhibit his desire if it is not his turn (frontal)? Thus, using these criteria, some features are overestimated and some features underestimated in terms of diagnostic importance.

The diagnosis of ADHD is made by the teacher and based on classroom performance. The physician must trust the history, especially since the child may be able to pull himself together in a one-on-one setting. If parents think the child has ADHD and the teacher does not, there are crucial emotional issues to be unraveled. There are a number of questionnaires available for parents and teachers, as well as the psychiatric interview method of diagnosis (*DSM-IIIR* definition). The most commonly used, Connors' teacher questionaire, is presented in Table 3. The child is rated on a scale of 0 to 3:0-none, 1-just a little, 2-pretty much, 3-very much. A score of over 15 on this short form puts the child in the ADHD range. This questionnaire has been validated against the DSM-IIIR definition of attention deficit disorder. There are two longer forms of Connors' questionnaire, both for parents and teachers. For equivocal situations or for titrating medication to particular aspects of behavior, these longer forms may sometimes be more useful.

The problem of diagnosis is highlighted by a study by Levine and colleagues. The diagnosis of ADHD for children with school problems was a unanimous yes by parents, teachers, and doctors in 9 percent of the cases, a unanimous no in 30 percent, and disagreed on in 61 percent. Some reasons for interobserver differences include diagnostic biases, social background effects, hidden personal agendas, varying observational skills, different attitudes towards questionnaires, and the effect of setting on ADHD.

Another problem with diagnosis is the issue of different types of ADHD. ADHD exists in isolation or with other LDs. Early speech and language impairment may be associated with an ADHD and LD combination at follow-up. Those with both LD and ADHD are at increased risk for behavior, mood, and anxiety disorders.

Attention deficit without hyperactivity may not be the same disease. One study showed that different personality characteristics were associated with attention deficit with and without hyperactivity. Those with hyperactivity were aggressive, had conduct disorders, evidenced bizarre behaviors, and were guiltless, very unpopular, and poor at academics. Those without

Table 3   Connors' Questionnaire Definition of Attention Deficit Hyperactivity Disorder

1. Restless in the squirmy sense
2. Demands must be met immediately
3. Distractibility or attention span a problem
4. Disturbs other children
5. Restless, always up and on the go
6. Excitable, impulsive
7. Fails to finish things he starts
8. Childish and immature
9. Easily frustrated
10. Difficulty in learning

From Connors CK. A teacher rating scale for use in drug studies with children. Am J Psychiatry 1969; 126:884; with permission.

hyperactivity were anxious, shy, socially withdrawn, poor at sports, unpopular, and poor at academics.

It is also not clear whether ADHD with and without conduct disorder is the same disease. Hyperactivity and conduct problems share half their variance on Connors' teacher rating scale. External validation with respect to cause, prognosis, and treatment response is required to clarify this issue.

There is clearly a residual type of ADHD (ADHD-RT) in adolescence and adulthood, which will occur in perhaps one-third of ADHD children. Aggressive, malicious children are more likely to have residual dysfunction. Wender developed criteria for the residual type, listed in Table 4. Wender also suggests the following exclusionary criteria for ADHD-RT: no schizophrenia or schizoaffective disorder; no current major mood disorder (but long situational dysphorias are commonly seen among the adults); no schizoid, schizotypal, borderline diagnosis, especially unstable and intense interpersonal relationships with idealization and devaluation, identity disturbances, intolerance of being alone, or physically self-damaging acts such as mutilation and suicidal gestures. These exclusionary criteria must be considered in the context of comparison with controls: 48 percent of adolescents and adults with a history of ADHD versus 8 percent of socioeconomically matched controls evidence antisocial behaviors, 32 percent versus 7 percent engage in substance abuse, 12 percent versus 5 percent suffer from alcoholism, and 58 percent versus 11 percent have been arrested. In addition there appears to be an increased risk of accidental death including motor vehicle accidents in those with ADHD.

EVALUATION

History

Historical features of ADHD, particularly in the younger child, include bad breath, dry skin, rash, red cheeks, bloated stomach, leg cramps, stuffy, runny nose, headache, and ear infections.

In addition to a genetic basis, a number of causes for ADHD are reported. Table 5 lists some of them.

Table 4   Utah Criteria for Attention Deficit Hyperactivity Disorder

*Childhood History of ADHD**
Fidgety, restless, always on the go, talks excessively
Attention problem
Behavior problem in school
Impulsivity
Overexcitability
Temper outburst

*Persistence of ADHD in Adulthood**
Persistent motor hyperactivity
Attention deficits
Affective lability
Inability to complete tasks
Hot temper, explosive short-lived outbursts
Impulsivity
Stress intolerance

*Must have first two characteristics and two of the remaining characteristics.

Physical Examination

A number of dysmorphic features reported in ADHD are listed in Table 1.

Neurologic Examination

The neurologic findings in the child with ADHD are similar to those in children with all types of LDs. There is an excess of soft neurologic signs. A number that are reliably found are listed in Table 2 of the chapter *Developmental Dyslexia*. Slow-rapid finger movements and excess overflow are particularly common in ADHD. As with other LDs, most investigators report a marked decline in number of soft signs after puberty. Methylphenidate is reported to diminish soft signs, independent of its effects on behavioral and attentional systems.

Laboratory Examination

Neither neuroimaging nor electroencephalogram (EEG) is necessary for the diagnosis of ADHD. Magnetic resonance imaging in ADHD patients is reported to show a smaller right frontal region and a thinned corpus callosum, especially the splenium. Nonspecific EEG abnormalities are reported, as in other LDs.

Neuropsychological Testing

Neuropsychological testing is used in ADHD to rule out other LDs, psychiatric problems (mania, depression, anxiety, psychosis), and to confirm the diagnosis. Low scores on the attentional triad of the Wechsler IQ scales—Digit Span, Coding, and Arithmetic—are found. Specific measures of attention that are useful in the ADHD patient are continuous performance tasks; matching familiar figures; paired associate learning; measures of right hemisphere visuo-perceptual functioning, including neglect; measures of aspects of attention (focussed, sustained, selective, alternating, divided); and

Table 5 Causes of Attention Deficit Hyperactivity Disorder

I. *Demographic Factors*
II. *Pre-perinatal*
    Drugs: cocaine, alcohol
    Prematurity, low birth weight
    Birth asphyxia
III. *Sequelae of Childhood Illnesses*
    Direct CNS disease: Reye's syndrome, meningitis, encephalitis
    Cardiac disease
    Autoimmune disorders
    Anemia
    Epilepsy
    Otitis
    Hyper- and hypothyroidism
IV. *Secondary to Metabolic Disorders*
V. *Secondary to Head Trauma*
VI. *Secondary to Toxins and Drugs*
    Lead
    Asthma medications
    Anticonvulsants

CNS = central nervous system.

Table 6 Measures of Frontal Functioning

	Initiate	*Sustain*	*Inhibit*	*Shift*
Wisconsin card sort	+	−	−	+
Continuous performance tasks	−	+	−	−
Reitan Trails A & B	−	+	−	−
Stroop Test	−	+	+	+
Matching familiar figures	−	−	+	−
Verbal fluency	+	+	+	+
Verbal learning	+	−	+	+
Rey figure copy	+	−	−	−

From Denckla M. ADHD-RT. J Child Neurol 1991; 6:S44; with permission.

Table 7 Summary of the Clinical Evaluation of the ADHD Child

Pediatrician
    Takes a history, asks the question
    Assesses for minor physical anomalies

Teacher
    Makes the diagnosis

Psychologist
    Confirms, checks IQ and for other learning disabilities

Psychiatrist
    Rules out mania, psychosis, depression, anxiety

Neurologist
    Discusses tics, Tourette's syndrome
    Discusses the issue of stimulants in the mentally retarded and those with seizures
    Treats and follows:
    Neither EEG or neuroimaging ordinarily indicated
    Baseline blood count and chemistry profile if planning to medicate
    Baseline ECG, follow-up ECG, and drug levels if using a tricyclic antidepressant

EEG = electroencephalogram, ECG = electrocardiogram.

Table 8 Approach to the Child with Attention Deficit Hyperactivity Disorder and Tourette's Syndrome

Careful personal and family history (tics, obsessive-compulsive disorder, learning disability)
Present the data fully
Examine carefully and serially
Drug choices:
    Stimulants
    Clonidine
    Stimulants-Haldol
    Tricyclic antidepressant

measures of frontal functioning. Aspects of frontal function measured by a variety of tasks are listed in Table 6. Swanson has recently shown that ADHD subjects perform as if covert attentional precesses are intact, but aspects of attention mediated by the frontal lobe are deficient.

Urion used a battery examining right hemisphere, frontal, and left hemisphere functions, including timed motor performance, timed naming (rapid automatized naming, alternating naming), Boston Naming Test, verbal fluency, and Rey complex figure copy. He suggests that medication response is predictable by neurologic subtype of ADHD. His data suggest that those with frontal deficits are likely to respond to stimulants and those with left hemisphere neuropsychological deficits respond to tricyclic antidepressants. Those with right hemisphere dysfunction are unlikely to be medication responders.

Table 7 lists the diagnostic and management roles of different practitioners. Special circumstances for the neurologist include the child with ADHD and Tourette's syndrome (Table 8). Mentally retarded children can have ADHD. Methylphenidate for treatment of ADHD in mentally retarded children has mixed effects. Improvement is seen in irritability, anxiety, mood, and activity. But in the same study, six of 27 developed tics and two of 27 became socially withdrawn. Children with seizures can have ADHD. Consideration should be given to a change of anticonvulsants, particularly if it is phenobarbital. Although stimulants lower seizure threshold, it can be used if needed.

SUGGESTED READING

Brumback RA. Childhood depression and medically treatable learning disability. In: Molfese D, Segalowitz S, eds. Brain lateralization in children. New York: Guilford Press, 1988:463.

Cantwell D. Association between ADHD and LD. J Learn Disabil 1991; 24:88.

Cantwell DP. Families with attention deficit disordered children and others at risk. J Chem Depend Treat 1988; 1:183–186.

Cantwell DP, Baker L. Differential diagnosis of hyperactivity. J Dev Behav Pediatr 1987; 8:159–165.

Comings D, Comings BA. Controlled study of Tourette's syndrome. I. ADD, learning disorders and school problems. Am J Hum Genet 1987; 41:742–760.

Connors CK. A teacher rating scale for use in drug studies with children. Am J Psychiatry 1969; 126:884–888.

Denckla M. ADHD-RT. J Child Neurol 1991; 6:S44.

Denckla MB, Rudel RD. Anomalies of motor development in hyperactive boys. Ann Neurol 1978; 3:231–233.

Feldman H, Crumrine P, Handen BL, et al. Methylphenidate in children with seizures and Attention-Deficit Disorder. Am J Dis Child 1989; 143:1081–1086.

Handen B, et al. Adverse side effects of Ritalin among mentally retarded children with ADHD. J Am Acad Child Adolesc Psychiatry 1991; 30:241–245.

Hinshaw SP. On the distinction between attentional deficits/hyperactivity and conduct problems/aggression in child psychopathology. Psychol Bull 1987; 101:443–463.

Hirtz D, Nelson K. Cognitive effects of antiepileptic drugs. In: Pedley T, Meldrum B, eds. Recent advances in epilepsy. New York: Churchill Livingstone, 1985.

Hynd G, Semrud-Clikeman M, et al. Corpus callosum morphology in ADHD. J Learn Disabil 1991; 24:141–147.

Kaplan BJ, McNicol J, Moghadam HK. Physical signs and symptoms in preschool-age hyperactive and normal children. J Dev Behav Pediatr 1987; 8:305–310.

Lahey BB, Schaughency EA, Strauss CC, Frame C. Are Attention Deficit Disorders with and without hyperactivity similar or dissimilar disorders? J Am Acad Child Psychiatry 1984; 3:302–309.

Lerer RJ, Lerer MP. The effects of methylphenidate on the soft neurological signs of hyperactive children. Pediatrics 1976; 57: 521–525.

Levine MD. The anser system. Cambridge, MA: Educators Publishing Service, 1981.

Levine MD, Busch B, Aufseeser C. The dimension of inattention among children with school problems. Pediatrics 1982; 70:387–395.

Nass R. Attention Deficit Disorder: Clin Pediatr (Phila) (in press).

Needleman HL, Schell A, Bellinger D, et al. The long-term effects of exposure to low doses of lead in childhood: An 11-year follow-up report. N Engl J Med 1990; 322:83-88.

Neuspiel D, et al. Cocaine and infant behavior. J Dev Behav Pediatr 1991; 12:55.

Nichols P, Chen TC. Minimal brain dysfunction: A prospective study. Hillsdale, NJ: Lawrence Ehrlbaum, 1984.

Sleator EK, Ullmann RK. Can the physician diagnose hyperactivity in the office? Pediatrics 1981; 67:13–17.

Touwen BCL, Prechtl HFR. The neurological examination of the child with minor central nervous system anomalies. London: Spastic International, 1970.

Ullman RK, Sleator EK, Sprague RL. Manual for the ADD-H Comprehensive Teacher's Rating Scale. AcTers. Champaign, Ill: MetriTech, 1988.

Urion D. Response to desipramine in ADHD is predicted by neurological subtype. Ann Neurol 1989; 30:481.

Wender P, et al. A controlled study of Ritalin in the treatment of ADD-RT in adults. Am J Psychiatry 1985; 142–145.

PERIPHERAL NERVE AND MUSCLE DISORDERS

PERIPHERAL NEUROPATHY

ERIC L. LOGIGIAN, M.D.

Strictly defined, disorders of peripheral nerve encompass the mono- and polyneuropathies. However, in caring for patients with peripheral neuropathy, one often has to consider a broader range of closely related disorders, those affecting the nerve cell bodies (neuronopathies), the dorsal and ventral roots (radiculopathies), and the plexi (plexopathies). Further, many generalized polyneuropathies appear to affect nerve and root (radiculoneuropathy); in others the cell bodies are at least partially implicated. This brief chapter focuses on the polyneuropathies, which from the viewpoint of diagnosis are the most challenging of this group of disorders.

As in all aspects of medicine, a systematic approach to polyneuropathy is required to (1) diagnose and thereby differentiate it from other, related disorders and (2) determine its cause or at least exclude treatable causes. Because peripheral nerve disease has on the one hand a relatively limited repertoire of clinical expression, but on the other hand hundreds of possible causes, it is the latter of these two goals that is most challenging. Still, both can usually be accomplished by carefully defining several key aspects of the patient's neuropathy (Table 1) with the help of several tools, the most important of which are the history, physical examination, and electrophysiologic studies. The key questions are:

1. What fiber types (sensory, motor, autonomic) are involved?
2. How is the neuropathy evolving in space?
3. How is it evolving in time?
4. What is its functional severity?
5. Are there clues to an inherited neuropathy?
6. Is there evidence of an underlying systemic disease, malnutrition, or exposure to neurotoxins (e.g., medicines, solvents)?
7. What is the physiology (e.g., axonal versus demyelinative) of the neuropathy?

Answers to these questions can be further refined by various laboratory tests and examination of family members. The clinician can then decide if knowledge of nerve histology would be useful enough to justify the performance of a nerve biopsy. A simplified paradigm illustrating this approach to polyneuropathy is shown in Figure 1.

FIBER TYPES

Signs and symptoms of a peripheral neuropathy reflect the fiber types (sensory, motor, and autonomic) that are affected by the disease process. Dysfunction of each fiber type results in "negative" and "positive" symptoms and signs (Table 2). As the history spontaneously unfolds, the nature of the symptoms tells us which fiber types are involved. Nevertheless, the clinician should probe for symptoms reflecting injury to each fiber type since patients may forget or overlook them. Inquiry into what the patient can or cannot do is often useful. For example, motor fiber involvement of distal limb muscles may cause trouble unscrewing jar lids from weakness of hand muscles or cause tripping when walking due to foot drop. Involvement of proximal limb muscles may cause trouble in reaching above the head to comb or dry the hair, getting out of a chair, or going upstairs. Sensory loss often leads to difficulty in fine motor tasks (out of proportion to weakness) such as in buttoning, zipping, knitting, or in maintaining balance, making it particularly difficult to walk in the dark or put on stockings while standing on one foot. Pain is a common sensory manifestation of peripheral neuropathy. One should determine its quality using the patient's own words, where it is centered, whether it radiates, what exacerbates or improves it.

The physical examination affords the opportunity to quantitate the negative deficits in the three fiber systems; positive motor or autonomic phenomena may also be observable. A few points should be emphasized. With respect to motor fibers, the clinician infers disease of this fiber population based on the presence of muscle atrophy and weakness. The presence of muscle atrophy is determined entirely by inspection, and its recognition requires some experience since one needs to take into account age, sex, and occupation. I pay particular

Table 1 Important Questions in the Evaluation of Polyneuropathy and the Tools to Answer Them

	History	Examination	Electrophysiology	Other Laboratory	Examination of Family Members	Biopsy
Fiber types?	+	+	+			
Spatial evolution?	+	+	+			
Temporal evolution?	+					
Severity?	+	+	+			
Hereditary cause?	+	+			+	
Systemic disease, malnutrition, toxins?	+	+		+		
Physiology?			+			+
Histology?						

attention to the tongue, spinati, deltoid and interossei muscles of the hand; the extensor digitorum brevis muscles of the feet, the calf, tibialis anterior, and quadricep muscles. Quantitating muscle strength is usually performed with the confrontational method, but in powerful leg muscles such as the hip abductors and ankle plantar flexors, more subtle weakness may be elicited by having the patient stand on one foot (to elicit pelvic tilt) and attempt to walk on tiptoes, respectively. With confrontational muscle testing, the 0 to 5 point Medical Research Council (MRC) scale is most useful for severe muscle weakness but not for more subtle weakness, which is graded as 4. This is because the MRC scale is nonlinear, and the range from 4 to 5 represents the upper 50 percent of the range of muscle force. For that reason, in patients with milder weakness I prefer to estimate muscle strength as a percentage of normal. In any case, I systematically test limb muscles along a proximal to distal axis from the shoulder and hip girdle muscles to those acting across the elbow and knee, to those acting at the wrist and ankle, and finally to the intrinsic hand and foot muscles. Most polyneuropathies selectively involve the longest nerve fibers and preferentially affect distal muscles, more in the legs than the arms. In the mildest cases, only the intrinsic foot muscles may be affected. In the severest, all muscles may be affected, including axial muscles innervated by short nerves such as the neck flexors and rectus abdominus.

With respect to sensory fibers, the two most useful bedside tests are sharp-dull discrimination (for small sensory fiber function) and vibratory sense (for the large fiber sensory system). One tries to establish areas of reduced sensation in symptomatic areas (usually the toes and fingers) relative to more proximal asymptomatic areas. Thus, one first shows that the patient can differentiate sharp from dull or a vibrating from a nonvibrating tuning fork in a proximal asymptomatic zone. Then the stimulus is applied to certain standardized distal sites (e.g., top of the great toe or top of the index finger) to determine threshold. If perception of the stimulus is diminished, it is moved proximally (e.g., toes to ankle to calf, or finger tips to wrist to elbow) to establish the point at which the stimulus is felt normally. The more proximal the point, the more severe the neuropathy. Since station, gait, and limb coordination are dependent on large fiber sensory feedback, the Romberg sign and ataxia of gait and limb can be manifestations of sensory neuropathy and should be specifically elicited when examining the peripheral nervous system.

The reflex examination is theoretically the most objective aspect of the examination of the peripheral nervous system and therefore is of great interest. The presence of tendon areflexia in symptomatic limbs strongly supports the diagnosis of neuropathy of either the sensory afferents or motor efferents subserving the reflex arc. The presence of a plantar extensor response in a patient with symptoms consistent with polyneuropathy suggests that the correct diagnosis may be a central nervous system (CNS) lesion at the level of the spinal cord or, less likely, the parasaggital area or the brain stem. However, it should be remembered that there are certain diseases in which both the CNS and peripheral nerves are affected. The most important of these is vitamin B_{12} deficiency.

The autonomic nervous system is difficult to assess even in the laboratory. At the bedside, one is generally limited to checking for orthostasis, for anhydrotic skin in the extremities, and for abnormal pupillary responses.

Most polyneuropathies involve all three fiber types, particularly the sensory and motor populations. At onset, though, the only abnormalities may be positive sensory phenomena. Given time, significant motor and autonomic fiber involvement may occur. Similarly, many static mild neuropathies that appear at the bedside to involve only sensory fibers show subtle but definite motor fiber involvement on electrophysiologic studies.

With more severe, longer-standing neuropathy, if only one fiber type appears to be involved, one of the neuronopathies should be a diagnostic consideration. Sensory neuronopathy may be a paraneoplastic manifestation of small cell carcinoma of the lung with elevated anti-Hu antibody, an autoimmune manifestation of Sjögren's disease, or a toxic manifestation of pyridoxine abuse. For motor fibers, the diagnosis of motor neuron disease of some type should be considered. An alternative diagnosis not to miss in a patient with only lower motor neuron findings is multifocal conduction block (with or without a high anti-GM1 titer), since these patients are treatable.

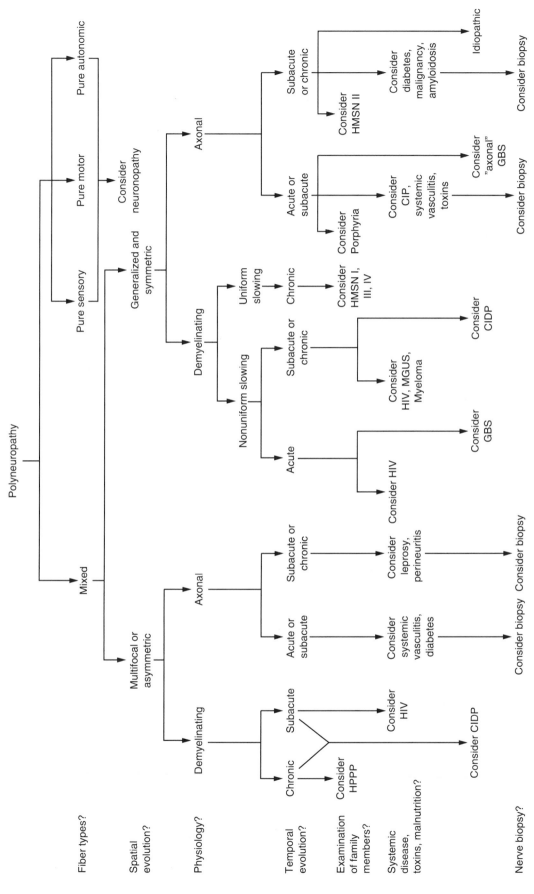

Figure 1 Algorithm for an approach to the diagnosis of polyneuropathy. HPPP = hereditary predisposition to pressure palsy, CIDP = chronic inflammatory demyelinating polyradiculoneuropathy, HIV = human immunodeficiency virus, GBS = Guillain-Barré syndrome, MGUS = monoclonal gammopathy of undetermined significance, HMSN = hereditary motor and sensory neuropathy, CIP = critical illness polyneuropathy. (Modified from Asbury AK, Gilliat RW. Peripheral nerve disorders. London: Butterworths, 1984; with permission.)

327

Table 2 Signs and Symptoms of Peripheral Nerve Disease

Negative	Positive
Motor	
Weakness, wasting, clumsiness, areflexia, hypotonia, deformities (pes cavus, kyphoscoliosis)	Muscle twitches (fasciculations, myokymia), cramps
Sensory	
Sensory loss, ataxia, clumsiness, areflexia, hypotonia	"Tingling," "pins and needles," "burning"
Autonomic	
Postural hypotension, loss of sweating, impotence, bowel and bladder symptoms	Hyperhidrosis, gustatory sweating
Trophic	Foot ulceration, Charcot arthropathy

SPATIAL EVOLUTION

One gathers information about the spatial distribution to determine first if the disease is localized to one body part (e.g., limb, trunk, cranial-innervated structure), as in a radiculopathy, mononeuropathy, or plexopathy, or if it is a more generalized process. If the disease is generalized, the next question is whether its pattern of evolution is asymmetrical-multifocal or symmetrical-diffuse. To determine this, I ask which body part was affected first, second, and so on to determine if the neuropathy evolved symmetrically or asymmetrically or if the pattern was unusual. For example, most acquired neuropathies present with a symmetrical sensory disturbance in the feet, which then "ascends" to the knees, followed by the fingertips, forearms, anterior chest wall, and top of head. Neuropathy that begins only in one leg, for example, or in both hands sparing the feet is more unusual and suggests an asymmetrical or multifocal process. The history is most important in making this distinction since cumulative multifocal deficits may eventually become confluent and appear on physical examination later in the course to be symmetrically diffusely distributed when in fact they accrued asymmetrically. Still, the physical examination often shows that some nerves are affected out of proportion to others by the presence of inter- and intra-limb asymmetries in muscle bulk, strength, cutaneous sensation, and reflexes. For example, median nerve motor and sensory functions may be more affected than those of the ulnar nerve on the same side or those of the median nerve on the other side.

Asymmetrical or multifocal polyneuropathy suggests the syndrome of mononeuropathy multiplex. This term is preferable to the less inclusive term *mononeuritis multiplex,* which refers to inflammatory causes of mononeuropathy multiplex. This syndrome has a differential diagnosis that includes many treatable forms of neuropathy, including vasculitic neuropathy, leprosy, multifocal conduction block, and chronic inflammatory demyelinating polyradiculoneuropathy (CIDP). Its recognition is therefore of key importance in the evaluation of patients with polyneuropathy.

Finally, in generalized symmetric polyneuropathy, there are some exceptions to the usual pattern of selective distal involvement. For example, in Guillain-Barré syndrome (GBS) or porphyric neuropathy, the girdle muscles may be as weak as or weaker than the distal limb muscles.

TEMPORAL EVOLUTION

One gathers information about the temporal evolution of signs and symptoms in parallel with the spatial data. Only the history can provide precise temporal information about the disease, although the physical and electrophysiologic examinations may provide some clues to disease chronicity. The two key points to ascertain are the time from onset to nadir or from onset to the current state if the nadir has not been reached and the "slope" of the descent: smooth, stepwise or relapsing-remitting. One can illustrate these three choices to the patient by "plotting them out" with the index finger in the air. Patients then have no trouble recognizing the temporal pattern their neuropathy most resembles.

Acute sensorimotor neuropathy with a time to nadir of less than 6 weeks is caused by only a few conditions, the most common being GBS. Others to consider are porphyric neuropathy, rapidly progressive vasculitic neuropathies, various acute toxic neuropathies (e.g., large ingestion of thallium or arsenic), and critical illness polyneuropathy (CIP). Severe subacute progressive or stepwise sensorimotor polyneuropathy with a time to nadir of 3 to 12 months has a broader differential diagnosis. The main treatable neuropathies to exclude are CIDP and vasculitic polyneuropathy. The former sometimes has a relapsing-remitting course.

SEVERITY

Negative and positive symptoms of peripheral nerve disease result in functional problems that may range in severity from annoying paresthesia, mild gait ataxia, or loss of hand dexterity that may produce no functional impairment to quadriplegia, deafferentation, or autonomic failure that leave the patient bedbound and helpless. In determining disease severity one should address both the "primary" symptoms and signs, such as degree of muscle weakness, and the patient's unique functional problems produced by the neuropathy, such as problems of daily living, or occupational difficulties. Thus the same polyneuropathy that is of minor severity for a sedentary executive could be debilitating for an athlete or a musician. The pace of the workup and the treatment will depend at least in part on the severity of the neuropathy.

INHERITED NEUROPATHY

Patients with inherited neuropathy may remain asymptomatic for decades before seeking medical attention. Such patients typically have signs of neuropathy on examination but are unaware of their neuropathy (or the neuropathy of family members) because of its slow progression and chronicity. When such a patient does finally seek medical attention, the clinician may assume that the neuropathy is acquired unless he or she pays attention to three clues. The first is that long-standing neuropathy may produce characteristic deformities of the foot (pes cavus) and of the spine (kyphoscoliosis). The second is that in comparison to most acquired neuropathies, typical hereditary sensorimotor neuropathy exhibits little in the way of positive sensory phenomena. Finally, examination of family members, even when asymptomatic, may reveal polyneuropathy.

SYSTEMIC DISEASE, MALNUTRITION, TOXINS

In the review of systems one probes for the presence of diabetes, connective tissue disease, underlying malignancy, infection, malnutrition, megavitaminosis, and exposure to drugs, alcohol, or toxins at the workplace. On physical examination, I pay attention to signs of malnutrition (cheilosis, tongue depapillation), skin rash, adenopathy, thyromegaly, joint swelling, breast masses, and stool guaiac.

Various blood studies are helpful in documenting the presence or absence of a systemic disease associated with neuropathy. In general, when history and physical exam do not provide a clue to the presence or absence of these diseases, the screening tests designed to detect their presence are usually negative. Certainly a fasting blood sugar should be obtained in any patient whose neuropathy is undiagnosed. However, given the vagaries of glucose tolerance testing, I choose not to order this test. Electrolytes, in particular creatinine and blood urea nitrogen, should be obtained. Vitamin B_{12} and a complete blood count should be obtained, particularly in patients with a predominantly sensory disturbance with or without corticospinal findings. Thyroid function tests are usually obtained, though I have yet to find them helpful. Similarly, detailed "connective tissue screens" in the absence of any symptoms or signs of connective tissue disease are rarely positive. Detailed testing to detect underlying neoplasia are usually fruitless. The exception is a patient with sensory neuronopathy and anti-Hu antibody in whom small cell carcinoma of the lung is likely. Otherwise, simple chest x-ray, breast exam, and stool guaiac testing is usually enough.

As many as 10 percent of patients with "idiopathic" sensorimotor polyneuropathy have a monoclonal spike on serum electrophoresis. In many cases, the monoclonal protein, referred to as monoclonal gammopathy of undetermined significance (MGUS), appears to cause the neuropathy. Because MGUS neuropathy is treatable, it is useful to obtain serum and urine protein and immunoelectrophoresis in a patient with otherwise idiopathic polyneuropathy. If a monoclonal paraprotein is found, then bone survey should be performed to look for osteosclerotic myeloma, and bone marrow biopsy

should be considered. The majority of such patients have no underlying hematologic disease. Approximately 50 percent of them have an IgG or IgA monoclonal protein, the remainder have IgM. In about half of the IgM patients, the IgM cross-reacts to myelin-associated glycoprotein (MAG); the other epitopes are not yet known. Patients with IgM monoclonal protein are more likely to have demyelinative physiology than are those with IgG or IgA, although there is a large overlap. A related group of patients are those with pure lower motor neuron involvement. They are sometimes found to have elevated titers to GM1 antibody, usually without a paraprotein. Particularly the subgroup of GM1 patients with conduction block on electrophysiologic studies improve with immunosuppressive therapy.

Although leprosy is the most common cause of neuropathy worldwide, in the Western hemisphere infectious causes of neuropathy are rare. The two to consider are infection with human immunodeficiency virus (HIV) and *Borrelia burgdorferi*. Early on in infection with HIV, GBS and CIDP can occur. Later, a painful sensory neuropathy may develop. In a patient with these kinds of neuropathies who is at risk for HIV, it is reasonable to obtain HIV titers. Lyme disease produces an acute, painful radiculoneuropathy, often in association with facial palsy and meningitis, in addition to a more chronic, milder sensory neuropathy. In patients with these syndromes who are exposed to the organism, it is reasonable to obtain a serum Lyme titer. Otherwise, Lyme disease testing is more likely to yield false-positives than true positives.

An underutilized test, in my opinion, is examination of cerebrospinal fluid (CSF). In a patient with a progressive, moderately severe to severe polyneuropathy in whom other studies are not particularly helpful, the CSF is useful in excluding cytoalbuminologic dissociation. This is seen most commonly in patients with diabetes or inflammatory demyelinating neuropathy. If CSF protein is very high and the patient does not have diabetes, the diagnosis of CIDP should be considered even if electrodiagnostic and nerve biopsy studies are indeterminant.

PHYSIOLOGY

The electrophysiologic examination is very useful in several respects. It helps to confirm the presence of polyneuropathy and differentiate it from other related disorders. It provides objective data concerning the severity, side-to-side symmetry, and chronicity of the neuropathy. Most importantly, physiologic studies are critical in determining whether the neuropathy meets criteria for demyelinative physiology. Further, it can often differentiate acquired from hereditary demyelinating neuropathy by the presence of nonuniform slowing of nerve conduction. Since the acquired demyelinating neuropathies include a relatively short list of treatable diseases (CIDP, some forms of MGUS neuropathy, multifocal conduction block, and osteosclerotic myeloma), physiologic studies are often central to the evaluation of polyneuropathy. Clues on the physical exam to distinguish demyelinating from axonal neuropathy are muscle weakness without atrophy and palpably thickened nerves.

There are some problems with electrophysiology. Unless special studies are performed, it may be negative in (1) the rare pure autonomic or "small fiber" sensory neuropathy, since routine electrophysiologic studies detect medium and large fiber abnormalities of the motor and sensory populations and (2) mild sensory neuropathy with only paresthesia and no negative symptoms, since routine sensory studies document only negative phenomena.

NERVE BIOPSY

It is obvious from the above approach that nerve biopsy is usually not performed to confirm nerve disease. The history, physical examination, and electrodiagnostic studies can almost always do that. Rather, nerve biopsy is performed in the few cases where vasculitic neuropathy is a diagnostic consideration. It may also be performed in a patient with a severe, chronically progressive neuropathy when the diagnosis remains uncertain despite complete workup. In such a case, one would be looking for an inflammatory or a demyelinating cause. Finally, biopsy is helpful in the very rare neuropathies due to leprosy, sarcoidosis, amyloidosis, and the leukodystrophies.

PROBLEMS AND PITFALLS IN DIAGNOSIS

Pseudoneuropathy

Taken one by one, almost all physical findings that we commonly consider to be indicative of neuropathy in fact are not. For example, distal muscle wasting and weakness are seen in the rare cases of distal myopathy or spinal muscular atrophy. Stocking sensory loss can be seen in patients with dorsal column lesions, as in spinal multiple sclerosis. Ankle areflexia can be seen in patients with spinal cord disease at the level of the conus. The bedside diagnosis of polyneuropathy is most secure when a number of these signs occur together in the absence of signs suggesting disease elsewhere. Even then it can be difficult to differentiate root from nerve disease clinically, as in a patient with spinal stenosis of the lumbosacral spine (e.g., polyradiculopathy) versus a patient with progressive sensorimotor polyneuropathy. Both may have distal sensory loss, muscle weakness, and ankle areflexia. Clinically, the two may be differentiated by the presence of pseudoclaudication or radicular back pain in spinal stenosis and distal "burning" pain in polyneuropathy. The electrophysiologic clue is the presence of normal sensory potentials in spinal stenosis and low-amplitude potentials in polyneuropathy.

Occasionally, a condition of acute cervical myelop-

athy, such as transverse myelitis, and spinal shock (e.g., flaccid areflexic paralysis) is confused with one of acute polyneuropathy, such as GBS. Clinically, the spinal cord patient is distinguished by the presence of a sensory and motor level, a brisk CSF pleocytosis, and the absence of demyelinative physiology.

Pseudostroke

Those unfamiliar with acute mononeuropathies of the radial or, less frequently the median, ulnar, or peroneal nerves may initially confuse them with plexus or root lesions and even stroke. Armed with an analytical approach and a knowledge of anatomy, the clinician recognizes that all the deficits are in the territory of one nerve. Still, as in most of medicine, there is no substitute for experience. One needs to see and think through such disorders at least once; thereafter they will not be missed.

Negative Family History

Hereditary neuropathy is very slowly progressive and does not have much in the way of positive sensory phenomena. Therefore, it may not be noticed by the patient (or by affected family members) until late in life. Particularly with a negative family history and the absence of pes cavus deformity, examination of family members may be very helpful in clinching the diagnosis of hereditary neuropathy.

Indeterminate Physiology

There are a fair number of patients with possible CIDP whose nerve conduction studies suggest but do not meet the criteria for demyelinative physiology. Since this neuropathy is often progressive, severe, and treatable, a nerve biopsy to carefully search for demyelinative histology with teased fiber analysis and a spinal tap to exclude a high CSF protein should be considered.

Underlying Diabetes

The most common cause of neuropathy in the Western hemisphere is diabetes. The spectrum of diabetic neuropathy is broad. It can present as a mononeuropathy multiplex or as a symmetrical polyneuropathy involving single or multiple fiber types. Therefore, when a patient has neuropathy and diabetes, it is often assumed that the two are related. Most of the time this is the case. However, I have seen patients with very mild diabetes and very severe progressive neuropathy who have some variant of CIDP. It is important to keep this in mind since some of these patients are responsive to immunosuppressive drugs.

Atypical Amyotrophic Lateral Sclerosis

In a similar vein, I have been fooled by patients with a distal sensory disturbance in the feet who have very severe progressive muscle wasting and weakness. Initially I assumed that these patients had a severe form of polyneuropathy, either CIDP or vasculitic neuropathy. Over time it became clear that they had amyotrophic lateral sclerosis with a coincidental minor sensory neuropathy of unclear cause.

Neuropathy in the Binge Drinker

Academically inclined physicians have doubted that alcohol causes neuropathy in the absence of malnutrition. Most physicians in the community take the contrary view, and over the years I have joined their ranks. I think that a predominantly sensory neuropathy usually affecting the feet can be caused by alcohol intake of moderate degree even in the presence of a normal diet.

Idiopathic Neuropathy

The most troublesome patient for me is the elderly patient with a relatively mild, stable, predominantly sensory, chronic polyneuropathy who does not have symptoms of diabetes or other systemic disease. The issue is always how fully to work these patients up, since in my experience I rarely discover the cause. My own approach is to do a complete physical examination; obtain electrodiagnostic studies to exclude demyelinative physiology; obtain stool guaiac, chest x-ray, and mammogram to help exclude common malignancies; and look for potentially reversible metabolic causes such as vitamin B_{12} deficiency, hypothyroidism, and diabetes. I usually do not take it much further than that unless the neuropathy progresses.

SUGGESTED READING

Asbury AK, Gilliat RW. Peripheral nerve disorders. London: Butterworths, 1984.

Barohn RJ, Kissel JT, Warmolts JR, Mendell JR. Chronic demyelinating polyradiculoneuropathy: Clinical characteristics, course, and recommendations for diagnostic criteria. Arch Neurol 1989; 46: 878–884.

Dyck PJ, Lais AC, Ohta M, et al. Chronic inflammatory polyradiculoneuropathy. Mayo Clin Proc 1975; 50:621–637.

Dyck PJ, Oviatt KF, Lambert EH. Intensive evaluation of referred unclassified neuropathies yields improved diagnosis. Ann Neurol 1981; 10:222–226.

Dyck PJ, Thomas PK, Griffin JW, et al, eds. Peripheral neuropathy. 3rd ed. Philadelphia:WB Saunders, 1993.

Kelly JJ, Kyle RA, O'Brien PC. Prevalence of monoclonal protein in peripheral neuropathy. Neurology 1981; 31:1480–1483.

Lewis RA, Summer AJ. The electrodiagnositic distinctions between chronic familial and acquired demyelinative neuropathies. Neurology 1982; 32:592–596.

Ropper AH, Wijdicks EFM, Truax BT. Guillain-Barré syndrome. Philadelphia:FA Davis, 1991.

Schaumberg HR, Berger AR, Thomas PK. Disorders of peripheral nerves. Philadelphia:FA Davis, 1991.

Zochodne DW, Bolton CF, Wells GA, et al. Critical illness polyneuropathy: A complication of sepsis and multiple organ failure. Brain 1987; 110:819–842.

BELL'S PALSY AND IDIOPATHIC CRANIAL NEURITIS

MARK B. BROMBERG, M.D., Ph.D.

The sudden onset of facial weakness, weakness of muscles innervated by other cranial nerves, or pain and dysesthesias about the head and neck can be frightening to the patient and can pose a diagnostic dilemma to the medical consultant. The patient is worried that this may represent a serious problem such as a stroke. The consultant wants to be certain of the diagnosis of idiopathic cranial neuritis to avoid extensive and unnecessary tests. The diagnosis of Bell's palsy or neuritis of another cranial nerve can be made at the bedside by a careful history and neurologic examination and exclusion of other lesion sites. A systematic evaluation will reduce the number of necessary laboratory tests and allow attention to those that can offer prognosis.

Idiopathic cranial neuritis may be a syndrome, with primary involvement of different cranial nerves but with a typical clinical course. Bell's palsy, for example, is caused by a lesion of the facial nerve, but additional cranial nerves are involved to lesser degrees. There are examples of neuritis of other cranial nerves, particularly one or more of the lower cranial nerves, which mimic the clinical course of Bell's palsy. Within this syndromic pattern there may be differences in cause and pathophysiology. Bell's palsy is the most common example of a cranial neuritis, and full epidemiologic data are available. For the other idiopathic cranial neuritides, the literature consists mostly of case reports and small series.

Since the diagnosis rests on recognition of the spectrum of dysfunction of each nerve, I will begin by presenting the clinical features of idiopathic cranial neuritis, using Bell's palsy as the prototypical example. I will then briefly review the causes and pathogenesis of each of the cranial neuritides, present guidelines for taking a thorough history and performing an adequate neurologic examination, and discuss appropriate laboratory tests, with attention focused on the use of electrodiagnostic testing. Finally, I will review the prognosis.

CLINICAL FEATURES

Facial Nerve (VII)

Although the description of unilateral facial weakness is attributed to Charles Bell in 1827, the disorder was recognized earlier, and sculptures of faces with characteristic asymmetric weakness are attributed to artists from the fifteenth century and earlier. The asymmetric appearance, accentuated by voluntary or emotional facial expression, has been likened to the face of the god Janus, with one side weeping and the other side laughing.

Bell's palsy is much more common than the other forms of cranial neuritis, but the reasons for this are not clear. The epidemiology of classic Bell's palsy is not diagnostically specific. The overall incidence is approximately 25 per 100,000 individuals, with a lower incidence in children and younger adults and a higher incidence in older adults. The median age is 40 years and the range is 1 to 91 years. The gender ratio varies with age but is close to equality. There is no racial predilection. Neither side of the face is affected with greater frequency.

The classic presentation of Bell's palsy is subacute onset of unilateral facial weakness. Symptoms can evolve overnight, over several hours, or occasionally over several days. Facial weakness may not be immediately apparent to the patient and might first be noted when looking in a mirror or may be recognized by others. Progression of weakness is usually rapid, over days and rarely over 1 to 2 weeks. The degree of facial weakness varies, from partial in one-third of patients, to complete in two-thirds. Bilateral involvement is extremely rare. A small number of patients have recurrent Bell's palsy, and in some the history indicates a familial predisposition to Bell's palsy.

Dysfunction of the trigeminal (V), glossopharyngeal (IX), and vagus (X) nerves is common and is an important diagnostic feature of Bell's palsy. Symptoms include hypesthesia or dysesthesia in the distribution of the trigeminal and glossopharyngeal nerves or the second cervical root. About half of patients note pain in the region of the mastoid process early in the course, frequently preceding the onset of weakness. One-third of patients describe abnormalities of taste. Hyperacusis, attributed to both stapedius muscle weakness and cochlear nerve dysfunction, is also observed, although less commonly. Tear production may be affected, with both excesses and inadequacies of flow.

Several symptoms and signs suggest an alternative diagnosis. Marked weakness of lower facial expression but normal ability to furrow the brow suggests an upper motor neuron pattern of facial weakness. This pattern of weakness is characteristically observed during voluntary smiling, whereas during emotional smiling the lower facial weakness lessens or resolves. Associated findings suggesting an upper motor neuron lesion above the level of the pons are weakness of limb strength, asymmetry of tendon reflexes, which initially may be reduced on the side of the weakness and later increased, and a plantar extensor response. Bilateral facial palsy may be part of a diffuse polyneuropathy, and symptoms of distal paresthesias and weakness and hyporeflexia or areflexia should be sought to support this localization. Progression of facial weakness over many weeks suggests an infiltrative process such as a tumor.

Vestibular Nerve (VIII)

An idiopathic neuropathy with primary involvement of the vestibular portion of the VIIIth cranial nerve has been described. Patients experience acute vestibular vertigo and symptoms referable to other cranial nerves. For example, three-quarters of patients have hypesthesia of facial sensation, two-thirds have hypesthesia of skin innervated by the second cervical nerve, and one-half have hypesthesia of the posterior pharyngeal wall. Half of patients have weakness of palatal elevation and the cricothyroid muscle. Three-quarters of patients report a recent upper respiratory tract infection. All of the patients in one series had complete resolution of symptoms within 4 weeks. One hypothesized mechanism is reactivation of herpes simplex infection.

This diagnosis excludes patients with cochlear hearing loss, verifiable by audiometry. When both the vestibular and auditory divisions are involved, or particularly when symptoms evolve slowly, a compressive lesion such as an acoustic neuroma should be considered.

Vagus Nerve (X)

Idiopathic neuropathy of the recurrent laryngeal nerve presents as hoarseness. This is a relatively common idiopathic palsy, accounting for approximately 30 percent of patients seen with vocal cord paralysis. The hoarseness is infrequently accompanied by dysphagia. Interestingly, males are affected twice as often as females. In addition, the left nerve is more commonly involved than the right, which is attributed to greater vulnerability due to its longer length. Occasionally, there is bilateral involvement. Rates of partial to full recovery are high, between 50 and 90 percent.

Recurrent laryngeal nerve paralysis occurs most commonly as a consequence of bronchial carcinoma or as a complication of thyroid surgery. Chest radiography or chest computed tomography scan is appropriate in smokers or those with other risk factors for lung cancer.

Spinal Accessory Nerve (XI)

There are rare reports of idiopathic and isolated weakness of the trapezius muscle referable to a lesion of the spinal accessory nerve. A common feature is moderate to severe unilateral shoulder pain at onset, with atrophy and weakness becoming apparent days later as the pain subsides. Clinical similarities have been noted between this disorder, Bell's palsy, and idiopathic brachial plexopathy. The outcome is variable.

Hypoglossal Nerve (XII)

Isolated idiopathic hypoglossal nerve palsies occur, although they are rare. The onset of unilateral tongue atrophy and weakness has been temporally associated with a common cold and may be preceded by an ipsilateral headache. The clinical findings are confined to the XIIth nerve and spontaneously reverse over several months.

In patients above the age of 50 years, temporal arteritis can present with headache and infarction of the tongue. Since this is a systemic disorder that may lead to sudden and irreversible blindness, it is important to obtain a sedimentation rate. If the sedimentation rate is elevated, temporal artery biopsy and treatment with corticosteroids are indicated.

Trigeminal Nerve (V)

Idiopathic cranial neuritis of upper cranial nerves is less common than involvement of the lower cranial nerves. A painless sensory trigeminal neuritis has been described, with exceedingly rare involvement of motor components of the nerve. The onset is usually sudden and rarely progresses over days. Unlike herpes zoster, which most commonly involves the first division, idiopathic trigeminal neuritis most frequently affects the second or third division, or both. The sensory loss is described as numbness, and the sense of taste is usually impaired. The neurologic examination is remarkable only for reduced perception to light touch. The corneal blink reflex is preserved. Prognosis is variable, with most patients achieving partial or complete recovery.

Trigeminal neuralgia or tic douloureux should not be confused with this painless condition, which occurs in various connective tissue disorders, such as systemic sclerosis (scleroderma), Sjögren syndrome, and mixed connective tissue disease. Therefore, careful review of systems and physical examination for involvement of other organs should be performed, as well as serologic testing when appropriate.

Oculomotor, Trochlear, and Abducens Nerves (III, IV, VI)

It is not clear how frequently isolated idiopathic neuritis occurs in these nerves. It has been described in children in the abducens nerve. Symptomatic involvement of these cranial nerves warrants a complete neuro-ophthalmologic evaluation since the differential diagnosis is broad and idiopathic afflictions are rare.

CAUSE AND PATHOPHYSIOLOGY

Bell's palsy and neuritis of the other cranial nerves are considered to be idiopathic once herpes zoster (Ramsay-Hunt syndrome), trauma (accidental and surgical), birth defects, otitis media, malignancy, marked hypertension, and diabetes mellitus are excluded. In Bell's palsy, the facial nerve is most likely damaged by edema, which arises from the initial insult and is exacerbated by the confines of the bony canal. Further increases in pressure lead to nerve ischemia, which begets more edema, and the cycle continues, resulting in demyelination with conduction block and axonal damage with wallerian degeneration. The cause remains obscure. Cold exposure of the face has long been discussed as a factor. Seasonal clustering of cases has been inconsistently reported. Various abnormalities of the immune system have been reported, suggesting cell-mediated immunity against peripheral nerve antigens. Strong arguments have been made for Bell's palsy being caused by initial or reactivated cytomegalovirus, herpes virus, or adenovirus infections. There are moderately strong associations with hypertension in children and with pregnancy.

The pathophysiology of neuritis of the other cranial nerves is less clear. When prompt recovery occurs (within days), an element of demyelination or conduction block is likely. When muscles are more chronically affected and examined by needle electromyogram (EMG) there is usually evidence for denervation reflecting axonal damage. Speculations about the cause of damage to the lower cranial nerves frequently focus on initial or recurrent viral infection. For neuritis of the spinal accessory nerve, the similarities with idiopathic brachial plexopathy are striking, but the cause of that form of neuritis is not known either.

CLINICAL DIAGNOSIS AND EVALUATION

The diagnosis of cranial neuritis rests with the recognition of cranial nerve involvement and can usually be made from the current and past medical histories. Because of undue attention to the primary deficit, involvement of other cranial nerves may go unrecognized. Key information to obtain from the history includes (1) involvement of multiple cranial nerves on the same side, (2) exclusion of diffuse symptoms suggesting a central nervous system lesion, and (3) exclusion of causally associated diseases. Establishing involvement of multiple cranial nerves is aided by taking an orderly inventory of the function of the cranial nerves (Table 1). Some forms of idiopathic cranial neuritis such as spinal accessory neuritis may occur in isolation.

The physical and neurologic examinations confirm the extent of cranial nerve involvement but also help to identify underlying causes. Table 2 lists physical and neurologic tests that accomplish both of these goals.

After a thorough history and physical examination, relatively few laboratory studies are necessary. Table 3 includes tests that are appropriate to order in every patient to identify the most frequent causes of cranial neuropathies. Many commonly ordered laboratory tests are rarely of diagnostic help except in special circumstances, which have been discussed. These include imaging studies of the cranium and brain, which are only indicated if there is a strong suspicion of a metastatic (known primary site) or primary tumor. An extensive

Table 1 Clinically Important Symptoms Commonly Produced in Idiopathic Cranial Neuritis

Cranial Nerves	Symptoms
III, IV, VI	Diplopia, unilateral ptosis
V	Facial numbness, heaviness, and dysesthetic sensations
	Dysgeusia
	Weakness of jaw closure and chewing
VII	Asymmetric facial appearance, especially with facial expression
	Dysgeusia
	Change in lacrimation
VIII	Vertigo
	Nystagmus
IX, X	Palatal numbness
	Hoarseness
	Dysphagia
XI	Asymmetric sternocleidomastoid and upper trapezius muscle weakness
XII	Asymmetric tongue weakness
	Dysarthria

Table 2 Clinical Tests Helpful in Evaluating Cranial Neuritis

General physical examination
  Vital signs for elevated temperature and marked hypertension
  Inspection of skin of head, neck, external ear canal, and oral pharynx for herpetic lesions
  Examination of tympanic membranes for otitis media
Neurologic examination to identify cranial nerve involvement
  Fullness of extraocular eye movements
  Facial sensation to light touch, and corneal response to light touch
  Bulk of masseter muscles and symmetry of effort to return mandible to midline after voluntary displacement
  Facial expression at rest and during voluntary activation, and fullness of eye closure
  Auditory acuity assessed by rubbing fingers, ticking watch, or a 512 Hz tuning fork
  Palatal elevation and palatal sensation to light touch with a Q-tip
  Sternocleidomastoid and trapezius muscle strength
  Deviation of tongue to protrusion, and weakness when pressing laterally against a tongue blade
Neurologic examination suggesting central nervous system involvement
  Weakness restricted to lower half of face
  Word finding difficulties
  Increased or asymmetric limb tone to passive manipulation
  Brisk or asymmetric deep tendon reflexes
  Presence of extensor plantar response

Table 3 Laboratory Tests Helpful in Identifying Specific Causes of Cranial Neuropathies

Fasting serum glucose for diabetes mellitus
Serum VDRL
Sedimentation rate for temporal (giant cell) arteritis
Serum Lyme titers when tick exposure is reasonable
Chest radiography for abnormalities supporting sarcoidosis or lung cancer

laboratory-based evaluation for a possible primary tumor is inefficient and is not a substitute for a thorough past medical history, review of systems, and general medical examination. If there is a strong suspicion of malignancy, then a focused battery of tests is reasonable. Cerebrospinal fluid is unremarkable and need be sampled only if a meningitis is suspected.

There is controversy about the role and timing of electrodiagnostic evaluation. This applies particularly to its use in assessing prognosis and managing therapy in Bell's palsy. It is worthwhile to review the range of nerve lesions and their demonstration on electrodiagnostic testing.

The least destructive lesion is to the myelin sheath. At a minimum, this slows impulse conduction across the lesion site, but this is usually asymptomatic and will not be brought to medical attention. A more severe degree of demyelination causes block of impulses across the lesion. The degree of paresis will be proportional to the number of blocked fibers in the nerve. Remyelination can proceed quickly, within days to weeks, and recovery will be complete. With damage of greater severity, there will be disruption of nerve fiber axons, resulting in wallerian degeneration. In this case the degree of paresis will be proportional to the number of damaged axons. Recovery of strength will depend upon growth of axons across the lesion site to the muscle, collateral sprouting of intramuscular branches from spared nerve fibers, or a combination of both processes.

In Bell's palsy, the lesion site is along the intracranial segment of the nerve, and most nerve conduction studies can only be carried out on the extracranial segment of the facial nerve. There are electrodiagnostic studies, such as the blink reflex, that can assess conduction along the intracranial segment, but they are less able to quantify the extent of the lesion. When a lesion causes only conduction block, the compound muscle action potential (CMAP) amplitude will be normal. It is most practical to compare the evoked amplitude of the affected side to that of the contralateral side. When the lesion involves axonal damage, the CMAP amplitude will be reduced in approximate proportion to the number of damaged axons. However, it is critical to appreciate that it takes 3 to 5 days for a damaged axon to stop conducting impulses and that the CMAP amplitude will be preserved during that time period (Fig. 1). Consequently, the amplitude provides information on the degree of axonal damage that occurred 3 to 5 days earlier. This prevents the effective use of serial nerve conduction studies to time surgical decompression of the bony canal.

During the same 3 to 5 day period that damaged axons are capable of conducting impulses to electrical stimulation, the needle EMG examination will be remarkable only for reduced motor unit recruitment, which will be proportional to the number of fibers with axonal damage plus those with conduction block. Only after 5 days will abnormal spontaneous activity in the form of positive sharp waves and fibrillation potentials occur (see Fig. 1). The amount of abnormal spontaneous activity, however, is not proportional to the number of damaged nerve fiber axons.

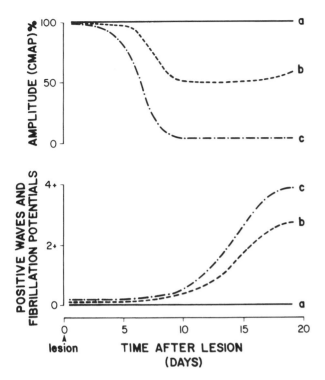

Figure 1 Representation of electrodiagnostic findings after facial nerve lesions of varying severity, plotted against time. *A,* Conduction block only; *B,* Conduction block and partial axonal degeneration; *C,* Complete axonal degeneration. *Top,* Compound muscle action potential (CMAP) amplitude as percentage of contralateral, unaffected side. *Bottom,* Presence and degree of abnormal spontaneous activity (fibrillation potentials and positive waves) recorded during needle electromyogram. (From Albers JW, Bromberg MB. Bell's palsy. In: Johnson RT, ed. Current therapy in neurologic disease. 3rd ed. Philadelphia: BC Decker, 1990:377; with permission.)

Electrodiagnostic studies of other cranial nerves are largely confined to needle EMG examination, looking for evidence of axonal damage. Most skeletal muscles can be studied, and common ones are masseter for trigeminal nerve, cricothyroid for vagus nerve, sternocleidomastoid and trapezius for spinal accessory nerve, and tongue for hypoglossal nerve. The spinal accessory nerve is accessible in the neck, and the trapezius CMAP amplitude can be compared to the contralateral side, as described for Bell's palsy.

PROGNOSIS

Prognostic features are best described for Bell's palsy. Patient age is inversely related to outcome, with patients over 35 doing poorly. Patients with greater facial weakness also have a poor outcome. Nerve conduction studies can be used as objective measures. The most helpful time to perform electrodiagnostic studies is 5 to 10 days after the clinical nadir of weakness. The most useful measure is the distal CMAP amplitude, compared to the normal side. If the amplitude is greater than 10 percent of normal, the long-term prognosis for a functionally acceptable outcome is good. Experience shows that if only 10 percent of fibers remain, they can undergo collateral sprouting to innervate enough denervated muscle fibers to restore acceptable facial function. In addition, a number of fibers usually cross the lesion and reinnervate muscle fibers.

An interesting phenomenon is frequently observed in association with regeneration of nerve fibers across the lesion site. A synkinetic response occurs, wherein a part of the face that should be relaxed will contract when another part is voluntarily activated. A common example is partial closure of an eye (winking) during smiling, although other less obvious associated facial movements occur. The usual explanation offered is that the regenerating fibers may reach the original target muscle or may follow other branches to different portions of the facial muscle.

Overall, complete recovery occurs in about half of patients. In this group, improvement begins within 10 days and is complete within 2 months. The half of patients with incomplete recovery begins to show improvement at 2 months and stabilize within 9 months. With careful study, residua are present in three-quarters of patients in the form of subtle synkinesis and mild weakness.

Prognosis for the other forms of cranial neuritis was discussed in their clinical descriptions.

SUGGESTED READING

Adour KK, Sprague MA, Hilsinger RL. Vestibular vertigo. A form of polyneuritis? JAMA 1981; 246:1564–1567.

Affi AK, Rifai ZH, Faris KB. Isolated, reversible, hypoglossal nerve palsy. Arch Neurol 1984; 41:1218.

Albers JW, Bromberg MB. Bell's palsy. In: Johnson RT, ed. Current therapy in neurologic disease. 3rd ed. Philadelphia: BC Decker, 1990:376.

Berry H, Blair RL. Isolated vagus nerve palsy and vagal mononeuritis. Arch Otolaryngol 1980; 106:333–337.

Blau JN, Harris M, Kennett S. Trigeminal sensory neuropathy. N Engl J Med 1969; 281:873–876.

Eisen A, Bertrand G. Isolated accessory nerve palsy of spontaneous origin. Arch Neurol 1972; 27:496–500.

Katusic SK, Beard CM, Wiederholt WC, et al. Incidence, clinical features, and prognosis in Bell's palsy, Rochester, Minnesota, 1968-1982. Ann Neurol 1986; 20:622–627.

METABOLIC MYOPATHY

ZIAD RIFAI, M.D.
ROBERT C. GRIGGS, M.D.

The metabolic myopathies consist of a group of disorders associated with genetically determined biochemical defects and characterized clinically by weakness or intermittent exercise-induced myalgias, cramps, and fatigue. In some of these disorders other organ systems may be involved. Age of onset and severity are variable. Different biochemical defects may have similar clinical manifestations. On the other hand, a single metabolic defect may be associated with a wide clinical spectrum. For diagnostic purposes, it is useful to divide the metabolic myopathies into two groups: dynamic disorders where exercise intolerance and myoglobinuria are the major manifestations, and static disorders where muscle weakness is the main symptom.

The chromosomal localization and gene product have recently been identified in virtually all metabolic myopathies, making genetic counseling and antenatal diagnosis feasible now or in the near future.

METABOLIC MYOPATHIES ASSOCIATED WITH EXERCISE INTOLERANCE

Recurrent episodes of muscle pain, cramps, and stiffness precipitated by exercise are the hallmark of these disorders. When severe, the muscle pain may be associated with muscle swelling, tenderness, and weakness. These findings reflect acute muscle fiber necrosis (rhabdomyolysis) and are associated with release into the serum of large amounts of myoglobin and creatine

Table 1 Differential Diagnosis of Recurrent Episodes of Exercise-Induced Muscle Pain and Myoglobinuria

Disorders of carbohydrate metabolism
  Myophosphorylase deficiency (McArdle's disease, type V glycogenosis)
  Phosphofructokinase deficiency (Tarui's disease, type VII glycogenosis)
  Phosphoglycerate kinase deficiency (type IX glycogenosis)
  Phosphoglycerate mutase deficiency (type X glycogenosis)
  Lactate dehydrogenase deficiency
  Phosphorylase b kinase deficiency

Disorders of fatty acid metabolism
  Carnitine palmityl transferase deficiency
  Long-chain acyl-coenzyme A dehydrogenase (LCAD) deficiency
  Short-chain hydroxyacyl-coenzyme A dehydrogenase (SCHAD) deficiency

Myoadenylate deaminase deficiency

X-Linked myopathy with abnormal dystrophin

Idiopathic

kinase (CK). In extreme situations, the urine becomes amber in color due to myoglobinuria. Consequently, acute tubular necrosis and renal failure may occur.

The metabolic causes of recurrent episodes of myoglobinuria include defects of carbohydrate metabolism, defects of fatty acid metabolism, and myoadenylate deaminase deficiency (Table 1). In about 50 percent of cases, however, a biochemical defect is not detected. Few of these patients are found to have an X-linked myopathy with abnormal dystrophin.

Disorders of Carbohydrate Metabolism

The syndrome of exercise intolerance and myoglobinuria has been associated with deficiencies of several enzymes involved in glycogen metabolism (see Table 1). Because glycogen is the main source of energy in the acutely exercising muscle, symptoms usually appear during intense physical activity.

Myophosphorylase Deficiency (McArdle's Disease)

McArdle's disease is usually inherited as an autosomal recessive trait and is restricted to skeletal muscle. Males are more often affected than females. As a child the patient may complain of fatigue and muscle aches, but severe exercise-induced painful contractures, often called "cramps" by the patient, associated with myoglobinuria usually do not become evident until adolescence or early adulthood. Pain typically starts during strenuous activity and is limited to the muscles that are being exercised. Rest may rapidly relieve the aching unless exercise is intense and prolonged, when pain may persist for several days. If the patient slows down at the first sign of fatigue, he or she may be able to sustain exercise at a slower pace for a longer period, the so-called second wind phenomenon.

Examination during a bout of rhabdomyolysis may reveal muscle swelling, tenderness, and weakness. In between episodes, the exam is normal. However, after repeated attacks of myoglobinuria, fixed proximal weakness may develop later in life.

Laboratory Tests. CK is usually elevated and increases manyfold after exercise. Myoglobin may be detected in the urine during severe episodes of muscle pain. The forearm exercise test, described in the next paragraph, shows minimal or no rise in venous blood lactate, indicating a block in the glycolytic pathway. Muscle biopsy demonstrates the absence of myophosphorylase by a histochemical reaction. Periodic acid-Schiff (PAS)–positive, glycogen filled subsarcolemmal blebs are usually present (Figs. 1 and 2). Necrotic and regenerating fibers can be seen following an episode of myoglobinuria. Biochemical analysis of a muscle biopsy specimen confirms the deficiency of myophosphorylase and usually demonstrates increased glycogen content.

Exhaustive Forearm Exercise Test. This test is helpful in narrowing the differential diagnosis in a patient presenting with exercise intolerance. A catheter is introduced retrogradely into an antecubital vein and

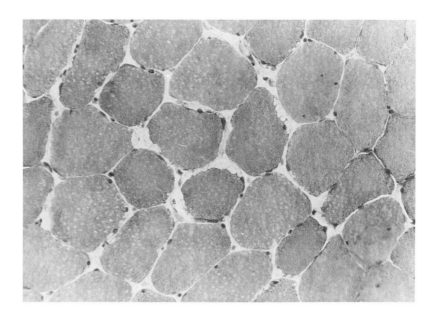

Figure 1 Myophosphorylase deficiency. Subsarcolemmal blebs (Modified Gomori trichrome, × 400).

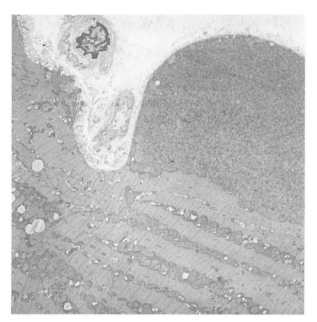

Figure 2 Myophosphorylase deficiency. Electron micrograph showing glycogen accumulation under the sarcolemma and between myofibrils (× 10,000).

connected to a three-way stopcock. Patency of the catheter is maintained with an infusion of normal saline. The side port is used to draw blood samples. The forearm muscles are exercised by squeezing a hand dynamometer to 50 percent of maximum grip strength until exhaustion (usually about 10 minutes). Ischemia, produced by inflating a sphygmomanometer cuff above arterial pressure, is often used but is unnecessary and can cause severe muscle necrosis. Blood samples obtained at baseline, immediately after exercise, and 1, 3, 5, and 10 minutes postexercise are analyzed for lactate and ammonia determinations. In a normal person, venous lactate increases three to five times with exercise, and ammonia doubles. Minimal or no rise in venous lactate indicates a block in the glycolytic pathway. Failure of ammonia to rise is associated with myoadenylate deaminase deficiency. Failure of either lactate or ammonia to increase may also indicate suboptimal exercise.

Phosphofructokinase Deficiency (Tarui's Disease)

The clinical presentation of Tarui's disease, an autosomal recessive disorder, is similar to that of McArdle's disease. Exercise-induced fatigue and cramps usually start in childhood. Severe episodes can be accompanied by nausea, vomiting, and myoglobinuria. Patients may have an associated mild hemolytic anemia due to reduction of the enzyme level in erythrocytes. During symptom-free intervals, the examination is normal.

Abnormal laboratory tests include an elevated CK and an increased reticulocyte count. Bilirubin and uric acid levels may also be elevated due to hemolysis. Venous lactate does not rise following forearm exercise. A histochemical stain of a muscle biopsy demonstrates the absence of phosphofructokinase. The enzyme deficiency is confirmed by a biochemical assay.

Other Defects of Glycolysis Associated with Exercise Intolerance

Deficiencies of phosphoglycerate kinase (PGK), phosphoglycerate mutase (PGAM), lactate dehydrogenase (LDH), and phosphorylase b kinase have been described in patients presenting with exercise-induced cramps, fatigue, and myoglobinuria. Inheritance of PGK deficiency is X-linked recessive. The other disorders are autosomal recessive. In each of these disorders, the specific enzyme deficiency is established by biochemical analysis of a muscle biopsy specimen.

Disorders of Fatty Acid Metabolism

Carnitine Palmityl Transferase Deficiency

Carnitine palmityl transferase (CPT) deficiency is the most common hereditary cause of myoglobinuria. The disorder is localized to chromosome 1 and is a recessive trait. Males are more frequently affected than females. CPT is an enzyme involved in shuttling fatty acids across the inner mitochondrial membrane. Its deficiency results in defective utilization of free fatty acids, which are the major source of energy during prolonged exercise. Therefore muscle pain and cramps usually start after low-intensity sustained exercise and may be associated with myoglobinuria. Fasting exacerbates the symptoms and may even precipitate an attack. The muscles may be swollen, tender, and weak during an episode of myoglobinuria. Severe attacks can be associated with respiratory failure. Patients are normal between episodes.

CK is usually normal but may increase dramatically following exercise. A normal rise of venous lactate and ammonia is observed after forearm exercise. The enzyme deficiency is demonstrated by a biochemical assay performed on a muscle biopsy specimen. Histologically, the muscle is usually normal.

Other Disorders of Fatty Acid Metabolism Associated with Recurrent Myoglobinuria

A syndrome of recurrent myoglobinuria and hypoglycemic encephalopathy, usually beginning in childhood or adolescence, has been associated with deficiency of two other enzymes involved in fatty acid metabolism: long-chain acyl-coenzyme A dehydrogenase (LCAD) and short-chain hydroxyacyl-coenzyme A dehydrogenase (SCHAD). Muscle weakness and cardiomyopathy can be present. The diagnosis is confirmed by biochemical analysis of a muscle biopsy specimen.

Myoadenylate Deaminase Deficiency

Myoadenylate deaminase deficiency occurs in about 1 percent of the population and has been identified in patients with exercise-induced pain and cramps. Some of these patients also have recurrent myoglobinuria. It is not always clear whether the enzyme deficiency is the cause of the symptoms or the association is coincidental. The examination is normal. Venous ammonia does not rise following forearm exercise, but lactate does. A muscle histochemical stain demonstrates the enzyme deficiency. The diagnosis is confirmed by a biochemical assay showing less than 5 percent residual enzyme activity.

METABOLIC MYOPATHIES ASSOCIATED WITH FIXED OR PROGRESSIVE WEAKNESS

Patients who present with fixed or progressive weakness, with or without other organ system involve-

Table 2 Inherited Metabolic Defects Causing Muscle Weakness

Disorders of carbohydrate metabolism
  Acid maltase deficiency (type II glycogenosis)
  Debrancher enzyme deficiency (type III glycogenosis)
  Brancher enzyme deficiency (type IV glycogenosis)
  Phosphorylase b kinase deficiency
  Phosphofructokinase kinase deficiency (late-onset)
  Myophosphorylase deficiency (fatal infantile form)

Disorders of lipid metabolism
  Muscle carnitine deficiency
  Systemic carnitine deficiency

ment, may have one of several identifiable metabolic defects. Age at onset and clinical severity are variable, reflecting the severity and distribution of the biochemical abnormality. This group of disorders includes defects of carbohydrate and lipid metabolism (Table 2).

Disorders of Carbohydrate Metabolism

Acid Maltase Deficiency (Type II Glycogenosis)

Acid maltase is a lysosomal enzyme involved in glycogenolysis. The gene for acid maltase is localized to chromosome 17. Deficiency of this enzyme is inherited as an autosomal recessive trait and is probably genetically heterogeneous. Phenotypically, a severe infantile form (Pompe's disease) and milder childhood and adult forms have been recognized.

The severe infantile form presents in the first few months of life with hypotonia, generalized weakness, and enlargement of the tongue, liver, and heart. Death occurs in infancy due to cardiorespiratory failure.

Patients with the milder childhood form have delayed motor milestones, proximal weakness, respiratory insufficiency, and muscles of a firm rubbery consistency. Calf enlargement can be present and may lead to an erroneous diagnosis of Duchenne dystrophy. Cardiomegaly and hepatomegaly are infrequent findings. Death usually occurs before the end of the second decade from respiratory failure.

The adult onset form presents in the third or fourth decade with slowly progressive proximal weakness affecting predominantly the pelvic girdle and mimicking limb girdle dystrophy or polymyositis. About one-third of patients have severe selective involvement of the respiratory muscles and may present with respiratory insufficiency. In these patients, restless sleep and early morning headaches may indicate impending respiratory failure.

The diagnosis of acid maltase deficiency should be considered in infants and children with weakness and organomegaly. The diagnosis should be suspected in adults presenting with limb girdle weakness, particularly when respiratory muscle weakness is disproportionately severe.

In all three forms, CK is elevated and the elec-

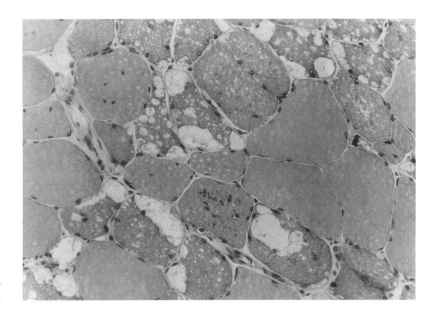

Figure 3 Acid maltase deficiency. Large vacuoles are seen in several fibers (H&E, × 400).

tromyogram (EMG) shows frequent spontaneous activity including myotonic and pseudomyotonic discharges. These are particularly prominent in the paraspinal muscles of adult patients. Myopathic, short duration, small motor unit potentials are recorded from the proximal muscles. In the infantile and childhood forms, the electrocardiogram (ECG) may show high-voltage QRS complexes and a short PR interval. Muscle biopsy reveals a vacuolar myopathy (Figure 3). The vacuoles are PAS- and acid phosphatase–positive. The vacuolar changes are most marked in the infantile form. The diagnosis of acid maltase deficiency is confirmed by biochemical analysis of a muscle biopsy specimen.

Debrancher Enzyme Deficiency (Type III Glycogenosis)

An infantile form and an adult onset form of debrancher enzyme deficiency, an autosomal recessive disorder, have been recognized. The infantile form presents with hepatomegaly and fasting hypoglycemia associated in some cases with hypotonia, weakness, and cardiomegaly. As the child grows older, the hepatic manifestations of the disease improve but the weakness may progress.

In the adult onset form, progressive weakness is the major symptom and may affect both proximal and distal muscles. The patient may also complain of fatigability, but myoglobinuria does not occur. The presence of associated cardiomyopathy and hepatomegaly is diagnostically useful. In some cases the disorder resembles a motor neuron disease.

CK is elevated. ECG shows biventricular hypertrophy. The EMG findings of frequent spontaneous activity and myopathic potentials are similar to those seen in acid maltase deficiency. Venous lactate production following forearm exercise is reduced. The muscle biopsy shows PAS-positive vacuoles. Biochemical anal-

ysis reveals increased glycogen content and confirms the enzyme deficiency.

Brancher Enzyme Deficiency (Type IV Glycogenosis)

Inheritance of brancher enzyme deficiency is autosomal recessive. In infants the disease presents with hepatosplenomegaly, hepatic failure, and growth retardation sometimes associated with weakness and cardiomegaly. Affected children do not survive beyond the first few years of life. In adults the enzyme deficiency may cause a limb girdle myopathy.

Recently brancher enzyme deficiency has been reported in some cases of adult polyglucosan body disease characterized by upper motor neuron dysfunction and peripheral neuropathy.

Other Disorders of Muscle Carbohydrate Metabolism Causing Weakness

Deficiency of phosphofructokinase or phosphorylase b kinase usually presents with exercise-induced myoglobinuria in adults. However, deficiency of either enzyme has also, rarely, been associated with a late onset myopathy characterized by progressive limb weakness. Myophosphorylase deficiency, a cause of exercise intolerance and myoglobinuria in adults, has also been identified as a cause of rapidly progressive fatal weakness in infants.

Disorders of Lipid Metabolism (Carnitine Deficiency Syndromes)

Carnitine plays an essential role in the metabolism of fatty acids by muscle fibers. Primary carnitine deficiency is inherited as an autosomal recessive trait and is associated with a lipid storage myopathy. The clinical manifestations are variable, but two forms can be recognized.

In systemic carnitine deficiency, carnitine content is reduced in plasma, heart, skeletal muscle, and liver. The disease presents in early childhood with episodes of hypoglycemic encephalopathy, metabolic acidosis, and evidence of liver damage. The episodes may resemble Reye's syndrome and can be precipitated by fasting. A progressive lipid storage myopathy involving cardiac and skeletal muscles is usually present. Untreated, the disease is fatal.

In muscle carnitine deficiency, the major manifestation is progressive limb weakness starting in childhood or occasionally in adulthood. Cardiac involvement may occur. Some patients also complain of exercise-induced muscle aches. Plasma carnitine is normal.

CK is normal or slightly elevated. EMG is myopathic. ECG may reveal biventricular hypertrophy or conduction abnormalities. Muscle biopsy shows large lipid droplets. The diagnosis is made by biochemical determination of muscle and plasma carnitine levels. Secondary causes of carnitine deficiency, such as renal failure, cirrhosis, and valproate therapy, should be excluded.

SUGGESTED READING

Dubowitz V. Metabolic and endocrine myopathies. In: Dubowitz V. ed. Muscle biopsy: A practical approach. ed 2. London: Bailliere Tindall, 1985:465.

Engel AG. Metabolic and endocrine myopathies. In: Walton J, ed. Disorders of voluntary muscle. ed 5. London: Churchill Livingstone, 1988:811.

Swash M, Schwartz MS. Metabolic myopathies. In: Swash M, Schwartz MS, ed. Neuromuscular diseases: A practical approach to diagnosis and management. ed 2. New York: Springer-Verlag, 1988:327.

Tein I, DiMauro S, De Vivo DC. Recurrent childhood myoglobinuria. Adv Pediatr 1990; 37:77–117.

Tonin P, Lewis P, Servidei S, DiMauro S. Metabolic causes of myoglobinuria. Ann Neurol 1990; 27:181–185.

MITOCHONDRIAL MYOPATHY

SALVATORE DiMAURO, M.D.

Mitochondrial myopathy is a restrictive term often used to label not only pure myopathies, but also a large and heterogeneous group of multisystem disorders due to mitochondrial dysfunction. These are more often called *mitochondrial encephalomyopathies,* also a restrictive term intended to stress the special vulnerability of brain and muscle to impairments of oxidative metabolism. In fact, all tissues with high dependence on oxidative metabolism tend to be involved clinically, and this provides useful diagnostic clues.

A further complicating and unique feature of mitochondrial diseases relates to the fact that mitochondria are the only organelles besides the nucleus that contain their own DNA (mtDNA), which encodes 13 polypeptides, all subunits of respiratory chain complexes. The dual genetic control of mitochondrial proteins, most of which are encoded by nuclear DNA (nDNA), and the need for intergenomic communication explain some of the complexity of mitochondrial genetics. Table 1 proposes a genetic classification and summarizes the general clinical and biochemical consequences of defects in nDNA, mtDNA, or in nDNA-mtDNA communication. These general principles are useful in assessing patients with suspected mitochondrial diseases, in interpreting the results of biochemical tests, and in planning molecular genetic analyses.

The extreme heterogeneity of clinical presentations makes it virtually impossible to describe unifying clinical criteria, but there are typical syndromes, and some symptoms are so common that they should raise the suspicion of mitochondrial dysfunction. I will consider myopathies and encephalomyopathies separately. Also, the emphasis of this review is on disorders of the respiratory chain, excluding defects of mitochondrial lipid metabolism, pyruvate metabolism, and the Krebs cycle.

MITOCHONDRIAL MYOPATHIES

Even in this subgroup, clinical heterogeneity is prevalent. When onset is in the neonatal period, with diffuse weakness (usually sparing extraocular and facial muscles) and respiratory insufficiency, a mitochondrial myopathy is an important diagnostic consideration, especially if the myopathy is accompanied by renal dysfunction (DeToni-Fanconi-Debre syndrome). The suspicion is confirmed if laboratory data show lactic acidosis, usually with abnormally elevated lactate/pyruvate ratio, and the muscle biopsy shows abnormal accumulation of mitochondria ("ragged-red fibers" [RRF] with the modified Gomori trichrome stain; dark-staining fibers with the succinate dehydrogenase [SDH] histochemical reaction; excessive numbers of subsarcolemmal and intermyofibrillar organelles by electron microscopy). There are at least three entities that present this way: (1) fatal infantile myopathy with cytochrome C oxidase (COX) deficiency; (2) benign infantile myopathy with reversible COX deficiency; and (3) fatal infantile myopathy with mtDNA depletion. All three diseases are transmitted by mendelian inheritance, apparently autosomal recessive, implying that the genetic defects are in nDNA. However, the two COX-

Table 1 Mitochondrial Diseases

	Site of Defect	Heredity	Clinical Features	Biochemistry
Group 1	Nuclear DNA (nDNA)			
	Tissue-specific gene	Mendelian	Tissue-specific syndrome	Tissue-specific monoenzymopathy
	Non–tissue-specific gene	Mendelian	Multisystemic disorder	Generalized monoenzymopathy
	Protein import controlling gene	Mendelian	?	?
Group 2	Mitochondrial DNA (mtDNA)			
	Point mutations	Maternal	Multisystemic, heterogeneous	Generalized monoenzymopathy (structural genes) Generalized multienzymopathy (tRNA genes)
	Deletions or duplications	Sporadic	PEO; KSS; Pearson	Generalized ($\pm$) multienzymopathy
Group 3	nDNA/mtDNA Communication			
	Multiple mtDNA deletions	Mendelian (AD)	PEO $\pm$ other features	Generalized multienzymopathy
	mtDNA depletion	Mendelian (AR)	Myopathy $\pm$ nephropathy; hepatopathy; encephalopathy	Tissue-specific multienzymopathy

Abbreviations: See footnote to Table 2.

deficient myopathies are attributed to defects in muscle-specific COX subunits (group 1 in Table 1), while the mtDNA depletion-myopathy is probably due to a defect of intergenomic communication (group 3 in Table 1). Biochemical analysis of muscle extracts shows isolated COX deficiency in both fatal and benign myopathies, but multiple respiratory chain defects in mtDNA depletion because all 13 subunits encoded by mtDNA are markedly decreased in this condition. If mtDNA depletion is suspected, confirmation may be provided by immunocytochemistry using anti-DNA antibodies (showing lack of reactivity in the cytoplasm contrasting with normal immunostain in nuclei) or by quantitative Southern blot analysis.

The differential diagnosis between fatal and benign COX-deficient myopathy is of crucial importance because the prognosis is very different. While patients with the fatal form show a relentlessly downhill course and die of respiratory failure within the first year, children with the benign myopathy, although they are critically ill in the first weeks or months of life, improve spontaneously and are usually normal by 2 or 3 years of age. The lactic acidosis also resolves in parallel with the clinical recovery. Histochemistry in repeat biopsies shows a return of COX activity in increasing number of fibers and this is confirmed by biochemistry. Immunocytochemistry using antibodies against individual COX subunits discriminates the benign from the fatal form in the first months of life, when they are clinically indistinguishable. There is lack of immunoreactivity only to COX subunit VIIa,b in the fatal myopathy, and to both subunit II and VIIa,b in the benign form.

Partial depletion of mtDNA in muscle causes a myopathy with slightly later onset and slower course than that accompanying severe mtDNA depletion. These children are normal until about 1 year of age, when

truncal and limb weakness appears, soon involving respiratory muscles and causing death at about age 3 years. Blood lactic acid may be normal, and early biopsies may show nonspecific changes, but RRF are seen in biopsies taken after severe weakness has developed.

Myopathies manifesting in older children or adults are characterized by intolerance to exercise and premature fatigue (without cramps) before permanent weakness sets in. Typically, these patients report feeling "wiped out" after walking a few blocks and need to rest frequently. Weakness is predominantly proximal and may involve respiratory muscles, but extraocular and facial muscles are usually spared. Blood lactic acid can be elevated at rest and increases excessively after even moderate aerobic exercise. Muscle biopsy shows RRF. A useful diagnostic test and a useful indicator of spontaneous progression or response to therapeutic trials is nuclear magnetic resonance spectroscopy with phosphorus-31 (^{31}P-NMRS). This provides an assessment of intracellular pH and of the ratio between phosphocreatine and inorganic phosphate (PCr/Pi). In mitochondrial myopathies, typically the PCr/Pi ratio (1) is lower than normal at rest, (2) decreases more than normal during exercise, and (3) returns to baseline more slowly than normal during recovery. Family history, when informative, suggests autosomal recessive inheritance. This clinical presentation has been described in patients with defects of complex I (NADH-coenzyme Q reductase), complex III (reduced CoQ-cytochrome C reductase), and complex IV (COX). The assumption is that the genetic defects involve nDNA-encoded, muscle-specific subunits in each of the three complexes.

A rare clinical presentation (described so far only in two patients) consists of severe nonthyroidal hypermetabolism and mild proximal weakness (Luft's disease).

The basal metabolic rate is markedly increased, but thyroid function tests are normal. Muscle biopsy shows RRF and capillary proliferation. Biochemical studies of mitochondria isolated from fresh muscle biopsies show loss of the physiologic control of respiration by phosphorylation (loose coupling).

Progressive external ophthalmoplegia (PEO) with ptosis and with or without proximal limb weakness should always raise the suspicion of a mitochondrial disease, which is confirmed by the presence of RRF in the muscle biopsy. Typically, RRF and some non-RRF are histochemically COX-negative. When present, lactic acidosis reinforces the diagnosis. If the patient is a sporadic case (that is, family history is negative), the most likely cause is a single deletion in mtDNA (group 2, Table 1). The deletion is detectable in muscle by Southern blot analysis, which shows two bands, corresponding to two populations of mtDNA (heteroplasmy). One band migrates normally and represents the normal-size (wild-type) mtDNA population. The other migrates faster and represents a population of smaller mtDNA molecules. Diagnosis requires genetic analysis of muscle because the deletion is often undetectable in blood cells, even using the extremely sensitive polymerase chain reaction. If present in tissues other than muscle, the deletion must affect a proportion of mtDNA molecules below the threshold needed to cause mitochondrial dysfunction and clinical expression. Biochemical studies in muscle extracts or isolated mitochondria may be difficult to interpret because of heteroplasmy. Activities of respiratory chain enzymes can be normal or variously decreased. The decrease usually affects those complexes that contain mtDNA-encoded subunits, such as I, III, and IV, while enzymes entirely encoded by nDNA, such as SDH or citrate synthase, have normal activities. This pattern, when observed, provides a clue that overall mitochondrial protein synthesis is impaired, a situation observed in mtDNA deletions, point mutations in tRNA genes, and in mtDNA depletion.

If family history is positive and suggests autosomal dominant transmission, the patient may have multiple mtDNA deletions. The Southern blot will show not just one, but multiple abnormal bands. This pathologic propensity of mtDNA to develop deletions is attributed to an nDNA error affecting intergenomic communications (group 3, Table 1). Although PEO and proximal weakness dominate the clinical picture, these patients may have additional symptoms, such as cataracts, hearing loss, and depression, and early death may ensue. Despite evidence of multisystem involvement, multiple deletions are not always detected in tissues other than muscle. Biochemical studies show variably severe defects of respiratory complexes containing mtDNA-encoded subunits, as described above.

If family history is positive and suggestive of maternal inheritance, the most likely underlying molecular defect is a point mutation at nucleotide (nt) 3243 (in the tRNA$^{Leu(UUR)}$ gene) of mtDNA, the same mutation that is more commonly associated with the MELAS syndrome (see below). Like patients with multiple deletions, patients with the MELAS mutation often have additional symptoms, such as hearing loss, seizures, or cerebellar signs. Biochemistry is of relatively little help in the diagnosis, as discussed.

MITOCHONDRIAL ENCEPHALOMYOPATHIES

The clinical classification of this group of disorders has raised a spirited controversy between "lumpers" and "splitters," which has centered on the three syndromes illustrated in Table 2 (KSS; MERRF; MELAS). My admittedly biased splitter's view is that this classification is useful at the bedside and has been largely verified by molecular genetic analysis. It is true, however, that some overlap exists, the most notable being PEO, which is the hallmark of mtDNA deletions but is also seen in a substantial number of patients with the MELAS mutation.

Also, many symptoms and signs are common to the three syndromes. Although nonspecific, they represent useful diagnostic clues to a mitochondrial causation. These include short stature, neurosensory hearing loss, dementia, renal tubular acidosis, and endocrine disorders such as diabetes and hypoparathyroidism.

Kearns-Sayre Syndrome

Kearns-Sayre syndrome (KSS) is defined by the invariant triad of (1) onset before age 20, (2) PEO, and (3) pigmentary retinopathy, plus at least one of the following: heart block, cerebellar syndrome, or cerebrospinal fluid (CSF) protein above 100 mg per deciliter. Prognosis is poor, even after placement of a pacemaker. The course is progressively downhill, and most patients die in the third or fourth decade. Muscle biopsy shows RRF and COX-negative fibers. As discussed above, biochemistry usually shows combined defects of respiratory chain complexes containing mtDNA-encoded subunits, but normal data do not exclude the diagnosis, which is established by Southern blot analysis showing a single mtDNA deletion. The deletion can be detected in blood in most patients, but negative results require confirmation in muscle. The disease is sporadic. Mothers of patients are normal, and the few affected women who have reproduced have had normal children.

Myoclonic Epilepsy with Ragged Red Fibers

Myoclonic epilepsy with RRF (MERRF) is characterized by (1) myoclonus or myoclonic epilepsy, (2) ataxia, and (3) myopathy with RRF. It is important to keep in mind, however, that clinical heterogeneity is typical of mtDNA mutations, and the disease may be fully expressed in only a few members of a given family, whereas other maternal relatives may show only some symptoms or may be completely asymptomatic. Eliciting the family history when maternal inheritance is suspected requires meticulous attention to apparently minor symptoms in matrilinear relatives, such as short

Table 2 Flow-chart for the Differential Diagnosis of Mitochondrial Encephalomyopathies

Clinical Findings		Family History	Laboratory Findings	Cranial MRI	Muscle Biopsy	Biochemistry	Molecular Genetics
MYOPATHY:							
Exercise intolerance			LA (exercise)		RRF	I; III; IV	
	Sporadic		LA (±)		RRF;COX – *	I + III + IV	Single mtDNA deletions
PEO	AD		LA	"Leuko-dystrophy"	RRF;COX – *	I + III + IV	Multiple mtDNA deletions
	maternal		LA		RRF;COX – *	I + III + IV	"MELAS mutation" (nt 3243)
Fatal infantile myopathy	AR		LA; L/P ↑; (Fanconi)		RRF;COX –	IV	nDNA (?)
Benign infantile myopathy	AR (?)		LA; L/P ↑		RRF;COX –	IV (reversible)	nDNA (?)
Nonthyroidal hypermetab.	Sporadic		BMR ↑		RRF	"Loose coupling"	
ENCEPHALOMYOPATHY:							
PEO Retinopathy Heart block } KSS	Sporadic		LA;CSF prot. > 100 mg/dl	"Leuko-dystrophy"	RRF;COX – *	I + III + IV	Single mtDNA deletions
Myoclonus Ataxia Seizures Dementia Short stature } MERRF	Maternal		LA		RRF;COX – *	I + III + IV	mtDNA point mutation (tRNA^{Lys}; nt8344; nt8356)
Episodic vomiting Cortical blindness Hemiparesis Hemianopia Hearing loss } MELAS	Maternal		LA	Focal lesions (post. cortex)	RRF;SSV	I + III + IV	mtDNA point mutation (tRNA$^{Leu(UUR)}$; nt3243; nt3271)
Devel. regression Dystonia	AR		LA; L/P ↑	Symmetrical lesions		IV	nDNA(?)
Nystagmus } Leigh syndrome	XR		LA; L/P normal	Symmetrical lesions		PDHC (E1α)	Various mutations at Xp22.1
Optic atrophy Abnormal breathing	Maternal		LA (±)	Symmetrical lesions		ATPsynthase (?)	mtDNA point mutation (ATPase 6; nt8993)
Visual loss	LHON	Maternal (M > F)					Various mtDNA point mutations (ND1;ND4;cyt b;COXIII)
Neuropathy Ataxia RP } NARP		Maternal				ATPsynthase (?)	mtDNA point mutation (ATPase 6; nt8993)

PEO = progressive external ophthalmoplegia; RP = retinitis pigmentosa; KSS = Kearns-Sayre syndrome; MERRF = myoclonus epilepsy and ragged-red fibers; MELAS = mitochondrial encephalomyopathy, lactic acidosis, and strokelike episodes; LHON = Leber's hereditary optic neuropathy; NARP = neuropathy, ataxia, retinitis pigmentosa; AD = autosomal dominant; AR = autosomal recessive; XR = X-linked recessive; M = male; F = female; LA = lactic acidosis; L/P = lactate-pyruvate ratio; CSF = cerebrospinal fluid; BMR = basal metabolic rate; RRF = ragged-red fibers; COX = cytochrome C oxidase (The asterisk indicates that the COX fibers are distributed in a mosaic pattern.); SSV = strongly SDH-reactive vessels; I, III, and IV refer to respiratory chain complexes; PDHC = pyruvate dehydrogenase complex; nt = nucleotide

stature, hearing loss, or migrainous headache. These may be telltale signs of mild mitochondrial dysfunction. Patients with MERRF usually have lactic acidosis, and muscle biopsy shows RRF and COX-negative fibers. Biochemical studies of muscle show combined, partial defects of respiratory chain complexes, especially COX. Most patients with MERRF harbor a point mutation at nt 8344, in the tRNA^{Lys} gene of mtDNA. Another mutation in the same gene (at nt 8356) has been found in two families. The mutation is detectable in blood cells, which facilitates diagnosis and genetic counseling.

MELAS

Mitochondrial encephalomyopathy, lactic acidosis, and strokelike episodes (MELAS) is highlighted by the strokelike episodes and, in their absence, may be difficult to recognize clinically. We define MELAS by the following criteria: (1) strokes, with computed tomography (CT) or magnetic resonance imaging (MRI) evidence of focal brain abnormalities, (2) lactic acidosis, RRF, or both, and (3) at least two of the following: focal or generalized seizures, dementia, recurrent headache, or vomiting. As implied by the acronym, most patients have lactic acidosis. Muscle biopsy shows RRF, many of which are COX-positive. A characteristic but not absolutely specific morphologic feature is the high reactivity of intramuscular vessels with the SDH stain. The majority of patients with typical MELAS have a mutation at nt 3243, in the tRNA$^{Leu(UUR)}$ gene of mtDNA. A second mutation in the same gene (at nt 3271) is found in a minority of patients. As in the case of MERRF, many maternal relatives of MELAS patients have few or no symptoms. Therefore, all mutations associated with typical MERRF and MELAS should be looked for, even in patients with nonspecific features of mitochondrial dysfunction and evidence of maternal inheritance. The mutation is usually, but not invariably, detected in blood cells.

Leigh Syndrome

Leigh syndrome (subacute necrotizing encephalomyelopathy) is a disease of infancy or childhood (rarely of adulthood) characterized by psychomotor regression, ataxia, optic atrophy, ophthalmoplegia, nystagmus, dystonia, tremor, pyramidal signs, and respiratory abnormalities. The characteristic neuropathologic lesions are symmetric areas of necrosis involving preferentially midbrain, pons, basal ganglia, thalamus, and optic nerves. These lesions can be demonstrated as characteristically distributed signal abnormalities by cranial CT or MRI scans, thus allowing premortem diagnosis. Microscopically, there is cystic cavitation, vascular proliferation, neuronal loss, and demyelination. Lactic acidosis is common, but muscle biopsy does *not* show RRF and is usually normal or nonspecifically altered. There are three major known causes of Leigh syndrome (see Table 2): (1) pyruvate dehydrogenase complex (PDHC) deficiency; (2) COX deficiency; and (3) a point mutation at nt 8993 in the ATPase 6 gene of mtDNA (the NARP mutation, see below). Clinically, the three forms are similar, but patients with PDHC deficiency or the NARP mutation tend to have earlier onset, in the first weeks or months of life, while patients with COX deficiency may be normal for the first year. Also, retinitis pigmentosa, when present, is characteristic of the NARP mutation. Inheritance is autosomal recessive or X-linked recessive in PDHC deficiency, autosomal recessive in COX deficiency, and maternal in NARP. Maternal relatives of patients with Leigh syndrome and the NARP mutation can be asymptomatic or can show a multisystem disorder characterized by neuropathy, ataxia, and retinitis pigmentosa (NARP). The earlier onset and more severe Leigh phenotype is apparently due to the very high percentage of mutant genomes in these patients. Biochemical data are diagnostic in PDHC and COX deficiency. Cultured fibroblasts can be used, but it

is important to remember that in some patients with COX deficiency, liver and fibroblasts have normal enzyme activity. COX histochemistry in muscle biopsies from patients with COX deficiency shows decreased stain in all fibers, including the intrafusal fibers of muscle spindles and the smooth muscle of intramuscular vessels.

DIAGNOSTIC GUIDELINES

Although the clinical and biochemical heterogeneity and the genetic complexity of mitochondrial diseases complicate the differential diagnosis, a tentative flowchart can be proposed to aid the clinician (Table 2). From the *clinical* point of view, exercise intolerance, severe infantile myopathy, developmental regression, loss of vision at a young age, and any of the symptoms and signs listed in Table 2, in isolation or in combinations suggesting KSS, MERRF, MELAS, or NARP, should raise the suspicion of a mitochondrial cause. A family history suggestive of maternal inheritance buttresses the diagnosis and indicates a defect in the mitochondrial genome, but family history may suggest mendelian transmission or be negative.

The most useful laboratory test is blood lactate at rest and after exercise. The lactate/pyruvate ratio is a good indicator of the site of the metabolic block. A normal ratio suggests a defect of PDHC. A high ratio points to a defect in the respiratory chain. In patients with encephalopathy, lactate and pyruvate may be more severely altered in CSF than in blood, where occasionally the levels may even be normal. Normal blood and CSF lactate concentrations make the diagnosis of mitochondrial disease less likely but do not exclude it. In patients with encephalomyopathies, cranial CT and MRI scans may show characteristic signal abnormalities: diffuse white matter lucency in KSS, focal lesions involving preferentially the posterior cortex in MELAS, focal symmetric lesions in basal ganglia, thalamus, periaqueductal gray matter, and cerebellum in Leigh syndrome, calcification of basal ganglia in KSS and MELAS. Muscle biopsy is a crucial diagnostic tool, not only in patients with myopathies but also in those with predominant brain involvement. The presence of RRF by Gomori trichrome or by the more sensitive SDH stain is strong evidence of mitochondrial disease. Electron microscopic alterations in the absence of RRF should be interpreted with caution. Lack of RRF, however, is not incompatible with mitochondrial disease. For example, no RRF are seen in Leigh syndrome or NARP.

Biochemical analysis of mitochondrial enzymes may reveal a specific and severe enzyme defect, such as PDHC or COX in Leigh syndrome. Partial combined defects of respiratory chain complexes containing mtDNA subunits suggests mtDNA deletions, mtDNA depletion, or mutations in mitochondrial tRNA genes. Normal biochemistry is not incompatible with a mitochondrial cause. It can be explained by heteroplasmy of mtDNA mutations or by a defect in a pathway not explored routinely. In multisystem disorders, biochemical analysis of cultured fibroblasts can provide the answer, but tissue-specific syndromes (myopathies, cardiopathies) may be due to tissue-specific isoforms of mitochondrial enzymes and require specific biochemical analysis of the affected tissue.

Molecular genetic analysis of mtDNA has become a diagnostic requirement for a large number of syndromes associated with mtDNA alterations, including PEO with RRF, KSS, MERRF, MELAS, NARP, Leber's hereditary optic neuropathy (LHON), fatal infantile mitochondrial myopathy with mtDNA depletion, mitochondrial myopathy and cardiopathy (MyMiCa). Ascertainment of mtDNA mutations is crucially important for genetic counseling.

RESOURCES

Biochemical analysis of muscle biopsies can be provided by Genica Pharmaceuticals Corporation, Two Biotech Park, 373 Plantation Street, Worcester, MA 01605 (1-800-394-4493).

Molecular genetic analysis of mtDNA is provided, among other laboratories, by:

H. Houston Merritt Clinical Research Center for Muscular Dystrophy and Related Diseases, 4-420 College of Physicians & Surgeons, 630 West 168th Street, New York, NY 10032 (212-305-3533), or

Emory Molecular Diagnostics Laboratory, Department of Genetics & Molecular Medicine and The Emory Clinic, Room 423, 1462 Clifton Road, Atlanta, GA 30322 (1-800-727-8309).

SUGGESTED READING

DiMauro S. Mitochondrial encephalomyopathies. In: Rosenberg RN, Prusiner SB, DiMauro S, et al, eds. The molecular and genetic basis of neurological disease. Boston: Butterworth-Heinemann, 1993:665.

Morgan-Hughes JA. Mitochondrial diseases. In: Mastaglia FL, Walton JN, eds. Skeletal muscle pathology. Edinburgh: Churchill Livingstone, 1992:367.

Symposium: Mitochondrial encephalomyopathies. Brain Pathol 1992; 2:111–162.

Wallace DC. Diseases of the mitochondrial DNA. Annu Rev Biochem 1992; 61:1175–1212.

MUSCULAR DYSTROPHY

JAMES M. GILCHRIST, M.D.

Muscular dystrophy is not a disease but rather a category of diseases united by hereditary, progressive destruction of muscle. While much work remains, the edifice of ignorance surrounding these diseases is starting to crumble under the attack of molecular biology and genetics. Nearly all of the better-defined muscular dystrophies have been assigned chromosomal locations,

Table 1 Muscular Dystrophy, Mode of Inheritance, and Chromosomal Location

Duchenne muscular dystrophy (XR)	Xp21
Becker muscular dystrophy (XR)	Xp21
Emery-Dreifuss muscular dystrophy (XR)	Xq28
Myotonic dystrophy (AD)	19q13.3
Oculopharyngeal muscular dystrophy (AD)	
Fascioscapulohumeral muscular dystrophy (AD)	4q35-qter
Limb-girdle muscular dystrophy 1 (AD)	5q
- -	- - - - -
Limb-girdle muscular dystrophy 2 (AR)	15q
Distal myopathies (AD, AR)	
Humeroperoneal muscular dystrophy (AD)	
Congenital muscular dystrophy (AR)	
Fukuyama muscular dystrophy (AR)	
Scapuloperoneal muscular atrophy (AD, XR)	
Severe childhood muscular dystrophy (AR)	

XR = x-linked recessive, AD = autosomal dominant, AR = autosomal recessive.

three have had the disease gene identified, and two have had the abnormal protein determined. Table 1 lists the muscular dystrophies: The nosology for several of the syndromes remains cloudy. The disorders to be discussed in this chapter are listed above the dotted line; those below will not be further considered.

The differential diagnosis for the muscular dystrophies includes essentially all disorders in which muscle is affected. The differential for each type of muscular dystrophy is much narrower because each has specific and characteristic features, with the exception of limb-girdle muscular dystrophy (LGMD).

DUCHENNE AND BECKER MUSCULAR DYSTROPHY

Duchenne (DMD) and Becker (BMD) muscular dystrophy are allelic disorders arising from defects in a gene on the X chromosome coding for a large structural protein called dystrophin. If a deleted or duplicated gene fragment disturbs the codon reading frame, little or no dystrophin is produced and the severe form, DMD, results. If the reading frame is preserved, dystrophin of abnormal molecular weight and quantity is produced, resulting in a milder form, BMD. Boys become symptomatic for DMD around 5 years of age, become wheelchairbound by 10 to 12 years, and die in their early 20s. BMD symptoms, while milder, are similar and reach the same milestones a decade or so later. The ability to assay for dystrophin has allowed for the diagnosis of rare dystrophinopathies with symptomatology not previously associated with BMD, including myoglobinuria, cramps, and focal myopathy. DMD-BMD affects only males, but females are carriers of the disease and uncommonly manifest a form of muscular dystrophy much milder than either DMD or BMD, beginning in the third or fourth decade.

The history and physical examination of DMD-BMD are quite distinctive, and the diagnosis can be made with confidence based on clinical characteristics and a few simple biochemical tests. Though the muscle damage is present from birth, it is uncommon for patients to present to the physician before the age of 4 or 5 years unless there is a pre-existing family history of DMD. While the toddler may be slow to reach motor milestones, growth of normal muscle tends to exceed the rate of muscle destruction and significant parental concern is not raised until socialization of the child reveals his relative disability. Boys with early DMD-BMD tend to be shy, a bit slow mentally (the IQ curve is shifted about 20 points to the left), and have a subtle but discernible pelvic waddle to their gait. Calves are almost always quite prominent, and hypertrophy can be seen less commonly in other muscles. A Gower sign upon attempting to rise from the floor is a helpful clue to the presence of proximal weakness. On direct muscle strength testing, patients have proximal weakness greater in legs than arms. As the disease progresses, weakness involves virtually all skeletal muscles, though calf size usually remains large from fat and fibrous replacement, leading to pseudohypertrophy. The gait deteriorates, with afflicted boys developing a more pronounced waddle and lordosis as compensation for toe-walking from Achilles tendon contracture. As the boy's strength and balance deteriorate, he becomes less ambulatory and eventually loses the ability to stand alone. Once wheelchairbound, contractures of shoulder, arm, hip, and knee develop, and scoliosis becomes prominent.

From birth the creatine kinase (CK) level is significantly increased, often being greater than 10,000 IU. Myoglobinuria is rare. Other muscle enzymes are also greatly increased in the serum, including glutamic oxaloacetic transaminase (SGOT) and aldolase. The presence of a typical clinical picture and a high CK value is very suspicious for DMD-BMD. The confirmatory test is to measure dystrophin in the muscle, though it could be argued that assay for gene deletion or duplication using lymphocyte DNA is a less invasive and simpler initial step. As mentioned above, dystrophin is absent in DMD, and abnormal in size and amount in BMD. This requires a piece of skeletal muscle but is pathognomonic for the disease. Deletion or duplication of the dystrophin gene is found in 70 percent of cases of DMD-BMD. Lack of either gene defect does not exclude DMD-BMD, but the presence of either confirms DMD-BMD. Unfortunately, deletion-duplication analysis does not tell which muscular dystrophy the patient has, and since the prognosis differs greatly, the more invasive route of muscle biopsy remains the favored confirmatory test. If available, needle biopsy of muscle is sufficient for dystrophin analysis, but it does not present much opportunity for morphologic study.

In the past, electromyography (EMG) and histochemical examination of muscle were cornerstones of DMD-BMD diagnosis, but neither are necessary today. Given the age of the patients, I would not recommend EMG unless another diagnosis is considered. Histochemical and morphologic changes of muscle are usually characteristic, and while not necessary to the diagnostic evaluation if dystrophin is analyzed, they do offer a window through which to observe the pathophysiology of the disease. The classic histologic changes include degeneration and loss of muscle fibers, fiber size variation, abnormal enlargement or atrophy of fibers, endomysial fibrosis, and adipose and connective tissue replacement. Posterobasal fibrosis of the heart is very common in DMD, less so in BMD, and the most common electrocardiogram changes are tall R waves in V_1 with an increased R:S ratio, shortened P-R interval, and deep Q waves in V_{5-6}.

EMERY-DREIFUSS MUSCULAR DYSTROPHY

Emery-Dreifuss muscular dystrophy (EDMD) is also X-linked, thus affecting males only, but otherwise is a completely different disorder from DMD-BMD. The constellation of signs is so unique as to be diagnostic when found, especially if the family history is positive. EDMD is characterized by onset in childhood of a slowly progressive proximal myopathy affecting most severely the humeral (biceps, triceps) muscles. Tendon contractures are an early feature, affecting joints not usually so afflicted, such as the neck, elbows, shoulders, hips, knees, ankles, and spine. The heart is also affected with the typical but otherwise rare cardiac syndrome of atrial standstill, which can result in sudden death. Calf hypertrophy is not present.

There is no confirmatory test. The standard muscle evaluation of CK, EMG, and muscle biopsy serves to further strengthen the clinical suspicion and exclude other diseases. CK levels range from mild elevation to 10 times normal. The EMG shows a typical myopathic pattern, most prominent in affected but not severely atrophic muscles, of small, brief, polyphasic motor unit potentials, along with fibrillations and positive waves indicative of myodegeneration. Muscle biopsy is also not specific but is indicative of myopathic disease, showing increased fiber size variability with atrophic and hypertrophic fibers, myonecrosis, internal nuclei, split fibers, and increased endomysial connective and adipose tissue. The ECG typically shows a slow junctional rhythm, though other abnormalities may be seen, including partial or complete atrioventricular conduction block and atrial fibrillation.

DNA markers have localized the disease to the Xq28 region of the X chromosome, and linkage analysis can be performed to determine either prenatal or presymptomatic genetic status. This requires living affected family members and is not useful in the diagnosis of the symptomatic patient.

MYOTONIC DYSTROPHY

Myotonic dystrophy, also known as dystrophica myotonica, myotonica atrophica, and Steinert's disease, is a multisystem disorder causing grip, percussion, and electrical myotonia, limb, facial, and pharyngeal skeletal muscle weakness, esophageal, gut, and uterine smooth muscle weakness, cardiac conduction abnormalities, endocrine dysfunction, frontal balding, cataracts, hearing loss, and mental retardation. Myotonic dystrophy is inherited as an autosomal dominant trait and, though 100 percent penetrant, shows marked variation in expression and age of onset, from intrauterine to middle age, most commonly becoming symptomatic in the second to fourth decades.

In the past, diagnosis depended upon a positive family history, the presence of clinical or electrical myotonia, and any of the other features listed above. It is not a difficult diagnosis to make if kept in mind. Where a diagnostic evaluation is most difficult is in the asymptomatic member of a family with myotonic dystrophy who is seeking genetic counseling. If that patient displays weakness or clinical myotonia, the diagnosis is likely and can be confirmed by finding electrical myotonia on EMG. If the clinical examination is normal, then I proceed to EMG and ophthalmologic evaluation. Electrical myotonia on EMG makes the diagnosis highly probable. If myotonia is not found but the patient has the typical lens changes, the diagnosis is likely. Early lens findings are specific and include multicolored, iridescent dustlike opacities distributed in the subcapsular layers of the lens. In the past, the diagnostic trail ended there. But recently investigators discovered that the disease was associated with triplet nucleotide repeats inserted into the affected gene on chromosome 19. Fewer than 40 repeats is normal; more than 100 repeats is diagnostic of myotonic dystrophy. This test uses lymphocyte DNA and requires only a small amount of blood. The ECG may be normal but more often reveals first-degree atrioventricular (A-V) block and left axis deviation. Bundle branch block, bradycardia, and higher degrees of A-V block indicate more severe cardiac involvement and necessitate a more thorough cardiac evaluation.

OCULOPHARYNGEAL MUSCULAR DYSTROPHY

Oculopharyngeal muscular dystrophy (OPMD) is an autosomal, dominantly inherited trait, which does not manifest until the fourth or fifth decade of life. It is among the milder forms of muscular dystrophy and frequently remains undiagnosed. As its name implies, the major effects are upon the ocular muscles, especially lid elevation, and the pharyngeal muscles. Patients often first appear because of dysphagia, though ptosis usually precedes pharyngeal involvement. Dysarthric speech may also be apparent or develop subsequently. Extraocular muscle involvement is usually mild and not a source of patient complaint. Patients often have a classic "nose in the air" appearance as they attempt to see out from under the ptotic lids. Facial and limb weakness is less common and infrequently disabling, though seen often enough in Muscular Dystrophy Association (MDA) clinics where these patients are likely to seek medical attention. A family history of problems swallowing and of droopy lids is frequently elicitable and brings the diagnosis to the fore.

OPMD patients have a wider differential than the previously discussed muscular dystrophies, including myotonic dystrophy, myasthenia gravis, and mitochondrial myopathy. There is no specific genetic test for OPMD, and the diagnosis is dependent upon the EMG and muscle biopsy. The CK level is normal or mildly elevated, and the ECG should be unremarkable.

The EMG is again consistent with a myopathy, showing small, brief, polyphasic motor unit potentials, but it is just as important in what it does not show. Myotonia is absent, making myotonic dystrophy unlikely. Single fiber EMG or repetitive stimulation should be part of the EMG examination and, if normal, excludes myasthenia gravis. OPMD patients may have mildly abnormal single fiber EMG, so an abnormal result is not helpful. A normal Tensilon test or acetylcholine receptor antibody may also be helpful in excluding myasthenia gravis, especially if the family history is obscure. The muscle biopsy is important for three features, two present and one absent. Cytoplasmic and nuclear inclusions, and rimmed vacuoles are present in most if not all patients with OPMD. These inclusions are 7 to 10 nm in diameter, smaller than the 12 to 18 nm inclusions seen in inclusion body myositis (IBM), and may be pathognomonic for OPMD. Rimmed vacuoles are seen in the majority of patients with OPMD but are also seen in other disorders, including IBM. The missing feature is ragged red fibers, indicative of mitochondrial myopathy.

FASCIOSCAPULOHUMERAL MUSCULAR DYSTROPHY

Fascioscapulohumeral muscular dystrophy (FSH) is another autosomal, dominantly inherited trait with a variable penetrance. Many affected patients have mild facial weakness, which patients either never notice or do not feel is serious enough to merit medical attention. Patients who do seek care are often more symptomatic, with shoulder, arm, and leg weakness. Because they often have no overt family history, the diagnosis may be missed. A careful family history, including examination of parents if possible, is very important to establishing this diagnosis.

The physical examination is the most specific part of the evaluation for FSH. CK measurement, EMG, and muscle biopsy are all abnormal but in a nonspecific way, consistent with any myopathic process. Facial weakness is a constant, even in the mildest affected carriers of the disease gene. Ptosis and extraocular weakness are not present, and dysarthria and dysphagia are uncommon unless the patient is severely affected. The primary limb muscles affected are the shoulder and upper arm muscles, resulting in scapular winging, pseudowebbing of the neck, horizontal clavicles (versus the normal downward angle from acromion to sternum), and reversal of the axillary fold. The shoulders slope dramatically from the neck and curve inward toward the midline, giving a caved-in appearance to the chest. There is atrophy of muscles overlying the scapula and the humerus. Distal strength is normal. The legs can also be affected, with pelvifemoral muscles weak more so than the lower leg. Calf hypertrophy is not seen. Cardiac disease is not a component of FSH dystrophy, and the ECG should be unremarkable.

LIMB-GIRDLE MUSCULAR DYSTROPHY

LGMD has been a much maligned entity of late because its diagnostic features are nonspecific and it is largely a diagnosis of exclusion. As such, the diagnosis has been likened to that of a trash receptacle, though I prefer recycling container, because several other diagnostic entities have been culled from LGMD, including BMD, EDMD, spinal muscular atrophy, and mitochondrial myopathy. Of late, support for LGMD as a real nosologic entity has emerged from molecular genetics. Both autosomal dominant (LGMD1) and autosomal recessive (LGMD2) forms of LGMD have been linked to chromosomal DNA markers, though the syndrome clearly remains heterogeneous. LGMD1 and LGMD2 differ only in inheritance pattern.

Unlike the already discussed muscular dystrophies, in which specific clinical, pathologic, electrophysiologic, or biochemical clues abound, LGMD is bereft of such assistance. Diagnosis depends upon ruling out related and similar-appearing disorders. The differential diagnosis includes other muscular dystrophies, spinal muscular atrophy, mitochondrial myopathy, connective tissue disorders, vasculitis, amyloidosis, sarcoidosis, polymyositis-dermatomyositis, inclusion body myositis, congenital myopathies, endocrine myopathies such as hypo- and hyperthyroidism, hypo- and hyperadrenalism, hypermagnesemia, and hypokalemia, metabolic myopathies including McArdle's disease, acid maltase deficiency, carnitine deficiency, periodic paralysis, myasthenic syndromes, toxic myopathy, and infectious myopathy, to name a few.

The age of onset of LGMD can be from late childhood to middle age, though most commonly symptoms begin in the late teens to mid-30s. The progression is slow, with an extended life expectancy. The disease most often manifests initially as proximal leg weakness, with patients complaining of problems running, climbing stairs, or walking up hills. The upper arms usually do not weaken for several years, or until the legs are more severely affected. Eventually, distal muscles of legs and arms may become weak but only over the course of many years. From onset of symptoms to wheelchair, which is not an immutable sequence, takes approximately 20 years. A rather discrete form appears in people in their 50s and 60s with a more rapid progression to wheelchair within 5 to 10 years. I have found absent ankle reflexes and Achilles tendon contractures an early feature in the majority of patients classified as LGMD, which is again not specific but uncommonly found in adult onset spinal muscular atrophy. Facial weakness, skin rash, myotonia, and cardiomyopathy are not found as part of LGMD. Calf hypertrophy and scapular winging are occasionally seen. The patient should be queried about other medical problems, alcohol intake, medications, HIV risk factors, and family history.

The CK is often elevated though not to the levels found in DMD-BMD, usually in the realm of two to five times normal. Other biochemical tests should be unremarkable, including thyroid function, serum electrolytes, and connective tissue disease screens. If the history is suggestive of a glycogen storage disorder (e.g., exercise intolerance, contractures, or prominent cramping), then an ischemic exercise test assessing venous lactate and ammonia should be considered. The EMG in LGMD is consistent with a myopathic process; that is, small, brief, polyphasic motor unit potentials and occasional fibrillations and positive waves. Myotonia is absent. The ECG should be normal unless concurrent disease exists. The muscle biopsy is indicative of a dystrophic process, with variable fiber size, central nuclei, fiber splitting, muscle fiber degeneration and atrophy, and endomysial tissue replacement with fibrosis and adiposity. The biopsy is more helpful for what it does not show and the diseases it thus excludes: fiber type grouping or type atrophy (SMA), ragged red fibers (mitochondrial myopathy), inclusions (IBM, OPMD, toxic and infectious myopathies), vacuoles (IBM, toxic myopathy, and periodic paralysis), inflammatory infiltrates (polymyositis, dermatomyositis, IBM, and infectious myopathy), glycogen (McArdle's, acid maltase), or lipid (carnitine deficiency) accumulation, amyloid or vasculitis. In addition, assay for dystrophin should be performed and will be normal in LGMD.

APPROACH TO DIAGNOSIS

An algorithm for the diagnosis of muscular dystrophy is shown in Figure 1. As with all of medicine, the diagnosis of muscular dystrophy must start with a thorough history and physical examination. Age of symptom onset, family history, concurrent medical problems, alcohol intake, medications, and the symptoms themselves will help sort out whether a muscular dystrophy is likely and, if so, which one. The physical examination should be designed to assess distribution of weakness and to look for the peculiarities of each of the muscular dystrophies: for example, calf hypertrophy, tendon contractures, focal or regional limb or facial weakness and atrophy, myotonia, and cardiac or ocular

Progressive Weakness

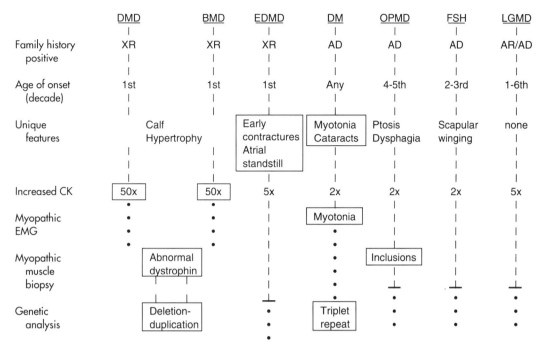

Figure 1 Algorithm for diagnosis of muscular dystrophy. Boxes indicate that finding can be diagnostic; dots indicate that step can usually be skipped. (DMD = Duchenne muscular dystrophy, BMD = Becker muscular dystrophy, EDMD = Emery-Dreifuss muscular dystrophy, DM = dystrophica myotonia, OPMD = oculopharyngeal muscular dystrophy, FSH = fascioscapulohumeral muscular dystrophy, LGMD = limb-girdle muscular dystrophy, XR = X-linked recessive, AD = autosomal dominant, AR = autosomal recessive, CK = creatine kinase, EMG = electromyogram)

involvement. Blood tests must include a CK measurement and should include tests to rule out other diseases with known propensity for muscle involvement, as mentioned above. An EMG should be performed after the blood work if the CK does not indicate DMD-BMD. Muscle biopsy, including dystrophin analysis, is the next step and should be done if the diagnosis remains uncertain. In the case of myotonic dystrophy, the muscle biopsy is usually not necessary, but blood for triplet repeat analysis may well be. An ECG should be obtained on all patients suspected of DMD, BMD, myotonic dystrophy, and EDMD. To the trained eye, many of the muscular dystrophies can be diagnosed by careful observation, sometimes while the patient sits in the waiting room.

SUGGESTED READING

Brooke MH. A clinician's guide to neuromuscular disease. 2nd ed. Baltimore: Williams & Wilkins, 1986.

Emery AEH. Duchenne muscular dystrophy. Oxford: Oxford University Press, 1987:25–91.

Engel AG, Banker BQ. Myology. Chapters 37–40, 43. New York: McGraw-Hill, 1986:1185–1296, 1327–1348.

Harper PS. The muscular dystrophies. In: Scriver CR, Beudet AL, Sly WS, Valle D, eds. The metabolic basis of inherited disease. 6th ed. New York: McGraw-Hill, 1989:2869.

Harper PS. Myotonic dystrophy. 2nd ed. Philadelphia: WB Saunders, 1989:13–78.

MYASTHENIA GRAVIS

JAMES M. GILCHRIST, M.D.

Myasthenia gravis is an autoimmune disorder in which polyclonal antibodies are directed against the postsynaptic acetylcholine receptor of the neuromuscular junction. The disease is characterized by fatigable weakness involving ocular, facial, pharyngeal, respiratory, and limb skeletal muscles. Pain and sensory disturbance are not part of the symptom complex. There is a bimodal incidence, affecting older males and younger females.

HISTORY AND EXAMINATION

The clinical history and examination of the patient with myasthenia gravis is often typical and highly suggestive if solicited by a prepared and suspicious physician. Confirmation of the clinical diagnosis rests on pharmacologic, electrodiagnostic, and immunologic grounds. A history of fluctuating symptoms, particularly following exercise of the weak muscle, is quite compelling, especially when paired with a typical distribution of weakness. Nearly 85 percent of patients with myasthenia gravis present with involvement of ocular muscles, half having signs and symptoms limited to those muscles. Indeed, in 15 percent of patients, the disease never spreads beyond the ocular area. Diplopia is the most common symptom in ocular myasthenia gravis, resulting from paresis of one or several extraocular muscles. Double vision can fluctuate dramatically over days or weeks, and even from minute to minute, in severity and direction. Diplopia is worsened by use of the affected muscles, and sustained horizontal and vertical gaze for 30 to 45 seconds is often sufficient to elicit worsening of symptoms. Red lens testing should be performed in all patients with suspected myasthenia gravis, even those without complaints of double vision, to delineate the affected extraocular muscles. It is not unusual to discover asymptomatic ocular involvement, which may serve to bring an otherwise blurry clinical picture into focus.

Ptosis is the other classic sign of ocular myasthenia gravis, which the patient may not complain about unless vision is obscured. On the other hand, severe ptosis may obscure diplopia by occluding one eye. Fluctuation is again common and may involve rapid shifts between normal and abnormal and from eye to eye. This latter sign is felt by some to be pathognomonic. Ptosis often worsens as the day progresses but can be present upon awakening. Sustained upgaze for 2 minutes is an easy maneuver for demonstrating the fatigable nature of the ptosis, and the length of time before ptosis develops or worsens can be used as a quantitative measure of disease activity and therapeutic response. Weakness of eye closure is another frequent finding.

The bulbar and facial muscles are also commonly involved, with complaints of dysphagia, dysphonia, and dysarthria frequently elicited. Asking patients to count backward from 100 is a simple provocative test that lends itself well to tape recording for later comparisons. These symptoms also fluctuate over time and in relation to chewing, swallowing, and talking. Weakness of the neck, especially in flexion, and of limb muscles, again with a varying course exacerbated by use, is typical of generalized myasthenia gravis. Limb weakness is most evident in proximal muscles and can be asymmetric.

DIAGNOSTIC TESTS

Tensilon Test

Acetylcholine is the neurotransmitter of the neuromuscular junction. It is metabolized by acetylcholinesterase, an enzyme blocked by a category of drugs called anticholinesterases, which thus prolongs the time each acetylcholine molecule ligates with the acetylcholine receptor, increasing the number of contracting muscle fibers and hence, strength. Edrophonium (Tensilon) is a short-acting anticholinesterase used as a diagnostic test for myasthenia gravis. Occasionally, neostigmine is used in the same role when its longer duration of action (approximately 1 hour) is needed, such as in infants. Given intravenously, Tensilon can quickly but briefly reverse the signs of myasthenia gravis. The emphasis is on signs, not symptoms. The Tensilon test is very useful and specific when performed correctly but is fraught with false-positives when patient symptoms of fatigue or weakness are used as markers of improvement, rather than actual testing of strength. Before administering Tensilon, one or several easily examined weak muscles should be chosen as benchmarks of response and then tested after each increment of Tensilon is given. If, in the judgment of the physician, some or all of those muscles definitely get significantly stronger, the test is positive. Otherwise, it is negative. Any test that is not obviously positive should be declared negative.

Performance of the test is simple, but some precautions are in order. In elderly patients especially, monitoring of the heart rate is important, and parenteral atropine should be readily available. I do not utilize the Emergency Department or an electrocardiograph when I do Tensilon tests, though some physicians do. The examination space should include a place for the patient to lie down should they exhibit some of the muscarinic side effects of Tensilon, which include the symptomatology of vasovagal syncope. Many physicians prefer to pair the giving of Tensilon with a placebo, but I find this unnecessary if one objectively tests weakness by direct examination of the muscle. Tensilon comes as a 10 mg per milliliter solution. I use 10 mg and prefer to use a 1 ml tuberculin syringe. After inserting a butterfly intracath into a forearm vein and flushing with saline, I inject 1 mg of Tensilon and flush again with saline. Physical improvement should be evident within 1 to 2 minutes. If there is no improvement in strength, I then inject 3 mg of Tensilon and flush. If no improvement is found upon examination after 3 to 5 minutes, I inject the final 6 mg. If there is no improvement, it is a negative Tensilon test. Obviously, if strength improves significantly with 1 or 3 mg doses, the test is declared positive and further doses are not given. I find this method lessens the number of patients with undesirable muscarinic side effects. In addition, it is possible to overshoot the benefit of Tensilon since giving 10 mg all at once may cause worsening of weakness from cholinergic overdose. A Tensilon test performed in this fashion should be a highly useful indicator of myasthenia gravis, while a negative test argues against, but does not exclude, myasthenia gravis. False-positives do occur, even in the most proficient hands: for example, in patients with amyotrophic lateral sclerosis (ALS), cranial neuritis, diabetic palsies and sphenoid ridge, parasellar or cavernous sinus masses.

Antibody Assays

Fortunately, the diagnosis of myasthenia gravis does not rest exclusively upon the Tensilon test. Antiacetylcholine receptor antibodies (antiAchR) can and should be assayed in any patient suspected of having myasthenia gravis. Several antibody assays exist, but the most commonly available assay measures what is often referred to as a binding antibody. Depending upon the source, between 70 and 90 percent of patients with generalized myasthenia gravis will have positive titers, though the rate is only 50 to 60 percent in ocular myasthenia gravis. It has been hypothesized that normal titers detected in early myasthenia gravis (up to 1 year) may occur because all the antiAchR are bound. Thus, a normal test should be repeated at a later date if the diagnosis remains in question. On occasion I have sent serum to a research laboratory for those patients with a negative binding antibody assay but an otherwise typical picture of myasthenia gravis, to look for blocking and modulating antiAchR.

AntiAchR are specific for myasthenia gravis, and a positive assay indicates the disease is present. However, the level of antibody is not indicative of disease severity and is of limited use as a serial indicator of progression or response. In the pregnant woman, high levels of antiAchR put the fetus at higher risk for antenatal or neonatal myasthenia gravis and necessitate closer monitoring.

Electrophysiologic Tests

There are several electrophysiologic measures of the abnormal neuromuscular transmission seen in myasthenia gravis. The two of greatest clinical value are repetitive nerve stimulation and single fiber electromyography (SFEMG). The easiest to perform and most readily available is repetitive stimulation. At low frequencies (2 to 5 Hz), a decrementing response will be seen in patients with myasthenia gravis. The test can be performed on muscles of the hand, arm, face, and leg and is most likely to be abnormal in proximal or facial muscles, though it is technically easiest and least painful to perform in hand muscles. If SFEMG is not available, I would recommend repetitive stimulation of a nerve to a hand muscle and, if normal, proceeding to repetitive nerve stimulation to a proximal and a facial muscle. This method is said to have a 75 percent yield, though my experience is closer to 50 percent. Again, the test is not specific for myasthenia gravis; it can be abnormal in other disorders of neuromuscular transmission such as Lambert-Eaton myasthenic syndrome (LEMS) and botulism, as well as ALS, neuropathy, radiculopathy, and myopathy.

SFEMG is the most sensitive test available for diagnosing abnormal neuromuscular transmission and is abnormal in 99 percent of cases of myasthenia gravis. It, too, is not specific, being abnormal in any neuropathic or myopathic disorder disturbing neuromuscular transmission. Abnormal results should be correlated with the clinical picture and a routine EMG study. SFEMG requires more specialized equipment and expertise and is not as generally available as repetitive stimulation, but in the difficult case resistant to other diagnostic attempts, it is irreplaceable.

In my practice, I obtain SFEMG on every patient suspected of having myasthenia gravis, even when other modalities are abnormal. SFEMG quantitatively measures neuromuscular transmission at individual motor endplates by measuring jitter. Jitter is the variability in time between consecutive discharges of a muscle fiber and is a normal part of synaptic transmission. Jitter increases as neuromuscular transmission falters, and impulse block occurs when neuromuscular transmission fails. The amount of jitter and impulse blocking correlates well with clinical severity of myasthenia gravis and is an excellent objective measure of disease progression. I find SFEMG quite useful in differentiating those patients with progression of disease from those with complaints referrable to other causes. Anticholinesterase drugs for the most part do not affect the diagnostic sensitivity of SFEMG for myasthenia gravis, but I recommend that patients stop them the day before the study.

DIFFERENTIAL DIAGNOSIS

Occasionally, even a seemingly typical clinical and laboratory pattern of myasthenia gravis can result in an incorrect diagnosis. Certain intracranial masses can mimic ocular myasthenia gravis, even causing abnormal Tensilon and electrophysiologic tests. Therefore, I find it prudent to obtain a magnetic resonance imaging of the head to rule out masses in and about the superior orbital fissure and sellar region in those patients with strictly ocular involvement, with or without a positive Tensilon test, and normal antibody assay and SFEMG. Other disorders that must be differentiated from myasthenia gravis include LEMS, oculopharyngeal muscular dystro-

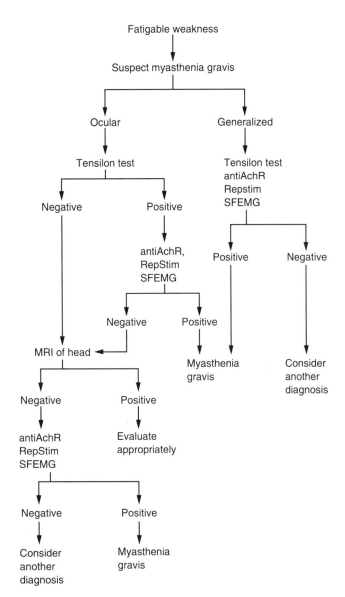

Figure 1 A general flow chart for evaluating the patient presenting with complaints suggestive of myasthenia gravis. (AntiAchR = antiacetylcholine receptor antibody test, Rep-Stim = repetitive nerve stimulation, SFEMG = single fiber electromyography, MRI = magnetic resonance imaging.)

phy, myotonic dystrophy, and mitochondrial myopathy (e.g., chronic progressive external ophthalmoplegia).

A diagnosis of myasthenia gravis may be the clue to diagnosis of other maladies as well. Thyroid disease is frequently encountered in the newly diagnosed myasthenic, both because dysthyroidism worsens symptoms of myasthenia gravis and because autoimmune diseases occur with increased frequency in myasthenia gravis, itself an autoimmune disease. Thyroid function tests, antinuclear antibody, and rheumatoid factor should be obtained as a minimum screen, and expanded depending on clinical presentation. Thymoma occurs in 15 percent of patients with myasthenia gravis and should be looked for in all newly diagnosed patients. A chest film will delineate any large mediastinal mass but is inadequate to exclude the presence of thymoma. Computed tomography (CT) of the chest should be performed in all cases where thymectomy will not be performed otherwise. Even in patients who will have surgery, most chest surgeons will want a CT scan before thymectomy. Intravenous contrast increases the yield of chest CT to identify thymoma, but the dye can exacerbate myasthenia gravis and its routine use should be avoided. Only 30 percent of patients with myasthenia gravis alone have an elevated titer of antistriated muscle antibodies, compared with 85 percent of patients with both myasthenia gravis and thymoma. I usually obtain this test as well and pay particular attention to the mediastinal imaging of those patients with an elevated titer. My general approach to those patients is outlined in Figure 1.

SUGGESTED READING

Daroff RB. The office Tensilon test for ocular myasthenia gravis. Arch Neurol 1986; 43:843–844.

Drachman DB, ed. Myasthenia gravis: Biology and treatment. Ann N Y Acad Sci 1987; 505:472–565.

Engel AG. Acquired autoimmune myasthenia gravis. In: Engel AG, Banker BQ, eds. Myology. New York: McGraw-Hill, 1986:1925.

Moorthy G, Behrens MM, Drachman DB, et al. Ocular pseudomyasthenia or ocular myasthenia 'plus': A warning to clinicians. Neurology 1989; 39:1150–1154.

PERIODIC PARALYSES AND RELATED MYOTONIC DISEASES

LAWRENCE J. HAYWARD, M.D., Ph.D.
ROBERT H. BROWN Jr., D.Phil., M.D.

Recent studies have implicated defective skeletal muscle voltage-sensitive ion channels in the pathogenesis of the periodic paralyses, myotonia congenita, and related diseases. This review summarizes these findings and provides a clinical approach to the diagnosis of myotonic disorders. The primary focus of this review is to discuss current findings related to the periodic paralyses, though brief remarks are included to contrast the clinical and genetic aspects of periodic paralysis with those of myotonia congenita and myotonic dystrophy.

THE PERIODIC PARALYSES AND PARAMYOTONIA CONGENITA

Clinical Features

The major symptom in the periodic paralyses is recurrent weakness that may be severe and that occurs without changes in consciousness, sensation, or heart function (Table 1). The disease was first reported over a century ago. By the 1930s, many individuals with this disease were shown to have low serum potassium levels during paralytic attacks and responded favorably to oral potassium. Other families were subsequently described in which the paralytic episodes developed concurrently either with hyperkalemia or normal serum potassium levels.

Hypokalemic and hyperkalemic periodic paralysis share several clinical features. In both diseases, attacks are brief, lasting from minutes to hours, may be frequent, and can be triggered by resting after a period of exertion. In both disorders, electromyography (EMG) during weakness reveals that affected muscles are depolarized and electrically silent. For both conditions, the carbonic anhydrase inhibitor acetazolamide or its derivatives are effective prophylactic treatments.

Hyperkalemic and hypokalemic periodic paralysis differ in several respects. Hyperkalemic paralysis begins in early childhood, while the hypokalemic form does not develop until puberty. In hyperkalemic paralysis, attacks are initiated by fasting and may be terminated by carbohydrate intake. Conversely, in hypokalemic paralysis, excessive carbohydrates may precipitate attacks.

Most patients with hyperkalemic paralysis develop

LJH is supported by the Muscular Dystrophy Association and by NIH Training Grant 5T32-NS07340-04. RHB receives generous support from the CB Day Investment Company, the Muscular Dystrophy Association, and NIH grant 5R01-AR41025-02.

myotonia, a form of muscle stiffness due to persistent electrical excitation of the muscle membrane. This is almost never present in hypokalemic paralysis. In most myotonic patients, this stiffness is worse in the cold. In the related disorders, myotonia congenita and paramyotonia congenita, myotonia is *the* major clinical symptom. In paramyotonia congenita, cooling may cause frank muscle paralysis. However, serum potassium levels are normal during such episodes. In most forms of myotonia, repetitive contractions reduce muscle stiffness, while in paramyotonia, repeated contractions paradoxically accentuate the stiffness, hence the name *para*myotonia.

Both hyperkalemic and hypokalemic paralysis are inherited as autosomal dominant traits. In hypokalemic but not hyperkalemic paralysis, penetrance is greater in males. Paramyotonia congenita is usually dominant, whereas myotonia congenita may be either dominant (Thomsen's disease) or recessive (Becker's type).

The periodic paralyses, myotonia congenita, and paramyotonia congenita are not characterized by muscle degeneration and are therefore said to be "nondystrophic." However, in either type of periodic paralysis, patients with frequent paralytic episodes develop irreversible proximal muscle weakness over time. These nondystrophic myotonias differ from myotonic dystrophy (Steinert's disease), which is characterized by myotonia and rather uniform, disabling, distal muscle deterioration.

Microscopic studies of affected muscle may be normal. After frequent attacks of periodic paralysis, microscopy may reveal vacuolated fibers with tubular aggregates. This degenerative pathology most likely contributes to irreversible proximal limb weakness in some individuals.

MOLECULAR BASIS OF PERIODIC PARALYSIS

As summarized in Figure 1, a growing family of sodium channel mutations underlie hyperkalemic periodic paralysis, paramyotonia congenita, and some variants of myotonia congenita. These mutations may be loosely grouped based on phenotype and location within the channel. The mutations causing well-defined hyperkalemic periodic paralysis (two human, one equine) are located toward the cytoplasmic ends of the membrane-spanning regions in domains II and IV. By contrast, five mutations correlated with a paramyotonia congenita phenotype are located either within the III-IV cytoplasmic loop or toward the extracellular ends of S3 and S4 alpha helices in channel domain IV. One mutation causes a mixed hyperkalemic paralysis-paramyotonia phenotype, varying between affected individuals within a family. This is located toward the inner or cytoplasmic membrane surface. Another mutation produces marked, chronic muscle stiffness suggestive of myotonia congenita in some but not all family members. This is located in a cytoplasmic loop associated with transmembrane segment S6 in domain II.

Table 1 Clinical and Genetic Features of the Periodic Paralyses and Related Myotonic Disorders

| | Periodic Paralyses | | | | | |
| | Hypokalemic | Myotonias | | | | |
		Hyperkalemic (Gamstorp, 1956)	Paramyotonia Congenita (Eulenburg, 1886)	Myotonia Congenita (Thomsen, 1876)	Generalized Myotonia (Becker, 1971)	Myotonic Dystrophy (Steinert, 1909)
Clinical Features						
Episodic weakness	Yes	Yes	Rarely	No	No	No
Progressive weakness,	+	+	+	+/−	+/−	+ + +
muscles affected	Proximal	Proximal	Proximal	Proximal	Proximal	Distal
Onset age	Puberty	Early childhood	Infancy	Childhood	Late childhood	Early adult‡
Attack duration	Hours to days	Minutes to days	Minutes to days			
Interictal interval	Hours to days	Minutes to days	Minutes to days			
Triggers weakness	Cold, rest after exercise, carbohydrates	Cold, rest after exercise, fasting, potassium	Cold, rest after exercise, fasting			
Ameliorates weakness	Potassium, sustained exercise, acetazolamide	Carbohydrates, sustained exercise, acetazolamide	Carbohydrates, sustained exercise, acetazolamide			
Myotonic stiffness	−	+ +	+ + +	+ + +	+ + +	+ +
Ameliorates myotonia		Mexiletine	Mexiletine	*	*	*
Systemic involvment	−	−	−	−	−	+ + +§
Genetic Features						
Inheritance pattern	AD	AD	AD	AD	AR	AD
Chromosomal location	?	17q	17q	7q	7q	19q
Defective gene	?	Na^+ channel	Na^+ channel	Cl^- channel†	Cl^- channel	Myotonin

+/−, rarely, + = occasionally, + + = frequently, + + + = invariably present, AD = autosomal dominant, AR = autosomal recessive
*Quinine or phenytoin may be beneficial in some patients.
†A Na^+ channel mutation has been described for some individuals with a similar phenotype.
‡Most commonly, though infants of affected mothers may be floppy.
§Includes cardiac dysrhythmias, subcapsular cataracts, frontal balding, testicular atrophy, and mental deficiency.

DIAGNOSTIC APPROACHES

Periodic Paralyses

The primary approach to diagnosis of the periodic paralyses is careful clinical evaluation, bearing in mind the features as listed in Table 1. In hypokalemic periodic paralysis, it is important to document a low serum potassium level during paralytic attacks. In cases where there is clinical uncertainty, provocative tests may be helpful. These may be performed by administering oral glucose (5 g per kilogram, to a total of 100 g, or intravenous glucose up to 3 g per kilogram over 1 hour if oral glucose does not provoke an attack). If necessary, insulin may be given intravenously up to 0.1 units per kilogram at 30 and 60 minutes into the glucose infusion. Patients should be monitored by an electrocardiogram and observed for at least 12 hours. The serum potassium should be measured every 15 to 30 minutes for 3 hours. Muscle biopsy of these patients usually shows myopathic changes and vacuolated fibers, though the appearance may be normal.

In hyperkalemic periodic paralysis, the clinical features are again primary. The potassium level is usually elevated during an attack, although it can be normal in some patients. Clinical and EMG evidence of myotonia is usually present. This disorder may be diagnosed by amplifying DNA obtained from a blood sample using polymerase chain reaction (PCR)–based techniques to document the presence of mutations in the skeletal muscle sodium channel. Muscle enzymes such as creatine kinase may be elevated, and following chronic damage, muscle biopsy may show vacuolated fibers, tubular aggregates, central nuclei, and fibrosis. Cautious provocative testing may be performed using *oral* potassium (1 mEq per kilogram). The serum potassium peaks at 90 to 180 minutes following ingestion. Intravenous potassium should *not* be given.

The diagnosis of paramyotonia congenita also depends heavily on the clinical features outlined in Table 1. The critical diagnostic element is provocation of either myotonia or weakness on exposure to cold. In paramyotonia congenita, the EMG reveals myotonia of resting muscles at room temperature following percussion or movement of the needle. Spontaneous activity (fibrillation) appears upon limb cooling to 30°C. Further cooling abolishes this activity and often provokes paralysis. Another early EMG manifestation with cooling may be loss of amplitude of the compound muscle action potential. As in hyperkalemic periodic paralysis, the diagnosis of paramyotonia congenita may be confirmed by PCR-based documentation of sodium channel muta-

A

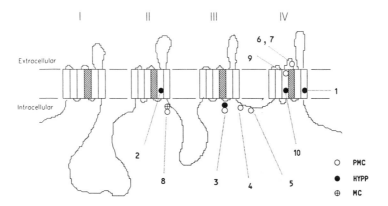

B

	Mutation	Position	Domain	Phenotype	Author
1.	Met --> Val	1592	IV, S6	HYPP	Rojas et al., '91
2.	Thr --> Met	704	II, S5	HYPP	Ptacek et al., '91c
3.	Ala --> Thr	1156	III, S4-5	HYPP/PMC	McClatchey et al., '92b
4.	Gly --> Val	1306	III-IV loop	PMC	McClatchey et al., '92a
5.	Thr --> Met	1313	III-IV loop	PMC	McClatchey et al., '92a
6.	Arg --> His	1448	IV, S4	PMC	Ptacek et al., '92a
7.	Arg --> Cys	1448	IV, S4	PMC	Ptacek et al., '92a
8.	Ser --> Phe	804	II, S6	PMC/MC	McClatchey et al., '92b
9.	Leu --> Arg	1433	IV, S3	PMC	Ptacek et al., '92b
10.	Phe --> Leu	1419	IV, S3	HYPP*	Rudolph et al., '92

*equine

Figure 1 Sodium channel alpha subunit and location of mutations in hyperkalemic periodic paralysis (HYPP), paramyotonia congenita (PMC), and myotonia congenita (MC). *A,* depicts the alpha subunit polypeptide composed of four homologous domains (I-IV), each containing six membrane-spanning helices (S1-S6). In the functional state, the four domains are believed to aggregate to form a tetrameric channel. The channel pore may be lined by the extracellular loops between S5 and S6 in each domain. Upon depolarization, the channel is activated by movement of S4 segments (*hatched* segments) in each domain; these four S4 segments are positively charged and may serve as voltage sensors. Inactivation probably entails movement of the intracytoplasmic loop between domains III and IV into the cytoplasmic vestibule of the channel pore. *B,* Mutations causing HYPP, PMC, and MC phenotypes are designated, by *closed, open,* and *hatched circles,* respectively. References above for specific mutations appear in Brown, 1993.

tions using DNA from a blood sample. The muscle biopsy may show myopathic changes.

Related Myotonic Disorders

In autosomal dominant myotonia congenita, myotonia is prominent clinically and on EMG. There are no dystrophic findings. The known mutation within the chloride channel gene or other mutations may be detected by PCR-based DNA diagnostic methods. Muscle biopsy may show absence of type 2B fibers or mildly increased fiber size. In the recessive Becker's form, muscle hypertrophy may be prominent.

The clinical presentation of myotonic dystrophy usually includes evidence of multisystem disease, such as subcapsular cataracts in almost all patients, cardiac conduction defects in 70 percent, frontal balding, testicular atrophy, insulin-resistant diabetes, mental deficiency, and personality changes. Sagging of the jaw and atrophy of facial muscles may be prominent. DNA analysis to evaluate abnormal CTG repeats may be important for both diagnostic and prognostic reasons since the size of the repeats may correlate with disease severity. The EMG shows classic myotonic discharges as well as myopathic features. Muscle biopsy may reveal fiber size variability, fibrosis, central nuclei, and ring fibers. Serum muscle enzymes may be slightly elevated, and serum IgG may be reduced.

DISCUSSION

The periodic paralyses and myotonias are an emerging family of primary muscle disorders that have until recently been diagnosed by clinical and EMG features. It is now evident that some of these disorders share fundamental defects in membrane excitability resulting from mutations in skeletal muscle ion channels or their modulators. In many instances, rapid, blood-based DNA analysis may confirm the diagnosis of a specific muscle ion channel mutation. As more affected families are studied, the range of natural mutations will become better defined. An analysis of the molecular biology of each mutation should illuminate not only the disease phenotype but also biophysical properties of specific subregions of sodium and chloride channels.

SUGGESTED READING

Brooke, MH. Disorders of Skeletal Muscle. In: Neurology in Clinical Practice. Bradley WG, Daroff RB, Fenichel, GM and Marsden CD eds. Boston: Butterworth-Heinemann, 1991:1843.

Brown RH Jr. Molecular basis for hyperkalemic periodic paralysis and related diseases. Curr Neurol 1993; 13:111–132.

Cannon SC, Brown RH Jr, Corey DP. A sodium channel defect in hyperkalemic periodic paralysis: Potassium induced failure of inactivation. Neuron 1991; 6:619–626.

Cannon SC, Brown RH Jr, Corey DP. Theoretical reconstruction of myotonia and paralysis caused by incomplete inactivation of sodium channels. Biophys J 1993; 65:270–288.

Catterall W, Scheuer T, Thomsen W, Rossie S. Structure and modulation of voltage-gated ion channels. Ann NY Acad Sci 1991; 625:174–180.

Engel AG. The periodic paralyses. In: Engel AG, Banker BQ, eds. Myology. New York: McGraw-Hill, 1986:1843.

Fontaine B, Khurana TS, Hoffman EP, et al. Hyperkalemic periodic paralysis and the adult muscle sodium channel alpha-subunit gene. Science 1990; 250:1,000–1,002.

George AL Jr, Crackower MA, Abdalla JA, et al. Molecular basis of Thomsen's disease (autosomal dominant myotonia congenita). Nature Genetics 1993; 3:305–310.

Ptacek LJ, Johnson KJ, Griggs RC. Genetics and physiology of the myotonic muscle disorders. N Engl J Med 1993; 328:482–489.

Riggs JE. The periodic paralyses. Neurol Clin 1988; 6:485–498.

Streib EW. Differential diagnosis of myotonic syndromes. Muscle Nerve 1987; 10:603–615.

BOTULISM

MICHAEL CHERINGTON, M.D.

The presentation of botulism in its classic form is the unmistakable pattern of descending muscle weakness in a previously healthy person, occurring several hours after ingestion of contaminated food. If the physician is unaware of this pattern, the diagnosis may be missed or delayed, particularly in mild cases or when only one patient presents at the office or hospital. The first symptoms are consistent with dysfunction of bulbar musculature with blurred vision, dizziness, diplopia, dysphagia, and dysarthria. This is followed by descending weakness and breathing difficulties. When two or more cases are brought to the clinician's attention, the correct diagnosis is likely to be quickly established. When a single case appears at the physician's office or outpatient clinic, other diagnostic possibilities are often considered. The differential diagnosis usually includes the Guillain-Barré syndrome, myasthenia gravis, and the Lambert-Eaton myasthenic syndrome (LEMS). Although each of these possibilities may resemble botulism, they can usually be differentiated by careful clinical assessment and appropriate laboratory studies.

CLINICAL PICTURE

In most cases the correct diagnosis of these disorders of neuromuscular transmission and peripheral nerve conduction can be strongly suspected on clinical grounds alone. In the typical case the clinical presentation of botulism is sufficiently characteristic to be diagnosed with near certainty on the basis of history and physical examination. The onset of bulbar symptoms after eating suspect food, followed by a pattern of descending weakness, should distinguish cases of botulism from Guillain-Barré syndrome, which usually presents with a pattern of ascending weakness. The Miller Fisher variant of Guillain-Barré syndrome, with prominent ocular and bulbar abnormalities, may present a more difficult diagnostic puzzle. Electrophysiologic studies (see subsequent section) can be most valuable in localizing the site of lesion either at the neuromuscular junction, consistent with botulism, or at the level of the peripheral nerve, which would be consistent with Guillain-Barré syndrome. Patients with food-borne botulism may present with gastrointestinal symptoms, such as nausea, vomiting, diarrhea, cramps, and constipation. They may also demonstrate involvement of the autonomic nervous systemm with dryness of the mouth, paralytic ileus, and, in some cases, pupillary abnormalities.

The clinical hallmark of myasthenia gravis is pathologic fatigue reversed by anticholinesterase medication. The short-term improvement following intravenous edrophonium chloride is often dramatic in myasthenic patients. The clinical improvement after edrophonium chloride in patients with botulism is usually less impressive, although there are reported exceptions to these observations. The time course of the illness should also alert the neurologist to the possibility of botulism. Botulism usually strikes a previously healthy individual 24 to 48 hours after eating contaminated food, while myasthenic syndromes are usually subacute or chronic. LEMS and myasthenia gravis are often associated with neoplastic diseases or other autoimmune diseases. Myasthenia gravis and thymoma are known to occur in the same patient. LEMS often occurs in patients who have small-cell carcinoma of the lung. Serologic testing for acetylcholine receptor antibody is an important tool in the diagnosis of myasthenia gravis. It is positive in over 80 percent of myasthenic patients. When combined with single fiber electromyogram (EMG) studies, confirmation of the diagnosis of myasthenia gravis has been reported to be as high as 90 percent or more. In some cases of LEMS, serum antibodies to voltage operated calcium channels are found.

In each of these three disorders of neuromuscular transmission (botulism, myasthenia gravis, LEMS), mentation and sensation are usually unaffected. Weakness or fatigue are the prominent neurologic problems. Deep tendon reflexes can be depressed in LEMS as well as in severe botulism.

ELECTROPHYSIOLOGIC STUDIES

Electrophysiologic studies are frequently helpful in establishing the correct diagnosis when the clinical diagnosis is still in doubt. Repetitive supramaximal motor nerve stimulation techniques are easily done, and each of these disorders is characterized by a different

Table 1 Changes in Amplitude of Compound Muscle Action Potential in Response to Supramaximal Nerve Stimulation

	Single Stimulus	2/Sec	After 10 Sec Isometric Exercise
Myasthenia gravis	Normal	Decrement	Decrement
LEMS	Small	Decrement	Increment
Botulism	Small	Decrement (variable)	Increment (variable)

Table 2 Electrodiagnostic Findings in Botulism

Normal motor conduction velocities and distal latencies
Normal sensory latencies
Small CMAP amplitude in affected muscle
Increment in CMAP amplitude with rapid repetitive nerve stimulation or after exercise (variable)
Decrement in CMAP amplitude with slow repetitive nerve stimulation (variable)
Short-duration, low-amplitude MUAPs on needle EMG study
Increased jitter and blocking on single fiber EMG

CMAP = compound muscle action potential, MUAP = motor unit action potential, EMG = electromyogram.

pattern (Table 1). In myasthenia gravis, the size of the action potential in the rested muscle is usually normal but decreases with repetitive nerve stimulation at slow rates. In LEMS and botulism, the rested muscle action potentials are typically reduced but increase following activation by volitional isometric exercise. Patients tolerate activation by 10 seconds of isometric exercise much better than supramaximal repetitive nerve stimulation at rates of 50 per second. In LEMS, the potentiation is marked and can be found in almost any muscle chosen. In botulism, the potentiation is not as dramatic and may not be found at all. The only electrical abnormality may be a markedly reduced evoked muscle action potential. Furthermore, in botulism, unlike LEMS, the electrical abnormality may be found in some muscles but not in others (Table 2). In both botulism and LEMS, the lesion is in the presynaptic region of the neuromuscular junction. Single fiber EMG in botulism reveals increased jitter and blocking, which is less marked after activation by isometric exercise or rapid repetitive nerve stimulation. In the few cases of botulism that have been studied with intracellular microelectrodes, there is a marked reduction in the release of quanta of acetylcholine as compared to normals after a single nerve action potential. These physiologic findings are consistent with the speculation that the toxin interferes with the release of acetylcholine from the nerve terminal.

FORMS OF BOTULISM

In the food-borne type of botulism, the symptoms begin several hours or days after ingestion of the contaminated food. The diagnosis is definitely established when the patient's serum is tested for mouse-killing power, and the toxin (usually A, B, or E) is identified with antiserum neutralization. Often the mouse lethality bioassay is negative when the diagnosis is delayed and the blood sample is obtained too late. In that case, one should test the suspect food if it is still available. Stool specimens should be examined for the presence of either the clostridial bacteria or the toxin. Neither should be present in a healthy adult individual, because normal intestinal flora are a barrier to intestinal colonization by *Clostridium botulinum*. State health departments and the Centers for Disease Control in Atlanta are helpful in directing the laboratory evaluations.

A more rarely reported form of botulism is known as wound botulism or endogenous botulism (Table 3). The clinical presentation, again, is one of a descending paralysis beginning in the bulbar territory. However the source of the toxin is not exogenous contaminated food but toxin-producing clostridial bacteria introduced in a wound, surgical or traumatic. In recent years, wound botulism has been reported in drug abusers. In patients who present with the pattern of a descending weakness, and where a history of eating contamined food is absent, look for a wound or abscess in the skin or intranasal sinus. The diagnosis is confirmed if the organism can be cultured from the wound material. If not, a presumptive diagnosis can be made with the help of electrophysiologic studies.

In 1976 a new form of botulism was discovered and named infant botulism. Since this discovery, more cases of infant botulism are reported each year than any other form. Infant botulism results from the production of toxin by the *Clostridium* organism inhabiting the intestinal tract. In normal adults and children, the normal intestinal flora are hostile to the clostridial bacteria, but in a small number of infants the toxin-producing bacteria are able to take hold. The patient is typically an infant under 6 months of age who presents with a weak cry and suck, ocular palsies or ptosis, poor head control, and generalized weakness and hypotonia. The diagnosis is confirmed by isolating the organism and toxin from fecal specimens. Electrophysiologic studies are often most helpful before microbiologic laboratory results are

Table 3 Clinical Classification of Botulism

Classic form: food-borne
Infantile form
Wound botulism
  Traumatic or surgical
  Drug abuse
    Intravenous
    Nasal
Hidden form

available. Expected findings include a small evoked muscle action potential after single supramaximal nerve stimulation and, in some cases, potentiation of muscle potentials after activation. The needle EMG examination reveals abundant, small, low-amplitude motor unit action potentials.

The rarest form of botulism, known as the hidden form, occurs in adult patients who have not consumed contaminated food or had a wound. They are patients who harbor the clostridial bacteria in their intestinal tract, similar to the infant form. These adult patients usually have some abnormality of the gastrointestinal tract, often postsurgical, which allows the toxin-producing organism to gain hold. The diagnostic procedures are those used in infant botulism: microbiologic evaluation of fecal and blood specimens and electrophysiologic studies.

SUGGESTED READING

Arnon SS. Infant botulism: Anticipating the second decade. J Infect Dis 1986; 154:205–210.

Cherington M. Botulism: Ten year experience. Arch Neurol 1974; 30:432–437.

Cherington M. Botulism. Semin Neurol 1990; 10:27–31.

Hughes JM, Blumenthal JR, Merson MH, et al. Clinical features of types A and B food-borne botulism. Ann Intern Med 1981; 95:442–445.

Pascuzzi RM, Kim YI. Lambert-Eaton syndrome. Semin Neurol 1990; 10:35–41.

Pickett JB, Berg B, Chaplin E, Brunstetter-Shafer MA. Syndrome of botulism in infancy: Clinical and electrophysiologic study. N Engl J Med 1976; 295:770–772.

Swift TR. Disorders of neuromuscular transmission other than myasthenia gravis. Muscle Nerve 1981; 4:334–353.

THORACIC OUTLET SYNDROME

JOHN R. PARZIALE, M.D.
EDWARD AKELMAN, M.D.

Thoracic outlet syndrome (TOS) is an often misdiagnosed cause of neck, shoulder, and arm disability. Neurovascular compression is more frequent in the interscalene triangle, costoclavicular space, or beneath the pectoralis minor, although any cause of shoulder girdle malalignment may produce a localized area of brachial plexus compression. Compression in this area may lead to arm pain, paresthesias, and numbness. A careful history and physical examination are essential to proper diagnosis. Diagnostic testing may be used to differentiate TOS from other causes of upper extremity numbness and pain.

Neurovascular compression attributed to TOS has been described as occurring in up to nine anatomic locations, with the three most common being the interscalene triangle (scalenus anticus syndrome), between the first rib and the clavicle (claviculocostal syndrome), and between the pectoralis minor and the thoracic cage (pectoral syndrome). These three clinical syndromes have several common characteristics, including onset frequently related to muscular spasm, brachial plexus traction due to shoulder depression, and local musculoskeletal trauma to neurovascular structures. A cervical rib, long transverse process at the cervical spine, clavicular fracture or anomaly, bifid first rib, or fusion of the first and second ribs has been identified in 20 percent of TOS patients in one series. A history of trauma was seen in 21 percent of the patients with surgically treated TOS in another series. Nerve compression at a distal site may be found in up to 44 percent of TOS cases, indicating that a "double crush" phenomenon may cause increased susceptibility to more proximal symptoms.

EPIDEMIOLOGY

TOS is seen much more commonly in women than men, with a 2 or 3 to 1 ratio. TOS is seen most commonly in persons in their late teens through their 30s. Patients who are diagnosed at a later age usually have had long-standing symptoms with an incorrect initial diagnosis. Leffert has described the classic TOS patient as a woman with an asthenic habitus, drooped shoulders, and a large bosom.

Certain occupations that require shoulder abduction and external rotation of the glenohumeral joint may lead to onset of this syndrome. Secretaries, computer operators, and bench workers may be at risk. A second group of young patients at risk may be those with hypertrophic musculature, seen in occupations that involve heavy lifting or hyperabduction of upper extremities. Weightlifters, jackhammer operators, electricians, and carpenters have been described with TOS. Patients with local trauma, such as malunions or nonunions of clavicular fractures, may be at risk. Congenital anomalies, such as cervical ribs or muscular congenital bands, may increase the effects of poor posture or local trauma causing TOS.

Patients usually complain of symptoms at night or in the early morning, after prolonged sitting with neck extension and lateral rotation or bending. Patients note that symptoms may occur with lifting or hyperabduction of the shoulder. Patients present with a history of a daily living activity or work that requires elevation of the humerus above the horizontal. These patients state that lifting their arms above their heads worsens their symptoms. After the patients bring their arms down to their sides, their symptoms decrease. Patients most commonly complain of supraclavicular shoulder pain with radiation into the medial upper arm and forearm into the fourth and fifth digits. A careful history will usually note patients complaining of hand weakness. Their symptoms may be increased by cervical motion and headaches. Patients less commonly complain of vascular compression symptoms such as a cool, pale hand or a swollen upper extremity. In patients with these symptoms due to intermittent arterial or venous compression, a careful history should be taken regarding traumatic events or work history.

In a study of 473 patients with TOS, symptom duration ranged from 4 weeks to 12 years, with an average of 18 months; 10 percent of patients had bilateral symptoms, and, in 4 percent, symptoms appeared on the contralateral side even after surgery.

EXAMINATION

An examination of these patients should include a thorough neurologic, musculoskeletal, and vascular examination. Upon inspection, atrophy may be noted, particularly in the first dorsal interosseous and hypothenar muscles of the hand and, less frequently, in the forearm, triceps, or trapezius. Inspection from behind may note scapular drooping on the affected side. The range of motion of the cervical spine, shoulder, elbow, and wrist should be carried out in both active and passive phases. Sensory examination should include two-point discrimination, light touch and proprioception, and response to cold and warm stimuli. Muscular examination should note reflex changes at the biceps, triceps, and brachioradialis muscles. Tests for upper motor neuron dysfunction, such as the Hoffman reflex examination, should be performed. Each vascular examination should include evaluation of pulses in the resting positions, and dynamic maneuvers should be carried out, including Adson's and Wright's tests.

Adson's maneuver is a test to identify the reduction or obliteration of the radial artery pulse due to compression by muscles at the interscalene triangle. The examiner abducts and externally rotates the patient's shoulder with the arm extended. The patient's cervical spine is then rotated so that the patient's chin faces the hand on the examined side. The patient is then asked to inspire deeply and hold his breath. With a deep inspiration, the subclavian artery may be compressed between the pectoralis muscle and the chest wall. The combination of these maneuvers contracts the interscalene space, leading to a reduction in the pulse pressure of the radial artery. A modified Adson's test, with rotation to the contralateral side, may be performed at the same time.

Wright's maneuver is an important test. Leffert has described this test as positive in 97 percent of his patients with TOS. Wright's maneuver is carried out by abducting the shoulder and externally rotating the humerus with the head and chin in a neutral position.

Other physical examination tests are valuable in establishing TOS. These have included the Roos test or the 3-minute elevation arm exercise test, in which early fatigability or heaviness develops in the involved arm, with gradual onset of numbness and tingling in the hand before 3 minutes. Direct pressure applied at the interscalene triangle or below the pectoralis minor muscle may elicit pain or paresthesias radiating down to the medial aspect of the hand. It is important to note that these maneuvers are considered positive only when neurologic symptoms are reproduced, not if only a pulse is obliterated. Many normal patients will have obliteration of pulse with these maneuvers.

Examination of the hand should be carefully directed toward the ulnar-innervated intrinsic muscles. These muscles are involved in the early phases of TOS, and it is not until long-term compression or the double crush syndrome occurs that thenar muscular changes are seen. Careful testing of sensibility in the medial forearm and in the ulnar digits of the hand may detect early findings.

DIFFERENTIAL DIAGNOSIS

There are many other conditions to consider in the differential diagnosis of TOS. Cervical strap muscle tendonitis, tendonitis of the biceps or medial wrist flexors, and generalized fibromyalgia may produce pain in the same general distribution of TOS. Cervical radiculopathy as well as ulnar neuropathy may present with paresthesias, pain, and hypothenar and intrinsic muscle wasting. Carpal tunnel syndrome may cause nocturnal paresthesias, waking a patient at night. The subclavian steal syndrome, characterized by reduction in pulses in the affected arm with exercise, may lead to coldness and pain. An apical lung tumor may, via pressure, mimic the symptoms of TOS.

DIAGNOSTIC TESTS

A full investigation of TOS requires that other diagnoses be excluded. Roentgenographic examination of the cervical spine, chest, and shoulder assesses for cervical rib, apical lung tumor, or arthritis. Electrodiagnostic examination has greater specifity than sensitivity for diagnosing TOS. Although most TOS patients present with neuritic symptoms, nerve conduction studies are of limited value in detecting demyelination in the area of the neck and upper chest. Explanations for this problem include the wide variability of normal range for median and ulnar nerve conduction velocities across this area, the doubling of right/left differential in the region as compared with nerve conduction velocities across the elbow and from elbow to wrist segments, and difficulty in localizing the point of compression. When nerve damage has progressed to the point of axonal pathology, quantitative electromyographic studies of ulnar and median innervated small hand muscles may reveal changes compatible with chronic denervation. EMG will help rule out confounding diagnoses, such as cervical radiculopathy, carpal tunnel syndrome and ulnar nerve compression at the elbow.

In our opinion, somatosensory evoked potential responses do not appreciably increase the sensitivity of electromyographic tests. There have been several published reports of the diagnostic utility of F-wave responses. Depending on the degree of Wallerian degeneration, sensory action potentials may be reduced in amplitude in digit 5 as compared with digit 3, and this may be a helpful adjunct to the diagnosis of TOS.

Arteriography may be useful in localizing a site of vascular compression. Arteriographic studies can differentiate between intrinsic and extrinsic causes of compression and indicate whether the obstruction is fixed or intermittent. These studies may be more useful in patients with large cervical ribs and in patients who have previously had unsuccessful first cervical rib resections.

In the evaluation of the cervical spinal cord, magnetic resonance imaging has largely replaced myelography for the diagnosis of cervical disk prolapse, syringomyelia, or disc herniation. Contrast studies with gadolinium will identify neoplasm and differentiate between scar and disk material.

Biopsy of the anterior scalene muscle performed during TOS surgery may demonstrate a transformation from mixed type I and type II fibers to predominantly type I muscle. This may confirm the diagnosis of TOS.

COMMENTS

TOS is not an easily diagnosed disorder. It is essential for the clinician to rule out causes such as cervical disk disease, radiculopathy, tendonitis, lung tumors, and nerve compression at the elbow and wrist. The diagnosis of TOS is clinical, and there is no consistently reproducible diagnostic test. It is important to identify those patients who present with a long neck, slouched posture, and weak cervical muscles because their treatment may differ substantially from that of the athletic patient with hypertrophied and spastic cervical musculature.

SUGGESTED READING

Cailliet R. Neck and arm pain. 2nd ed. Philadelphia: FA Davis, 1989:137.

Dale WA. Thoracic outlet compression syndrome. Arch Surg 1982; 117:1437–1445.

Huffman JD. Electrodiagnostic techniques for and conservative management of thoracic outlet syndrome. Clin Orthop 1986; 207:21–23.

Karas SE. Thoracic outlet syndrome. Clin Sports Med 1990; 9:297–310.

Kelly TR. Thoracic outlet syndrome: Current concepts of treatment. Ann Surg 1979; 190:657–662.

Lord JW. A critical re-appraisal of diagnostic and therapeutic modalities for thoracic outlet syndromes. Surg Gynecol Obstet 1989; 168:337–340.

Machleder HI, Moll F, Verity MA. The anterior scalene muscle in thoracic outlet syndrome. Arch Surg 1986; 121:141–144.

Rob CG, Standeven A. Arterial occlusion complicating thoracic outlet compression syndrome. BMJ 1958; 2:709.

Roos DB. Transaxillary approach for first rib resection to relieve thoracic outlet syndrome. Ann Surg 1966; 163:354–358.

Roos DB. Experience with first rib resection for thoracic outlet syndrome. Ann Surg 1971; 173:429–442.

Roos DB. Congenital anomalies associated with thoracic outlet syndrome. Am J Surg 1977; 132:771.

Roos DB. Essentials and safeguards of surgery for thoracic outlet syndrome. Angiology 1981; 32:187–193.

Selke FW, Kelly TR. Thoracic outlet syndrome. Am J Surg 1988; 156:54–57.

Wood VE, Biondi J. Double-crush nerve compression in thoracic outlet syndrome. J Bone Joint Surg 1990; 72-A:85–87.

CHRONIC FATIGUE SYNDROME

ROBERT G. MILLER, M.D.

Chronic fatigue syndrome is the currently accepted term for a constellation of symptoms that center around excessive fatigability. A number of other terms have been used to describe this condition, including postviral fatigue syndrome, myalgic encephalomyelitis, epidemic neuromyasthenia, Icelandic disease, and the Royal-Free Hospital syndrome. The term *chronic fatigue syndrome* is preferable because it implies no identified cause for this disorder. Some controversy still exists about the diagnosis. Recently, objective clinical criteria have been published to clarify the diagnosis, but the criteria for diagnosis have not as yet been subjected to a controlled prospective study such as that carried out with fibromyalgia.

Patients who have excessive fatigue should be suspected of having this condition, but other causes of fatigue must be carefully considered. The precise nature of the fatigue is a major issue, and in this respect a thorough history is of critical importance. Patients with true muscular fatigability, such as myasthenia gravis, complain of reduced muscular endurance that occurs with sustained or repeated activity involving certain muscle groups. By contrast, patients with the chronic fatigue syndrome usually have four different types of fatigue, and most patients complain of all four types. First, patients usually have a generalized lack of energy, which is present particularly upon rising in the morning and often prompts them to seek rest or sleep during the day. In some cases, there is a clear-cut similarity to the biologic symptoms of depression, and many patients also have constipation, disturbed sleep pattern, low energy, and low spirits as well. However, a significant percentage of patients do not appear to have signs of clinical depression. The second type of fatigue is reduced muscular endurance in activities that used to be performed easily and can no longer be carried out or can be executed only in part. The third component of fatigue in these patients is a delayed recovery after physical exertion. Patients typically report that it takes many days to recover after some form of physical exercise. Finally, many patients complain of mental fatigue, which includes difficulty with memory and impaired concentration that is aggravated by intense intellectual activity. A careful dissection of the symptom of fatigue in terms of these different aspects often helps.

Many patients have other symptoms besides fatigue (Table 1). Generalized myalgia and arthralgia are very common. Other symptoms include disturbed sleep pattern, sometimes with hypersomnia, headache, painful lymph nodes, sore throat, fever or chills, and some neuropsychological abnormalities such as excessive irritability, confusion, forgetfulness, inability to concentrate, and trouble thinking clearly. All of these symptoms are considered part of the list of minor criteria for the diagnosis. The major criteria include new debilitating fatigue that reduces activity below 50 percent of the prior level and does not resolve within 6 months of onset and with a period of bed rest. It is imperative that other conditions which may cause fatigue should be thoroughly evaluated, such as metabolic muscle disease, neuromuscular junction disturbances, central nervous system disorders, and underlying metabolic or endocrinologic abnormalities.

On examination, such patients may have physical evidence of a low-grade temperature, a nonexudative pharyngitis, and palpable or tender lymph nodes in the cervical or axillary region. The remainder of the general physical examination is usually normal.

The neurologic examination may disclose some "giving way" weakness, but there is usually no objective abnormality of mental function, cranial nerves, tendon reflexes, strength, or sensation.

I make a point of evaluating muscular endurance

Table 1 Diagnostic Criteria for Chronic
Fatigue Syndrome*

Major Criteria
    Exclude systemic cause
    New onset of persistent or relapsing severe fatigue for 6 months

Minor Criteria
    Headache
    Sleep disturbance
    Psychological symptoms
    Migratory joint pains
    Unexplained muscle weakness
    Myalgias
    Sore throat
    Painful lymph nodes
    Fatigue prevents usual activity
    Symptoms began abruptly
    Fever

Physical Findings
    Low-grade fever
    Nonexudative inflamed pharynx
    Palpable or tender cervical or axillary lymph nodes

*Must fulfill (1) both major criteria *and either* (2) six or more of the minor criteria and two or more of the physical criteria or (3) eight or more of the minor criteria.

using clinical bedside tests that provide some quantitative measure of fatigue. I employ the outstretched arm time, which should exceed 2 minutes, the ability to hold the head off the bed when supine, which should normally be greater than 30 seconds, holding the leg at 45 degrees when supine, which normally is at least 1 minute, and the ability to carry out 20 deep knee bends. The patient who can easily perform all of these tests is not likely to have a clinically significant disorder of neuromuscular transmission or muscle function. Patients with a mitochondrial disorder or metabolic myopathy may show not only marked fatigability in carrying out these tests, but a striking elevation of heart rate during this modest form of exercise.

LABORATORY FINDINGS

I usually order the following laboratory studies: serum creatine kinase, thyroid function, complete blood count, serum lactate, metabolic panel, and erythrocyte sedimentation rate. When the symptoms sound convincingly muscular, I carry out electrodiagnostic studies to further evaluate a neuromuscular cause of fatigability. I start with routine electromyographic (EMG) study of symptomatic muscles. Low-frequency discharges of motor units in symptomatic muscles imply incomplete effort and sometimes are also associated with intermittent recruitment and limited effort, all of which is consistent with "giving way" weakness. The EMG study is particularly helpful in ruling out a myogenic or neurogenic cause of weakness or fatigue. Nerve conduction studies are performed on at least one motor and sensory nerve to rule out a neuropathy or a polyradiculopathy.

Superimposed maximal nerve stimulation with recording of muscular force can also be employed during an isometric contraction to evaluate the degree of voluntary effort. Added force in response to electrical stimulation during a maximal voluntary contraction documents the presence of incomplete voluntary effort and is often present in patients with chronic fatigue syndrome.

I also carry out repetitive nerve stimulation to evaluate for myasthenia gravis or the myasthenic syndrome. This is done both before and after exercise using standard protocols. In addition, I perform 20 Hz stimulation for 50 seconds to evaluate energy metabolism within muscle. In patients with myophosphorylase deficiency, there is a decremental response of greater than 25 percent during this stimulation protocol. In normal subjects, there is no decrement greater than 25 percent. This protocol is uncomfortable, but with adequate preparation and explanation, most patients can tolerate the discomfort. It is imperative to completely immobilize the limb during this stimulation.

Patients who might be candidates for muscle biopsy undergo exercise testing of forearm muscles in our laboratory, using a ramp protocol that begins with 10 percent of maximum voluntary contraction in the finger flexors and increases each minute by an additional 10 percent until excessive fatigue or contracture. We use no blood pressure cuff because of the risk of myoglobinuria in patients with a defect in glycogen metabolism. Early excessive lactic acid formation occurs in patients with mitochondrial dysfunction, and no formation of lactate suggests a defect in glycogen metabolism. We simultaneously obtain blood for serum ammonia in order to screen for myoadenylate deaminase deficiency in patients who may present with myalgia and fatigue. The forearm exercise test is useful in planning the biochemical analysis of muscle biopsy tissue.

We perform muscle biopsy in patients with excessive fatigue when there is some abnormality in any of the above tests or the clinical impression suggests an underlying myopathy. In patients with chronic fatigue syndrome, the muscle biopsy is usually normal, disclosing no deposits of lipid or carbohydrate as one might see with carnitine deficiency or a glycolytic defect. We carefully evaluate the trichrome stain for mitochondrial abnormalities and use electron microscopy for a thorough evaluation of the mitochondria.

DIFFERENTIAL DIAGNOSIS

Patients with myasthenia gravis usually describe only fatigability in specific muscle groups brought out by sustained or repeated activity. These abnormalities are usually readily demonstrable upon endurance testing and can be reversed with pharmacologic intervention (pyridostigmine or edrophonium, for example). Patients with the myasthenic syndrome may have myalgia as well as limb fatigability, and electrophysiologic tests are particularly helpful in evaluating both of these neuromuscular transmission defects. Patients with metabolic muscle diseases, particularly myophosphorylase or phosphofructokinase deficiency, complain of easy fatigue in exercised muscles, and there is usually a history of both pigmenturia and painful muscle contracture induced by exercise. By contrast, patients with a defect of lipid metabolism such as carnitine palmitoyl transferase deficiency have symptoms only with prolonged exercise (usually greater than 45 minutes of sustained activity), particularly after fasting. These patients develop stiffness and pain in the muscles and episodes of myoglobinuria. In such patients, all diagnostic studies are normal except for muscle biopsy, which may show lipid droplets, and a biochemical enzyme analysis is necessary for diagnosis.

Fatigue may also complicate a number of other neurologic conditions, including chronic inflammatory demyelinating polyradiculoneuropathy. This is usually easily detected by electrodiagnostic studies where nerve conduction velocity is markedly slowed along with dispersion and conduction block. Patients with amyotrophic lateral sclerosis frequently complain of excessive fatigue, but there are usually obvious lower motor neuron or upper motor neuron signs, or both, by the time fatigue becomes a symptomatic problem. Fatigue is the most common complaint of patients with multiple sclerosis, but other symptoms and signs are usually sufficient to raise the clinical suspicion of the diagnosis. Patients with post-polio syndrome also complain of significant pain and fatigue, but the history of polio and the absence of any other associated condition is critical in establishing the basis for this condition. Patients with human immunodeficiency virus infection frequently complain of fatigue during the advanced phase of the illness. Most patients have both myalgia and fatigue, but frequently manual muscle testing discloses no weakness and tests of muscular endurance are normal. This symptom of fatigue is probably constitutional since quantitative tests of muscle function have been normal and most patients have no objective evidence of pathologic muscular fatigability on standard testing. The same is true of patients with cancer who have malaise and generalized fatigue but usually no neuromuscular dysfunction.

Patients with depression have excessive fatigue, and upwards of 70 percent of patients with chronic fatigue syndrome have either anxiety or depression or both. Thus some investigators have suggested that the chronic fatigue syndrome is probably a psychophysiologic disorder. This may well be true for some patients, particularly when the cases are clustered in an epidemic. However, at least 30 percent of patients have no obvious psychological disturbance, so that it cannot be considered a sine qua non for this disorder.

Thus, for the diagnosis of chronic fatigue syndrome, both of the major diagnostic criteria and at least six of the minor criteria must be fulfilled. These patients should have normal muscular endurance on clinical testing, normal blood studies, normal electrodiagnostic studies, and normal forearm exercise tests and muscle biopsies when appropriate. I provide substantial reassurance about the relatively benign nature of the diagnosis and the strong tendency toward spontaneous improvement in the majority of patients. I recommend treatment with amitriptyline and a program of modest, graduated aerobic exercise to repair the deconditioning present in most patients.

SUGGESTED READING

Behan P, Behand W. Postviral fatigue syndrome. Crit Rev Neurobiol 1988; 4:157–162.
Boissevain MD, McCain GA. Toward an integrated understanding of fibromyalgia syndrome: I. Medical and pathophysiological aspects. Pain 1991; 45:227–238.
Holmes GP, Kaplan JE, Gantz NM, et al. Chronic fatigue syndrome: A working case definition. Ann Intern Med 1988; 108:387–389.
Kent-Braun JA, Sharma KR, Weiner MW, et al. Central basis of muscle fatigue in chronic fatigue syndrome. Neurology 43:125–131.
Komaroff AL, Goldenberg D. The chronic fatigue syndrome: Definition, current studies and lessons for fibromyalgia research. J Rheumatol 1989; 16(suppl 19):23.
Rosen SD, King JC, Wilkinson JB, Nixon PG. Is chronic fatigue syndrome synonymous with effort syndrome? J R Soc Med 1990; 83:761–764.
Shafran SD. The chronic fatigue syndrome. Am J Med 1991; 90:730–739.

POST-POLIO SYNDROME

DAVE HOLLANDER, M.D., FRCP(C)
THEODORE L. MUNSAT, M.D.

The development of the Salk and Sabin polio vaccines and the subsequent introduction of widespread vaccination programs has led to the virtual disappearance of acute poliomyelitis in the United States and other industrialized countries. This disease, which formerly terrorized parents and physicians alike, has become so rare that most physicians currently in practice have never seen a case of paralytic polio. Although the great epidemics, with polio wards full of patients and attendant fear and panic among the population, are but memories today, living testimony to these terrible epidemics endures in thousands of polio survivors. It is estimated that in the United States alone, there are more than 500,000 polio survivors. Most, with the tenacity and drive for which polio victims are renowned, have overcome serious physical impairments and become fully participatory members of society. In the past decade, however, it has become apparent that in a significant proportion of these patients, late sequelae of polio may develop. These symptoms, commonly known as the post-polio syndrome (PPS), typically occur some 30 years after the original bout of polio. Their appearance is yet another challenge in the lives of polio survivors.

SYMPTOMS AND CLINICAL FINDINGS

PPS is conservatively estimated to develop in 25 percent of polio survivors, but the true figure may in fact be much higher. The core of the PPS consists of the triad of fatigue, pain, and progressive weakness. About one-third of patients with PPS display all these symptoms. Other, less common features include the development of fasciculations and new muscle atrophy. The risk of developing these late sequelae is related to the severity of the initial illness. Patients with severe polio are at greatest risk, and severely affected muscles are more likely to develop late weakness than clinically spared muscles. Nonetheless, even patients with mild polio may develop typical PPS.

Fatigue in PPS may be mild and limited to individual, previously affected muscle groups or may be generalized. Such generalized fatigue may be severe and overwhelming, developing even after minimal exertion. The pain of PPS is musculoskeletal and may be related to several factors. Most common are joint pains, particularly in large weight-bearing joints. These pains are mechanical in nature, arising as a result of the unbalanced forces and stresses placed over the years on joints, tendons, and ligaments that have been called upon to compensate for muscle and limb weakness. Frank, degenerative arthritis may develop in such joints. Also common are muscle pains. These are exertion induced and are presumably related to the limited exercise capacity of previously denervated muscles, especially if these muscles have an added burden imposed upon them by weakness in other muscle groups. Pain may also develop as a consequence of nerve or root entrapment. Degenerative disk disease of the spine or scoliosis may result in radiculopathies. Compressive neuropathies, such as ulnar neuropathy and carpal tunnel syndrome, may secondarily develop as a consequence of the long-term use of braces and crutches. These various pain syndromes are not by themselves diagnostic of PPS but may be considered part of the syndrome when associated with other neuromuscular symptoms.

Muscle weakness is the final element of the classic triad in PPS. New weakness may develop in any muscle group, even in those that previously appeared to be unaffected. This reflects the usually widespread invasion of the neuraxis by the polio virus. Even though only some limbs may appear to have been affected, there is in fact more generalized, subclinical motor neuron involvement. The new weakness of PPS is typically very slowly progressive, with strength decline estimated to be on the order of 1 percent per year. Even so, there may be

significant functional consequences. Patients who had previously been ambulatory may now be forced to use assistive devices, and the ability to perform other activities of daily life may become impaired. Respiratory symptoms may develop in patients who had previous involvement of respiratory muscles. Frank muscle atrophy may develop in a minority of patients.

The examination findings in patients with PPS are, for the most part, similar to those seen in polio patients without late sequelae. Muscle atrophy, weakness, and areflexia are typically present, although in patients who had very mild polio, muscle bulk may appear intact. The weakness need not be limited to the amyotrophic limbs. Fasciculations may be present, and there may be atrophy of muscles that were originally unaffected. Upper motor neuron findings are extremely uncommon but may occur, presumably as a consequence of the meningoencephalitis associated with the original polio infection. Before ascribing these findings to polio, other possible causes such as cervical myelopathy or stroke must be ruled out, especially if the upper motor neuron signs are prominent. Bulbar findings are rare. Sensory changes are absent except as a secondary phenomenon, such as in cases of nerve entrapment.

DIAGNOSIS

The diagnosis of PPS is primarily a clinical one. Laboratory tests serve to confirm the diagnosis but are not, in and of themselves, diagnostic. The most useful tests are electromyography (EMG) and muscle biopsy. Nerve conduction studies demonstrate reduced compound muscle action potentials in affected muscles but are otherwise normal. The needle component of the EMG may demonstrate widespread active and chronic denervative changes, even in muscles seemingly unaffected. As previously discussed, this is a consequence of the more widespread subclinical involvement at the time of the original infection. The active changes consist of fibrillation potentials and positive sharp waves. Fasciculations may also be present. The chronic changes are due to denervation and subsequent reinnervation of muscle fibers. Motor unit potentials may be enlarged and prolonged, and there may be an increase in the number of polyphasic motor unit potentials. Recruitment is reduced. Single fiber EMG studies demonstrate increased fiber density and jitter, and blocking.

Muscle biopsies may show a mixture of myopathic and neurogenic changes. The former consist of variation in fiber size, central nuclei, fiber splitting, and increases in connective tissue. The latter consist of fiber type grouping, group atrophy (suggestive of chronic denervation), and small angulated fibers (suggestive of acute denervation). Similar EMG and biopsy findings may be seen in polio patients who do not suffer any of the late sequelae, thereby limiting the diagnostic usefulness of these tests. Their chief usefulness lies in confirming the diagnosis of PPS in cases where a clear antecedent history of polio is not available.

Diagnostic criteria for PPS have been suggested. These consist of a history of acute polio and subsequent recovery, with a prolonged period of functional stability (greater than 10 to 20 years) followed by the development of new neuromuscular symptoms. In such cases, the diagnosis of PPS is straightforward. Care must be taken not to overdiagnose PPS. The development of musculoskeletal pain alone does not necessarily constitute PPS; such pains may develop in any patient with chronic disability from whatever cause. For this reason, there should be evidence of new neuromuscular symptoms, such as weakness and fatigue. In some cases, the initial symptoms, particularly if restricted to one limb, may resemble a radiculopathy or peripheral neuropathy. Imaging studies of the spine may be helpful in deciding whether a radiculopathy is present. It is often difficult to diagnose radiculopathies by EMG in the face of the widespread denervative changes that may already be present as a consequence of the initial polio infection. Entrapment neuropathies, on the other hand, may often be diagnosed by EMG studies.

Further diagnostic pitfalls arise in patients with no known history of polio. Diagnoses such as chronic inflammatory demyelinating polyneuropathy and myasthenia gravis may be entertained in some of these patients. In such cases, the EMG studies are extremely important in ruling out these diagnoses. The picture of new onset weakness, possibly associated with fasciculations and new atrophy, and without sensory involvement, may be mistakenly diagnosed as early amyotrophic lateral sclerosis (ALS). Although the diagnosis of ALS requires the presence of both upper and lower motor neuron findings, many cases initially present with just lower motor neuron findings and may resemble PPS. In those rare instances of PPS associated with upper motor neuron findings, the similarity to ALS is, of course, even greater. EMG and muscle biopsy are not helpful in distinguishing between these two entities, since similar changes may be seen in both conditions. In such cases, it is the slow rate of progression, the lack of development of significant bulbar and respiratory symptoms, and the failure to develop upper motor neuron signs that ultimately point to the diagnosis of PPS. Conversely, we have seen polio patients who have subsequently developed ALS. In these cases, the reverse features, rapid progression and development of bulbar and respiratory symptoms and upper motor neuron signs, have led to the diagnosis of ALS.

PROGNOSIS

Little can be done at this time to prevent the progression of weakness in PPS, although clinical trials of neurotrophic agents are being planned and hold out some hope for the future. Patients should be reassured that progression is slow and rarely life-threatening. The exception to this is in patients who have previously had significant respiratory involvement. Such patients may have minimal respiratory reserve and may decompensate years after their initial illness. They may require ventilatory support, especially at night.

Even for the majority of patients who do not develop respiratory symptoms, however, deficits and loss of function will occur, often necessitating adjustments in life-style. This loss of function can be especially disheartening to polio patients who have had to overcome major disabilities in the past, often by pushing themselves to the very limits of their ability. They may now become profoundly depressed or, alternatively, may undertake unreasonably strenuous rehabilitation programs, which may, if anything, aggravate their symptoms. Often their symptoms, which by their very nature may be mild and vague early on, are not taken seriously by others, and it is a relief just to be able to speak with an understanding doctor. Patient management in PPS requires a thoughtful, supportive approach on the part of the treating physician.

SUGGESTED READING

Dalakas M, Illa I. Post-polio syndrome: Concepts in clinical diagnosis, pathogenesis, and etiology. In: Rowland LP, ed. Amyotrophic lateral sclerosis and other motor neuron diseases. New York: Raven Press, 1991; 495.

Jubelt B, Cashman NR. Neurologic manifestations of the post-polio syndrome. Crit Rev Neurobiol 1987; 3:199–220.

Munsat TL, ed. Post-polio syndrome. Boston: Butterworth-Heinemann, 1991.

MOVEMENT DISORDERS

CHOREA

LISA M. SHULMAN, M.D.
WILLIAM J. WEINER, M.D.

The presence of excessive, extraneous body movements is often readily apparent to the clinical observer, while the classification of the movement disorder and the implications for the differential diagnosis are more elusive. Chorea refers to involuntary, nonrhythmic, brief, and unsustained movements that appear to flow from one body part to another in random sequence. The characteristic movements of chorea are nonrepetitive and unpredictable. Even though randomness of the movements is essential to diagnose chorea in clinical practice, there is some tolerance for applying the term *chorea* to movements that are more repetitive and stereotypical. For example, the repetitive oral-buccal-lingual movements, or "piano-playing hands," of tardive dyskinesia (TD) are in contrast to the brief, flitting movements in Huntington's disease (HD), yet both are termed *choreic.*

Physicians have a tendency to diagnose all hyperkinetic movements as chorea. Rapid, nonrhythmic, involuntary movements are also seen in myoclonus, tics, and dystonia. The diagnosis of chorea is complicated by the fact that early chorea is often subtle. There is an acceptable range of spontaneous movements among normals that is quite variable and is influenced by a number of factors such as personality, mood, and environment. The patient is usually unaware of the excessive movement. Although choreiform movement appears as if it would cause subjective discomfort, this is rarely reported. Family members and the physician are often more disturbed and distracted by the patient's chorea.

The onset of chorea is usually insidious, although there are exceptions, as in structural lesions of the basal ganglia and drug-induced chorea, which may present more acutely. The patient often accommodates to the chorea by consciously or subconsciously incorporating the involuntary movement into the normal flow of spontaneous movement. Thus a sudden flexion of the arm is transformed into a hand gesture during speech or an opportunity to fix the hair, while a shoulder or leg movement will lead to an adjustment of body position.

Aside from social embarrassment, chorea may not cause functional disability until it is far advanced. Early in its course the patient may appear unusually clumsy or sloppy. Food stains on the clothes, runs in ladies' stockings, poorly applied make-up, or a generally disheveled appearance may be early clues.

Facial chorea—consisting of grimacing, blinking, eyebrow raising, forehead wrinkling, chewing, puckering, and tongue protrusions—may often go unnoticed until the movements cause disability. Frequent oral-buccal-lingual movements may cause injury to the tongue or inner cheek due to inadvertent biting or abrasions. Frequently the patient reports difficulty maintaining dentures in the mouth, as well as interference with chewing, swallowing, and speech production. Respiratory dyskinesias may occur, particularly in TD, resulting in interference with prosody of speech, involuntary spitting, and difficulty eating.

Generalized chorea is often characterized by brief flitting movements of the fingers, toes, wrists, and ankles, head jerking, shoulder shrugging, trunk jerking or arching, and pelvic rocking or thrusting. The overall impression may be that of general fidgetiness, but a careful history will often reveal a progressive pattern of clumsiness with increasing incoordination. Superimposed chorea during performance of tasks requiring dexterity and during ambulation may cause the patient to be uncharacteristically prone to accidents.

Historical clues will guide your thinking when prioritizing the differential diagnosis. Consider the age at onset of the movement disorder. Has the course been static, episodic, progressive, or remitting-exacerbating? Are there aspects of the past medical history that may be associated with the appearance of a movement disorder, such as cerebral ischemic or traumatic injury, recent streptococcal throat infection, or toxic exposure? Explore the drug history in detail, especially the use of neuroleptics, metoclopromide, prochlorperazine, amoxapine, antiparkinsonian agents, amphetamines, anticonvulsants, oral contraceptives, and illicit substances.

Supported in part by a grant from the National Parkinson Foundation.

Changes in personality, behavior, and school or work performance are often most accurately reported by relatives and friends and may be reliable indicators of cognitive or psychiatric impairment.

The characteristics of the movement disorder are studied from the moment the patient is initially greeted through the interview and neurologic examination. In this manner the effects of stress, mood, activity, and rest on the movements may be observed. The location, rhythmicity, speed, frequency, amplitude, and predictability of the dyskinesias should all be noted. Other discriminating features include suppressibility of the involuntary movement, interference with tasks requiring coordination, and association with other types of movement disorders. Bizarre movements that disappear with distraction or worsen on inspection in a patient with multiple somatizations or the potential for secondary gain may indicate a psychogenic cause.

Although the range of conditions that can precipitate chorea is remarkably broad, the pathogenesis of the movement disorder in every case is believed to involve dysfunction of the basal ganglia. The basal ganglia play a complex and multifaceted role in the production of movement, including the initiation of movement, the perpetuation of desired movement, and the suppression of unnecessary intrusive movements. Disinhibition of the thalamus precipitates excessive choreiform movement and may be caused either by underactivity of primarily gamma-aminobutyric acid–ergic striatopallidal-subthalamic pathways (Huntington's disease) or overactivity of dopaminergic nigrostriatal pathways (TD, levodopa-induced dyskinesia). Generally speaking, sizable subcortical lesions are less likely to result in chorea than neurodegenerative, metabolic, or pharmacologic processes.

The identification of a choreiform movement disorder does not hold the diagnostic specificity of the pill-rolling resting tremor of Parkinson's disease or the Kayser-Fleischer rings of Wilson's disease. A remarkable range and variety of pathologies can underlie choreic movement, including metabolic, endocrine, infectious, neoplastic, immunologic, traumatic, and iatrogenic disorders. In-depth discussion of the intricacies of differential diagnosis is beyond the scope of this chapter. Instead, we present an approach to evaluating the patient presenting with chorea relative to the associated clinical findings (Table 1). Representative disorders are highlighted in each section, chosen on the basis of their prevalence, reversibility, or notoriety. Accompanying tables outline further examples for reference. Not uncommonly, a disorder may be found on more than one table. For example, HD may initially present with either

neurologic or psychiatric symptoms and therefore must be considered in both of these clinical settings.

CHOREA PRESENTING IN THE SETTING OF OTHER NEUROLOGIC DEFICITS

The clinician must scrutinize the patient presenting with chorea for further evidence of neurologic dysfunction (Table 2). Alterations of facial expressivity, the spontaneity and speed of movement, motor tone, finger dexterity, coordination, gait, and postural stability are fundamental expressions of disruption of the basal ganglia pathways. Other hyperkinetic movement disorders such as tremor, myoclonus, ballismus, athetosis, and dystonia may coexist with choreiform movement. Abnormalities of cognition, behavior, speech, and oculomotor function and the presence of pathologic reflexes frequently accompany extrapyramidal signs.

The presence of hemichorea-hemiballismus is often a clue to an underlying structural lesion. Ballism is characterized by irregular, violent, flinging movements of the limbs, primarily due to contraction of the proximal muscles, while chorea consists of random, smaller amplitude movements of both the distal and proximal musculature. While hemichorea or hemiballism may occur separately, they are usually found in combination. The difference between chorea and ballism is more

Table 1 Clinical Classification of Chorea

Chorea presenting in the setting of other neurologic deficits
Chorea presenting in psychiatric illness
Chorea presenting in systemic illness
Chorea presenting in isolation

Table 2 Chorea Presenting in the Setting of Other Neurologic Deficits

Drugs	Infectious diseases
Anticonvulsants: phenytoin, carbamazepine, ethosuximide, phenobarbital	Bacterial (encephalitis, abscess) Creutzfeldt-Jakob disease
Antiparkinsonian agents: levodopa-carbidopa, bromocriptine, pergolide, amantadine, selegiline, anticholinergics	Viral (HIV, encephalitis lethargica)
Neuroleptics	Neoplasia
Stimulants	Primary brain tumor
Steroids	Metastatic brain tumor
Intoxications	Cerebrovascular disease
Alcohol	Arteriovenous malformation
Carbon monoxide	Basal ganglia infarction
Heavy metal poisoning	Intracerebral hemorrhage
	Migraine
Hereditary disorders	Miscellaneous
Hallervorden Spatz disease	Head trauma
Huntington's disease	Multiple sclerosis
Joseph's disease	Multiple system atrophy
Neuroacanthocytosis	Neurosurgical intervention
Olivopontocerebellar atrophy	Perinatal injury (cerebral
Wilson's disease	palsy, kernicterus)
	Psychogenic movement
Metabolic disorders	disorder
Electrolyte disorders	
Hepatic encephalopathy	
Hormonal dysregulation	
Nutritional deficiency	
Uremic encephalopathy	

descriptive than pathophysiologic. They appear to represent different levels of severity on a clinical spectrum. Accordingly, hemiballismus often evolves into hemichorea as it resolves.

Hemiballism is usually associated with contralateral lesions of the subthalamus. However, it has also been described with injury of the contralateral caudate, putamen, globus pallidus, and thalamus. Stroke is the most common cause, but other structural lesions such as arteriovenous malformation, venous angioma, abscess, primary or metastatic tumor, multiple sclerosis, head trauma, and neurosurgical complications may be the cause. More diffuse central nervous system (CNS) insults, including hyperglycemic nonketotic states, encephalitis, tuberculous meningitis, and lupus cerebritis, have also precipitated a unilateral hyperkinetic disorder. Additionally, hemichorea-hemiballism has been reported in association with levodopa administration, phenytoin intoxication, and oral contraceptive use.

The most common scenario is the onset of hemichorea or hemiballism in an elderly patient with risk factors for cerebral vascular disease, such as hypertension, diabetes mellitus, cardiovascular disease, or hypercholesterolemia. The onset of the movement disorder may either be abrupt at the time of the vascular insult or appear gradually while the initial neurologic deficits wane. Neuroimaging, preferably magnetic resonance imaging (MRI), is indicated to detect an acute or subacute infarction and confirm the diagnosis.

The involuntary movements of hemiballism may be forceful, with significant potential for self-injury, aspiration, or exhaustion. Padding of bed rails and the use of gentle restraints is often necessary. Fortunately, in most cases the movement disorder spontaneously regresses over a period of weeks or months. In the interim, haloperidol, reserpine, and clonazepam are generally the most effective agents. Periodically, neuroleptic administration should be discontinued to reevaluate the movement disorder and the need for continued pharmacotherapy.

The involuntary movements induced by levodopa therapy in Parkinson's disease are likely to be the most common type of choreiform disorder confronted in the practice of clinical neurology. Chronic levodopa administration is associated with the onset of dyskinesias in approximately 50 percent of patients with Parkinson's disease after 2 years of therapy, and about 80 percent after 5 years. The dyskinesias first appear as mild fidgety movements that often go unnoticed by the patient and family. There may be very subtle nodding movements of the head, an appearance of restlessness of the extremities, sinuous movements of the hands and feet, and adventitious mouthing or chewing motions. Although most patients prefer the dyskinetic "on" state to the akinetic, rigid "off" state, with time the movements may become so severe as to be the predominant problem.

Choreodystonic or choreoathetoid movements, ballism, myoclonus, stereotyped movements, focal dystonia, and akathisia may all occur in this setting. Most commonly, the timing of the dyskinesias corresponds with the period of time when the patient experiences levodopa's therapeutic effect, and they are thus referred to as peak-dose dyskinesias. Other patients experience dyskinesias during periods of pronounced drug level fluctuations. These diphasic dyskinesias occur shortly after levodopa administration, followed by a period of relative quiescence, and reoccur late in the dosing interval as the blood level falls.

Involuntary movements related to levodopa administration tend to be most troublesome in patients most severely affected with Parkinson's disease who demonstrate a significant clinical response to dopaminergic therapy. Early onset patients have been observed to be particularly at risk. Interestingly, chronic levodopa administration to "normal subjects" does not induce dyskinesias. Therefore, it is reasonable to conclude that these involuntary movements are produced by the interaction of levodopa with an abnormal substrate. Dyskinesias generally appear first on the side of the body most affected by the illness.

The pathogenesis of levodopa-induced movements remains unclear. Contributory factors may include the duration of illness, the daily dose or cumulative exposure to levodopa, the pulsing of levodopa concentrations, or the production of levodopa metabolites. Dopamine agonists alone in levodopa naive patients rarely cause involuntary movements. It would be advantageous if a therapeutic window existed where antiparkinsonian effects could be obtained without the induction of dyskinesia. Unfortunately, in practice it is rarely possible to identify a dose or dosing schedule of levodopa that separates out the therapeutic and adverse effects.

CHOREA PRESENTING IN THE SETTING OF PSYCHIATRIC SYMPTOMS

The coupling of behavior and cognition with regulation of movement is strikingly demonstrated by the ubiquitous presence of movement disorders precipitated by antipsychotic agents, as well as psychiatric disturbances induced by dopaminergic agents (Table 3). While the neural pathways mediating these effects appear to be distinct (mesocorticolimbic pathways for psychiatric effects and basal ganglia pathways for motor function), the neurotransmitters and receptors are clearly intermixed. Although pharmacologic agents and dosing schedules exist that produce the desired antipsychotic or motor effect, the therapeutic window is small. Many patients receiving neuroleptic drugs develop signs of motor dysfunction, and a significant number of patients receiving long-term dopaminergic therapy exhibit psychiatric symptoms.

The delayed onset of an involuntary movement disorder following neuroleptic exposure was first recognized and described in the late 1950s, several years after the introduction of chlorpromazine, the first neuroleptic agent. The prerequisites for a diagnosis of TD are a history of at least 3 months of neuroleptic exposure, the presence of involuntary movements, and the absence of

Table 3 Chorea Presenting in the Setting of Psychiatric Symptoms

Drugs
  Anticholinergics
  Anticonvulsants
  Antiparkinsonian agents
  Heterocyclic antidepressants (amoxapine)
  Lithium
  Neuroleptics
    phenothiazines (chlorpromazine, thioridazine)
    butyrophenones (haloperidol)
    thioxanthenes (thiothixene)
    benzamides (metoclopramide)
  Stimulants
    amphetamines, methylphenidate, pemoline, cocaine

Intoxications
  Alcohol
  Carbon monoxide
  Heavy metal poisoning (mercury, manganese)
  Toluene (glue sniffing)

Metabolic disorders
  Adrenal dysfunction
  Hepatic encephalopathy
  Nutritional deficiency (pellagra)
  Thyroid dysfunction
  Parathyroid dysfunction
  Pituitary dysfunction
  Uremic encephalopathy

Hereditary disorders
  Huntington's disease
  Porphyria
  Wilson's disease

Miscellaneous
  Psychogenic movement disorders
  Schizophrenia with stereotyped behavior

other conditions that might produce a movement disorder. The simplicity of these criteria obscures the difficulty that may be encountered when considering this diagnosis.

The clinician's initial contact with the patient who presents for evaluation of suspected TD usually follows the onset of involuntary movements. Therefore, one must rely on history alone to ascertain if any movement disorder existed prior to the administration of neuroleptics. Because there is no reliable way to discriminate among disparate choreiform disorders by observation alone, it may be difficult to distinguish TD from benign spontaneous chorea (oral-buccal-lingual dyskinesias of the elderly) or the numerous disorders that may present with both motor and psychiatric symptoms (e.g., Wilson's disease, HD, metabolic encephalopathy).

Furthermore, neuroleptics may have been introduced to treat a pre-existing movement disorder, such as the tics of Tourette's syndrome, hemiballismus resulting from infarction, or any of the choreiform disorders. In the absence of thorough documentation, optimally with the use of videotape prior to neuroleptic use, the pre-existing condition may be inseparable from the newly reported findings. Of course, acute dystonic

reactions, acute transient dyskinesias, and parkinsonism may also result from treatment with antipsychotics and must be distinguished from TD because the management of these varying conditions is distinct.

The involuntary movements of TD are choreic; however, they are often less random and unpredictable and more stereotypic and repetitive than the movements of classic chorea. Stereotyped movements are particularly characteristic of oral-buccal-lingual dyskinesias, which are often the earliest and sometimes the sole feature of TD. Fine, vermicular movements of the tongue progress to to-and-fro lateral movements and then to twisting or curling tongue movements with bulging of the cheek and involuntary tongue protrusions. Limb dyskinesias may also be stereotypic, with twisting, wiggling movements of the fingers and toes, foot tapping, and marching in place. Athetosis, dystonic posturing, and akathisia are often intermixed with the chorea of tardive syndromes.

The cumulative incidence of TD has been reported to be 5 percent after 1 year of neuroleptic exposure, 19 percent after 4 years, and 40 percent after 8 years. The most reliable risk factors are age and gender. The mean prevalence of TD is three times greater in patients over 40, and most studies have found a higher incidence of TD in women than men. Other suggested risk factors include type of neuroleptic agent, dose and duration of treatment, exposure to multiple neuroleptics, drug-free intervals, concurrent antiparkinsonian treatment, type of primary psychiatric illness, and pre-existing brain injury. It is generally accepted that involuntary movements may emerge within a 3 to 6 month period following the discontinuation of neuroleptic agents and still be attributed to TD.

It is difficult to clearly characterize the natural history of TD. The onset is usually insidious, and the symptoms are often complicated by adjustments and variations in medication regimens from patient to patient. Long-term data indicate that after a period of progression, the movements begin to stabilize or gradually improve, even in patients continuing on neuroleptics. In a minority of cases, the dyskinesias persist. It is unclear at this time whether this is actually permanent TD or persistent dyskinesias in that group of individuals who are predisposed to develop spontaneous dyskinesias.

Since the treatment of TD is difficult and often inadequate, the major emphasis is on prevention. The indications for long-term antipsychotic treatment must be clearly established and regularly reevaluated. Neuroleptics should be administered in the lowest possible dosage, with low-potency preparations used when feasible. Reversal of TD is most likely to occur when neuroleptics are discontinued at the earliest sign of the appearance of the movement disorder.

The clinical triad of chorea, dementia, and family history should immediately trigger the thought of HD. HD is a chronic progressive neurodegenerative disorder transmitted as an autosomal dominant trait with 100 percent penetrance. The onset of symptoms is usually between 35 and 40 years of age, although there is actually a wide range, with a small percentage of cases presenting in childhood or in old age.

The initial symptoms may be either the insidious onset of choreic movement or the subtle signs of early cognitive changes. In most patients, these findings occur simultaneously and progress concurrently. The movement disorder is characterized by a random flow of brief, adventitious movements in a generalized distribution. Involvement of the muscles of facial expression and the upper extremities may predominate initially.

Personality changes, irritability, aggressiveness, sexual promiscuity, inattention, apathy, and poor judgment are early manifestations of cognitive decline. A wide variety of psychiatric symptomatology has been described. However, the common thread is development of a progressive dementia. Depression is common, with suicide responsible for 7 percent of the deaths of HD patients.

Communication is often affected by a progressive dysarthria, word-finding difficulty, or alterations in the prosody of speech produced by choreic involvement of respiratory or articulatory musculature. Oculomotor function is impaired, with loss of smooth pursuit, slow hypometric saccades, and gaze impersistence. A characteristic gait develops, which is distinguished by a widened base and swaying movements of variable cadence that convey a dancing quality. There is a loss of finger dexterity and an impersistence of sustained movement that causes an inability to maintain tongue protrusion, eye closure, or hand grip ("milk-maid's grip"). Hyper-reflexia and Babinski signs may be elicited.

The nonstereotyped, unpredictable flow of choreic movement, motor impersistence, oculomotor disturbances, and progressive course are the major features that assist the clinician in distinguishing HD from TD. Additional differential diagnoses that merit attention include Creutzfeldt-Jakob disease, Wilson's disease, familial Alzheimer's disease with myoclonus, benign familial chorea, Tourette's syndrome, schizophrenia with stereotyped movements, and Parkinson's disease treated with levodopa.

Childhood onset, known as the Westphal variant, is associated with more parkinsonian features, recurrent seizures, and rapid progression. HD with late onset is exemplified by a choreic disorder with more moderate cognitive decline. Advanced HD is characterized by the tragic picture of severe dysarthria, dysphagia, and dementia, with postural instability and loss of ambulation. Parkinsonian and dystonic features may become increasingly prominent as the chorea subsides. The duration of disease is generally 10 to 20 years, with death caused by aspiration pneumonia, sepsis, nutritional deficiency, accidental injury, or suicide.

The finding of a progressive choreic disorder of insidious onset in conjunction with a progressive dementia and a corroborative family history is the sine qua non of the diagnosis of HD. Family history may be lacking due to family secrecy, the perceived stigma of mental illness, ignorance regarding the fate of family members, and uncertain paternity. Late onset of symptoms and mild cases may also be obstacles to diagnosis.

Supportive evidence can be obtained with computed tomography (CT), MRI, or positron emission tomography (PET). Atrophy of the caudate nucleus and the cerebral cortex is often demonstrated on CT and MRI. PET scans using fluorodeoxyglucose have revealed reduced glucose metabolism in the caudate.

Now that the gene responsible for HD has been identified, each case may be genetically confirmed. Novel pharmacologic approaches and even gene therapy may become possible. A genetic test for HD continues to pose an ethical dilemma that must be approached on an individual basis.

CHOREA PRESENTING IN THE SETTING OF SYSTEMIC ILLNESS

Chorea is an uncommon accompaniment to a wide and heterogeneous range of systemic disorders (Table 4). It appears more likely that individual patients who manifest chorea in such diverse settings share some predisposing factor, such as pre-existing brain injury or genetic predisposition, rather than each disorder having a unique effect on the neural pathways of the basal ganglia.

Among the primary systemic diseases, the emergence of choreic movements is most often encountered in systemic lupus erythematosus (SLE). Nonetheless, chorea occurs in only 2 percent of these patients. Involuntary movement is seen early in the course of the disease in most cases and may precede the diagnosis of SLE in 21 percent of patients. Chorea may be present in either a generalized or hemidistribution, and often occurs in an episodic and recurrent pattern.

The pathogenesis of chorea in SLE is unknown. Postmortem examination has revealed CNS vasculitis in only a small proportion of cases, and cerebrospinal fluid analysis is usually normal. A majority of SLE patients with chorea have antiphospholipid antibodies in their serum. These are a heterogeneous group of antibodies (lupus anticoagulant, anticardiolipin antibodies, false-positive serology for syphilis) that are associated with hypercoaguability.

A subgroup of patients who are antiphospholipid antibody–positive but have insufficient clinical or serologic features to be classified as SLE carry the diagnosis of primary antiphospholipid antibody syndrome (APAS). Chorea has been reported with APAS along with the more common manifestations of recurrent arterial or venous thrombosis, spontaneous abortions, arthralgias, Raynaud's phenomenon, and thrombocytopenia.

The episodic nature of the choreic movement in both SLE and APAS may reflect the remitting-exacerbating course of these illnesses, although a clear relationship between the chorea and the activity of the underlying disease has not been demonstrated.

Table 4 Chorea Presenting in the Setting
of Systemic Illness

Drugs
  Anticonvulsants
    carbamazepine, phenytoin (seizures, neurogenic pain
      syndromes)
    ethosuximide, phenobarbital
  Antiparkinsonian agents
    amantadine (flu prophylaxis)
    anticholinergics
    bromocriptine (pituitary dysfunction)
  Neuroleptics
    chlorpromazine (intractable hiccoughs)
    haloperidol (acute agitation)
    metoclopramide (gastrointestinal motility disorders)
  Opiates (methadone)
  Oral contraceptive pills
  Steroids (autoimmune disease, COPD)
  Stimulants
    aminophylline (COPD)
    amphetamine, methylphenidate, pemoline, caffeine (chronic
      fatigue)
    cocaine
  Miscellaneous
    amoxapine, antihistamines, cimetidine, cyclizine, diazoxide,
      digoxin, isoniazid, lithium, methyldopa, prochlorperazine,
      reserpine, triazolam, tricyclic antidepressants

Intoxications
  Alcohol
  Carbon monoxide
  Heavy metal poisoning
  Toluene (glue sniffing)

Metabolic-Endocrine Disorders
  Addison's disease
  Chorea gravidarum
  Hyperthyroidism
  Hypocalcemia
  Hypoglycemia-hyperglycemia
  Hypomagnesemia
  Hyponatremia-hypernatremia
  Hypoparathyroidism-hyperparathyroidism
  Nutritional deficiency (beriberi, pellagra)
  Pseudohypoparathyroidism

Hereditary disorders
  Disorders of amino acid metabolism
  Disorders of carbohydrate metabolism
  Disorders of lipid metabolism
  Hepatolenticular degeneration-Wilson's disease
  Huntington's disease
  Joseph's disease
  Neuroacanthocytosis
  Porphyria

Neoplasia
  Metastatic brain tumor

Systemic illness
  Antiphospholipid antibody syndrome
  Bacterial endocarditis
  Behçet's disease
  Henoch-Schonlein purpura
  Hepatic failure
  Periarteritis nodosa
  Polycythemia vera
  Renal failure
  Sarcoidosis
  Sydenham's chorea (poststreptococcal)
  Systemic lupus erythematosus
  Viral encephalitis (HIV, influenza, measles)

Miscellaneous
  Multiple trauma with basal ganglia injury

COPD = chronic obstructive pulmonary disease, HIV = human immuno-deficiency virus.

Metabolic disorders including hormonal dysregulation and electrolyte abnormalities may be associated with the onset of choreic movement. Chronic metabolic disorders, with slowly progressive electrolyte disturbances that often go unnoticed, more commonly predispose to chorea than acute events. Choreiform dyskinesias have been reported with hyperthyroidism, although an exaggerated physiologic tremor is far more common in this setting. Both dopamine receptor antagonists and treatment of the underlying condition will relieve the movement disorder.

Sydenham's chorea (SC), polyarthritis, and carditis are manifestations of rheumatic fever (RF), the sequelae of an untreated antecedent group A streptococcal pharyngeal infection. The widespread use of antibiotics for strep throat has been accompanied by a sharp decline in the prevalence of both RF and SC, and they are now uncommon. Chorea is a delayed symptom of RF. Onset is usually 1 to 6 months after the initial infection, when other manifestations, such as polyarthritis and fever, have usually subsided. In one-third of the cases, the recognition of chorea prompts the discovery of carditis, which otherwise may remain undetected.

The age at onset of SC is generally between 5 and 15 years, with greater incidence in females. The emergence of chorea may be either abrupt or insidious and is often accompanied by emotional instability, confusion, or speech disturbance. The movement disorder may progress for a few weeks and then usually completely resolves over 3 to 6 months. Chorea may later reoccur with reinfection or may be triggered by provocative drugs, such as phenytoin, oral contraceptive pills, or alcohol, or metabolic changes such as pregnancy or hypernatremia.

Streptococcal antibody titer (antistreptolysin O test), erythrocyte sedimentation rate, and C-reactive protein, which are uniformly elevated in acute RF, may be declining or low if the interval between the acute infection and the chorea is greater than 2 months. The movement disorder is self-limiting.

CHOREA PRESENTING IN ISOLATION

Since choreic movement may be the initial and sole manifestation of an array of disorders, the presentation of chorea of unknown cause should prompt a carefully planned diagnostic investigation (Table 5). Particular attention to the medication history may be required to elicit details that may seem unimportant to the patient, such as recent metoclopramide use for a gastrointestinal disorder, or routine administration of oral contraceptives. Reassurance regarding issues of confidentiality is often necessary to obtain a detailed history of substance abuse.

With time, follow-up evaluations may reveal evolution of the movement disorder with emergence of new medical, neurologic, or psychiatric features that establish the diagnosis. In the absence of any associated findings on examination or laboratory evaluation, con-

Table 5 Diagnostic Investigation of Chorea of Unknown Cause

Primary evaluation
  History
    Present illness; past medical, neurologic, and psychiatric history;
      current and past medications; substance abuse; occupational
      history; family history
  Examination
    Medical, neurologic, and psychiatric
  Laboratory
    Complete blood count with platelet count
    Chemistry profile
      Electrolytes, liver function tests, renal function tests, calcium,
      magnesium
    Erythrocyte sedimentation rate
    HIV testing
    Thyroid function tests
    Toxicology screen
    CT imaging or MRI scan of the brain

Individualized evaluation
  Angiotensin converting enzyme level
  Anticardiolipin antibodies
  Anticonvulsant levels
  Antinuclear antibody titer
  Antistreptolysin O titer
  Blood smear for acanthocytes
  Ceruloplasmin, serum copper, 24 hour urinary copper
  Chest radiography
  EEG
  ECG
  Heavy metal screen
  Lactate and pyruvate levels
  Lithium level
  Liver biopsy
  Lysosomal enzymes
  Organic and amino acids
  Slit lamp evaluation
  VDRL

HIV = human immunodeficiency virus, CT = computed tomography,
MRI = magnetic resonance imaging; EEG = electroencephalogram,
ECG = electrocardiogram; VDRL = Venereal Disease Research Laboratories.

Table 6 Chorea Presenting in Isolation

Drugs
  Amphetamines
  Anabolic steroids
  Caffeine
  Cocaine
  Oral contraceptives

Intoxications
  Alcohol
  Carbon monoxide
  Manganese
  Mercury
  Toluene (glue sniffing)

Hereditary disorders
  Benign familial chorea
  Paroxysmal dystonic choreoathetosis
  Paroxysmal kinesigenic choreoathetosis

Miscellaneous
  Edentulous dyskinesias
  Psychogenic movement disorder
  Senile chorea
  Spontaneous oral-buccal-lingual dyskinesias of the elderly

sider the possibility of benign familial chorea, senile chorea, spontaneous oral-buccal-lingual dyskinesias, or a paroxysmal choreic disorder (Table 6).

Benign familial chorea is distinguished by early onset and a nonprogressive course. Senile chorea is notable for the absence of family history and onset after 65 years of age. Neither of these disorders is associated with cognitive impairment. Repetitive oral masticatory movements, inseparable from the oral-buccal-lingual dyskinesias following neuroleptic use, may occur spontaneously in approximately 10 percent of the elderly. Edentulousness has been reported to be a predisposing factor. The lines between these different classifications remain indistinct, although the number of affected people is notable. The cause of these dyskinesias is unknown. It has been suggested that perhaps the elderly are susceptible to a "developmental chorea" that simply reflects aging of the basal ganglia or, alternatively, that late onset chorea represents a delayed, mild form of HD.

Recurrent episodic choreic movement with totally quiescent intervening periods is characteristic of the paroxysmal dyskinesias. Paroxysmal kinesigenic choreoathetosis (PKC) is triggered by sudden movement, with attacks lasting seconds to a few minutes. Consciousness is preserved throughout the episode. Although the electroencephalogram is usually normal, the movement disorder is often successfully treated with anticonvulsant agents.

Paroxysmal dystonic (nonkinesigenic) choreoathetosis (PDC) is precipitated by stress, fatigue, caffeine, or alcohol. The episodes are longer, lasting minutes to hours. PDC is more difficult to treat than the kinesigenic form, but may respond to benzodiazepines or acetazolamide. Both PKC and PDC usually begin in childhood and adolescence and may be either familial, sporadic, or symptomatic. Differential diagnoses include partial seizures, drug-induced dyskinesias, and metabolic disorders.

Following a thorough and well-planned clinical investigation, a number of patients with chorea will continue to defy precise diagnosis. In these cases, the guiding principles of management are periodic follow-up with reevaluation, the judicious use of neuroleptic medications solely for disabling chorea, and routine withdrawal of neuroleptics to reassess the need for continued therapy.

SUGGESTED READING

Hyde TM, Hotson JR, Kleinman JE. Differential diagnosis of choreiform tardive dyskinesia. J Neuropsychiatry Clin Neurosci 1991; 3:255–268.

Kurlan R, Shoulson I. Differential diagnosis of facial chorea. Adv Neurol 1988; 49:225–237.

Lang AE. Movement disorder symptomatology. In: Bradley WJ, Daroff

RB, Fenichel GM, Marsden CD, eds. Neurology in clinical practice. Boston: Butterworth-Heinemann, 1991:315.

Lang AE. Movement disorders: Approach, definitions and differential diagnosis. In: Lang AE, Weiner WJ, eds. Drug-induced movement disorders. Mt. Kisco, NY: Futura, 1992:1.

Nutt JG. Dyskinesia induced by levodopa and dopamine agonists in patients with Parkinson's disease. In: Lang AE, Weiner WJ, eds.

Drug-induced movement disorders. Mt. Kisco, NY: Futura, 1992:257.

Shoulson I. On chorea. Clin Neuropharmacol 1986; 9(suppl 2): 585–599.

Weiner WJ, Lang AE. Movement disorders: A comprehensive survey. Mt. Kisco, NY: Futura, 1989.

DYSTONIA

CYNTHIA L. COMELLA, M.D.

DEFINITION AND RECOGNITION

Dystonia is defined as "a syndrome of sustained muscle contractions, frequently causing twisting and repetitive movements or abnormal postures." The sustained movements typical of dystonia are distinct from other movement disorders, such as chorea, tics, or tremor. Chorea is characterized by rapid movements occurring randomly and flowing from one movement to another, often involving the distal limbs or face. Tics are patterned, stereotyped quick jerks, such as eye blinks, or slower, more sustained movements, such as forcible jaw opening, referred to as dystonic tics. Tremor is characterized by rhythmic oscillations resulting from either alternating or simultaneous contraction of agonist-antagonist muscle pairs. Tremor may sometimes be present in a dystonia patient as an additional distinct movement disorder or may be secondary to the dystonia itself. Dystonic tremor characteristically affects the body area(s) affected by dystonia and is usually maximal with forced voluntary movement opposite to the direction of the dystonia.

Historically, the syndrome of dystonia has sometimes erroneously been thought to be a psychogenic disorder. Subsequently, the idea that dystonia is a manifestation of either psychiatric dysfunction or malingering has been largely abandoned and the neurologic basis of this disorder has been established. Although dystonia is recognized as a neurologic disorder, patients may still be referred to orthopedic or psychiatric colleagues by a physician unfamiliar with this syndrome.

Dystonia may present to the physician in a variety of ways. Typically the onset of symptoms is gradual. Initially, involuntary muscle spasms may occur only with action of the involved area and may be intermittent. As time passes the symptoms may be more continuous, often persisting at rest. The functional impact of dystonia on an individual patient varies depending on the severity, body area involved, and adaptability of the patient. Some patients find dystonia a nuisance but experience no more serious consequences. Others are disabled by their symptoms and may be handicapped by the involuntary movements or associated pain. The severity of the dystonia may fluctuate over time and may spread to involve adjacent body regions. In many patients, symptoms may stabilize 5 years after onset, but periods of stress or illness exacerbate symptoms. Remissions lasting from days to years occur in about 20 percent of adults, but recurrences are frequent, and permanent remissions are rare.

CLASSIFICATION

Clinically, dystonia may be classified in several ways (Fig. 1). A frequently used scheme includes classification by cause, age of onset, and pattern of body involvement. Classification by cause divides dystonia into primary and secondary forms. Primary dystonia has no discernible underlying cause and may affect either adults or children. Primary dystonia may be either hereditary or sporadic.

Classification by Cause

Primary, Inherited Dystonia

Classic inherited torsion dystonia (ITD) is autosomal dominant with a reduced penetrance of 30 to 40 percent. The DYT1 gene causing ITD has been mapped to the long arm of chromosome 9 and, through linkage analysis, has been narrowed to 20 possible gene candidates. This gene is responsible for ITD in Ashkenazi Jewish families as well as some non-Jewish families. This syndrome typically begins in childhood, with early involvement of the limbs, in particular the foot, and may generalize.

In addition to classic ITD, there are several types of variant ITD. Autosomal dominant, dopa-responsive dystonia (DRD), with onset in childhood, is a syndrome marked by diurnal variation such that symptoms typically are best in the morning and worst in the evening. Patients with DRD may have dramatic, sustained benefit from treatment with small doses of levodopa. Another inherited dystonia is Lubag, an X-linked syndrome typically affecting Filipino males in their fifth decade, combining dystonia with parkinsonism.

Other dystonias may appear as both inherited and sporadic disorders. Myoclonic dystonia, combining myoclonus and dystonia, may be familial and may be quite responsive to alcohol. Paroxysmal dystonia is dystonia that intermittently appears in an otherwise normal individual, either triggered by movement (kinesigenic) or independent of movement (nonkinesigenic).

Primary Sporadic Dystonia

The sporadic form of dystonia, in which no family history is found, tends to begin in adulthood and usually affects a limited body distribution. Although fluctuating in severity, sporadic dystonia rarely generalizes. Recent evidence has suggested that a genetic component may be present even in sporadic dystonia.

Secondary Dystonia

Secondary dystonia results from an underlying cause. Perinatal asphyxia, vascular or structural cerebral lesions, acute drug-induced dystonic reactions, tardive dystonia, underlying metabolic diseases, encephalitis, and perhaps peripheral trauma are all possible causes of secondary dystonia. Clinical clues that dystonia may be due to an underlying disorder include cognitive impairment, additional non-neurologic abnormalities on physical examination or laboratory tests, or evidence of more widespread neurologic dysfunction. The onset of dystonic symptoms at age 50 years or younger requires an evaluation for Wilson's disease. Wilson's disease is an autosomal recessive disorder of altered copper metab-olism, which may present with predominant dystonic symptoms. Appropriate treatment reverses this otherwise disabling and progressive disease.

Rarely, a patient may present with "dystonia" that is nondystonic. Atlantoaxial subluxation is an example of such a disorder in which the abnormal posture of the head and neck is the result of a local process. Clues to the diagnosis of this condition are the sudden onset of symptoms, intense neck pain, and almost complete restriction of head and neck movement. Another disorder associated with abnormal postures of the head and neck of non-neurologic origin is Sandifer's syndrome, a disorder occurring mostly in children and associated with hiatal hernia.

Classification by Age of Onset

In this category, dystonia is divided by age of onset into childhood (0 to 12 years), adolescence (13 to 20), and adulthood (over 20 years). Childhood onset hereditary dystonia usually begins with limb involvement, often with an inversion of the foot occurring at first during walking or running. Childhood onset dystonia tends to generalize to involve other body areas and may become a disabling disorder by early adulthood with contortions of the limbs, neck, and trunk. Despite incapacitation of the body, cognition and awareness remain intact.

In contrast to childhood onset, the dystonia beginning in adulthood usually involves only single (focal dystonia) or contiguous (segmental dystonia) body areas. The majority of those afflicted with adult onset dystonia do not experience a generalization of the dystonia.

Classification by Body Distribution

Finally, dystonia is classified by pattern of body involvement. Focal dystonia is the most restricted, affecting only one body area. Isolated involvement of eyes (blepharospasm), neck (cervical dystonia), jaw (oromandibular dystonia), larynx (spasmodic dysphonia), and arm (writer's cramp) are examples of focal dystonia. Segmental dystonia refers to involvement of two or more contiguous body areas. Examples include neck and trunk dystonia (axial dystonia), face and neck (cranial), one arm and trunk (brachial), and one leg and trunk (crural). Multifocal dystonia describes involvement of two noncontiguous body areas. Hemidystonia is a dystonia involving only one side of the body, most commonly arising from a vascular or other structural lesion in the contralateral basal ganglia. Generalized dystonia is a combination of crural dystonia with dystonia of another body area.

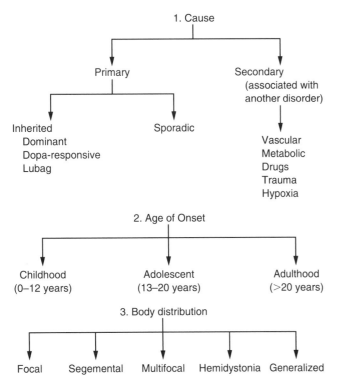

Figure 1 Classification of dystonia by cause, age of onset, and affected body areas.

CLINICAL FEATURES

Cervical Dystonia

The most common adult onset focal dystonia evaluated in referral centers is cervical dystonia (spasmodic torticollis). Cervical dystonia (CD) results from involuntary contractions of the neck muscles (Fig. 2). Depending upon the muscles affected, a variety of different head postures occur. There may be turning of the head to right or left (torticollis), tilting of the head toward the shoulder (laterocollis), forward flexing with tilting of the chin toward the chest (anterocollis), a backward extending of the head (retrocollis), or a lifting of a shoulder (shoulder elevation). Movement of the neck on the shoulders can also occur, causing sagittal or lateral shifting of the neck. CD can appear as a sustained abnormal posture of the head and neck or, if muscles with opposite actions are affected, as a tremor-like head movement. In some patients, CD may be quite painful, often in the posterior neck area. Occasionally the abnormal head position may cause a nerve root compression resulting in radicular symptoms. Many patients with CD describe voluntary maneuvers, or "tricks," that can transiently improve CD symptoms. This phenomenon is also referred to as a "geste antagoniste." For some patients, it may be touching the chin or the back of the head (Fig. 3). Others have more exotic gestures, such as wrapping a towel around the head or reaching over and pulling on the opposite ear. Before the recognition of dystonia as a neurologic disorder, the presence of these gestures was considered evidence of a psychiatric origin for dystonia. Although the mechanism by which these gestures improve dystonic symptoms is not understood, the frequency of such gestures in patients with CD suggests that sensory input may play a role in the underlying disorder. Further evidence that external factors influence the symptoms of dystonia is the occurrence of post-traumatic dystonia, in which an injury to a body area precedes the appearance of dystonia in that same area.

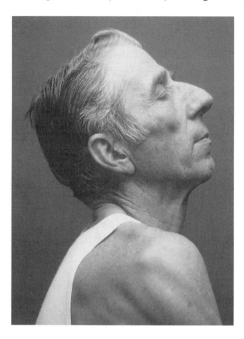

Figure 2 Prominent retrocollis with involvement of bilateral cervical paraspinal muscles.

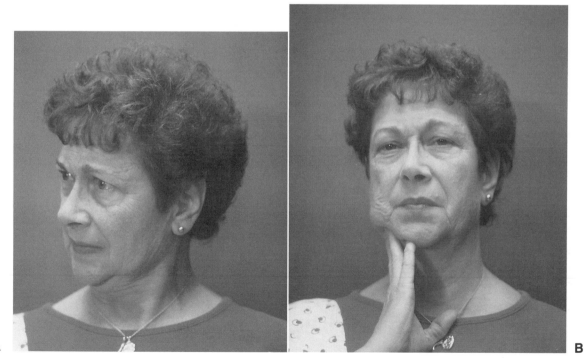

Figure 3 Demonstration of a common "trick" in cervical dystonia. *A,* At rest, an involuntary turn of the head to the right. *B,* The beneficial effect of a touch to the right cheek.

Blepharospasm

Dystonic spasms of the orbicularis oculi muscles (blepharospasm) is another common focal dystonia. The symptoms of blepharospasm usually begin insidiously with an increase in eye blinking. There may be a sensation of grittiness or irritation in the eyes prior to the onset of the involuntary spasms. Initially symptoms may predominate in one eye, but with progression both eyes are usually involved. Eventually, in some patients, tonic spasms of forced eyelid closure may cause virtual blindness as a result of the inability to overcome the spasms and open the eyes. Symptoms may be exacerbated by attempting to watch television, read, or drive. Bright lights or wind are other common aggravating factors. With forceful spasms, the patient may not be able to spontaneously open the eyes. Like patients with CD, however, those with blepharospasm may find that a touch to the side of the face or movement of the jaw can facilitate overcoming the spasms and allow the eyes to open.

Oromandibular Dystonia

Involuntary spasms of the muscles of the jaw, lower face, or tongue are referred to as oromandibular or lower facial dystonia. When combined with blepharospasm, the syndrome is referred to as Meige's or Breughl's syndrome (Fig. 4). The lower facial spasms may involve one or more of the following: the platysma muscle, facial muscles, muscles of mastication, or the genioglossus (tongue) muscle. Involvement of these muscles may present as involuntary grimacing, snarling, frowning, forced jaw opening, spasms of jaw closing, or tongue protrusion. In addition to the unacceptable social aspects of this focal dystonia, problems with swallowing or speech are frequent, adding a substantial functional disability. In jaw closing dystonia, dentition may be a particular problem, with the continuous gnashing causing chipping or breakage of the teeth.

Spasmodic Dysphonia

Spasmodic dysphonia is a focal dystonia involving the laryngeal muscles. The most frequent type of spasmodic dysphonia is the adductor type in which the vocal cords involuntarily spasm together. These spasms tend to occur when vocalization is attempted, resulting in an irregular choked, strained sound. Less frequently, the vocal cords may spasm apart (abductor), causing a breathy, hoarse sounding voice. In like manner to the other dystonias, patients may observe that simple maneuvers such as whispering or singing improve symptoms. As with the other focal dystonias, at the onset of the disorder the symptoms may be intermittent, perhaps occurring only under stressful situations. If symptoms are continuous and severe, speech may become impossible. In particular, talking on the telephone may be difficult. Although the vocal characteristics of this disorder are fairly distinct, a thorough evaluation of the larynx is advised to eliminate the possibility of other laryngeal disorders.

Other Focal Dystonias

Focal dystonia of the limbs may present in a variety of ways (Fig. 5). The most common primary limb dystonia is writer's cramp. In this disorder the dystonia becomes apparent with the manual task of writing. At rest and with other types of activity, the hand and arm appear normal. While writing, an involuntary flexion or

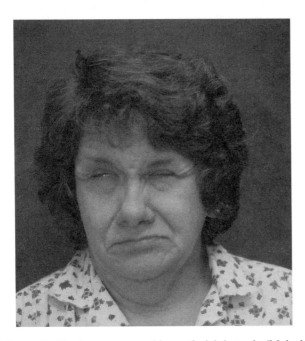

Figure 4 Blepharospasm and lower facial dystonia (Meige's syndrome).

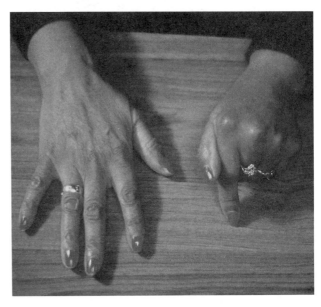

Figure 5 Dystonia of left hand at rest with extension of the index finger and flexion of the other fingers and thumb.

extension of the wrist and fingers occurs. The act of writing becomes labored and, in some, even impossible, while other activities including typing or writing on a blackboard may be completely unimpaired. These patients have been misdiagnosed as having carpal tunnel syndrome, orthopedic conditions, or a psychological malady but in fact have a neurologic disorder. Patients with writer's cramp may use tricks, such as writing with a thick pen or with a different hand posture, in order to alleviate the symptoms. Sometimes patients accommodate by learning to write with the other hand. Similarly, action-induced hand dystonia may be observed associated with specific occupations. Some musicians have been completely disabled by involuntary movements of their hand occurring only when attempting to play a specific musical instrument and not with any other activity.

Dystonia of the trunk is the result of involuntary contractions of paraspinal or prevertebral muscles, causing a bending of the trunk. This may appear as an arching of the back, a leaning to one side, or a forward flexion at the waist. Truncal dystonia is frequently associated with cervical dystonia and may arise as tardive phenomenon, a potentially permanent sequelae of chronic neuroleptic exposure.

CAUSE AND PATHOPHYSIOLOGY

The cause and pathophysiology of dystonia remain elusive. Observations in secondary dystonia, in particular hemidystonia, have suggested that the basal ganglia and its connections are the likely anatomic sites of pathology. Electrophysiologic studies, including long latency reflexes and blink reflex recovery curves, have suggested that a loss of central descending inhibition on brain stem nuclei may be one of the pathophysiologic mechanisms for dystonia. Although quantitative studies of brain neurochemistry in a limited number of brains of dystonic patients have not been consistent, pharmacologic trials have implicated multiple neurotransmitters, including acetylcholine and dopamine, as possible modulators of clinical symptomatology.

DIAGNOSTIC TESTS

The diagnosis of dystonia relies on the neurologic examination and visual recognition of the disorder. There are no laboratory tests to confirm the diagnosis. Brain imaging, blood tests, and other laboratory evaluations are obtained to look for secondary dystonia. The number of tests obtained depends upon the individual patient and the degree of clinical suspicion of secondary dystonia. I will order magnetic resonance imaging of the brain, blood chemistries including liver enzymes, blood counts including microscopic evaluation for acanthocytes, erythrocyte sedimentation rate, thyroid function tests, and neuropsychological assessment of cognitive function. In the appropriate patient as emphasized previously, Wilson's disease is an important diagnosis to consider. Screening tests for Wilson's disease include a serum copper, ceruloplasmin, and ophthalmologic slit-lamp examination for Kayser-Fleischer rings. Abnormalities on screening tests should be vigorously pursued.

With recent advances in genetic testing for dystonia and the availability of new, effective symptomatic therapies, familiarity with the clinical features and ability to diagnose dystonia are now essential.

SUGGESTED READING

Fahn S. Concept and classification of dystonia. Adv Neurol 1988; 50:1–8.

Fahn S, Marsden CD, Calne DB. Classification and investigation of dystonia. In: Marsden CD, Fahn S, eds. Movement disorders 2. London: Butterworth, 1987:332.

Jankovic J, Leder S, Warner D, Schwartz K. Cervical dystonia: Clinical findings and associated movement disorders. Neurology 1991; 41:1088–1091.

Marsden CD. Investigation of dystonia. Adv Neurol 1988; 50:35–44.

McGeer EG, McGeer PL. The dystonias. Can J Neurol Sci 1988; 15:447–483.

Ozelius L, Kramer P, deLeon D, et al. Strong allelic association between the torsion dystonia gene (DYT1) and loci on chromosome 9q34 in Ashkenazi Jews. Am J Hum Genet 1992; 50:619–628.

Suchawersy O, Calne DB. Non-dystonic causes of torticollis. Adv Neurol 1988; 50:501–508.

Weiner WJ, Lang AE. Idiopathic torsion dystonia. In: Weiner WJ, Lang AE. Movement disorders: A comprehensive survey. Mt. Kisco, NY: Futura, 1989: 347.

TREMOR

KAPIL D. SETHI, M.D., M.R.C.P. (U.K.)

Tremor is an approximately rhythmic, roughly sinusoidal involuntary movement that is usually classified according to disease or to the behavior with which it occurs. Correct recognition of the type of tremor is important because it has implications for diagnosis, prognosis, and therapy. Tremor can be physiologic. This "normal tremor" is present in all body parts. Pathologic tremors most commonly affect the hands but may involve other areas of the body including head, leg, and voice.

Clinically the most useful way of classifying tremor is according to the behavior (rest, action, tasks) with which it usually occurs (Table 1).

Rest tremor occurs when the body part is in repose. It is most frequently seen in the setting of parkinsonism, including Parkinson's disease. Action tremor is any tremor that occurs during voluntary muscle contraction and includes both postural and kinetic tremor. One form of kinetic tremor is terminal kinetic tremor, traditionally called intention tremor. Static tremor is a poor term, referring to tremor present when there is no voluntary movement, and includes rest tremor and postural tremor. This term should be avoided. Task-specific tremors occur during specific behaviors such as writing (primary writing tremor) or standing (orthostatic tremor).

Tremors can be studied electrophysiologically by using a variety of transducers. Miniature uniaxial accelerometers are the most popular devices and give sufficient information for clinical use.

PHYSIOLOGIC TREMOR

Physiologic tremor is barely seen with the unaided eye. It is symptomatic only during activities that require extreme precision. Usually it is an 8 to 12 Hz oscillation. Physiologic tremor may be exaggerated by fatigue, anxiety, and some medications (Table 2). This is termed enhanced physiologic tremor (EPT).

EPT has the frequency of physiologic tremor. It is absent at rest and present on posture. It is present but not exaggerated during movement. EPT results from synchronization of the motor unit discharges due to enhanced reflex feedback from the periphery. Commonly this is a result of increased systemic adrenergic activity. It is common in anxiety states and in a variety of metabolic disorders including thyrotoxicosis, pheochromocytoma, and hypoglycemia. Catecholamines and xanthines induce EPT by direct peripheral receptor stimulation. Withdrawal of drugs such as beta blockers, morphine, or alcohol can produce tremor by increasing the activity of the peripheral adrenergic receptors. This type of tremor improves with beta adrenergic receptor blocking agents such as propranolol.

Severe muscle fatigue from prolonged intense muscle contraction, as from climbing rocks, can result in tremor resembling clonus (Rock Climber's Tremor).

Table 1 Classification of Tremor

Physiologic tremor	Normal
	Enhanced physiologic tremor (EPT)
Pathologic Tremor	
Rest tremor	
Action tremor	Postural tremor
	Kinetic tremor
	Terminal kinetic tremor (intention tremor)
Task-specific tremor	Primary writing tremor
	Orthostatic tremor

Table 2 Conditions Enhancing Physiologic Tremor

Anxiety
Fatigue
Drugs
   theophylline
   catecholamines
   caffeine
   steroids
   amphetamines
Withdrawal of alcohol or opioids
Thyrotoxicosis
Pheochromocytoma
Hypoglycemia

REST TREMOR

Most frequently, rest tremor is seen in Parkinson's disease or drug-induced parkinsonism. This tremor is present at rest and disappears or markedly attenuates with action. It usually involves upper or lower limbs but may involve the chin, jaw, and tongue. Typically the movements include pronation and supination of the forearm and rhythmic movements of the thumb across the fingers, called "pill rolling." Usually this tremor has a frequency of 4 to 6 Hz. Electromyographic (EMG) studies have shown that agonist and antagonist muscles are activated alternately in this type of tremor. Other signs such as bradykinesia or cogwheel rigidity are usually present. This tremor may be markedly asymmetric at onset. It is not unusual to see unilateral rest tremor in early cases of Parkinson's disease.

Occasionally, the tremor reappears when the hands are outstretched, where it usually has the same frequency as the rest tremor. Other types of tremors may be seen in Parkinson's disease as well. These tremors are usually intermediate or high-frequency (8 to 11 Hz) and are present on action. It has been shown that the cogwheel phenomenon (palpable tremor with movement of the joint) is related to postural tremor rather than rest tremor.

Myorhythmia refers to 1 to 3 Hz slow tremor that

occurs along with palatal movement (palatal myoclonus). It is much slower than the rest tremor of Parkinson's disease and is seen in brain stem strokes, demyelinating disease, Whipple's disease, and other conditions affecting the brain stem.

ACTION TREMORS

Postural Tremor

Postural tremor occurs in a variety of conditions. Enhanced physiologic tremor is predominantly a postural tremor. The most common postural tremor other than EPT is essential tremor (ET).

Essential Tremor

ET is a common disorder with an autosomal dominant mode of inheritance. However, a family history is found in only 50 percent of cases. The tremor may appear from childhood to late life (senile tremor) and runs a slowly progressive course. This tremor is also called benign ET, a term to be avoided because the condition is not always benign. Patients may suffer from considerable embarrassment and functional disability.

Typically ET presents as a distal postural tremor of the upper extremities. It is absent at rest. It is usually most evident at the end of a goal-directed movement. ET involves the upper extremities and head more frequently than the legs or the voice. Unlike in Parkinson's disease, the jaw and the tongue are rarely involved. The neurologic examination apart from the tremor is normal except for mild cogwheeling, which is present in patients who are anxious and tense. It must be stressed that cogwheeling is not synonymous with the diagnosis of Parkinson's disease and can be seen in anxious patients even without essential tremor. Table 3 lists some differences between ET and Parkinson's disease.

Essential tremor typically improves with alcohol or beta blockers. Marsden et al have divided essential tremor into four types. Type one refers to the typical 8 to 12 Hz tremor that is indistinguishable from enhanced physiologic tremor. Type two refers to a slightly slower frequency tremor of 5 to 7 Hz. Type three refers to severe disabling tremor of large amplitude and low frequency often involving many body parts. Type four refers to association with other neurologic disorders, such as dystonia, peripheral neuropathy, and essential myoclonus.

Cerebellar Postural Tremors

Although the most characteristic cerebellar tremor is terminal kinetic tremor, otherwise known as intention tremor, purely postural tremor can occur in cerebellar disease. The most severe type has traditionally been called rubral tremor. The term *rubral tremor,* while ingrained in medical literature, should be avoided because it implies a clinicoanatomical correlation that does not exist. It refers to a severe postural tremor of about 3 to 5 Hz that may persist at rest and is markedly exaggerated by goal-directed movements. It is usually associated with cerebellar outflow lesions, such as lesions of the superior cerebellar peduncle. In several pathologically studied cases, lesions are either not present in the red nucleus or are irrelevant. This tremor has also been called midbrain tremor. Severe cerebellar postural tremor may be found in demyelinating disease, brain stem infarction, brain tumor, or head trauma (see below).

Table 3 Differentiation Between Parkinson's Disease and Essential Tremor

	Parkinson's Disease	*Essential Tremor*
Age group	Usually older	Any age (most frequently middle age)
Family history	Usually negative	Usually positive
Parts of body involved	Hands > legs > jaw > tongue	Hands > neck > voice > legs
Type of tremor	At rest and on maintained posture	During maintained posture and terminal kinetic — not at rest
Frequency	Rest 4–6 Hz Postural 7–12 Hz	6–12 Hz
Other neurologic signs	Bradykinesia Forward flexion of trunk Postural instability Masked facies Cogwheeling	No bradykinesia Normal posture No postural instability No masked facies Cogwheeling rarely
Gait	Slow shuffling Decreased arm swing Freezing	Normal
Pharmacology	Responds to levodopa, dopamine agonists, and anticholinergics	Responds to propranolol and primidone
PET scan	Striatal fluorodopa uptake decreased	Normal PET scan

PET = positron emission tomography.

Mild Postural Cerebellar Tremor

This tremor is less well defined than the severe variety. This tremor is more rapid, up to 10 Hz. The conditions giving rise to severe postural cerebellar tremor may lead to mild postural cerebellar tremor as well. However, the response to drugs may be different. The severe postural variety often responds to isoniazid, whereas the mild one does not.

Postural Tremor in Peripheral Neuropathy

Tremor occurs in heredity peripheral neuropathy, such as heredity motor sensory neuropathy (HMSN) type 1 and occasionally in HMSN type 2. Cases with predominant tremor are given the label Roussy-Levy syndrome. Acquired neuropathy may also give rise to tremor, particularly paraproteinemic IgM neuropathy. Tremor may occur transiently at any stage from onset to recovery. The tremor improves as the neuropathy improves with treatment. The tremor is not related to the degree of proprioceptive loss. Beta blockers usually do not improve this tremor. Tremor may also be seen in the recovery phase of Guillain-Barré syndrome. Rarely, tremor occurs with other acquired neuropathies such as diabetic, uremic, or porphyric neuropathy.

Terminal Kinetic Tremor (Intention Tremor)

Intention tremor is characterized by increasing rhythmic oscillations as a target is approached, and is perpendicular to the direction of movement. Once the target is reached, the tremor stops. In contrast, postural action tremor continues even when the target is reached because postural maintenance is required to remain on the target. EMG activity in antagonist muscles alternates during cerebellar intention tremor, the frequency ranging from 3 to 5 Hz. Terminal kinetic tremor must be differentiated from dysmetria, which means "wrong distance," since patients with dysmetria may have irregular tremulous movements when approaching a target. Intention tremor occurs in many cerebellar diseases.

TASK-SPECIFIC TREMOR

Primary Writing Tremor

Primary writing tremor is the prototype of a task-specific tremor. It appears only with handwriting or certain other skilled manual tasks. It is not seen with all skilled tasks and is not produced with posture. Primary writing tremor is focal and is often misdiagnosed. There is some debate over whether primary writing tremor represents a form of dystonia or is a variant of essential tremor. In some patients the tremor is jerky and resembles myoclonus, but there is usually no evidence of cortical hyperexcitability. In some families, writer's cramp, a focal dystonia, may coexist with primary writing tremor.

Vocal Tremor

There are rare patients who appear to have isolated tremor while speaking. There is no tremor of other parts of the body. Some of these patients have a variant of essential tremor since they have a positive family history of tremor and the tremor improves with alcohol. In other patients, this tremor may be associated with spasmodic dysphonia and may be a manifestation of focal dystonia. This area needs further clarification.

Orthostatic Tremor

Heilman described orthostatic tremor in patients with tremor only while standing. This tremor disappeared while walking and did not occur with voluntary activation of the leg muscles. Some of these patients have tremor in the arms. Orthostatic tremor may represent a variant of essential tremor. Orthostatic tremor may occur in patients with thyrotoxicosis and improve with treatment of thyrotoxicosis. This tremor is of high frequency (18 to 20 Hz) and pharmacologically is different from essential tremor in that it may respond to clonazepam (4 to 6 mg per day).

OTHER TREMORS

Drug-Induced Tremor

In addition to the aggravation of physiologic tremor by certain drugs, other drugs may *produce* tremor. Antipsychotic drugs, in addition to producing drug-induced parkinsonism, may produce a tremor that is predominantly postural and responds to dopamine depletors such as tetrabenazine or reserpine. This response distinguishes the postural tremor from rest tremor induced by these drugs. This "tardive tremor" is an uncommon side effect of neuroleptic drugs. Tricyclic antidepressants may aggravate tremor. Tremor occurs in up to 15 percent of patients receiving sodium valproate, there being a poor correlation between tremor amplitude and serum drug levels. MPTP (1 Methyl-4-Phenyl, 1-2-3-6 Tetra-tryclopyridine) produces typical parkinsonian rest tremor in humans and primates. Lithium causes cerebellar ataxia as well as postural and intention tremors, particularly in toxic dosages.

Wilson's Disease

Wilson's disease may cause tremor as the only manifestation. However, the tremor is often associated with other movement disorders and psychiatric disturbances. The tremor has classically been called "wing-beating tremor" and is shown with shoulders abducted to 90 degrees and the elbows flexed. However, wing-beating tremor is an uncommon manifestation of Wilson's disease.

Post-Traumatic Tremor

Tremor occurs as a consequence of head injury, appearing a few weeks to months after the injury. The tremor is typically present on posture and is made worse by intention. In this respect it resembles the midbrain or cerebellar outflow tremor often erroneously called rubral tremor. Such patients may respond to beta blockers. Occasionally they require stereotaxic thalamotomy.

Tremor and Dystonia

Tremor and dystonia frequently coexist. While in some patients with dystonia typical essential tremor occurs, in others the tremor is more irregular and is made worse by the patient's attempts to correct the dystonic posture. The tremor may improve with sensory tricks, such as touching the cheek lightly to correct torticollis.

Psychogenic Tremor

Psychogenic tremor is not uncommon. Such tremor may have features of rest and action tremor. These tremors can be paroxysmal or continuous, unilateral or bilateral, and may be associated with other movement disorders or hysterical manifestations. The tremor typically attenuates on distraction and has varying frequencies on accelerometry. In contrast, organic tremor has a relatively fixed frequency but may have varying amplitude. In addition, psychogenic tremor may respond to placebo injection or psychotherapy.

Paroxysmal Tremors

Paroxysmal tremors are rare and may be associated with ataxia. Such events are dramatic, and tremor may involve the entire body. Paroxysmal tremor-ataxia may respond to acetazolamide.

SOME CONDITIONS MIMICKING TREMOR

Hereditary Chin Quivering

This autosomal dominant condition results in irregular movements of the chin, which may be rapid or slow and resemble dystonia. These can be brought on by anxiety and are benign. The movements are not rhythmic enough to be classified as tremor.

Oscillatory Myoclonus

Oscillatory myoclonus, also called rhythmic myoclonus, is jerky and not sinusoidal. The condition can be inherited and involves trunk or extremity muscles.

Asterixis (Flapping Tremor)

Although this has been called flapping tremor, the condition is a result of lapses in maintained posture and is classified as a negative myoclonus. The movements are not rhythmic enough to be called tremor but, when frequent, may impart a tremulous appearance.

Shuddering Attacks

This condition is found in children having a family history of essential tremor. The attacks consist of sudden violent body shaking of short duration. Some of these children later develop essential tremor.

SUGGESTED READING

Biary N, Cleeves L, Findley L, Koller W. Post-traumatic tremor. Neurology 1989; 39:103–106.

Elble R. Physiologic and essential tremor. Neurology 1986; 36:225–231.

Findley LH. Tremors: Differential diagnosis and pharmacology. In: Parkinson's disease and movement disorders. Jankovic J, Tolosa E, eds. Baltimore: Urban & Schwarzenberg, 1988:243.

Findley LH, Capildeo R. Movement disorders: Tremor. New York: Oxford University Press, 1984.

Hallet HM. Differential diagnosis of tremor. In: Handbook of clinical neurology. Vinken PV, Bruyn GW, Klawans HC, eds. Vol 49. Amsterdam: Elsevier, 1986:583.

Heilman KM. Orthostatic tremor. Arch Neurol 1984; 41:880–881.

Jedynal CP, Bonnet AM, Agid Y. Tremor and idiopathic dystonia. Mov Disord 1991; 6:230–236.

Koller W, Lang A, Vetere-Overfield B., et al. Psychogenic tremors. Neurology 1989; 39:1094–1099.

NEUROLEPTIC MALIGNANT SYNDROME AND OTHER NEUROLEPTIC TOXICITIES

JOSEPH H. FRIEDMAN, M.D.

This chapter covers the neurologic complications of the drugs that block dopamine receptors. Although most of these are antipsychotics, other drugs, such as metoclopramide (Reglan) for gastric motility and prochlorperazine (Compazine) for nausea, may also cause the same adverse effects.

Antipsychotic drugs are also called neuroleptics, meaning "gripping the nerve," and have a wide spectrum of adverse effects. The easiest way to categorize the neurologic side effects is chronologically. There are acute effects that tend to occur early and then remit, acute effects that may persist while the drug is being used, and tardive syndromes, which occur late.

ACUTE EFFECTS

Akathisia and Acute Dystonic Reactions

The earliest neuroleptic adverse effects are akathisia and acute dystonic reactions. Akathisia, meaning "not to sit," refers to a sense of inner restlessness that forces the patient to move in order to attain some relief. The sensation is extremely uncomfortable and has been described by nonpsychotic individuals as an "alien force" taking control, forcing the patient to move. In its classic form, patients are unable to remain seated for more than a few seconds. They must stand up to either walk or march in place. The problem is that many of the patients who suffer from this are not able to communicate adequately. Generally the problem occurs in young schizophrenic patients started on high-potency neuroleptics such as haloperidol, but it may occur in patients of any age on any dopamine receptor blocker. Nonpsychotic patients can register their reaction and may describe jitteriness or extreme anxiety and an uncomfortable sensation in their legs that forces them to move. The bulk of the affected population is psychotic, however, and received the neuroleptic in order to control disturbed behavior and thought processes. It is therefore often difficult for the subjects to describe this unpleasant reaction. The treating physician may, quite reasonably, assume that the patent's increasing agitation reflects increasing psychosis that necessitates more neuroleptic. The cycle may continue for long periods of time before the true nature of the restlessness becomes apparent. This problem is thought to be a major reason why psychotic patients refuse to take their medications. Akathisia is a problem that should always be considered when patients become more agitated after drug treatment begins. It should also be considered when patients have a seemingly paradoxical response to drugs and suffer worsening psychosis as medication is increased. Any patient receiving neuroleptics who cannot sit without rocking, shifting position, or standing or who cannot stand without marching in place should be considered to have akathisia.

Acute dystonic reactions are involuntary muscle spasms that cause prolonged abnormal postures. These spasms may or may not be painful and usually involve the cervical or cranial muscles. The spasms persist for about 20 to 30 minutes and remit for variable periods of time before recurring. Patients may experience torticollis, with the neck turned to one side, or retrocollis, with the neck extended, jaw clenching, tongue protruding, or combinations of these. Oculogyric crises refer to involuntary conjugate deviation of the eyes, usually up and to one side. This may occur in addition to torticollis. During the attack the patient can sometimes overcome the postural abnormality, but only for short periods after which the abnormal posture resumes. Typically the same abnormality recurs; that is, the head persistently turns to the same side during each recurrence of the particular dystonic reaction. One does not see a patient develop an acute dystonic reaction with torticollis remitting after a few minutes to develop dystonia in another part of the body. On rare occasions such a sequence does occur, however. I have witnessed alternating unilateral jaw spasms as an acute dystonic reaction. One must also know that generalized acute dystonic reactions may occur in which the whole body is involved, including axial muscles.

To establish a diagnosis of acute dystonic reaction requires a history of medication exposure. Sometimes in the emergency room patients deny drug ingestion because they have obtained the drug surreptitiously, not knowing what they were taking. A response to therapy should be considered confirmatory of the diagnosis. Nearly 100 percent of cases remit completely within 5 to 10 minutes of an intravenous bolus of benztropine or diphenhydramine. Acute dystonia can be distinguished from idiopathic dystonia by the onset, which is over minutes rather than days to years. The acute dystonic postures last several minutes and then resolve. Again, a history of drug exposure must be present.

Neuroleptic Malignant Syndrome

Chronologically, the next syndrome one encounters is the neuroleptic malignant syndrome (NMS). This usually occurs within about 2 weeks after initiation of a neuroleptic but for unclear reasons can also occur after years on a stable dose. The patient typically develops the cardinal signs of high fever, altered mental state, and extreme rigidity. Fevers are generally greater than 101°F and may be over 108°F. The extrapyramidal syndrome that typically occurs is rigidity but has been described as tremors in some reports. This rigidity refers to severe, persistent muscle contraction rather than the passive tone increase present in parkinsonism. While persistent contraction is also the hallmark of dystonia, these patients usually do not have the typical dystonic postures of torticollis, opisthotonus, or inverted feet. Thus the patient may look severely parkinsonian but be so rigid that the tested limb cannot be flexed. These patients are usually obtunded, but delirium or confusion may be seen. The diagnostic problem involves the lack of a confirmatory laboratory test, the wide spectrum of possible presentations, and the interrelationships between the features of the illness. For example, when a young, otherwise healthy person is placed on a neuroleptic for psychosis and shortly thereafter becomes extremely stiff, febrile to 103°F, and lethargic, the diagnosis is fairly simple. On the other hand, in an elderly patient newly placed on a neuroleptic for behavioral problems due to dementia, fever from any cause is likely to cause delirium or obtundation and worsening of drug-induced parkinsonism. Consider too the clinical problem of the patient on a neuroleptic with acquired immunodeficiency syndrome who presents with elements of this syndrome and one can appreciate the problems caused by overlapping syndromes.

Laboratory studies in NMS may reveal elevated serum muscle enzymes and a leukocytosis. With high serum creatine phosphokinase (CPK) levels, indicating a large amount of muscle necrosis, serum myoglobin will be elevated. This in turn causes a positive urine dipstick test for blood, which may be a harbinger of renal failure secondary to myoglobinuria.

Physiologic changes in NMS can be difficult to interpret. Tachypnea, profuse diaphoresis, and tachycardia are common but are also seen nonspecifically with fever. Many physicians believe that serum CPK elevations are synonymous with NMS, but this is clearly not true. Diagnosis is more difficult in patients with mild symptoms or only two of the three cardinal features. When a patient on a neuroleptic has a moderate fever, how much of the increased tremor or rigidity and altered sensorium can be ascribed to the fever alone? If a patient, especially an elderly one, is very rigid, perhaps from an acute dystonic reaction, could there be an aspiration pneumonia? Could an elevated CPK be due to trauma? Was the patient lying on the ground immobile for a few hours, causing muscle crush?

Since the diagnosis of NMS rests on clinical grounds, and since the disorder has a presumed mortality of 20 percent untreated, it behooves us to always consider the diagnosis in febrile patients on neuroleptics. It must always be considered a diagnosis of exclusion. Infectious causes of fever must always be in the differential diagnosis, no matter how straightforward the syndrome appears.

If an acute generalized dystonic reaction is on the differential diagnostic list, a trial of intravenous treatment is mandatory. A positive response confirms the diagnosis and excludes NMS. A negative response should trigger a treatment protocol for NMS while the search for an infectious cause continues.

Far less common syndromes to consider when diagnosing NMS are lethal catatonia, a poorly charac-terized entity, and a recently described serotonergic syndrome of mental status changes, agitation, tremors, myoclonus, diaphoresis, and occasionally fever due to an interaction between monoamine oxidase inhibitors and serotonin-enhancing drugs.

Drug-Induced Parkinsonism

Drug-induced parkinsonism (DIP) usually develops insidiously over the first several weeks of neuroleptic exposure. The severity of the syndrome is highly variable, depending in part on the neuroleptic, the dose, and the patient's age. The syndrome exactly mimics idiopathic Parkinson's disease (PD) but, as with early PD, may manifest with only some of the cardinal features. In my own experience a decrease in blink rate, subtle facial masking, and decreased arm swing while walking are the most common features in the mild form. Just as in PD, the presentation is variable, with some patients having prominent rest tremors of fingers, arm, jaw, and feet, and others having none. The extreme form of the DIP may mimic catatonia, especially if tremor is not significant.

Any patient who appears parkinsonian and has been exposed to neuroleptics must be presumed to have DIP unless the exposure was insignificant or in the distant past. It is commonly not recognized that DIP, like PD, may be asymmetric and that the parkinsonian effects of neuroleptics far exceed the serum half-lives of the drugs. DIP has been reported to persist over 18 months after drug discontinuation, and persistence of parkinsonian signs for 6 months is common.

The difficulty in diagnosis generally occurs in older patients who have been on a fixed neuroleptic dose for decades without adverse effects and then develop signs of parkinsonism. Is it PD unmasked early by the dopamine receptor blockage, or is this simply increased sensitivity of an aging brain to the drug? Only by stopping the offending agent and observing the patient over the next year or more will the diagnosis become clear. The presence or absence of a response to antiparkinson medications is not helpful in distinguishing the syndromes.

LATE EFFECTS

The tardive syndromes, often lumped together under the term *tardive dyskinesias* (TD), actually refer to a set of syndromes that can be distinct or present in highly variable combinations. These occur after "long-term" exposure to neuroleptics. In most cases the exposure has been years. Rarely, the syndrome appears to develop in weeks. By convention, a 3 month exposure to neuroleptics is the minimum necessary to classify a syndrome as tardive for the purposes of a research study.

The most common tardive syndrome is persistent involuntary writhing tongue, accompanied by purpose-less jaw and lip movements. These are frequently not recognized by the patient. The movements cannot be distinguished from the normal movements made when the mouth is dry or when dentures fit poorly. Many edentulous people also constantly chew and move their tongues. Finally, a syndrome of oral-lingual chorea has been recognized as being fairly common in the elderly who have never been exposed to neuroleptics. This is considered a form of senile chorea. Tardive dyskinesias may involve any body region. Usually one sees arm or leg in addition to oral, buccal, and lingual chorea, but it may occur in isolated body parts sparing the mouth and face. The movements are choreic (that is, random and jerky) in nature, athetoid (that is, slow and vermiform), or choreoathetoid, a combination of the two. Usually the movements are mild, often incorporated into semipurposeful movements and not recognized by the patient. They can be functionally disabling in severity, however, in addition to being socially embarrassing.

When severe, TD can be impossible to distinguish from Huntington's disease (HD). HD always causes dementia after a time and usually causes some degree of extraocular movement dysfunction. At a single point in time it may be impossible to distinguish TD from HD, but with time HD always worsens, with progression of dementia, chorea, and a prominent dysarthria, not common in TD. Wilson's disease is a rare syndrome that should be considered in young patients with severe TD.

There are other, less common tardive syndromes that are important to recognize because they may be treatable or should at least prompt a reassessment of neuroleptic use.

Tardive akathisia refers to a persistent syndrome of restlessness that, like acute akathisia, causes patients to move. Unlike acute akathisia, which is frequently seen in association with DIP, tardive akathisia is frequently seen in association with TD. Diagnosis can be difficult due to communication problems, as with acute akathisia, because many of the patients are psychotic. Complicating this may be a generalized form of TD that makes the patient appear restless and thus suffer from "pseudoakathisia." In psychotic patients who truly are restless, need to march in place when standing, and can't sit still,

the issue often revolves around whether the psychosis is driving the restlessness or the restlessness represents akathisia that is driving the psychosis. In both the acute and tardive forms of akathisia, which respond quite differently to pharmacologic interventions, one must also consider the possibility that extraneous drugs such as cocaine and amphetamine are complicating the picture, as well as drug withdrawal syndromes.

Tardive dystonia refers to a persistent abnormal posture, which develops after chronic neuroleptic use without other apparent explanation. Usually it involves the neck, but it can be generalized or focal, causing isolated blepharospasm or limb dystonia. It is often associated with the more common TD. In patients under age 40 with unilateral or isolated limb involvement, it must be distinguished from Wilson's disease and rare structural lesions of the brain or spinal cord.

Finally, neuroleptics can cause extremely complex mixtures of disorders with simultaneous tics, akathisia, dystonia, dyskinesias, and even elements of parkinsonism. In fact, the more complex the disorder, the more likely it is to reflect a neuroleptic-induced syndrome.

SUGGESTED READING

Braude WM, Barnes TRE, Gore SM. Clinical characteristics of akathisia. Br J Psychiatry 1983; 143:134–150.

Hardie RJ, Less AJ. Neuroleptic-induced Parkinson's syndrome: Clinical features and results of treatment with levodopa. J Neurol Neurosurg Psychiatry 1988; 51:850–854.

Kang UJ, Burke RE, Fahn S. Natural history and treatment of tardive dystonia. Mov Disord 1986; 1:193–208.

Kurlan R, Hamill R, Shoulson I. Neuroleptic malignant syndrome. Clin Neuropharmacol 1984; 7:109–120.

Mann SC, Caroff SN, Bleier H, et al. Lethal catatonia. Am J Psychiatry 1986; 143:1374–1381.

Sternbach H. The serotonin syndrome. Am J Psychiatry 1991; 148:705–713.

Van Putten T. The many faces of akathisia. Compr Psychiatry 1975; 16:43–47.

Weiner W, Lange AE, eds. Drug induced movement disorders. Mt. Kisco, NY: Futura, 1992.

GAIT DISORDER

LEWIS R. SUDARSKY, M.D.

Gait is a fundamental motor skill and a distinctive feature of the individual. Abnormality of gait may be the presenting feature of a neurologic disease at any age. Gait disorder is particularly common among the elderly, resulting in loss of functional status and increased risk for fall-related injury. By age 80, one person in four will use assistive devices while walking. Injury due to falls is

an important source of morbidity and mortality among older Americans. Despite the frequency with which these problems are encountered, gait and balance disorders sometimes present a particular challenge in diagnosis.

A strategy for the evaluation of gait disorders must examine a large search space, a long list of possible diagnoses. There is not a uniquely specific diagnosis for each patient. Gait problems are sometimes multifactorial, particularly in the elderly. There may be comorbidity from arthritis, and the gait is highly sensitive to minor degrees of orthopedic deformity. Still, I am optimistic in the evaluation of patients still ambulatory that the causal factors in the decline of walking skill can be successfully identified. Roughly one patient in four will have a treatable disorder.

Our basic strategy includes observation of the failing gait, a functional assessment that does not always reveal the diagnosis but helps to define the problem. Is the patient describing a disorder of motor control, a disturbance of balance, or is the gait primarily limited by pain and arthritic change? The neurologic exam is used to narrow the differential diagnosis by localizing the deficit. Finally, we consider the use of diagnostic tests, standard neurophysiology and magnetic resonance imaging (MRI), as well as specialized investigations like platform posturography and gait analysis.

CHARACTERIZATION OF ABNORMAL GAIT

Gait can be broken down into two component tasks: locomotion and balance. Locomotor control in animals depends on a spinal pattern generator under the direction of locomotor centers in the brain stem and diencephalon. Primates are not capable of spinal "fictive locomotion" and are more reliant on higher level motor control. Bipedal ambulation stresses the integration of balance with locomotion. Cerebellar and vestibular control of the upright posture depends on sensory afferent information from the visual system, the vestibular labyrinth, and proprioceptive input from the lower limbs and trunk. There is normally a healthy redundancy of afferent information, but dynamic balance may be compromised if these sensory systems are degraded by disease. The diversity of disorders seen clinically reflects the large anatomy involved in the production of a stable and efficient gait.

Observation of the failing gait calls on skill in pattern recognition. Certain features are distinctive, particularly the festinating gait of Parkinson's disease (PD). Freezing and start hesitation are less specific. Patients with spastic paraparesis from spinal disease walk with a stiff-legged circumduction and bounce. Cerebellar patients have excess lateral instability of the trunk, erratic foot placement, and a marked decompensation when attempting to walk on a narrow base. All too often the changes are nonspecific, and many failing gaits are fundamentally similar. Characteristic abnormalities are blurred and overwhelmed by nonspecific adaptive responses and defense reactions. The base of support is widened, stride length is reduced, and the period of double support time (normally around 20 percent) is extended. Anxiety and fear of falling may further color the performance. This unfortunate reality limits the utility of any approach based entirely on observation and descriptive analysis.

THE SEARCH FOR A CAUSE

The principal focus of the evaluation is to determine the cause of the disorder. Table 1 reviews some of the common causes of gait disorder in a neurologic referral

Table 1 Classification of Gait Disorder According to Cause in 75 Patients

	1980–1982	1990	Total	Percent
Myelopathy	8	6	14	18.4
Parkinsonism	5	2	7	9.2
Hydrocephalus	2	3	5	6.6
Multiple infarcts	8	5	13	17.1
Cerebellar degeneration	4	1	5	6.6
Sensory deficits	9	6	15	19.7
Toxic-metabolic	3	0	3	3.9
Psychogenic	1	2	3	3.9
Other	3	0	3	3.9
Unknown cause	7	1	8	10.5

Data for 1980–1982 patients from Sudarsky L, Ronthal M. Gait disorders among the elderly patients: A survey study of 50 patients. Arch Neurol 1983; 40:740. Twenty-five additional patients are from 1990. Presented at II European Congress of Gerontology, Madrid 1991.

practice. The data reflect patients over 65 referred to the neurologist for an undiagnosed disorder of gait. Patients with major arthritic limitation, previously known PD, and paralyzing stroke were excluded, as were patients on neuroleptic drugs. This series of cases provides a framework for review of the common disorders and the diagnostic issues they present.

Myelopathy

Often unrecognized by internists and generalists, myelopathy from cervical spondylosis contributes to gait disorders among the elderly. Studies of prevalence in a general autopsy population suggest that the problem is increasingly common with advanced age. Spondylitic bars and ligamentous hypertrophy narrow the canal, causing mechanical compression and vascular compromise. The core clinical features are spastic paraparesis, together with mild standing imbalance and bladder instability (urgency, frequency). Neck pain and radiculopathy are often absent, though some patients complain of "numb clumsy hands." The condition is typically associated with a spastic or spastic-ataxic gait. An occasional patient will experience a discrete worsening in relation to an injury or fall.

MRI has improved the ease of diagnosis, though clinical correlation with the degree of spinal compression is quite imprecise. Plain films with flexion and extension sometimes reveal abnormal mobility about protruding bars when deformation of the cord is not dramatic on MRI. The natural history is quite variable. Some patients apparently stabilize, while others progress. There is no consensus on the role of spondylosis surgery in the older patient.

We have seen a few patients over 60 with myelopathy from vitamin B_{12} deficiency and now obtain B_{12} levels routinely in patients with this presentation.

Parkinsonism

PD is common, affecting 1.5 percent of the population over 65. The flexed attitude in posture and the festinating gait are distinctive. Older patients sometimes present with axial rigidity and gait disorder, without tremor or slowness in the upper limbs. Nearly one-fourth of patients presenting with a bradykinetic-rigid syndrome turn out to have something other than idiopathic PD. The list of causes includes progressive supranuclear palsy, striatonigral degeneration, and corticobasal ganglionic degeneration. These diagnoses should be considered, particularly in patients presenting with postural instability and in those unresponsive to levodopa.

Drug-induced parkinsonism is increasingly recognized in ambulatory practice as a cause of impaired gait and balance. It is particularly common in a chronic care setting. Neuroleptic drugs are known to impair postural support responses and contribute to the risk for falls. The disorder often takes 2 to 3 months to resolve after the offending medication has been discontinued.

Late-Life Hydrocephalus

Since normal pressure hydrocephalus (NPH) was described by Adams, Fisher, and Hakim 25 years ago, there has been a sense that NPH is uncommon as a cause of reversible dementia. Hydrocephalus in the elderly more often presents with gait disorder as the salient feature. The gait is slowed with start hesitation, and patients walk with feet "stuck to the floor." The pathophysiology is not well understood. There is presumably a disconnection of cortical modulation. Among patients presenting with this type of frontal gait disorder (gait apraxia), it is not unusual to find ventricular enlargement by computed tomography (CT) or MRI. A dynamic test is necessary to confirm the presence of hydrocephalus. Gait improves more consistently than mental function after shunting.

Vascular Disease and Gait

Neurologic deficits from stroke often contribute to gait impairment, particularly if there is an element of lower limb paralysis or ataxia. Acutely, stroke can compromise postural control without causing paralysis if the lesion involves the lateral thalamus (thalamic astasia) or upper brain stem tegmentum (central vertigo).

Some patients with vascular disease present with a progressive disorder of gait *without* a clear-cut history of stroke. Parkinsonian features may be correlated with basal ganglia lacunes, evident by CT or MRI. Some patients with chronic hypertension have ischemic lesions of the deep white matter, so-called Binswanger disease. Diagnosis should not be based solely on the radiologic picture, which is somewhat nonspecific. The clinical syndrome consists of mental change, dysarthria, pseudobulbar affect, hyperreflexia in the limbs, and a shuffling gait. Patients have difficulty with gait initiation and turns, and a variable degree of imbalance. The pathophysiology of gait impairment is probably similar to that in hydrocephalus.

Cerebellar Disorders

The ataxic gait is characterized by lateral instability of the trunk, erratic foot placement, a widened stance, and decompensation of balance when attempting to walk tandem. Inherited and sporadic forms of cerebellar degeneration are described in late life. Olivopontocerebellar atrophy (OPCA) is the most commonly recognized syndrome, but other types are described. Molecular markers may someday help with the classification of inherited ataxia. For the present, atrophy of the cerebellum and brain stem can be appreciated by CT or MRI.

Other causes of cerebellar atrophy include toxins (alcohol, possibly phenytoin) and paraneoplastic cerebellar degeneration. Chronic alcoholics with anterior vermis atrophy experience primarily truncal ataxia.

Sensory Ataxia and Impaired Balance

Many patients present with chronic imbalance due to a disorder of sensory afferent systems. Balance depends on high-quality information from the visual system, the vestibular system, and proprioceptive afferents. When this information is lost, standing balance is impaired and gait instability results. Some patients perceive imbalance and adopt a cautious gait. Others lurch about with gross sensory ataxia and an erratic stride, which put them at particular risk for falls. Somatosensory deficits sufficient to compromise balance can be appreciated using Romberg's test and looking at stance on one leg. Most such patients have peripheral neuropathy affecting large fiber afferents. In the absence of other sensory deficits, neuropathy needs to be moderately severe before gait and balance are impaired. Patients with bilateral vestibular deficits may lack vertigo, and physiologic testing is often required to confirm the clinical impression.

Other Causes Common Enough to Mention

It is important to recognize motor manifestations of toxic and metabolic encephalopathies because these disorders are relatively common and usually treatable. Patients with metabolic encephalopathy often display an insecure gait and may fall over backward if displaced. This phenomenon is particularly dramatic with uremia and hepatic failure, in which asterixis may impair stance. Sedative drugs, especially neuroleptics and long-acting benzodiazepines, affect postural reflexes and increase the risk for falls.

A few elderly patients presenting with gait disorder have a mass lesion: primary central nervous system tumor or metastatic cancer. Subdural hematoma should be ruled out in the patient with subacute evolution and a history of falls.

Psychogenic Gait Disorder

Functional disturbance of gait can typically be recognized without costly tests, though obtaining a confirmatory normal CT is good practice in older patients. Psychomotor retardation may be evident in the gait of a depressed person. Hysterical gait disorders are not confined to the young. Several distinctive patterns have been described: astasia-abasia, unnatural slowness, extreme caution ("walking on ice"). These disorders are usually not subtle, and a dramatic cure is sometimes possible.

Gait Disorder Without Identifiable Cause

In up to 15 percent of patients, there is no obvious diagnosis after a careful evaluation and workup. These cases are sometimes called *essential senile gait,* though it is unlikely that they represent a true morbid entity.

NEUROIMAGING AND OTHER DIAGNOSTIC TESTS

MRI has been a major advance in the evaluation of patients with gait disturbance. Topography of cerebellar degeneration can be appreciated by MRI, while it may be inapparent by CT. MRI is an excellent screening test for hydrocephalus, and MRI-based studies of cerebrospinal fluid flow may prove useful as a dynamic test. MRI is invaluable in examining cerebral infarcts, which contribute to gait disorder. The issue of clinical correlation is more controversial with respect to white matter abnormality (leukoaraiosis). Masdeu and others have suggested a relationship between white matter disease in the elderly and disorders of gait and postural control. MRI is a sensitive investigation, and the appearance of excess water on the T2 imaging study is both common and nonspecific. Pathologic correlation has been problematic when the lesions are slight. Experience suggests that the phenomenon may be relevant to gait disorder in elderly patients when the lesions are extensive and confluent in the frontal centrum semiovale.

Standard neurophysiologic investigations such as nerve conduction velocity, somatosensory evoked potentials, and electronystagmography are occasionally useful in the evaluation of the patient with sensory ataxia. Platform tests of balance are very useful descriptively and provide a good functional assessment for patients receiving physical therapy, but they provide little aid in differential diagnosis.

Gait analysis technology has matured since the first efforts of Murray and others to characterize gait changes in the elderly. Still, the diagnostic utility of kinematic studies is limited because distinctive characteristics of the disorder are masked by nonspecific adaptations. Until more sophisticated pattern recognition is incorporated into the computer software, these studies will continue to be less informative than the observations of an experienced clinician.

SUGGESTED READING

Elble RJ, Hughes L, Higgins C. The syndrome of senile gait. J Neurol 1992; 239:71–75.

Fisher CM. Hydocephalus as a cause of disturbances of gait in the elderly. Neurology 1982; 32:1358–1363.

Lempert T, Brandt T, Dietrich M, Huppert D. How to identify psychogenic disorders of stance and gait. J Neurol 1991; 238: 140–146.

Masdeu JC, Wolfson L, Lantos G, et al. Brain white matter changes in the elderly prone to falling. Arch Neurol 1989; 46:1292–1296.

Murray MP, Kory RC, Clarkson BH. Walking patterns in healthy old men. Gerontology 1969; 24:169–178.

Raibert MH, Sutherland IE. Machines that walk. Sci Am 1983; 248:44–53.

Sabin T. Biologic aspects of falls and mobility limitations in the elderly. J Am Geriatr Soc 1982; 30:51–58.

Sudarsky L, Ronthal M. Gait disorders among the elderly patients: a survey study of 50 patients. Arch Neurol 1983; 40:740–743.

Sudarsky L, Simon S. Gait disorder in late-life hydrocephalus. Arch Neurol 1987; 44:263–267.

Thompson PD, Marsden CD. Gait disorder of subcortical arteriosclerotic encephalopathy: Binswanger's disease. Mov Disord 1987; 2:1–8.